Body Composition
Health and Performance in Exercise and Sport

Body Composition
Health and Performance
in Exercise and Sport

Edited by
Henry C. Lukaski

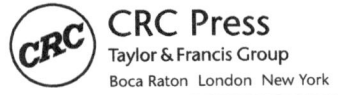

CRC Press
Taylor & Francis Group
Boca Raton London New York

CRC Press is an imprint of the
Taylor & Francis Group, an **informa** business

First published 2017 by CRC Press

Published 2019 by CRC Press
Taylor & Francis Group
6000 Broken Sound Parkway NW, Suite 300
Boca Raton, FL 33487-2742

First issued in paperback 2021

ISBN 13: 978-1-03-209682-7 (pbk)
ISBN 13: 978-1-4987-3167-6 (hbk)

Library of Congress Cataloging-in-Publication Data

Names: Lukaski, Henry Charles, editor.
Title: Body composition: health and performance in exercise and sport/
    [edited by] Henry Lukaski.
Other titles: Body composition (Lukaski)
Description: Boca Raton : Taylor & Francis, 2017. | Includes bibliographical
    references and index.
Identifiers: LCCN 2016054140 | ISBN 9781498731676 (hardback : alk. paper)
Subjects: | MESH: Body Composition | Exercise | Sports
Classification: LCC RA781 | NLM QU 100 | DDC 613.7--dc23
LC record available at https://lccn.loc.gov/2016054140

Visit the Taylor & Francis Web site at
http://www.taylorandfrancis.com

and the CRC Press Web site at
http://www.crcpress.com

Contents

SECTION I   Body Composition Assessment

SECTION II   Physical Activity and Body Composition

SECTION III   Body Composition in Sports and Occupations

SECTION IV Moderating Factors

Editor

Henry C. Lukaski, PhD, is an adjunct professor in the Department of Kinesiology and Public Health Education, University of North Dakota. He earned his undergraduate education at the University of Michigan and Eastern Michigan University, and earned his master of science and doctoral degrees in physiology with a minor in nutrition from The Pennsylvania State University where he was a National Institutes of Health (NIH) pre-doctoral trainee in human biology and a research collaborator at Brookhaven National Laboratory. He was a postdoctoral research associate at the U.S. Department of Agriculture, Agricultural Research Service, Grand Forks Human Nutrition Research Center then served as supervisory research physiologist, research leader, and assistant center director. He is and has been a member of numerous editorial boards of peer-reviewed scientific journals in the fields of human nutrition, exercise science, sports nutrition, and applied physiology, has served as a member of NIH, Department of Defense, National Aeronautics and Space Administration, U.S. Public Health Service program and grant review boards and advisor to the Food and Drug Administration, Institute of Medicine (Food and Nutrition Board Military Nutrition Committee), World Health Organization, Pan American Health Organization, National Collegiate Athletic Association, U.S. and International Olympic Medical Committees, international scientific organizations, sports nutrition community, and the biomedical industry. He has authored more than 145 peer-reviewed research publications, 45 book chapters, 160 abstracts and short communications, coedited special issues of professional publications on body composition and sports nutrition, and made more than 240 invited presentations in the United States, Europe, and Central and South America. He is an international authority in the field of interactions among diet and physical activity on body structure, function, and health, and is recognized internationally as a leader in development and validation of methods for the assessment of human body composition. Dr. Lukaski was elected to Fellowship in the American College of Sports Medicine, Human Biology Council, and the Society of Nutrition for Latin America.

Contributors

Mark G. Abel
Department of Kinesiology and Health
Promotion
University of Kentucky
Lexington, Kentucky

Tim Ackland
School of Sport Science
Exercise & Health, University of Western
Australia
Perth, Australia

Jennifer Bea
Department of Medicine & Nutritional
Sciences
The University of Arizona
Tucson, Arizona

Tyler A. Bosch
Educational Technology Innovations
College of Education and Human
Development
University of Minnesota
Minneapolis, Minnesota

Andrea M. Brennan
School of Kinesiology and Health Studies
Queen's University
Kingston, Ontario, Canada

and

School of Physical Education
University of Guelph
Guelph, Ontario, Canada

Martin Burtscher
Department of Sport Science
University of Innsbruck
Innsbruck, Austria

Lynn Cialdella-Kam
Department of Nutrition
School of Medicine
Case Western Reserve University
Cleveland, Ohio

Manuel J. Coelho e Silva
Faculty of Sport Science and Physical
Education
University of Coimbra
Coimbra, Portugal

Paul O. Davis
First Responder Institute
Washington, DC

and

Emergency Responders, Inc.
Silver Spring, Maryland

Donald R. Dengel
School of Kinesiology
University of Minnesota
Minneapolis, Minnesota

and

Department of Pediatrics
University of Minnesota Medical School
Minneapolis, Minnesota

Michaela C. Devries
Department of Kinesiology
University of Waterloo
Waterloo, Ontario, Canada

Joshua Farr
Division of Endocrinology
Mayo Clinic
College of Medicine
Rochester, Minnesota

Col. Karl E. Friedl
U.S. Army Research Institute of
Environmental Medicine
Natick, Massachusetts

David H. Fukuda
Sport and Exercise Science
Institute of Exercise Physiology and Wellness
University of Central Florida
Orlando, Florida

Hannes Gatterer
Department of Sport Science
University of Innsbruck
Innsbruck, Austria

Scott Going
Department of Nutritional Sciences
The University of Arizona
Tucson, Arizona

Brittany P. Hammond
School of Kinesiology and Health Studies
Queen's University
Kingston, Ontario, Canada

and

School of Physical Education
University of Guelph
Guelph, Ontario, Canada

Jay R. Hoffman
Sport and Exercise Science
Institute of Exercise Physiology and Wellness
University of Central Florida
Orlando, Florida

Kristina L. Kendall
Department of Digital Publishing
Bodybuilding.com
Boise, Idaho

Henry C. Lukaski
Department of Kinesiology and Public Health
    Education
University of North Dakota
Grand Forks, North Dakota

Robert M. Malina
Department of Kinesiology and Health Education
University of Texas at Austin
Austin, Texas

and

School of Public Health and Information
    Sciences
University of Louisville
Louisville, Kentucky

and

Department of Kinesiology
Tarleton State University
Stephenville, Texas

Melinda M. Manore
Nutrition and Exercise Sciences
School of Biological and Population
    Sciences
Oregon State University
Corvallis, Oregon

Catarina N. Matias
Exercise and Health Laboratory
CIPER, Faculty of Human Kinetics
University of Lisbon
Lisbon, Portugal

Ronald J. Maughan
School of Medicine
University of St Andrews
Fife, United Kingdom

Jordan R. Moon
Clinical Department
ImpediMed, Inc.
Carlsbad, California

Sara Y. Oikawa
Department of Kinesiology
McMaster University
Hamilton, Ontario, Canada

Stuart M. Phillips
Department of Kinesiology
McMaster University
Hamilton, Ontario, Canada

Christiana J. Raymond
School of Kinesiology
University of Minnesota
Minneapolis, Minnesota

Robert Ross
School of Kinesiology and Health Studies
and
School of Medicine
Queen's University
Kingston, Ontario, Canada

and

School of Physical Education
University of Guelph
Guelph, Ontario, Canada

Diana A. Santos
Exercise and Health Laboratory, CIPER
Faculty of Human Kinetics
University of Lisbon
Lisbon, Portugal

Luis B. Sardinha
Exercise and Health Laboratory, CIPER
Faculty of Human Kinetics
University of Lisbon
Lisbon, Portugal

Kai Schenk
Department of Sport Science
University of Innsbruck
Innsbruck, Austria

Susan M. Shirreffs
School of Medicine
University of St Andrews
Fife, United Kingdom

Analiza M. Silva
Exercise and Health Laboratory,
  CIPER
Faculty of Human Kinetics
University of Lisbon
Lisbon, Portugal

Arthur Stewart
School of Health Sciences
Centre for Obesity Research &
  Epidemiology
Robert Gordon University
Aberdeen, United Kingdom

Jeffrey R. Stout
Sport and Exercise Science
Institute of Exercise Physiology
  and Wellness
University of Central Florida
Orlando, Florida

Section I

Body Composition Assessment

1 Body Composition in Perspective

Henry C. Lukaski

CONTENTS

1.1 INTRODUCTION

Estimation of body composition is a cornerstone of human nutrition assessment for health care providers, clinical researchers, and epidemiologists. Similarly, determination of fat-free mass, muscle mass, fat mass, and bone quantity and quality is an ongoing topic of interest and practice in the multidisciplinary area of exercise science (Thomas et al. 2016). Awareness and curiosity about the use and interpretation of body composition measurements are extensive and persist among coaches, nutritionists, physical therapists, athletic trainers, and physically active people. Interested persons include not only competitive and recreational athletes but also individuals engaged in physically demanding occupations. For an individual, however, discussion of body composition assessment may elicit concerns related to the rationale and implications of such testing: what is measured (fat, lean, and muscle) and why (e.g., performance enhancement, eligibility for competition, selection and retention for employment, or physical appearance)? Measurement of body composition is escalating into health surveillance with the global assessment of risk for cardiometabolic disease (e.g., obesity and adipose tissue [AT] distribution), appraisal of the impact of increased physical activity with and without concurrent restriction of energy intake on the manifestation and consequences of endocrine dysfunction including bone mass and density or increased jeopardy of musculoskeletal injury, as well as any benefits or detriments of physical training on wellness, growth, and development of youth. These expanding emphases on the inclusion of body composition measurements, particularly in conjunction with physical activity or training and encompassing health-related consequences, contribute to a rationalized, outcome-based model of body composition assessment. These broad interests advance body composition assessment from a descriptive tool to an innovative model that integrates body structure, function, and health (Figure 1.1). This chapter outlines the fundamentals of this practical construct of body composition.

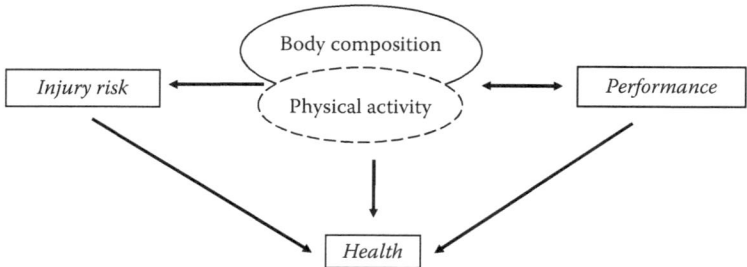

FIGURE 1.1   General model of interaction of physical activity and body composition on health, injury risk, and performance.

1.2   BODY COMPOSITION OF ATHLETES

The history of human body composition begins circa 400 BC with Hippocrates, who theorized health as the balance of the four body fluids, and expands into the early Greek concept that the components of the immediate environment (earth, water, fire, and air) are the basic constituents of the human body. Wen et al. (2005) chronicled the contributors and their accomplishments in body composition science since the 1850s, including the progression of methods, models, and applications in various fields of inquiry including anthropology, medicine, nutrition, and physiology. Stewart (2012) augmented this narrative and focused on the history, concepts, and application of body composition assessment in exercise and work. He highlighted the contribution of the Greek sculptor, Polykleitos (460–410 BC), who is credited with the first association of the ideal body shape with physical function in his classic work, *Doryphorus*, the spear bearer, and acknowledged this work as the origin of the field of anthropometry. Ancient Greek civilization contributed more tangibly to the field of body composition research with the discovery by Archimedes (287–212 BC) that the mass of water displaced when an object is submerged can be used to determine the specific gravity of that object. This crucial observation led to the densitometric method to assess body fatness.

An initial product of body composition research with physically active individuals was the characterization of body fatness (percent body fat) by sport and gender. These reports emphasized the percent body fat levels of adult athletes and reported them as sport-specific group averages and ranges of values for women and men (Buskirk and Taylor 1957; Novak et al. 1968; De Garay et al. 1974; Fleck 1983; Wilmore 1983; Buskirk and Mendez 1984; Lukaski 1997). Overall, body fatness tended to be greater among female compared to male athletes and this trend continued within a specific sport. Also, participants in sports that required weight classifications or utilized predominantly endurance activity tended to have lower average body fatness than participants in other sports. Wilmore (1983) posited that the range of body fatness by gender for a sport could serve as one component of an athlete's physiological profile, and it could be used by aspirant athletes to compare to elite performers to individualize training and dietary recommendations.

1.3   BODY STRUCTURE AND FUNCTION

The 1940s and 1950s were the formative years of body composition research as related to physical activity. A.R. Behnke provided the impetus to advance body composition research by first reporting that differences in body composition were related to significant differences in physical function. Weltham and Behnke (1942) observed that male professional athletes, compared to male civilians and Navy personnel, were classified as overweight (91 vs. 68 kg, respectively) according to standard weight for height tables and, hence, were designated as "unfit for military service and at an increased risk for life insurance." Body densities were greater for the athletes compared to the non-athletes

(1.080 vs. 1.056 g/cc, respectively) indicating that body fatness was less for the athletes. The male athletes, however, had very high levels of physical fitness that was incongruous with the classification of unfit for military service and denial of life insurance. This crucial finding established that body composition assessment, and densitometry per se, could distinguish "big and muscular from big and fat" bodies (Behnke et al. 1942). Dupertuis et al. (1951) and others (Bolonchuk et al. 1989; Siders et al. 1993) later demonstrated that body build or physique, characterized by the principal components of somatotype, was directly related to body composition and performance.

Concurrently, Behnke (1942) reported that retention of inhaled nitrogen by experienced undersea divers depended on body fatness. Because inhaled nitrogen is nearly five times more soluble in fat than water or blood, this finding provided a physiological explanation for the debilitating condition of nitrogen narcosis afflicting some Navy divers. This important finding provided the first indication of an association between body composition (body fatness) and physiological function (excess nitrogen retention), albeit adverse.

1.3.1 BODY FAT

Body composition generally affects cardiorespiratory performance and function. The classic work of E.R. Buskirk demonstrated that maximal oxygen consumption was highly dependent on the fat-free mass of a diverse group of men whose usual physical activity ranged from sedentary to trained endurance athletes (Buskirk 1954; Buskirk and Taylor 1957). Among sedentary male students, body fatness did not affect maximal oxygen consumption values when expressed per unit fat-free mass. In contrast, maximal oxygen uptake was significantly reduced when expressed per unit body weight. Thus, excess weight (e.g., fat) not related to energy production (e.g., fat-free mass) increased the energy cost of performing work during exercise on a treadmill.

Body fatness, however, impairs weight-dependent physical performance. The results of fitness tests of speed and endurance (50-yd sprint and 12-min run, respectively) and power (vertical jump) of women and men were adversely affected by body fatness (Cureton et al. 1979). The men had less fat and performed better than the women on each of the physical fitness tests. The rate of decline in performance as related to body fatness, notably, was similar for the women and the men and indicated that the negative effect of body fatness on weight-dependent activities was independent of gender. Excess body fat is detrimental to performance of weight-supported physical activities regardless of whether the activity is vertical (e.g., jumping) or horizontal (e.g., running) because body fat does not contribute to the production of force that is needed to move the body (Miller and Blyth 1955; Boileau and Lohman 1977; Harman and Frykman 1992; Malina 1992).

Increased levels of body fat, however, may be advantageous in certain activities. As noted by Sinning (1996), contact sports that require the absorption of force or momentum (e.g., American football or Sumo wrestling) may benefit from strategically distributed AT. Similarly, activities that require prolonged exposure in cold water gain an advantage from the buoyancy and insulative characteristics of body fat.

1.3.2 FAT-FREE MASS

Fat-free mass is beneficial in physical activities that require development and application of force (Boileau and Lohman 1977; Harman and Frykman 1992). Generalizations regarding fat-free mass and performance should be tempered with awareness of the needs for muscle mass in sport-specific functions. Activities that require strength and power (e.g., throwing and pushing) and include body movement should optimize muscle mass and, hence, fat-free mass (Slater and Phillips 2011; Stellingwerff et al. 2011). Sports with weight classes, however, should maximize power relative to body weight or size for performance (e.g., combat sports, rowing) with caution to avoid excessive minimization of body weight and fatness (e.g., diving, gymnastics, and endurance sports) (Sundgot-Borgen and Garthe 2011; Sundgot-Borgen et al. 2013).

Relationships between body composition and work-specific performance emphasize the benefit of fat-free mass. Extensive studies of military personnel reveal that fat-free mass is positively correlated with military-specific assessments of aerobic capacity and muscular strength (Harman and Frykman 1992). Body fatness, interestingly, does not predict performance of military tasks unless extreme values are considered (Friedl 2012). Excess adiposity, however, can limit performance in the field that requires work in restricted areas or prolonged aerobic activity, largely due to the negative effects of excess weight (fat) on the energy requirement for movement, and possible limitations associated with impaired thermoregulatory function (Friedl 2004).

1.4 BODY COMPOSITION, PERFORMANCE, AND HEALTH

The relationships among body size and structure, performance and health are interrelated (Figure 1.1). Some sports favor individuals with body sizes, shapes, and composition that, when taken to extremes, can be conducive to health disturbances. Conversely, some individuals with excess adiposity engage in physical activity to change AT distribution and improve health that can be viewed as a form of performance. Other individuals may be required to maintain standards of body composition and physical performance for retention in employment.

1.4.1 PUBLIC SAFETY EMPLOYMENT

Public service occupations include law enforcement, firefighting, and emergency services. Women and men who serve in public safety occupations are required to undertake physically demanding tasks. Thus, physical fitness, which includes work capacity (strength and endurance) and body composition, is a factor in successful completion of employment-related tasks (Moulson-Litchfield and Freedson 1986). Decrements in physical fitness predict an increased risk of injury and chronic disease (Pope et al. 1999; Jahnke et al. 2013).

Consistent with the findings from studies involving athletes, body composition affects the outcomes of physical performance assessments of public safety personnel. Dawes et al. (2016) found that skinfold-based estimates of body fat were negatively correlated with performance of weight-supported activities whereas lean body mass was positively related to strength tests of law enforcement officers. Similarly, performance of simulated work-specific tasks (e.g., carrying weight comparable to rescue or protective equipment) was adversely affected by increased body weight (BMI) and body fat (Michaelides et al. 2011). Increased body size can limit body movement and impair the execution of emergency procedures that can place an emergency responder at an increased risk of injury.

1.4.2 EXTREME LEANNESS

Body weight and composition can be important performance-moderating variables in certain sports (Ackland et al. 2012). Participants in weight-sensitive sports may be at risk for extreme food restriction and clinical disordered eating behaviors (ED) to achieve specific low body weights deemed appropriate for competition (Manore et al. 2007; Sundgot-Borgen et al. 2013). Consequences of restricted food intake that result in low energy availability (LEA) may include nutritional deficiencies (macro- and micronutrient), increased risk of infections, endocrine disturbances leading to amenorrhea in women (Sundgot-Borgen and Garthe 2011; Sundgot-Borgen et al. 2013), impaired bone health (quantity and quality of bone) as well as adverse disruptions of other physiological systems in women and men (Joy et al. 2016; Tenforde et al. 2016).

The performance consequences of ED and LEA depend on the age of initiation of these factors, rate of weight reduction, duration of the LEA, use of additive means for weight loss, and the pathology of ED. Functional impairments include a decrease in aerobic capacity and muscular strength due to altered cardiovascular function and concurrent loss of muscle mass, dehydration, and electrolyte imbalance. Descriptions of performance decrements attributed to body composition change may be confounded by dubious estimates of body composition. This limitation contributes to concerns related to proposals for minimally acceptable levels of body fatness that impact measures of performance and health (Sundgot-Borgen and Garthe 2011; Ackland et al. 2012; Sundgot-Borgen et al. 2013).

1.4.3 Hydration

Hydration is a complex physiological condition that includes total body water, its distribution, and the concentration of the major electrolytes (osmolality). It may be classified as under- or hypohydration, normal or euhydration, and over- or hyperhydration. The simplicity of these designations belies the controversy in establishing the criterion biological indicators and threshold values to classify the hydration status of an individual (Maughan 2012). There is no universally accepted standard for classification of hypohydration or dehydration (Cheuvront et al. 2010). Reduction in body weight is a noninvasive, commonly used indicator whereas plasma or serum osmolality, saliva osmolality, and various urine parameters are more invasive and should be obtained under controlled conditions (Cheuvront and Kenefick 2014). Weight loss exceeding 2.5% is one indicator of hypohydration because it reflects a 3% deficit in body water that equates to significant reductions in plasma volume and increases in plasma osmolality levels (Sawka et al. 2015). Such water deficits and alterations in electrolyte concentrations are associated with impaired aerobic, strength, and power performances that are exacerbated in a hot environment (Cheuvront and Kenefick 2014).

Emerging, but not definitive, evidence suggests that hypohydration, may also adversely affect cognition and other mental functions. Adan (2012) noted that hypohydration, characterized by body weight loss exceeding 2%, impairs performance of tasks that require attention, psychomotor skills, and immediate memory skills whereas the performance of long-term, working memory tasks and executive functions are better preserved, especially if moderate exercise is the cause of dehydration. Benton and Young (2015) concluded that dehydration, indicated by a 2% or greater decrease in body mass, impairs mood, decreases perception of alertness and promotes self-reported fatigue. Muñoz et al. (2015) observed that total daily water intake was a significant predictor of mood in a large sample of healthy young women. The magnitude of the variance in predicting altered mood states associated with total daily water intake, however, was modest (<11%) after controlling for known factors that affect mood (e.g., exercise, caffeine, and macronutrient intakes). Benton et al. (2016) reported that mild dehydration, described as a 1% decrease in body weight, has functional consequences including significant reductions in attention and memory and increases in anxiety among adults.

1.4.4 Injury Risk

Individuals who engage in physical training are likely to incur musculoskeletal injury. Two factors contribute to an increased relative risk of injury. Extremes of body weight, assessed with BMI, and body fatness predict increased risk of injury among military recruits and law enforcement officers (Jones et al. 1992; Jahnke et al. 2013). Aerobic fitness or endurance also predicts risk of injury with less fit women and men at greater risk of injury (Jones et al. 1992; Pope et al. 1999).

1.4.5 Health Risk

Epidemiological surveys reveal, and clinical research confirms, that body composition is related to risk of cardiometabolic (obesity, insulin insensitivity, and type 2 diabetes) and cardiovascular diseases. Excess accumulation of fat or AT in adults, evidenced with BMI values exceeding 30 kg/m^2, is a risk factor positively associated with morbidity and mortality for cardiovascular and other chronic diseases independent of gender and age (Poirier et al. 2006). However, increased BMI only partially explains some of this increased risk. Accretion of AT in the abdomen, specifically in the visceral (VAT) as compared to subcutaneous region (SAT), is a unique phenotype associated with the greatest health risk (Després 2012; Bastien et al. 2014). Whereas magnetic resonance imaging is the reference method to determine estimated VAT and SAT in clinical research, abdominal circumference is a valid surrogate for practical assessment of VAT (Kuk et al. 2005). Caloric restriction and exercise, independently and in combination, reduce the volume of VAT and SAT in obese adults (Ross et al. 2000).

Because the origin of cardiovascular disease can begin early in life, there is a growing interest in determining the effects of increased physical activity on amelioration of obesity and risk-related AT distribution of children. Whereas energy restriction can be used to attenuate obesity in adults, it poses a potential problem in children because excessive dieting may adversely affect growth and development. Thus, exercise is an attractive modality because it also is critical for growth and development of children (Malina et al. 2004).

Aerobic exercise decreases total body fat and facilitates a favorable distribution of abdominal AT in children (Atlantis et al. 2006; Kelley and Kelley 2013). Interestingly, aerobic and resistance exercise independently enable loss of body fat and abdominal AT in obese adolescents (Monteiro et al. 2015). Resistance exercise may be additionally important because it specifically stimulates musculoskeletal development in adolescents. Noteworthy is the direct benefit of resistance, as compared to aerobic, exercise on bone in youth with evidence that gains in bone quality and quantity may persist during adulthood (Tan et al. 2014).

1.5   EMPIRICAL MODEL OF BODY COMPOSITION, FUNCTION, AND HEALTH

Burgeoning information links body composition, a component of physique, as a shared factor influencing performance, health, and injury risk (Figure 1.2). Increased body size and shape, as evidenced with an increased BMI and enlarged waist circumference, are risk factors for cardiometabolic disease, and can adversely affect weight-supported performance. Similarly, increased body fat is adversely related to endurance performance whereas increased fat-free mass and muscle mass are associated with increased power and strength particularly in weight classification activities. Emerging evidence identifies differences in muscle quality and function (e.g., distribution of mass and strength) in the upper versus the lower body, ipsilateral versus contralateral regions and opposing areas (e.g., anterior and posterior) of major muscle groups (e.g., shoulder, trunk, upper and lower

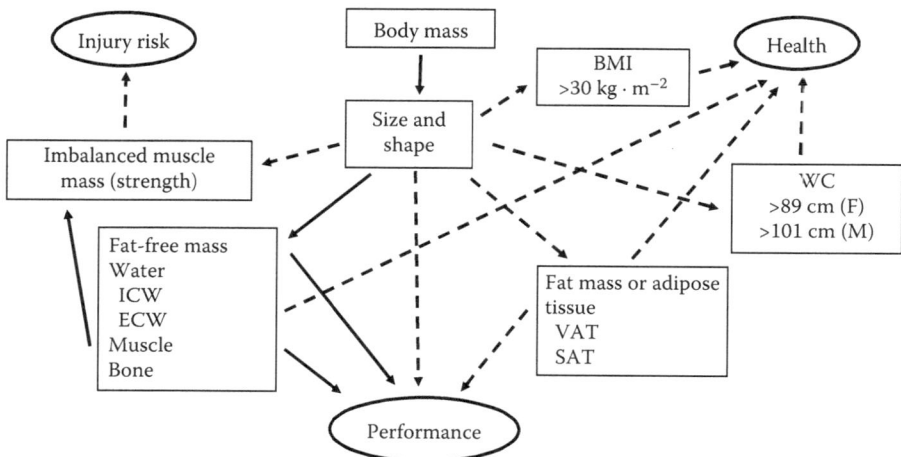

FIGURE 1.2 Integrated model of body composition variables affecting health, injury risk, and performance. Solid lines designate beneficial effects and interrupted lines indicate adverse effects. BMI = body mass index; WC = waist circumference; F = female; M = male; VAT = visceral adipose tissue; SAT = subcutaneous adipose tissue; ICW = intracellular water; ECW = extracellular water.

leg) as indicators of an elevated risk of injury and probable constraints to optimal performance and health.

Environmental and behavioral factors can impact body size and composition, health, injury hazard, and performance. Unwarranted physical activity and dietary restriction to achieve excessive and unnecessary weight loss among female and male athletes can impair health, bone quality, and performance. Similarly, failure to adequately maintain fluid intake and balance during periods of physical training or occupational demands can markedly decrease physical and probably cognitive functions. Beneficial effects of physical activity to reduce total fat and localized AT of adults and youth result in improvements in cardiorespiratory function, muscle strength and endurance, and, in certain situations, bone mass and quality.

Body composition, as a component of physique, is one factor in the physiological profile of an individual. Reliance on body composition alone to predict performance is inappropriate because of the fundamental contributions of mediating influences including metabolic capacity, skill, psychological attributes, and genetics, which influence some of these factors. Proper understanding of the possible limitations of assessments of fat-free mass, muscle mass, and percent body fat is needed for interpretation of test results. Specifically, interindividual variability and errors of the method (technical and biological) impact the validity of any body composition measurement. These factors need to be considered in relation to proposed changes in compositional variables for anticipated improvements in performance and health. Thus, body composition assessments broadly describe characteristics and highlight physical areas to emphasize in development of individualized training and dietary intervention. Importantly, body composition per se does not predict performance for an individual but only identifies traits related to the performance of others; it can be a useful guide to monitor effectiveness of preparation to improve performance and health.

REFERENCES

Ackland, T. R., T. G. Lohman, J. Sundgot-Borgen et al. 2012. Current status of body composition assessment in sport: Review and position statement on behalf of the ad hoc research working group on body composition health and performance, under the auspices of the I.O.C. Medical Commission. *Sports Med* 42:227–49.

Adan, A. 2012. Cognitive performance and dehydration. *J Am Coll Nutr* 31:71–8.

Atlantis, E., E. H. Barnes, and M. A. Singh. 2006. Efficacy of exercise for treating overweight in children and adolescents: A systematic review. *Int J Obes (Lond)* 30(7):1027–40.

Bastien, M., P. Pirier, I. LemBieux, and J. P. Després. 2014. Overview of epidemiology and contribution of obesity to cardiovascular disease. *Prog Cardiovasc Dis* 56:369–81.

Behnke, A. R. 1942. Physiologic studies pertaining to deep sea diving and aviation, especially in relation to the fat content and composition of the body: The Harvey Lecture, March 19, 1942. *Bull N Y Acad Med* 18:561–85.

Behnke, A. R., B. G. Feen, and W. C. Welham. 1942. The specific gravity of healthy men: Body weight divided by volume as an index of obesity. *J Am Med Assoc* 118:495–8.

Benton, D., K. T. Jenkins, H. T. Watkins, and H. A. Young. 2016. Minor degree of hypohydration adversely influences cognition: A mediator analysis. *Am J Clin Nutr* 104:603–12.

Benton, D. and H. A. Young. 2015. Do small differences in hydration status affect mood and mental performance? *Nutr Rev* 70(Suppl. 2):S128–31.

Boileau, R. A. and T. G. Lohman. 1977. The measurement of human physique and its effect on physical performance. *Orthop Clin North Am* 8:563–81.

Bolonchuk, W. W., C. B. Hall, H. C. Lukaski, and W. A. Siders. 1989. Relationship between body composition and the components of somatotype. *Am J Hum Biol* 1:239–48.

Buskirk, E. R. 1954. Relationships in man between maximal oxygen uptake and components of body composition. PhD thesis. Minneapolis, MN: University of Minnesota.

Buskirk, E. R. and J. Mendez. 1984. Sports science and body composition analysis: Emphasis on cell and muscle mass. *Med Sci Sports Exerc* 16:584–95.

Buskirk, E. R. and H. L. Taylor. 1957. Maximal oxygen uptake and its relation to body composition, with special reference to chronic physical activity and obesity. *J Appl Physiol* 11:72–8.

Calavalle, A. R., D. Sisti, G. Mennelli et al. 2013. A simple method to analyze overall individual physical fitness in firefighters. *J Strength Cond Res* 27:769–75.

Cheuvront, S. and R. Kenefick. 2014. Dehydration: Physiology, assessment, and performance effects. *Comp Physiol* 4:257–85.

Cheuvront, S. N., B. R. Ely, R. W. Kenefick, and M. N. Sawka. 2010. Biological variation and diagnostic accuracy of dehydration assessment markers. *Am J Clin Nutr* 92:565–73.

Cureton, K. J., L. D. Hensley, and A. Tiburzi. 1979. Body fatness and performance differences between men and women. *Res Q* 50:333–40.

Dawes, J. J., R. M. Orr, C. L. Siekaniec, A. A. Vanderwoude, and R. Pope. 2016. Associations between anthropometric characteristics and physical performance in male law enforcement officers: A retrospective cohort study. *Ann Occup Environ Med* 28:26.

De Garay, A. L., L. Levine, and J. E. L. Carter. 1974. *Genetic and Anthropological Studies of Olympic Athletes*. New York: Academic Press.

Després, J. P. 2012. Body fat distribution and risk of cardiovascular disease: An update. *Circulation* 126(10):1301–13.

Dupertuis, C. W., G. C. Pitts, E. F. Osserman, W. C. Welham, and A. R. Behnke. 1951. Relation of specific gravity to body build in a group of healthy men. *J Appl Physiol* 3:676–80.

Fleck, S. J. 1983. Body composition of elite American athletes. *Am J Sports Med* 11:398–403.

Friedl, K. E. 2004. Can you be large and not obese? The distinction between body weight, body fat, and abdominal fat in occupational standards. *Diab Technol Ther* 6:732–49.

Friedl, K. E. 2012. Body composition and military performance—Many things to many people. *J Strength Cond Res* 26(Suppl 2):S87–100.

Harman, E. A. and P. N. Frykman. 1992. The relationship of body size and composition to the performance of physically demanding military tasks. In: *Body Composition and Physical Performance: Applications for the Military Services*, eds. B. M. Marriott and J. Grumstrup-Scott, 105–18. Washington, DC: National Academy Press.

Jahnke, S. A., W. S. Poston, C. K. Haddock, and N. Jitnarin. 2013. Obesity and incident injury among career firefighters in the central United States. *Obesity* 21:1505–8.

Jones, B. H., M. W. Bovee, and J. J. Knapik. 1992. Associations among body composition, physical fitness, and injury in men and women Army trainees. In *Body Composition and Physical Performance: Applications for the Military Services*, eds. B. M. Marriott and J. Grumstrup-Scott, 141–74. Washington, DC: National Academies Press.

Joy, E., A. Kussman, and A. Nattiv. 2016. 2016 update on eating disorders in athletes: A comprehensive narrative review with a focus on clinical assessment and management. *Br J Sports Med* 50:154–62.

Kelley, G. A. and K. S. Kelley. 2013. Effects of exercise in the treatment of overweight and obese children and adolescents: A systematic review of meta-analyses. *J Obes* 2013:783103.

Kuk, J. L., S. Lee, S. B. Heymsfield, and R. Ross. 2005. Waist circumference and abdominal adipose tissue distribution: Influence of age and sex. *Am J Clin Nutr* 81:1330–4.

Lukaski, H. C. 1997. Body composition in exercise and sport. In *Nutrition in Exercise and Sport*, ed. I. Wolinsky, 621–44. Boca Raton, FL: CRC Press.

Malina, R., C. Bouchard, and O. Bar-Or. 2004. *Growth, Maturation, and Physical Activity*, 2nd Ed., Champaign, IL: Human Kinetics.

Malina, R. M. 1992. Physique and body composition: Effects on performance and effects on training, semistarvation and overtraining. In *Eating, Body Weight and Performance in Athletes*, eds. K. D. Brownell, J. Rodin, and J. H. Wilmore, 94–114. Champaign, IL: Human Kinetics.

Manore, M. M., L. C. Kam, and A. B. Loucks. 2007. The female athlete triad: Components, nutrition issues, and health consequences. *J Sports Sci* 25(Suppl 1):S61–71.

Maughan, R. J. 2012. Investigating the associations between hydration and exercise performance: Methodology and limitations. *Nutr Rev* 11(Suppl 2):S128–31.

Michaelides, M. A., K. M. Parpa, L. J. Henry, G. B. Thompson, and B. S. Brown. 2011. Assessment of physical fitness aspects and their relationship to firefighters' job abilities. *J Strength Cond Res* 25:956–65.

Miller, A. T. and C. S. Blyth. 1955. Influence of body type and body fat content on the metabolic cost of work. *J Appl Physiol* 8:139–41.

Monteiro, P. A., K. Y. Chen, F. S. Lira et al. 2015. Concurrent and aerobic exercise training promote similar benefits in body composition and metabolic profiles in obese adolescents. *Lipids Health Dis* 14:153. doi: 10.1186/s12944-015-0152-9.

Moulson-Litchfield, M. and P. S. Freedson. 1986. Physical training programs for public safety personnel. *Clin Sports Med* 5:571–87.

Muñoz, C. X., E. C. Johnson, A. L. McKenzie et al. 2015. Habitual total water intake and dimensions of mood in healthy young women. *Appetite* 92:81–6.

Novak, L. P., R. E. Hyatt, and J. F. Alexander. 1968. Body composition and physiologic function of athletes. *J Am Med Assoc* 205:764–70.

Poirier, P., T. D. Giles, G. A. Bray et al. 2006. Obesity and cardiovascular disease: Pathophysiology, evaluation, and effect of weight loss. *Arterioscler Thromb Vasc Biol* 26:968–76.

Pope, R. P., R. Herbert, J. D. Kirwin, and B. J. Graham. 1999. Predicting attrition in basic military training. *Mil Med* 164:710–4.

Ross, R., D. Dagnone, P. J. Jones et al. 2000. Reduction in obesity and related comorbid conditions after diet-induced weight loss or exercise-induced weight loss in men. A randomized, controlled trial. *Ann Intern Med* 133:92–103.

Sawka, M. N., S. N. Cheuvront, and R. W. Kenefick. 2015. Hypohydration and human performance: Impact of environment and physiological mechanisms. *Sports Med* 45(Suppl 1):S51–60.

Siders W. A., H. C. Lukaski, and W. W. Bolonchuk. 1993. Relationships among swimming performance, body composition and somatotype in competitive collegiate swimmers. *J Sports Med Phys Fitness* 33:166–71.

Sinning, W. E. 1996. Body composition in athletes. In *Human Body Composition*, 1st Ed., eds. A. F. Roche, S. B. Heymsfield, and T. G. Lohman, 257–74. Champaign, IL: Human Kinetics.

Slater, G. and S. M. Phillips. 2011. Nutrition guidelines for strength sports: Sprinting, weightlifting, throwing events, and body building. *J Sports Sci* 29(S1):S67–77.

Stellingwerff, T., R. J. Maughan, and L. M. Burke. 2011. Nutrition for power sports: Middle-distance running, track cycling, rowing/canoeing/kayaking, and swimming. *J Sports Sci* 29(S1):S79–89.

Stewart, A. D. 2012. The concept of body composition and its application. In *Body Composition in Sport, Exercise and Health*, eds. A. D. Stewart and L. Sutton, 1–19. New York: Routledge.

Sundgot-Borgen, J. and I. Garthe. 2011. Elite athletes in aesthetic and Olympic weight class sports and the challenges of body weight and composition. *J Sports Sci* 29(S1):S101–14.

Sundgot-Borgen, J., N. L. Meyer, T. G. Lohman et al. 2013. How to minimise the health risks to athletes who compete in weight-sensitive sports review and position statement on behalf of the Ad Hoc Research Working Group on Body Composition, Health and Performance, under the auspices of the IOC Medical Commission. *Br J Sports Med* 47:1012–22.

Tan, V. P., H. M. Macdonald, S. Kim et al. 2014. Influence of physical activity on bone strength in children and adolescents: A systematic review and narrative synthesis. *J Bone Miner Res* 29:2161–81.

Tenforde, A. S., M. T. Barrack, A. Nattiv, and M. Fredericson. 2016. Parallels with the Female Athlete Triad in male athletes. *Sports Med* 46:171–82.

Thomas, D. T., K. A. Erdman, and L. M. Burke. 2016. American College of Sports Medicine Joint Position Statement. Nutrition and Athletic Performance. *Med Sci Sports Exerc* 48:543–68.

Weltham, W. C. and A. R. Behnke. 1942. The specific gravity of healthy men: Body weight ÷ volume and other physical characteristics of exceptional athletes and of naval personnel. *JAMA* 118:498–501.

Wen, S., M.-P. St-Onge, Z. Wang, and S. B. Heymsfield. 2005. Study of body composition: An overview. In *Human Body Composition*, 2nd Ed., eds. S. B. Heymsfield, T. G. Lohman, Z. Wang, and S. B. Going, 3–14. Champaign, IL: Human Kinetics.

Wilmore, J. H. 1983. Body composition in sport and exercise: Directions for future research. *Med Sci Sports Exerc* 15:21–3n1.

2 Assessment of Human Body Composition

Methods and Limitations

Hannes Gatterer, Kai Schenk, and Martin Burtscher

CONTENTS

2.1 INTRODUCTION

The assessment of the human body composition is a useful practice in various fields, including medicine, nutrition, and sports sciences (Ackland et al. 2012; Fosbøl and Zerahn 2015). Individuals participating in regular and/or intense physical activity (recreation, competition, and occupation) have an interest in body composition as it relates to key components, such as lean or fat-free mass, muscle mass, and fatness, that can be associated with function, performance, and health (Ackland et al. 2012). Measurement of human body composition requires an understanding of the basic principles and limitations of the wide variety of methods and techniques available. This information enables a realistic assessment of body components that allows for characterization and identification of changes in response to training and other interventions (van Marken Lichtenbelt et al. 2004).

Assessment of human body composition utilizes different models that rely on specific chemical components and distinctive physical characteristics of the healthy body (Lukaski 1987). The most commonly applied model in sports is the two-component model that consists of fat mass (FM) and fat-free mass (FFM) (van Marken Lichtenbelt et al. 2004; Ackland et al. 2012; Fosbøl and Zerahn 2015). It relies on certain assumptions, including a constant hydration of the fat-free body and a constant bone-to-muscle ratio that have been questioned (Womersley et al. 1976). Awareness of interindividual differences in bone mineral density and hydration associated with growth, physical training, and aging led to the development of the three-component (fat, lean content, and bone, or fat, water, and non-fat solids) and four-component (water, protein, lipids, others) models that

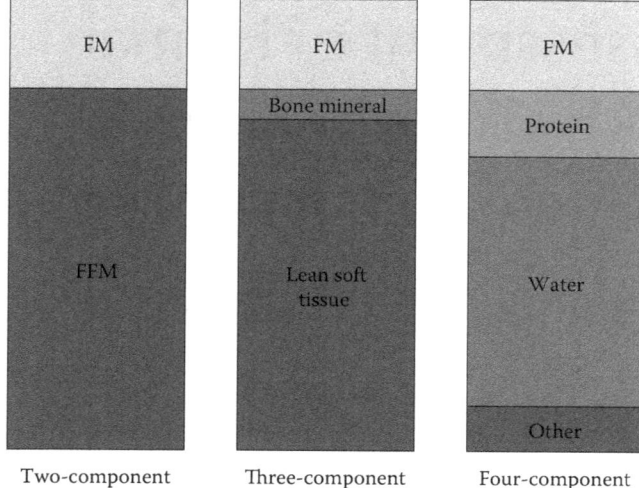

FIGURE 2.1   Main body component models. FM, fat mass; FFM, fat-free mass.

differentiated body fractions to account for interindividual differences in the components of the fat-free body (Figure 2.1) (Ellis 2000; Ackland et al. 2012; Fosbøl and Zerahn 2015; Heymsfield et al. 2015).

Numerous methods are available for the assessment of human body composition. They include simple techniques applicable for use in the field or non-laboratory settings such as weight, standing height, anthropometry (skinfold thicknesses and body circumferences), and bioelectrical impedance analysis (BIA). In contrast, more complex methods are limited to the controlled environment of a laboratory and require sophisticated equipment and trained technical support personnel and range from isotope dilution, densitometry, whole-body plethysmography, and radiological methods with increased risk due to exposure to ionizing radiation (Heymsfield et al. 1997). Despite the plethora of available methods and techniques, there is consensus that an absolute standard or reference method for human body composition is lacking. Whereas there is growing support for some radiological methods for use in validation studies of new and indirect methods because of their high precision and acceptable accuracy, their general availability is very restricted (Earthman 2015). Thus, all individual methods follow an indirect approach and are not entirely free from error (Withers et al. 1999; Earthman 2015). Comparisons among newly proposed methods rely on validation with multicomponent model assessments (Nana et al. 2015). Whereas the validity of body composition assessment can be ascertained with group comparisons to an accepted reference method, the practical question remains the precision of an estimate for an individual.

The main aim of this chapter is to describe the physical bases of the methods for the assessment of body composition and outline the characteristics of each technique focusing on validity, applicability, and precision of estimation of a body component for an individual.

2.2   VALIDITY AND APPLICABILITY

Validity and applicability are critical issues when describing measurement methods. In most body composition studies, validity encompasses the concepts of accuracy and precision besides others (Earthman 2015). Precision refers to the degree of agreement among repeated measurements for a specific method, that is, how variable are repeated measurements. The magnitude of precision is generally reported as the coefficient of variation (CV), given as percent value and calculated as standard deviation (SD) expressed as a percent of the mean of repeated measurements (CV = [SD/mean] × 100%) (Earthman 2015). Another expression of precision is the intraclass (ICC) or simple correlation coefficient. The ICC measures the relative homogeneity within groups in ratio to the total variation and is calculated as between subject variability/(between subject variability + error) (Weir 2005; Currell and Jeukendrup 2008).

Accuracy differs from precision because it indicates the closeness of agreement between two assessment methods, that is, how close a measured value is to the "true" value. Accuracy is determined with different statistical approaches. One method uses linear regression analysis between paired measurements in a group of individuals. It reports the correlation coefficient and standard error of the estimate (SEE) that indicates the variability of the data distributed around the line representing the data. Linear regression analysis is a basic approach that provides some insight to validity when a significant correlation coefficient and a small SEE are found. It also provides the total error (TE) calculated as the sum of squared differences between the practical estimate of reference and candidate methods, which is a similar indicator as SEE. Researchers use inferential statistics to secure a greater degree of examination of validity within a broad sample by using a paired t-test and can ascertain validity within subgroups (e.g., female and male, lean and obese) of the larger sample with analysis of variance (ANOVA) and appropriate post hoc test when a significant main effect is found. The most rigorous test of validity is the Bland–Altman analysis that generally follows an ANOVA. It is a graphical representation of the mean difference or bias between measured and predicted values that are shown as a function of the average value ([measured + predicted]/s) and includes the 95% confidence interval (CI) for the mean difference. Importantly, the Bland–Altman analysis shows the trend for bias with increasing body composition values expressed as the correlation coefficient and limits of agreement (LOA; e.g., 95% CI) that indicates the precision of an estimate for an individual (Earthman 2015; Fosbøl and Zerahn 2015). It is important to note that the true accuracy of any body composition method can be considered problematic, as no "gold standard" or "true" value is available. Thus, accuracy of an individual method can be established solely by comparing the results to the best-available reference method (Earthman 2015).

Applicability is a fundamental issue to consider when performing body composition analysis. Methods like anthropometry, skinfold thicknesses, and BIA are safe, simple, "portable," noninvasive, easy-to-perform, and relatively inexpensive methods that are popular in sports, but might lack accuracy under some circumstances (Prado and Heymsfield 2014). Conversely, complex methods (for example, hydrodensitometry, air displacement plethysmography [ADP], dual x-ray absorptiometry [DXA]) require very controlled and standardized conditions, specialized operator technical skills, high level of patient cooperation, and possible exposure to ionizing radiation, and are costly to operate but may be considered more accurate (Prado and Heymsfield 2014). Therefore, the choice of the body composition technique depends on the intended purpose, required accuracy and precision, and availability of the technique.

2.3 TECHNIQUES FOR THE ASSESSMENT OF BODY COMPOSITION

2.3.1 TWO-COMPONENT METHODS

2.3.1.1 Anthropometry

The most commonly recorded anthropometric data are body mass, standing height, specific body segment lengths, breadths and circumferences, skinfold thickness, and, currently, the measurement of subcutaneous fat with ultrasound (Bellisari and Roche 2005; Ackland et al. 2012; Pescatello et al. 2014; Fosbøl and Zerahn 2015; Müller et al. 2016b). Owing to their association with body components, all of these values, individually or in various combinations, can be used to estimate FM and FFM in a two-component model. It should be emphasized that all equations are specific to the population from whom the equation was derived and thus large estimation errors may occur with differing populations (e.g., in athletes). Nonetheless, anthropometric data in general can be provided by simple and feasible measurements outside laboratory conditions. As a consequence, anthropometry may be used on large samples to obtain national estimates of body composition and/or representative samples for investigating changes over time (Bellisari and Roche 2005). However, performing anthropometric measurements have to be trained in order to achieve high precision and reduce the intra- and interobserver variability (Fosbøl and Zerahn 2015).

2.3.1.1.1 Body Mass Index

Body mass index (BMI) is calculated from body mass and height (kg/m^2). BMI values are moderately correlated to body-fat percentage (%BF, $r = 0.6$–0.8) and can be used to estimate %BF with an intraindividual precision (SEE) of approximately ±5% (Gallagher et al. 2000; Bellisari and Roche 2005; Pescatello et al. 2014). To be meaningful for children and adolescents, the BMI must be compared to a reference standard that accounts for age and sex (Must and Anderson 2006).

The use of BMI to estimate changes in %BF after strength training in bodybuilders was associated with a mean estimated bias of +2.6%BF with LOA of approximately 3.7% compared to a four-component model, which showed changes of −1.6%BF and a range of −5.0% to 1.2% (van Marken Lichtenbelt et al. 2004). For FFM changes, mean bias was approximately −2.3 kg with LOA of approximately 3.8 kg compared to the four-component model with reported changes of +3.7 kg and a range of −0.6 to 7.7 kg (van Marken Lichtenbelt et al. 2004). Additionally, in judo athletes performing a weight loss program, an SEE for the determination of %BF changes of 1.9% was reported (compared to a four-component model) (Silva et al. 2009).

2.3.1.1.2 Circumferences

Measurements of body regions provide a general picture of body composition. Abdominal and limb circumferences show moderate correlation with body density ($r = -0.7$ and $r = -0.4$, respectively) and the accuracy of %BF estimation may be within 2.5%–4.4% if the subjects possess similar characteristics as the reference population (Tran and Weltman 1988, 1989; Bellisari and Roche 2005; Pescatello et al. 2014). Moreover, when compared to a four-component model, LOA ranging between +11.4% and −13.2% for %BF estimation were reported for a general healthy population (Clasey et al. 1999).

2.3.1.1.3 Skinfold Thickness

Assessment of subcutaneous adipose tissue measured by using a calibrated caliper is an accepted and frequently applied method to predict body density and body FM. There are described more than 19 sites for measuring skinfold thickness and well over 100 FM prediction equations exist (Ackland et al. 2012; Fosbøl and Zerahn 2015). The method is based on two basic assumptions: the amount of subcutaneous fat is proportional to the total amount of FM and the sites selected for measurement represent the average thickness of the subcutaneous tissue (Lukaski 1987; Pescatello et al. 2014). Both assumptions are questionable and may give rise to measurement errors. For example, sex, age, and race differences may exist in the exact proportion of subcutaneous to total FM (Pescatello et al. 2014). Additionally, even though the measurement method appears simple, substantial intra- and interobserver variability may exist (Fosbøl and Zerahn 2015). The reasons for this variability include variations in the selection/location of the measurement site and/or in the technique of grasping the skinfold, edema, or difficulties when measuring extremely lean or obese subjects (Pescatello et al. 2014; Fosbøl and Zerahn 2015). Skinfold thickness shows correlations in the range of $r = 0.7$–0.9 with %BF and a precision of within 5% can be attained by properly trained individuals (Lukaski 1987; Bellisari and Roche 2005). The accuracy of %BF prediction is approximately ±3.5% provided that appropriate techniques and equations are applied (Evans et al. 2005; Pescatello et al. 2014), but also SEE of ~5% and LOA ranging from 13% to 22%FM are reported when %BF was compared with four-component models (Durnin and Womersley 1974; Clasey et al. 1999; Ackland et al. 2012; Fosbøl and Zerahn 2015). In male and female athletes, SEE for %FM estimation in the range of 2.38%–3.16% and 3.02%–3.37%, respectively, were reported compared to underwater weighing (UWW) (Sinning and Wilson 1984; Sinning et al. 1985). When %BF and FFM changes after strength training were compared to a four-component model, a mean estimation bias of 0.3% and −0.3 kg was reported with LOA of approximately 3.5% and 2.3 kg, respectively (using the four-component model, the established changes for %FM were −1.6% with a range of −5.0% to 1.2% and for FFM +3.7 kg with a range of −0.6% to 7.7 kg) (van Marken Lichtenbelt et al. 2004). Additionally, for %BF changes, similar results were reported in judo athletes performing a weight reduction program with mean biases ranging from −0.1% to 0.1% (depending on the equation) and with LOA ranging from −3.4% to 3.6% when compared to a four-component model, which showed changes of −0.44 ± 2.17%BF (Silva et al. 2009). Furthermore, with physical training and nutritional interventions, mean biases for changes in %BF were 1.0 ± 2.0% and LOA of 3.6%–4.2% were reported in a weight reduction setting (Evans et al. 1999).

2.3.1.1.4 Ultrasound
An alternative method to measure subcutaneous adipose or FM uses the pulse-echo technique (Ackland et al. 2012). A short pulse (several wavelengths long) is applied, which propagates with the speed of sound through the tissues where it is partially reflected from dissimilar tissue interfaces and returns to the transducer as an echo (Bellisari and Roche 2005; Müller et al. 2016b). An advantage of ultrasound when compared to skinfold thickness measurement is the possibility to measure very obese subjects and at anatomical sites where skinfolds cannot be raised (Bellisari and Roche 2005; Fosbøl and Zerahn 2015). It was found that with ultrasound, differences of 2 mm of subcutaneous FM (of the sum from eight sites) can be distinguished reproducibly (95% of subcutaneous FM thickness sums were within ±1 mm) (Müller et al. 2016b). From a technical perspective, the accuracy of ultrasound subcutaneous FM thickness measurement is approximately 0.2 mm, if sound speed is set correctly (Müller et al. 2016b). Recently, appropriate measurement sites have been defined and standardization of measurement technique was provided for the ultrasound method (Müller et al. 2016b). However, equations for the estimation of total body FM are not yet available.

2.3.1.2 Bioelectrical Impedance Analyses and Bioimpedance Spectroscopy
Bioimpedance provides indirect information on body composition by measuring resistance (R), which is the opposition to the flow of an alternating current through intra- and extracellular ionic solution, and reactance (Xc), which is the capacitive component of tissue interfaces, cell membranes, and organelles of the body (Lukaski 2013). Impedance is the term used to describe the combination of R and Xc (Kyle et al. 2004a) and is determined by the vector relationship of impedance (Z) contributed by R and Xc (Chumlea and Sun 2005; Earthman 2015). The technique assumes that the body is cylindrical in shape and that the conductivity is constant throughout the conductor (Kyle et al. 2004a; Fosbøl and Zerahn 2015). The technique involves the application of a weak, alternating current throughout the body either with surface, contact electrodes placed on the foot and hand or fixed metallic electrodes of an impedance device directly in contact with the soles of the feet and/or palms of the hands (Duren et al. 2008; Earthman 2015; Fosbøl and Zerahn 2015). The electrical conduction in the body is related to the water and electrolyte distribution. While FFM (typically containing an assumed 73% water) easily conducts the current, FM and bone do not (Lukaski 1987; Ellis 2000; Kyle et al. 2004a; Earthman 2015). Additionally, different current frequencies may be applied by the devices. At low frequencies (i.e., 0–5 kHz), the current flows predominantly through the extracellular water as it does not penetrate the cell membrane that acts as insulator (Kyle et al. 2004a; Chumlea and Sun 2005). Thus, R at these frequencies represents the extracellular fluid (ECF) whereas no Xc is measured (Kyle et al. 2004a). With increasing frequency, the current also penetrates the cell membrane after a brief delay and enters the intracellular space; the delay at cell membrane enables measurement of capacitance or 1/reactance ($1/Xc$). At very high frequencies (i.e., >100 kHz), the current penetrates all body tissues, Xc is again minimized and R represents both intracellular and extracellular fluid (Kyle et al. 2004a; Chumlea and Sun 2005). With bioimpedance, FFM is estimated from different equations using one or more impedance variables (e.g., R, Xc, Z), standing height, body weight, and gender, and by assuming a constant hydration level of the FFM

(Earthman 2015). There exist also equations for the estimation of body FM (Kyle et al. 2004a), but FM can likewise be calculated by subtracting FFM from body weight. It is emphasized that all equations are derived from comparison with other body composition methods (e.g., DXA, densitometry) using regression analyses and are specific to the population under investigation.

2.3.1.2.1 Single-Frequency BIA

This technique generally uses a frequency of 50 kHz. As mentioned, at 50 kHz, the current passes through both intra- and extracellular fluid and thus measures are a weighted sum of intracellular and extracellular water (Kyle et al. 2004a).

2.3.1.2.2 Multiple-Frequency BIA

In contrast to single-frequency BIA, this method utilizes alternating currents at various combinations of three to five frequencies typically including at least one low (i.e., <5 kHz), several mid-level (e.g., 50, 100, 200 kHz), and one or more at high frequency (500 kHz to 1 MHz). In contrast to single-frequency BIA, multiple-frequency BIA theoretically allows the differentiation of estimations of both intracellular and extracellular water (Kyle et al. 2004a; Earthman 2015).

2.3.1.2.3 Bioimpedance Spectroscopy

Another approach is bioimpedance spectroscopy (BIS) that uses 50 or more frequencies ranging from very low (e.g., 1–5 kHz) to very high (e.g., 1000–1200 kHz) (Earthman 2015). The application of a current to the body with these frequency ranges yields an interrupted semicircle locus from which the Cole plot can be depicted by using nonlinear, least squares curve fitting (Figure 2.2) (Lukaski 2013). Values derived from the Cole plot (e.g., R_0, R_∞) are used to develop prediction equations for body composition estimates (Kyle et al. 2004a).

The precision of all impedance techniques (i.e., single- and multiple-frequency BIA and BIS) is very good, with 1%–2% variability for single- and multiple-frequency BIA and 2%–3% for BIS (Earthman 2015). Close adherence to recommended measurement protocols for bioimpedance measurements as outlined by Kyle et al. (2004b) is essential to minimize potential errors (Earthman 2015).

With bioimpedance, the SEE for FM estimation typically ranges between 3.8%–5% and 1.9–3.6 kg and for FFM between 1.8 and 3.6 kg for healthy adults and athletes (Stewart and Hannan 2000; Kyle et al. 2004a). Additionally, Fosbøl et al. reported a bias for %BF determination when compared to a four-component model of −10% to 5%, with LOA ranging up to ±8% in healthy adults (Fosbøl and Zerahn 2015). By using BIA to establish %BF and FFM changes after a strength training program, mean biases of 1.5% and −1.1 kg and LOA of approximately 6.2% and 5.2 kg, respectively, were reported compared to a four-component model with changes of −1.6% (range −5.0% to 1.2%) for %BF and +3.7 kg (range −0.6 to 7.7 kg) for FFM (van Marken Lichtenbelt et al. 2004). Additionally,

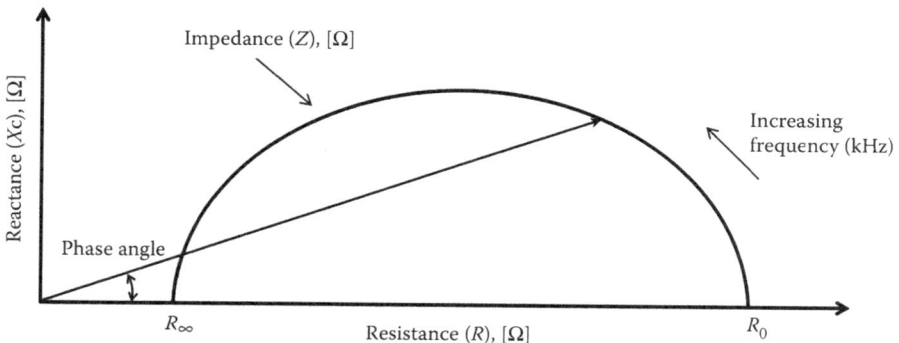

FIGURE 2.2 Example of the Cole plot. R_∞, resistance at infinity frequency; R_0, resistance at 0 frequency.

in a setting were body changes in judo athletes were investigated with BIS, the mean biases for FFM changes were −0.5 kg with LOA ranging from −3.36% to 2.59 kg when compared to a four-component model (Matias et al. 2012). Moreover, in obese women performing a weight reduction program including physical activity and a nutritional intervention, mean biases for %BF reductions were found to be approximately 0.8% ± 2.1%BF with LOA ranging between −3.6% and 4.8%, when compared to a four-component model (Evans et al. 1999).

It should be clearly noted that the accuracy of any impedance method depends on many variables, including the prediction model, sample specificity (use of prediction model in sample similar to that in which it was derived), and validity of BIA assumptions (constant hydration, standard body geometry) as outlined by Kyle et al. (2004b).

2.3.1.3 Hydrodensitometry and Air Displacement Plethysmography

2.3.1.3.1 *Hydrodensitometry or Underwater Weighing*

This method was developed by Behnke et al. (1942) in the 1940s and is based on a two-component model. UWW is used to determine body volume and, in combination with body weight, calculate whole-body density (Fosbøl and Zerahn 2015). The method requires that the body is fully submerged in water while subjects are required to completely exhale. The volume of water displaced or more commonly the body's weight underwater, combined with the laboratory weight is used to calculate body density (Lukaski 1987; Wagner and Heyward 1999; Ellis 2000; Fosbøl and Zerahn 2015). Based on the inverse relationship between fat and density, body density is used to calculate percent fat mass (%BF) from different equations as for example by using the equations proposed by Siri (1956) and Brozek et al. (1963). The method of UWW has some restrictions and limitations. UWW assumes a constant chemical composition and thus constant density of FM (i.e., 0.9007 g/mL) and FFM (i.e., 1.100 g/mL) (Lukaski 1987; Fosbøl and Zerahn 2015). These assumptions are open to question as it was shown that age, sex, ethnicity, and training status may influence the density of the FFM (Ackland et al. 2012; Fosbøl and Zerahn 2015). A further issue of UWW is the need to determine the residual lung volume that makes an approximately 1–2 L contribution to the measured body volume (Lukaski 1987). Estimation errors of residual lung volume in the order of 300–400 mL may add a further 3%–4% uncertainty in the %BF value (Ellis 2000). In addition to this technical issue, this method is rarely well tolerated by subjects because of the complete submersion of the body and the requirement to completely exhale (Wagner and Heyward 1999; Fosbøl and Zerahn 2015).

Overall, the precision of this method is high in regard to the determined body density ($r = 0.99$ for test retest conditions (Ward et al. 1978), trial-to-trial variation: 0.0015–0.0020 g/mL (Lukaski 1987; Going 2005), and an error for predicting %BF in the order of 2%–4% for the individual subject (using an adequate residual lung volume) (Lukaski 1987; Ellis 2000; Going 2005). However, LOA of also up to ±10% were reported when compared to a four-component model (Clasey et al. 1999). Additionally, when investigating changes due to strength training, van Marken Lichtenbelt et al. (2004) reported a mean bias of 0.1% and 0.1 kg with LOA of approximately 2.4% and 2.0 kg for changes in %BF and FFM, respectively, when compared to a four-component model with average changes in %BF of −1.6% (range: −5.0% to 1.2%), and in FFM of +3.7 kg (range: −0.6 to 7.7 kg) (van Marken Lichtenbelt et al. 2004).

2.3.1.3.2 *Air Displacement Plethysmography*

This method is considered an alternative to UWW and, in comparison to UWW, may be considered a more "comfortable" and better-tolerated method (Fosbøl and Zerahn 2015). The ADP system consists of two chambers (i.e., the measuring chamber where the subject is seated and a reference chamber) linked by a flexible diaphragm. By oscillations, the diaphragm produces volume and pressure changes in both chambers (Fosbøl and Zerahn 2015). The body volume is calculated from the relationship of pressure versus volume (Poisson's law) using corrections for thermally affected areas (close to the skin, clothes, and in the airway and lungs) (Ellis 2001; Fields et al. 2004). Body density is calculated in the same way as it is done for UWW and the same restrictions described for UWW persist for ADP. Nonetheless, UWW and ADP might yield somewhat different results. In female athletes, ADP significantly overestimated %BF by 8% when compared to UWW (Vescovi et al. 2002). Furthermore, mean bias in %BF estimation between ADP and UWW in male college football players was shown to be approximately 2% with LOA of ±4.5% (Collins et al. 1999). Besides, LOA also between methods in the order of −6.1% to 5.9% are reported for ADP (Biaggi et al. 1999).

Typically, the CV for sequential BF measurements in adults using ADP ranges from 0.3% to 4.5% (Fosbøl and Zerahn 2015). Compared to multicomponent methods, the bias of FM estimation ranges from 2% to 4% with LOA in the order of 2%–7% (total error for the %FM estimation: 2.7%–6%) in adults and children (Collins et al. 1999; Millard-Stafford et al. 2001; Going 2005; Fosbøl and Zerahn 2015).

2.3.1.4   Dilution with Isotopes

The isotope dilution technique is a method to measure total body water (TBW) and ECF. The basic principle of this technique is that the ratio of a tracer dose, administered orally or intravenous, to its concentration after dilution in the body, corresponds to the volume of distribution (Ellis 2000). Determination of the tracer concentration within the body involves blood or urine samples before and several hours after the administration of the tracer (Schoeller et al. 1980; Earthman 2015). It is assumed that the tracer is distributed only in body water or ECF for sodium bromide, which is rapidly and equally distributed in all liquid compartments (or in ECF) and that neither the tracer nor the body water is metabolized during equilibration (Schoeller 2005). The tracers are typically deuterium (^2H, a stable isotope of hydrogen) and ^{18}O-labeled water (^{18}O, a stable isotope of oxygen) for TBW determination in humans and sodium bromide for ECW determination (Schoeller et al. 1980; Earthman 2015). TBW can be used to estimate FFM and as a consequence also FM by assuming a relatively constant water content of the FFM (i.e., 73%) (Lukaski 1987; Wagner and Heyward 1999; Ellis 2000, 2001; Duren et al. 2008).

The precision of the TBW measurement when using deuterium or ^{18}O-labeled water amounts to 1%–2% (Schoeller 2005; Earthman 2015). The accuracy of TBW measurement depends on the correctness of the aforementioned assumptions and is about 1% (Schoeller 2005). For the estimation of FFM, a further loss of accuracy of about 2% has to be considered due to the uncertainty about the hydration constant (Schoeller 2005). For the %BF estimation, an error of 2% (~1.4 kg) (Ellis 2000) up to 3.6% (assuming no technical error in TBW measurement) is reported (Wagner and Heyward 1999). With respect to the ability to document changes after a strength training program, dilution methods showed a mean bias in %BF estimation of approximately 0.4% and for FFM of approximately −0.3 kg with LOA of approximately 3.1% and 2.5 kg, respectively, when compared to a four-component model (four-component model changes of −1.6%BF, range −5.0% to 1.2%, and FFM changes of +3.7 kg, range −0.6 to 7.7 kg) (van Marken Lichtenbelt et al. 2004).

2.3.2   Three-Component Method

2.3.2.1   Dual X-Ray Absorptiometry

DXA is a popular method for quantifying FM, lean soft tissue, and bone mineral mass (Duren et al. 2008; Fosbøl and Zerahn 2015). The technique passes low-dose x-rays of two different energies through the body and an image is created as the photon detector measures the differential attenuation of the low and high x-ray energy by the soft tissue (i.e., FM and lean soft tissue) and bone (Earthman 2015).

DXA has good precision with reports of CV for FM determination ranging from 0.8% to 2.7% (SEM of 0.39–0.5 kg) and for lean soft tissues in the range of 0.4%–1.3% (SEM 0.35–0.54 kg) (Hangartner et al. 2013; Earthman 2015; Fosbøl and Zerahn 2015). When compared to four-component models, the bias for %BF ranges from −3.8% to 2.8% with LOA of ±3% up to ±10% (Prior et al. 1997; Clasey et al. 1999; Wang et al. 2010; Fosbøl and Zerahn 2015). Nevertheless, SEE for %BF typically ranges between 2.5% and 3.5% (Prior et al. 1997; Lohman et al. 2000; Stewart and Hannan 2000; Wang et al. 2010). With DXA, changes in %BF and FFM after a strength training program may be documented with a mean bias of approximately −0.2% and 0.2 kg and with LOA of approximately 3.8% and 3.1 kg, respectively, when compared to a four-component model (four-component model changes of −1.6%BF, range −5.0% to 1.2%, and FFM changes of +3.7 kg, range −0.6 to 7.7 kg) (van Marken Lichtenbelt et al. 2004). Similar findings were reported in a weight loss setting in judo athletes where mean biases for %BF and FFM changes of 0.8% and −0.5 kg were reported with LOA ranging from 5.3% to −3.7% and 2.7 to −3.7 kg, respectively (four-component model changes of −1.22% ± 2.70%BF, and FFM changes of 0.07 ± 2.04 kg) (Santos et al. 2010). Additionally, in a weight reduction setting (training nutritional intervention), including obese women, mean biases for %BF changes of 1.3% ± 2.1% with LOA between −4.0% and 4.6% were reported (Evans et al. 1999).

The use of DXA to assess body composition of physically active people has gained acceptance internationally. One concern, however, has been the lack of a general procedure to implement DXA as well as reporting protocols for body composition. Hangartner et al. (2013) led a technical review group of the International Society for Clinical Densitometry (ISCD) and developed a standardized DXA measurement protocol (e.g., calibration of the DXA, patient position on the scan table and data reporting) that should be used in the assessment of body composition (lean soft tissue, fat and bone mineral content) of athletes (Hangartner et al. 2013).

Fundamental in serial measurements of athletes is knowledge of the least significant change (LSC) in DXA measurements of body composition. Nana et al. (2012) reported diurnal and lifestyle variation effects on DXA measurements among 31 physically active adults, who were measured five times over a 2-day period that included different conditions of diet (overnight fasting, usual food, and beverage consumption) and 8-h after physical activity. Initial duplicate measurements served as the baseline variability and showed that body weight from DXA varied by <300 g, lean mass by <180 g, and fat mass by <150 g. The measurements at the end of the day revealed an increase in DXA total mass of 500 g and in lean mass of 560 g with a concomitant decrease in fat mass of 120 g for the female participants. The differences for the male participants were similar, although the total mass increase was lower. The differences after breakfast consumption were, for males, an increase in DXA total body mass of 1110 g, in lean mass of 900 g, and in fat mass of 280 g. Although the females showed a smaller total body mass increase of only 530 g, their increase in fat mass was similar at 210 g. These findings provide an estimate of the LSCs from DXA to indicate meaningful effects of diet, activity, or other interventions among physically active adults. Among adults not regularly participating in physical training, the variability characterized as the combination of confounding lifestyle parameters is consistently larger than the LSC as calculated from the initial duplicate measurements for total mass and lean mass but not for fat mass. These LSCs are, for men and women, respectively, 400 and 290 g for DXA total body mass, 380 and 410 g for lean mass, and 290 and 350 g for fat mass (Hangartner et al. 2013).

2.3.3 Four-Component Methods

2.3.3.1 Computed Tomography and Magnetic Resonance Imaging

The imaging techniques, computed tomography (CT) and magnetic resonance imaging (MRI), are considered very accurate methods for the quantification of body composition on the tissue level (Ross and Janssen 2005; Fosbøl and Zerahn 2015). The applicability of CT is limited as CT is based on x-ray and the radiation dose for the whole-body composition analysis is substantial (Prado and Heymsfield 2014; Fosbøl and Zerahn 2015). MRI, in contrast to CT, does not use radiation and is based on the interaction between atoms and molecules in the magnetic field produced by the MRI device (Ross and Janssen 2005). A disadvantage of MRI is that this technique is time consuming and costly; thus, its availability is limited to specialized research facilities (Fosbøl and Zerahn 2015).

For CT, the reproducibility of sequential measurements of the visceral adipose tissue expressed as CV ranges from 0.6% to 12.3% and for MRI from 3.5% to 9.4% (Fosbøl and Zerahn 2015). The

TABLE 2.1

Summary of Precision and Accuracy of Methods to Estimate Body Composition in Physically Active People

Components	Method	Accuracy	Precision	Applicability	Reference
2 (FM and FFM)	Body mass index	%BF: SEE ±5%	%BF: $r = 0.6$–0.8	Simple but too inaccurate	Gallagher et al. (2000), Pescatello et al. (2014)
	Circumferences	%BF: TE 2.5%–4.4% (prerequisite: similarity to the reference population)	Body density: $r = -0.7$ to -0.4	Simple but too inaccurate	Tran and Weltman (1988, 1989), Pescatello et al. (2014)
	Skinfold caliper	%BF: SEE 3.5%–5%	%BF: $r = 0.7$–0.9 within 5%	Portable, simple, and inexpensive	Durnin and Womersley (1974), Lukaski (1987), Ackland et al. (2012), Fosbøl and Zerahn (2015)
	BIA/BIS	%BF: SEE 3.8%–5%	BIA: 1%–2% BIS: 2%–3%	Portable, simple, reproducible, and inexpensive	Kyle et al. (2004a) Earthman (2015), Fosbøl and Zerahn (2015)
	Hydrodensitometry (underwater weighing)	%BF: SEE 2%–4% TE up to 6%	Body density: test retest $r = 0.99$ Trial to trial: 0.0015–0.0020 g/mL	High cost and patient burden, laboratory setting	Ward et al. (1978), Lukaski (1987), Clasey et al. (1999), Ellis (2000), Going (2005)
	Air displacement plethysmography	%BF: SEE 2%–4%	CV: 0.3%–4.5%	Laboratory setting	Going (2005), Fosbøl and Zerahn (2015)
	Dilution with isotopes	%BF: TE 2%–3.6% (assuming no technical error in TBW measurement; accuracy of TBW: about 2%)	TBW: 1%–2%	High cost, laboratory setting	Wagner and Heyward (1999), Schoeller (2005), Earthman (2015)
3 (FM, lean soft tissue, bone)	Dual x-ray absorptiometry	%BF: SEE 2.5%–3.5%	CV FM: 0.8%–2.7%	Cost and time efficient, low radiation, laboratory setting	Prior et al. (1997), Lohman et al. (2000), Lohman and Chen (2005), Ackland et al. (2012), Earthman (2015)
4 (FM, bone, muscle, other)	Computer tomography (CT) and magnetic resonance imaging (MRI)	Volume measurements within ±5%	CV: visceral adipose tissue: CT: 0.6%–12.3%; MRI from 3.5% to 9.4%	High cost, laboratory setting CT: high radiation	Fosbøl and Zerahn (2015), Müller et al. (2016a)
4–6 (FM, water, protein, others)	Multicomponent models	%BF: SEE <1% TE up to 3%	1%–2%	High cost, laboratory setting	Wang et al. (2005), Ackland et al. (2012), Fosbøl and Zerahn (2015)

Note: %BF = percent body fat; CV = coefficient of variation; SEE = standard error of the estimate; TE = total error; TBW = total body water.

validity of volume measurements compared with cadaver analyses was reported to be within ±5% (Müller et al. 2016a).

2.3.4 MULTICOMPONENT MODELS

Multicomponent models combine two or more measurement methods outlined above. The objective is to reduce errors in estimating the body composition due to different assumptions inherent to each individual method. For example, measuring TBW reduces the error in a classical two-component model (i.e., FM and FFM) by including information on possible variations in hydration of the FFM (Fosbøl and Zerahn 2015). This yields a three-component model. Further subdividing FFM by including bone mineral mass leads to a four-component model (Fosbøl and Zerahn 2015) and so on. Of course, the measurement error of each technique included may lead to inaccuracies (Wang et al. 2005). Technical errors of the combined estimation of body volume, TBW, and bone mineral were reported to yield an error of about 1% in %BF (Ackland et al. 2012). Precision and accuracy of multicomponent models should be in the order of 1%–2% (Ackland et al. 2012) but different reports on validity exist. For %BF, the total error of measurement in four-, five-, and six-component models was found to range between 0.59% and 0.89% (Fosbøl and Zerahn 2015). Comparative studies between different multicomponent methods show an SEE for body fat <1% (Fosbøl and Zerahn 2015) and mean biases between approximately 1% and 2.1%BF (Heymsfield et al. 2015). Nonetheless, the error for estimating body fat mass with four- and six-component models has been reported to be as much as 2.7% and 3.4%, respectively (Wang et al. 2005).

2.4 CONCLUSION

Whereas the assessment of body composition can provide useful information for an individual athlete, it is emphasized that no individual or combined method exists that can be considered as an absolutely accurate measure of body fat, lean mass, or muscle mass. Each method relies on assumptions and/or calculations and is validated against reference methods that are not inherently free of error. For varying situations, different methods and models may be convenient and thus it is important to choose an appropriate method well balanced with regard to cost, time resources, validity, and applicability (Table 2.1). In sports, simple methods may be preferred (van Marken Lichtenbelt et al. 2004). Thus, coaches, athletic trainers, and athletes should make realistic and practical decisions whether the precision and the accuracy of the methods under deliberation adequately address the needs of the individual sports performer. The precision of most methods can be considered high if well-trained persons perform the measurements and appropriate models that translate body measurements to body composition variables are used. The accuracy of predicting FM and FFM depends on the method but, in general, ranges between 2% and 5%. Because changes in body composition occur with training, nutritional intervention, and recovery from injury, athletic practitioners need be aware that many methods have low mean biases (e.g., errors compared to reference methods); the wide LOA may limit the ability of some methods to detect biologically meaningful changes for an individual.

REFERENCES

Ackland, T. R., T. G. Lohman, J. Sundgot-Borgen et al. 2012. Current status of body composition assessment in sport: Review and position statement on behalf of the ad hoc research working group on body composition health and performance, under the auspices of the I.O.C. Medical Commission. *Sports Med* 42:227–49.

Behnke, A. R., B. G. Feen, and W. C. Welham. 1942. The specific gravity of healthy men: Body weight divided by volume as an index of obesity. *J Am Med Assoc* 118:495–8.

Bellisari, A. and A. Roche. 2005. Anthropometry and ultrasound. In *Human Body Composition*, eds. S. B. Heymsfield, T. Lohman, Z. Wang, and S. Going, 109–27. Champaign, IL: Human Kinetics.

Biaggi, R. R., M. W. Vollman, M. A. Nies et al. 1999. Comparison of air-displacement plethysmography with hydrostatic weighing and bioelectrical impedance analysis for the assessment of body composition in healthy adults. *Am J Clin Nutr* 69:898–903.

Brozek, J., F. Grande, J. T. Anderson, and A. Keys. 1963. Densitometric analysis of body composition: Revision of some quantitative assumptions. *Ann N Y Acad Sci* 110:113–40.

Chumlea, C. and S. Sun. 2005. Bioelectrical impedance analysis. In *Human Body Composition*, eds. S. B. Heymsfield, T. Lohman, Z. Wang, and S. Going, 79–88. Champaign, IL: Human Kinetics.

Clasey, J. L., J. A. Kanaley, L. Wideman et al. 1999. Validity of methods of body composition assessment in young and older men and women. *J Appl Physiol (1985)* 86:1728–38.

Collins, M. A., M. L. Millard-Stafford, P. B. Sparling et al. 1999. Evaluation of the BOD POD for assessing body fat in collegiate football players. *Med Sci Sports Exerc* 31:1350–6.

Currell, K. and A. E. Jeukendrup. 2008. Validity, reliability and sensitivity of measures of sporting performance. *Sports Med* 38:297–316.

Duren, D. L., R. J. Sherwood, S. A. Czerwinski et al. 2008. Body composition methods: Comparisons and interpretation. *J Diabetes Sci Technol* 2:1139–46.

Durnin, J. V. and J. Womersley. 1974. Body fat assessed from total body density and its estimation from skinfold thickness: Measurements on 481 men and women aged from 16 to 72 years. *Br J Nutr* 32:77–97.

Earthman, C. P. 2015. Body composition tools for assessment of adult malnutrition at the bedside: A tutorial on research considerations and clinical applications. *JPEN J Parenter Enteral Nutr* 39:787–822.

Ellis, K. J. 2000. Human body composition: *In vivo* methods. *Physiol Rev* 80:649–80.

Ellis, K. J. 2001. Selected body composition methods can be used in field studies. *J Nutr* 131:1589–95.

Evans, E. M., D. A. Rowe, M. M. Misic, B. M. Prior, and S. A. Arngrímsson. 2005. Skinfold prediction equation for athletes developed using a four-component model. *Med Sci Sports Exerc* 37:2006–11.

Evans, E. M., M. J. Saunders, M. A. Spano, S. A. Arngrimsson, R. D. Lewis, and K. J. Cureton. 1999. Body-composition changes with diet and exercise in obese women: A comparison of estimates from clinical methods and a 4-component model. *Am J Clin Nutr* 70:5–12.

Fields, D. A., P. B. Higgins, and G. R. Hunter. 2004. Assessment of body composition by air-displacement plethysmography: Influence of body temperature and moisture. *Dyn Med* 3:3.

Fosbøl, M. and B. Zerahn. 2015. Contemporary methods of body composition measurement. *Clin Physiol Funct Imaging* 35:81–97.

Gallagher, D., S. B. Heymsfield, M. Heo, S. A. Jebb, P. R. Murgatroyd, and Y. Sakamoto. 2000. Healthy percentage body fat ranges: An approach for developing guidelines based on body mass index. *Am J Clin Nutr* 72:694–701.

Going, S. 2005. Hydrodensitometry and air displacement plethysmography. In *Human Body Composition*, eds. S. B. Heymsfield, T. Lohman, Z. Wang, and S. Going, 17–33. Champaign, IL: Human Kinetics.

Hangartner, T. N., S. Warner, P. Braillon, L. Jankowski, and J. Shepherd. 2013. The official positions of the International Society for Clinical Densitometry: Acquisition of dual-energy x-ray absorptiometry body composition and considerations regarding analysis and repeatability of measures. *J Clin Densitom* 16:520–36.

Heymsfield, S. B., C. B. Ebbeling, J. Zheng et al. 2015. Multi-component molecular-level body composition reference methods: Evolving concepts and future directions. *Obes Rev* 16:282–94.

Heymsfield, S. B., Z. Wang, R. N. Baumgartner, and R. Ross. 1997. Human body composition: Advances in models and methods. *Annu Rev Nutr* 17:527–58.

Kyle, U. G., I. Bosaeus, A. D. De Lorenzo et al. 2004a. Bioelectrical impedance analysis-Part I: Review of principles and methods. *Clin Nutr* 23:1226–43.

Kyle, U. G., I. Bosaeus, A. D. De Lorenzo et al. 2004b. Bioelectrical impedance analysis-Part II: Utilization in clinical practice. *Clin Nutr* 23:1430–53.

Lohman, T. and Z. Chen. 2005. Dual-energy x-ray absorptiometry. In *Human Body Composition*, eds. S. B. Heymsfield, T. Lohman, Z. Wang, and S. Going, 63–77. Champaign, IL: Human Kinetics.

Lohman, T. G., M. Harris, P. J. Teixeira, and L. Weiss. 2000. Assessing body composition and changes in body composition. Another look at dual-energy x-ray absorptiometry. *Ann N Y Acad Sci* 904:45–54.

Lukaski, H. C. 1987. Methods for the assessment of human body composition: Traditional and new. *Am J Clin Nutr* 46:537–56.

Lukaski, H. C. 2013. Evolution of bioimpedance: A circuitous journey from estimation of physiological function to assessment of body composition and a return to clinical research. *Eur J Clin Nutr* 67(Suppl 1):2–9.

Matias, C. N., D. A. Santos, D. A. Fields, L. B. Sardinha, and A. M. Silva. 2012. Is bioelectrical impedance spectroscopy accurate in estimating changes in fat-free mass in judo athletes? *J Sports Sci* 30:1323.

Millard-Stafford, M. L., M. A. Collins, E. M. Evans, T. K. Snow, K. J. Cureton, and L. B. Rosskopf. 2001. Use of air displacement plethysmography for estimating body fat in a four-component model. *Med Sci Sports Exerc* 33:1311–7.

Müller, M. J., W. Braun, M. Pourhassan, C. Geisler, and A. Bosy-Westphal. 2016a. Application of standards and models in body composition analysis. *Proc Nutr Soc* 75:181–7.

Müller, W., T. G. Lohman, A. D. Stewart et al. 2016b. Subcutaneous fat patterning in athletes: Selection of appropriate sites and standardisation of a novel ultrasound measurement technique: Ad hoc working group on body composition, health and performance, under the auspices of the IOC Medical Commission. *Br J Sports Med* 50:45–54.

Must, A. and S. E. Anderson. 2006. Body mass index in children and adolescents: Considerations for population-based applications. *Int J Obes (Lond)* 30:590–4.

Nana, A., G. J. Slater, W. G. Hopkins, and L. M. Burke. 2012. Effects of daily activities on dual-energy x-ray absorptiometry measurements of body composition in active people. *Med Sci Sports Exerc* 44:180–9.

Nana, A., G. J. Slater, A. D. Stewart, and L. M. Burke. 2015. Methodology review: Using dual-energy x-ray absorptiometry (DXA) for the assessment of body composition in athletes and active people. *Int J Sport Nutr Exerc Metab* 25:198–215.

Pescatello, L., R. Arena, D. Riebe, and P. Thompson. 2014. *ACSM's Guidelines for Exercise Testing and Prescription* (9th Ed.), Philadelphia, PA: Lippincott Williams & Wilkins.

Prado, C. M. and S. B. Heymsfield. 2014. Lean tissue imaging: A new era for nutritional assessment and intervention. *JPEN J Parenter Enteral Nutr* 38:940–53.

Prior, B. M., K. J. Cureton, C. M. Modlesky et al. 1997. *In vivo* validation of whole body composition estimates from dual-energy x-ray absorptiometry. *J Appl Physiol* 83:623–30.

Ross, R. and I. Janssen. 2005. Computed tomography and magnetic resonance imaging. In *Human Body Composition*, eds. S. B. Heymsfield, T. Lohman, Z. Wang, and S. Going, 89–108. Champaign, IL: Human Kinetics.

Santos, D. A., A. M. Silva, C. N. Matias, D. A. Fields, S. B. Heymsfield, and L. B. Sardinha. 2010. Accuracy of DXA in estimating body composition changes in elite athletes using a four compartment model as the reference method. *Nutr Metab (Lond)* 7:22.

Schoeller, D. 2005. Hydrometry. In *Human Body Composition*, eds. S. B. Heymsfield, T. Lohman, Z. Wang and S. Going, 35–49. Champaign, IL: Human Kinetics.

Schoeller, D. A., E. van Santen, D. W. Peterson, W. Dietz, J. Jaspan, and P. D. Klein. 1980. Total body water measurement in humans with 18O and 2H labeled water. *Am J Clin Nutr* 33:2686–93.

Silva, A. M., D. A. Fields, A. L. Quitério, and L. B. Sardinha. 2009. Are skinfold-based models accurate and suitable for assessing changes in body composition in highly trained athletes? *J Strength Cond Res* 23:1688–96.

Sinning, W. E., D. G. Dolny, K. D. Little et al. 1985. Validity of "generalized" equations for body composition analysis in male athletes. *Med Sci Sports Exerc* 17:124–30.

Sinning, W. E. and J. R. Wilson. 1984. Validity of "generalized" equations for body composition analysis in women athletes. *Res Q Exerc Sport* 55:153–60.

Siri, W. E. 1956. The gross composition of the body. *Adv Biol Med Phys* 4:239–80.

Stewart, A. D. and W. J. Hannan. 2000. Prediction of fat and fat-free mass in male athletes using dual x-ray absorptiometry as the reference method. *J Sports Sci* 18:263–74.

Tran, Z. V. and A. Weltman. 1988. Predicting body composition of men from girth measurements. *Hum Biol* 60:167–75.

Tran, Z. V. and A. Weltman. 1989. Generalized equation for predicting body density of women from girth measurements. *Med Sci Sports Exerc* 21:101–4.

van Marken Lichtenbelt, W. D., F. Hartgens, N. B. Vollaard, S. Ebbing, and H. Kuipers. 2004. Body composition changes in bodybuilders: A method comparison. *Med Sci Sports Exerc* 36:490–7.

Vescovi, J. D., L. Hildebrandt, W. Miller, R. Hammer, and A. Spiller. 2002. Evaluation of the BOD POD for estimating percent fat in female college athletes. *J Strength Cond Res* 16:599–605.

Wagner, D. R. and V. H. Heyward. 1999. Techniques of body composition assessment: A review of laboratory and field methods. *Res Q Exerc Sport* 70:135–49.

Wang, Z., S. B. Heymsfield, Z. Chen, S. Zhu, and R. N. Pierson. 2010. Estimation of percentage body fat by dual-energy x-ray absorptiometry: Evaluation by *in vivo* human elemental composition. *Phys Med Biol* 55:2619–35.

Wang, Z., W. Shen, R. Withers, and S. Heymsfield. 2005. Multicomponent molecular-level models of body composition analysis. In *Human Body Composition*, eds. S. B. Heymsfield, T. Lohman, Z. Wang, and S. Going, 163–76. Champaign, IL: Human Kinetics.

Ward, A., M. L. Pollock, A. S. Jackson, J. J. Ayres, and G. Pape. 1978. A comparison of body fat determined by underwater weighing and volume displacement. *Am J Physiol* 234:94–6.

Weir, J. P. 2005. Quantifying test-retest reliability using the intraclass correlation coefficient and the SEM. *J Strength Cond Res* 19:231–40.

Withers, R. T., J. Laforgia, and S. B. Heymsfield. 1999. Critical appraisal of the estimation of body composition via two-, three-, and four-compartment models. *Am J Hum Biol* 11:175–85.

Womersley, J., J. V. Durnin, K. Boddy, and M. Mahaffy. 1976. Influence of muscular development, obesity, and age on the fat-free mass of adults. *J Appl Physiol* 41:223–9.

3 Assessment of Muscle Mass

Donald R. Dengel, Christiana J. Raymond, and Tyler A. Bosch

CONTENTS

3.1 INTRODUCTION: BACKGROUND

Skeletal muscle is by far the largest body component in adults (Heymsfield et al. 2015). In humans, skeletal muscle mass increases from less than a kilogram at birth (~25% of the total body mass), to approximately 30 kilograms in an adult male, or roughly 40% of the total body mass (Shephard 1991). By the age of 40, adults gradually lose skeletal muscle mass and that loss accelerates past the age of 70 (Heymsfield et al. 2015). Skeletal muscle varies in size, has structural and mechanical functions, and contributes significantly to the body's metabolic function.

Although the definitions for total body mass and fat mass are well agreed upon, skeletal muscle mass is often referred to as either fat-free mass or lean body mass, depending on the technique used to measure it. These two terms are used interchangeably, but they are not identical. Lean body mass, sometimes called lean soft tissue, is the sum of body water, total body protein, carbohydrates, non-fat lipids, and soft tissue mineral (Prado and Heymsfield 2014). In simpler terms, lean soft tissue is the total body mass minus fat and bone. Conversely, fat-free mass includes bone as well as skeletal muscle, organs, and connective tissue (Prado and Heymsfield 2014).

The use of the term "fat-free mass" or lean soft tissue is ultimately dependent upon the methodology used to measure skeletal muscle. Determination of body composition using a two-component model (e.g., water displacement) (Figure 3.1) divides the body into either fat mass or fat-free mass. On the other hand, determining body composition using a three-component model (e.g., dual x-ray absorptiometry [DXA]) can differentiate between fat mass, bone mass, and lean soft tissue mass (Figure 3.1).

This chapter will examine the various methods to determine skeletal muscle and will explore both the advantages and disadvantages of each method as outlined in Tables 3.1 and 3.2. In addition, this chapter will also examine methods to measure not only total skeletal muscle, but also regional skeletal muscle mass. Finally, we will discuss the relationship between skeletal muscle mass, muscle function, sports performance, and general health.

3.2 METHODS FOR DETERMINING BODY COMPOSITION

3.2.1 METHODS USING TWO-COMPONENT MODEL

Body composition measurement methods using a two-component model make the following two assumptions: (1) the composition of an individual's total body mass is either fat-free mass or fat mass, and (2) the density of these two components is constant throughout the body (Table 3.1). The flaws in these assumptions explain the inaccuracy of the two-component model since the inclusion of bone mass with lean soft tissue leads to an overestimation of skeletal muscle mass, and the density of these two components can differ in regions of the body. Several methods are available to measure skeletal muscle mass using a two-component model, ranging from simple, inexpensive field methods (e.g., skinfold thickness) to more complicated and expensive laboratory methods (e.g., air displacement). These methods vary in accuracy, but can be useful on a day-to-day basis.

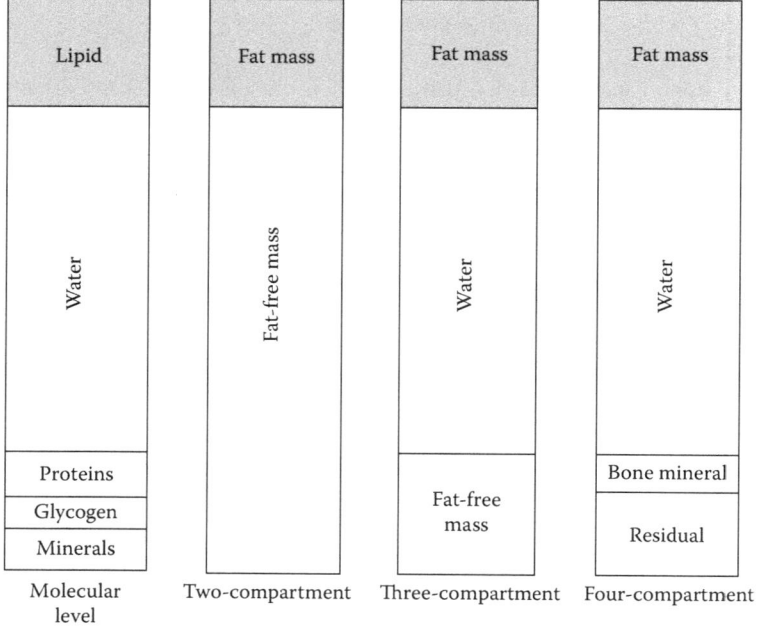

FIGURE 3.1 The molecular and tissue–organ levels of body composition. Lean mass components are depicted for both levels and for each of the compartment models at the tissue–organ level: two-compartment, three-compartment, and four-compartment. The sum of components at each level is equal to body weight, and lean components exclude lipid and fat components shaded in gray. Lean soft tissue excludes fat mass and bone mineral content, and fat-free body mass excludes only fat mass.

3.2.1.1 Anthropometry

Anthropometric techniques measure limb lengths, widths, and circumferences using a non-stretch tape measure and skinfold thickness at various sites using specially designed calipers. The measurement of skinfold thickness has for many years been an accepted predictor of total body fat. Numerous sites for measuring skinfold thickness have been described, and a number of prediction equations have been developed to calculate percent body fat (Wang et al. 2000). These prediction equations use skinfold thickness from several sites as well as sex, age, height, or weight (Bellisari and Roche 2005). The use of skinfold thickness to estimate percent body fat is based on the implicit assumption of a fixed relationship between subcutaneous adipose tissue in predefined anatomical locations and total body fat. This relationship is dependent upon various factors, including age, sex, and health status (Durnin and Womersley 1974; Lohman 1981; Baumgartner et al. 1991). Classical, but still frequently used, regression equations to predict fat mass, such as those proposed by Jackson and Pollock (1978) and Jackson et al. (1980), are derived from the measurement of body density by hydrodensitometry and the calculation of fat mass by the Siri equation (Siri 1956).

Simple skinfold calipers, which were developed in the 1930s, measure skinfold thickness at multiple sites on the body and represent the average total body thickness of subcutaneous adipose tissue (Roubenoff and Kehayias 1991; Roche et al. 1996). Skinfold calipers allow for convenient and relatively inexpensive field testing and a trained individual can collect reproducible results. Also, skinfold thickness at select sites can be used to estimate regional measures of fat-free mass and fat mass (Durnin and Womersley 1974; Lukaski 1987). Despite these advantages, anthropometric measures are highly susceptible to precision error (5%–10%) that is magnified when multiple individuals collect the measurements (Roubenoff and Kehayias 1991). Caliper placement, differences in measurement techniques, type of caliper used, and sites chosen increase the variability in this method. The skinfold method is inexpensive, portable, and noninvasive, and individuals with experience can produce reliable results, which explains its popularity as a method for measuring body composition (Table 3.1).

3.2.1.2 Body Volume/Density

Body volume can be measured by the displacement of water (hydrodensitometry) and more recently by the displacement of air. Hydrodensitometry, referred to as underwater weighing, was once considered the gold standard of body composition and still accurately measures body composition (3%–5% error). This method measures a subject's body weight on land and after being fully submersed under water. This method relies on maximal lung expiration while being weighed in water, but even with a maximal expiration, the lungs still retain air (residual volume). The residual volume can be estimated or measured to correct the measured body volume (Wilmore et al. 1980; Latin and Ruhling 1986). Body density is calculated from the measured body volume and weight. The density is then used to estimate fat mass using prediction equations (Siri 1956; Brozek et al. 1963). Fat-free mass is subsequently calculated by subtracting the fat mass from the total body mass. Hydrodensitometry requires a high degree of investigator expertise and subject compliance to obtain high precision and reliability (Roubenoff and Kehayias 1991) and it prohibits regional body composition assessment (Roubenoff and Kehayias 1991). The high cost of building and maintaining the underwater weighing tank limits the usefulness of this method.

Air displacement is a newer method of volume displacement. This method requires a subject to sit inside a sealed measuring chamber. The change in volume of air that the body creates inside the chamber is used to calculate body volume. The calculation of fat mass and fat-free mass is the same for hydrodensitometry. For most individuals, the air displacement method offers a less troublesome method of determining body composition. However, the disadvantages associated with this particular method are similar to those of hydrodensitometry, including its incapability of providing individual measures of isolated body regions (Table 3.1). Additionally, the cost of an air displacement device is expensive and requires a stable environment to assure its accuracy. Therefore, although

TABLE 3.1

Commonly Used Two-Component Models of Body Composition Assessment Techniques

Technique	Principle and Measurements	Advantages	Disadvantages	References
		Anthropometry		
Circumferences; lengths and breadths; skinfold thickness	Body mass, height, waist and hip circumferences, and geometry measured using calipers, scales, stadiometers, and tape. Skinfold thickness used to estimate FFM and muscle size.	Inexpensive, noninvasive, portable, and minimal training.	Assumptions: Constant SAT thickness in a limb cross-section; measurement sites represent average total body SAT thickness; constant FFM density. LM cannot be directly measured using calipers; LM estimations include intramuscular AT. Interobserver error; requires investigator expertise.	Heymsfield et al. (2015) Roche et al. (1996) Roubenoff and Kehayias (1991) Wells and Fewtrell (2006)
		Body Density and Volume		
Hydrodensitometry or underwater weighing (UWW)	BV measurements used to calculate Db via Archimedes' principle, comparing a subject's mass in air and under water. Provides estimations of FM and FFM.	Valid and reliable for the assessment of Db, FM, and %BF. Considered a reference method for Db measurements.	Assumptions: Known constant density of FM and FFM. Relies on Db, LM density, and residual lung volume estimation. FM and FFM cannot be regionally assessed. Requires: investigator expertise; patient cooperation; specialized laboratory; high cost.	Heymsfield et al. (2015) Prado and Heymsfield (2014) Roubenoff and Kehayias (1991) Wang et al. (2005)
Air displacement plethysmography (BOD POD)	Measures uncorrected BOD volume, thoracic gas volume (averaged over 3-s tidal breathing interval), computation of surface area artifact. Relationship between pressure and volume is used to determine BV and Db. Estimates FM, FFM.	Precise and accurate volume measurements. Noninvasive, quick, safe, comfortable, automated, accommodates various subject types (e.g., children, obese, elderly, disabled, tall). Db used in multicomponent model calculations.	Assumption: Known constant density of FM and FFM. FM and FFM cannot be assessed in isolated body regions. Low validity compared to hydrodensitometry.	Lee and Gallagher (2008) Siervo and Jebb (2010)

(Continued)

TABLE 3.1 (*Continued*)
Commonly Used Two-Component Models of Body Composition Assessment Techniques

Technique	Principle and Measurements	Advantages	Disadvantages	References
		Impedance		
Bioelectrical impedance analysis (BIA)	Based upon relationship between BV, body length, and body components (i.e., FM, FFM) and the impedance of each. Measures resistance and reactance from an electrical current and the body's impedance; electrical conductivity is greatest in tissues with high fluid and electrical content (i.e., FFM). Measures TBW; estimates FFM and FM.	Portable, low cost, noninvasive, reproducible, depends minimally on investigator skill, and requires little patient cooperation. After isotope dilution, may be considered reference method for body composition assessment in the field setting.	Assumptions: Hydration status is constant (73% of the body is water). Sensitive to physical activity, body temperature, hydration status, menstrual cycle. Unable to delineate regional anatomical boundaries. Validity dependent upon reference population prediction equations.	Esco et al. (2015) Garby et al. (1990) Heymsfield et al. (2015) Lukaski (1989) Segal et al. (1988) Siervo and Jebb (2010)

Note: FFM, fat-free mass; FM, fat mass; SAT, subcutaneous adipose tissue; LM, lean muscle mass; AT, adipose tissue; VAT, visceral adipose tissue; BV, body volume; Db, body density; %BF, percent body fat; TBW, total body water; ECW, extracellular water; BMC, bone mineral content; BMM, bone mineral mass.

the use of the air displacement method in measuring body composition may be more convenient than hydrodensitometry, more complex methods that offer a higher degree of accuracy are likely preferred in the laboratory setting.

3.2.1.3 Bioimpedance Analysis

Bioimpedance analysis (BIA) measures the body's impedance of a small electric current and is therefore sensitive to hydration status, functioning under the assumption that 73% of the body's fat-free mass is water (Segal et al. 1988; Lukaski 1989; Esco et al. 2015). Further, although multifrequency, eight-polar BIA has been shown (Anderson et al. 2012; Esco et al. 2015) to provide reproducible regional assessments of fat and fat-free masses in the arms, legs, and trunk, compared with more complex body composition methods (i.e., DXA), it is not possible to delineate regional anatomical boundaries (i.e., manual segmentation). This fact limits BIA's use in both clinical and laboratory settings (Esco et al. 2015). Additionally, the validity of body composition measurements performed by BIA is dependent upon whether the study participant matches the reference population (e.g., obese, elderly, children) from which the prediction equations are obtained (Roubenoff and Kehayias 1991; Buchholz et al. 2004; Fosbøl and Zerahn 2015). BIA has the advantage in that it depends minimally on investigator skill, is portable, and requires very little patient cooperation. This method does assume, however, that hydration status is constant and is sensitive to physical activity, body temperature, and menstrual cycle (Heymsfield et al. 2015) (Table 3.1). BIA provides another method to monitor body composition on a daily basis to determine any dramatic shifts and, using a standardized measurement protocol (e.g., hydration status), it is possible to obtain reliable results.

3.2.2 Methods Using Three-Component Model

Body composition measurement methods utilizing a three-component model make the assumption that the composition of an individual's total body mass can be divided into three distinct components: bone mass, lean soft tissue, and fat mass (Table 3.2). The delineation of fat-free mass into bone mass and lean soft tissue improves the accuracy of methods that utilize this model, but also increases the overall cost. Typically, these methods are laboratory or clinically based and cannot be used in a field setting. These methods are ideal for testing 2–4 times per year or to investigate a dramatic shift observed from a simpler method.

3.2.2.1 Ultrasound

Recent advances in ultrasound technology allow for its use in the measurement of skeletal mass. Ultrasound produces high-frequency sound waves that pass through the skin surface and reflect off underlying anatomical structures (e.g., skeletal muscle, adipose tissue, and bone). The transducer receives the wave reflections and converts them to an electrical signal to form a 2D image (Prado and Heymsfield 2014). The boundaries between tissues are determined on the ultrasound image and internal calipers are used to determine the thickness of the various tissues. The measurement of skeletal muscle via ultrasound is complicated by muscle compressibility, site selection, and the subject's hydration status (Mayans et al. 2012) and only produces a cross-sectional area of the site being measured. The similar acoustic impedance of skeletal muscle and adipose tissue lead to low resolution between the boundaries of these tissues, which can reduce the accuracy of the measurements (Wagner 2013). Overall, the use of ultrasound for determining lean soft tissue is expensive and requires a high degree of investigator expertise. Additional limitations include the potential presence of inherent artifacts (e.g., fascia) and the capability of providing only regional measures, instead of total body measures, of lean soft tissue (Wagner 2013) (Table 3.2). Thus, while ultrasound provides some increase in accuracy, and the ability to measure regional areas, a small region of interest and decreased resolution between muscle and fat limits its widespread use. Some interesting developments have been proposed to use ultrasound combined with muscle contraction to assess function and may provide a promising method in the future.

TABLE 3.2

Commonly Used Three-Component Models of Body Composition Assessment Techniques

Technique	Principle and Measurements	Advantages	Disadvantages	References
		Imaging and X-Ray Attenuation		
Dual-energy x-ray absorptiometry (DXA)	Uses x-ray beam attenuation of two different energies to differentiate between two components in each pixel: soft tissue and bone mass, or LM and FM when bone is not present. Gives total body and regional body BMC, FM, and LM measures (3-C model).	Quick, safe for repeated measures, noninvasive, high precision and accuracy of total body and regional quantification of BMC, FM, and LM. Reference method for the diagnosis of osteoporosis. Low ionizing radiation.	Measurement differences between and within manufacturers and software versions. Measurements influenced by tissue depth and hydration status. Not safe for pregnant women. High level of investigator expertise.	Lee and Gallagher (2008) Siervo and Jebb (2010)
Computed tomography (CT)	Uses x-ray attenuation to produce cross-sectional layers ("slices") depicting detailed images of the body, including AT, skeletal muscle, visceral organs, and brain tissue.	Noninvasive. Capable of assessing total body and regional composition and quantifying SAT, AT, LM, and bone tissue volumes.	High cost, low accessibility, long scan time, and requires investigator expertise. Size of scanning table limits ability to accommodate obese subjects. High ionizing radiation.	Delmonico et al. (2009) Modica et al. (2011) Roubenoff and Kehayias (1991) Siervo and Jebb (2010)
Peripheral quantitative computed tomography (pQCT)	Measures component-specific density, cortical bone parameters, skeletal muscle area, muscle density, and intramuscular adipose tissue. Provides cross-sectional area of muscle, fat, and muscle–bone unit in the upper and lower limbs.	Quick, portable, low investigator expertise, and small ionizing radiation. Allows volumetric scans of multiple regions of the body to assess bone (e.g., femur, tibia, forearm). Allows for muscle quality assessment.	Limited capability of accurate tissue measures compared with CT and MRI. No standardized scanning protocols have been developed.	Erlandson et al. (2016) Frost and Schoenau (2000) Lee and Gallagher (2008) Rauch et al. (2004) Schoenau et al. (2002)

(Continued)

TABLE 3.2 (Continued)
Commonly Used Three-Component Models of Body Composition Assessment Techniques

Technique	Principle and Measurements	Advantages	Disadvantages	References
Magnetic resonance imaging (MRI)	Uses magnetic fields and radio waves to depict detailed images of the following: AT, skeletal muscle, and visceral organs. Atomic protons are aligned in the magnetic field, activated by a radio frequency wave, and absorb and release energy. This energy is used to create cross-sectional images of tissues.	Noninvasive, excellent image resolution, no radiation. Capable of assessing total body and regional AT, LM, and bone tissue volumes. Accurately quantifies segmented FFM. Allows for automatic segmentation and manual delineation of tissues.	High cost, low accessibility, long scan time, and requires investigator expertise. Size of scanning table limits scanning of obese subjects. Cannot scan those with pacemakers or metal implants. Difficult to distinguish boundaries between tissue layers.	Fouladian et al. (2005) Modica et al. (2011) Mourtzakis et al. (2008) Shen and Chen (2008) Siervo and Jebb (2010)
Ultrasound	Primarily measures SAT and VAT; measurement of muscle and bone is being studied. Reflection of ultrasound waves from tissue in a beam's path transmitted through the skin. Amount of sound reflected is dependent on changes in acoustic impedance between fat–muscle or muscle–bone.	Noninvasive, quick, and high accuracy and precision of measurements with minimal tissue compression. Capable of assessing total body and regional SAT and VAT. No ionizing radiation.	High cost and requires high degree of investigator expertise. Measurement procedures and techniques are not yet standardized. Inherent artifacts (e.g., fascia) may be present on image produced.	Fanelli and Kuczmarski (1984) Wagner (2013)

Note: FFM, fat-free mass; FM, fat mass; SAT, subcutaneous adipose tissue; LM, lean muscle mass; AT, adipose tissue; VAT, visceral adipose tissue; BV, body volume; Db, body density; %BF, percent body fat; TBW, total body water; ECW, extracellular water; BMC, bone mineral content; BMM, bone mineral mass.

3.2.2.2 Dual X-Ray Absorptiometry

The most common three-component method of measuring body composition is DXA, which was first introduced in 1987. DXA is the most accurate and reliable body composition method that is widely used, particularly in clinical and laboratory settings, and has been validated against a four-component model. Originally based on the principle of bone densitometry, DXA technology has evolved over several decades. Early techniques used x-rays to examine known amounts of bone mineral density (i.e., the bone mineral content mass per unit of a particular area) in an aluminum phantom for validation purposes (Blake and Fogelman 1997).

DXA uses a narrow fan beam collimator to measure body tissue mass via the transmission of x-rays rather than gamma rays at two different frequencies (high and low), providing a quicker and safer body composition assessment with minimal ionizing radiation. Depending on an individual's body size, the amount of radiation exposure from DXA is 1%–10% of the radiation emitted by a chest x-ray or computed tomography (CT) scan (0.2–15 μSv vs. 250–2,700 μSv, respectively) or less than 1% of average annual total background radiation exposure (Lohman and Chen 2005; Lee et al. 2009). During a DXA scan, the two low-radiation x-rays pass through the body and are identified by a photon detector that measures the amount of energy absorbed by the subject's soft tissue and bone (Lohman and Chen 2005). The soft tissue is then subdivided into fat and lean soft tissue based on the empiric attenuation of both pure fat and bone-free soft tissue (Roubenoff et al. 1993). Therefore, the DXA gives us measures of three distinct components of bone mass, fat mass, and lean soft tissue, which improves its overall accuracy. Further, the DXA is quick and noninvasive, and can provide both total as well as regional estimates of the three components. Although the results of a DXA scan are highly correlated with cadaver analysis, their accuracy depends on factors such as patient's body size, machine calibration, DXA device, and software version used (Prado and Heymsfield 2014).

3.2.2.3 Computed Tomography

CT imaging has increased substantially in the clinical setting over the past few years. This increase is due in part to its accuracy and reliability. Clinically, CT is used more to evaluate lean soft tissue as a result of injury. In terms of body composition analysis, CT scanning is considered the gold standard for tissue–organ-level body composition analysis (Ross and Janssen 2005). The basic CT system consists of an x-ray tube and detector that rotate in a perpendicular plane to the subject. The x-ray beam is attenuated as it passes through tissue, and the images are reconstructed with mathematical techniques. Each pixel of the CT image is given a Hounsfield unit (HU) based upon tissue attenuation (related to electron density) that is colored white (Ross and Jenssen 2005). For example, water, which is more dense than air, is assigned an HU value of 0, while air is assigned an HU value of −1000. In addition, bone, skeletal muscle, and adipose tissue, as well as visceral organs, have specific HU ranges allowing for their identification (Ross and Janssen 2005). In the 1980s, Sjorstrom et al. (1986) and Sjorstrom (1991) introduced the concept of "total-body multicomponent CT," which allowed for the reliable body composition analysis of multiple body regions. Essentially, imaging "slices" can be taken at each of 22 body sites to examine total body and regional adipose tissue, lean body mass, bone, and other organ and tissue volumes. Currently, however, CT imaging is most commonly used to assess the amount of adipose tissue and skeletal muscle in a given region of the body. This is due to the fact that the radiation generated by CT imaging is high, and exposing healthy individuals to this high radiation dose for the purpose of conducting body composition research may be considered unethical (Ross and Jenssen 2005). Another limitation of CT imaging is the size of the patient in comparison to the size of the CT scanner. Obese patients may not fit into the CT scan field of view, thereby potentially compromising the image quaility of subcutaneous adipose tissue or skeletal muscle mass (Prado and Heymsfield 2014) (Table 3.2).

3.2.2.4 Peripheral Quantitative Computed Tomography

Recently, a mobile, less expensive CT scanner was developed to primarily measure bone mineral density and bone morphology in the radius and tibia, but its use in the assessment of skeletal muscle mass, among other measurements, has been realized (Prevrhal et al. 2008; Erlandson et al. 2016). Notably, this high-resolution peripheral CT scanner can provide information on the cross-sectional area of muscle and fat and of a muscle–bone unit in the upper and lower limbs. Additionally, information regarding bone geometry, skeletal muscle density, and intramuscular adipose tissue can be obtained, thereby providing muscle quality assessment (Frost and Schoenau 2000; Schoenau et al. 2002; Rauch et al. 2004; Erlandson et al. 2016). In detail, the scanned peripheral area of interest is determined by calculating the percentage of limb length from the line of reference (e.g., at the 66% tibia and 65% radius sites, respectively). However, the placement of the line of reference will change the total limb area that is scanned, making comparisons across studies difficult (Erlandson et al. 2016). Additionally, the use of peripheral quantitative computed tomography (pQCT) is attractive due to its shorter scan time, low degree of investigator expertise, smaller effective dose of ionizing radiation (<1 μSv) when compared with CT, and its capability of providing either single-slice or multislice 3D scan images (Engelke et al. 2008; Erlandson et al. 2016) (Table 3.2). Furthermore, recent pQCT models have been designed with a larger aperture diameter allowing for quantification not only of tissue measures within the lower leg and arm but also the upper leg and arm, thereby providing additional body composition information (Erlandson et al. 2016). Despite these advantages, pQCT is limited in its capability of accurately assessing soft tissue measures compared with CT and magnetic resonance imaging (MRI) (Erlandson et al. 2016). However, Sherk et al. (2011) found high correlations of muscle cross-sectional area, specifically at the mid-thigh level, using pQCT compared with MRI. Finally, although small, pQCT emits ionizing radiation—a characteristic that may limit its use for assessing individuals longitudinally in the research and performance settings—and standardized scanning protocols have not yet been developed (Erlandson et al. 2016).

3.2.2.5 Magnetic Resonance Imaging

Clinically, MRI like CT is used to evaluate lean soft tissue for injury or damage. Unlike CT imaging, MRI does not require the use of ionizing radiation but uses a powerful magnetic field to measure the interaction of hydrogen nuclei in the body. When hydrogen nuclei are placed in a strong magnetic field, they will align themselves in a known direction. A radio frequency pulse is then applied and subsequently absorbed by the hydrogen nuclei. When the hydrogen nuclei return to their aligned state, they release the energy in the form of a radio frequency, which is then used to generate the resulting images (Edelman et al. 2006).

Unlike CT scanning, MRI does not provide information on tissue density. Therefore, segmentation of different tissues must be performed by manual or automatic delineation based on either signal intensity or morphology (Arif et al. 2007; Shen and Chen 2008; Gray et al. 2011). Fully automated analysis methods are faster and more reproducible than methods dependent on manual delineation, but may introduce errors regarding accuracy of adipose tissue measurement (Arif et al. 2007). Most often, a semiautomatic approach is applied thereby taking advantage of time-saving and precise automated procedures but allowing manual correction to achieve accuracy (Shen and Chen 2008). MRI measurement of body composition has been validated in phantoms, animals, and human cadavers and shows good agreement (Fowler et al. 1991; Ross et al. 1991; Abate et al. 1994; Mitsiopoulos et al. 1998). However, MRI for whole-body composition measurements is time-consuming and costly. In addition, large individuals may have difficulty fitting into MRI scanners, and individuals who are claustrophobic may have difficulty with the procedure (Table 3.2).

3.2.3 Methods Using Four-Component Model

Multicomponent models of body composition have been developed. The most common of these multicomponent models is the four-component model, which requires the measurement of body volume (e.g., hydrodensitometry or air displacement plethysmography) total body water usually determined by the dilution with deuterium water (^2H_2O) and ^{18}O-labeled water ($H_2^{18}O$) (i.e., doubly labeled water) and bone mineral content (e.g., DXA) (Fosbøl and Zerahn 2015). The four-compartment model does not account for the mineral content of lean soft tissue (e.g., of soluble minerals and electrolytes), which is small, but it does contribute to the density of the component (Fosbøl and Zerahn 2015). In addition, five- and six-component methods are capable of determining body composition. Clearly, however, the utilization of the four-component model and other multicomponent models of body compositions require the use of multiple methods of body composition analysis, which not only increases the cost but the time needed to determine body composition. A comparison study between six-, four-, and three-component methods to measure body composition found bias of <1% body fat in healthy adults (Wang et al. 1998). This finding would suggest that limited accuracy is actually gained by the measurement of additional components beyond the three-component model, particularly when care is taken in the measurement protocol (e.g., same time of day, proper hydration). Given the cost and the time needed to make these extra measurements, the three-component model would appear to be the most practical choice in most clinical and research settings.

3.2.4 Urinary Markers

Two main urinary biomarkers are commonly used to estimate skeletal muscle mass in humans. Creatinine is a metabolite of creatine and approximately 98% of creatine in the body is found in muscle (Shephard 1991). The daily excretion of creatinine is approximately proportional to muscle mass (Cheek 1968; Grant et al. 1981; Heymsfield et al. 1983). Creatinine-based determinations of lean body mass can be altered if the subject being tested consumes meat or fish (Lykken et al. 1980). In addition, the collection of one or more 24-hour urine samples makes the use of creatinine-based estimates of skeletal muscle unattractive for use in humans.

Although urinary metabolites are noninvasive, safe, and inexpensive, they require a great deal of patient cooperation due to the fact that urine must be collected over a 24-hour period and the patient must refrain from consuming meat. More importantly, urinary metabolites only give a measure of total muscle cell mass but regional estimates of muscle cell mass are not possible (Table 3.1).

3.3 METHODS FOR DETERMINING REGIONAL MUSCLE MASS

Following the validation of total body composition, the need for regional body composition analysis to assess asymmetries or to provide a more detailed tissue composition analysis within particular body regions has been realized. Regional body composition analysis is useful in the evaluation of diseased or disabled individuals (i.e., cachexia, cancer), obesity intervention, athletic performance, and rehabilitation efforts. Burkhart et al. (2009) were among the first to examine DXA's reliability when segmenting the upper and lower extremities of the body to assess bone mass, fat mass, and lean soft tissue (i.e., regional composition measurements). More recently, Hart et al. (2015) assessed between-day inter- and intra-rater reliability of manually produced ROIs while segmenting body regions in the frontal view to examine bone and soft tissue (i.e., fat and lean muscle) masses. These studies demonstrated high inter- and intrarater reliability with small coefficients of variation in the postscan analysis of the upper and lower regions of the body.

Hart et al. (2015) also established successful DXA subject positioning for the upper and lower extremities in the traditional frontal view with coefficient of variation (CVs) of 1.6% or smaller for all scans, similar to previous studies (Pfeiffer et al. 2010). Standard subject positioning allows for maximum visibility of regional body composition, resulting in high inter- and intrarater reliability of DXA scan analysis of segmented lean soft tissue mass and fat mass quantification in the frontal view (Hart et al. 2015). Additional body positions have also been examined. Previous studies (Lambrinoudaki et al. 1998; Lohman et al. 2009) have examined DXA's reliability in providing reproducible values of total body fat mass and lean soft tissue mass measures—comparing supine-supine and supine-prone scans. Significant differences resulted between the supine and prone positions in total body measures of fat mass and lean soft tissue mass; thus, differences in subject positioning affect DXA body composition measurements due to slight changes in tissue depth and fat distribution between the two positions (Lambrinoudaki et al. 1998). Notably, these studies suggest that variations in body thickness seen within athletic populations and the distribution of bone and soft tissue may interfere with DXA's accuracy. It is therefore suggested that future studies examine additional methods of subject positioning, including that in the lateral view.

The assessment of ipsilateral regional differences in the appendicular skeleton (i.e., upper and lower limbs) may be more beneficial in examining injury risk and the rehabilitative process. Specifically, the ability to quantify lean tissue mass in ipsilateral, opposing regions of the body (i.e., anterior vs. posterior), to assess muscle quality via strength testing, and to examine muscle functionality in athletic populations, would allow for the development of more efficient and individualized strength training and rehabilitation programs. The development of these programs would allow for enhanced sports performance while minimizing reinjury risk. Additionally, the ability to examine longitudinal lean soft tissue mass changes (e.g., baseline/preinjury, postinjury/surgery, before returning to play, or at increments throughout the course of an athlete's career) in ipsilateral, opposing regions of the body is important as these changes affect the competitive performance of elite athletes. Lateral segmented longitudinal analysis of these measures would also provide greater insight into causes of injury (i.e., imbalances within regions) and the recovery process. Longitudinal analysis would further allow for the long-term evaluation of strength training and rehabilitation programs and assessment of nutritional interventions (Stewart 2001; Bilsborough et al. 2014).

3.4 SPORTS VALUE OF ASSESSING LEAN MUSCLE MASS

The assessment of lean mass has long been linked to sports performance. The overarching belief is that since fat mass does not contribute to function, maximizing lean mass will maximize performance. A limitation of this hypothesis is the assumption that lean soft tissue mass accumulation is continuous with increasing body mass. Even in highly trained athletes, a 1 kg (2.2 lbs.) increase in body weight is composed of 65%–70% lean tissue with the rest being fat and a small fraction of bone. Strikingly, above 114 kg (250 lbs.), this proportion shifts and every 1 kg increase is associated with 65%–70% increase in fat mass and only about 30%–35% lean mass (Figures 3.2 and 3.3). These data suggest limitations in lean soft tissue mass accumulation with increasing body weight, which may have to do with an individual's body frame and their ability to support extra lean mass. Also, nutrition and training during increased body weight accumulation plays a significant role as well, but the idea of strictly adding lean mass during weight gain is unlikely. This section will briefly review frame-sizing individuals to identify their ideal body type. We will examine the relationship between skeletal muscle mass, performance measures, muscle function, and injury. Finally, we will identify critical new directions for the application of lean mass, and body composition as a whole, as an identifier of future success.

3.5 FRAME-SIZING

Several body types exist in athletics that are beneficial for specific sports. While exceptions exist for every sport, generally certain body types are more advantageous than others. Identifying an individual's body type can shape training programs as well as expectations for each individual's training response. William H. Sheldon, PhD, MD first introduced somatotypes (body types) in the 1940s (Sheldon et al. 1940). The three basic body types are ectomorphs, endomorphs, and mesomorphs each with distinctive body characteristics. Ectomorphs are long and lean, they have little body fat and muscle mass (e.g., distance runners, basketball players). Endomorphs have both body fat and skeletal muscle (e.g., football linemen) and are typically rounder. Mesomorphs on the other hand are typically thicker with a large amount of muscle mass. The somatotype measurements use anthropometrics to provide a relative score of three numbers to describe each type (e.g., 711, 171, 117)—these numbers describe the level of endomorphy, mesomorphy, and ectomorphy, respectively

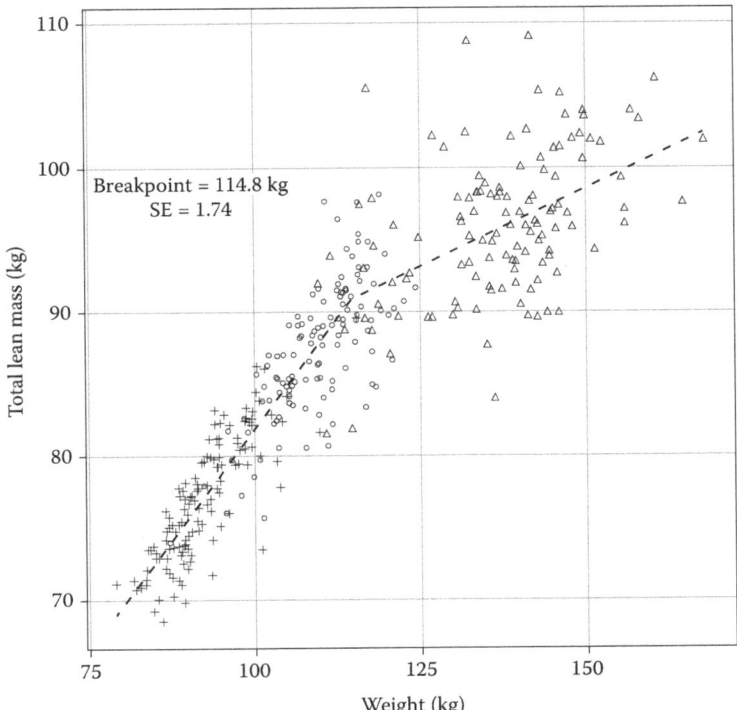

FIGURE 3.2 Total lean mass versus body weight with the change in slope at ~114 kg of body weight in linebackers, tight ends, running backs, quarterbacks, punters, and place kickers (open circles); offensive and defensive linemen (open triangles); wide receivers and defensive backs (plus symbol). (Adapted from Bosch, T. A. et al. 2014. *J Strength Cond Res* 28:3313–19.)

(Sheldon et al. 1940). Each area uses different values to estimate the level of each, endomorphy uses the sum of three skinfolds (triceps, subscapular, and supraspinale) corrected for height—the higher the sum, the higher the endomorphy score. Mesomorphy is estimated based on height, breadths of the humerus and femur, and girths of the biceps (flexed and relaxed) and calf. The girths are corrected for body fat using skinfold measurement. Ectomorphy is estimated based on height, weight, and the height–weight ratio. At the heart of this method are several assumptions, the key being the Trunk Index, or the ratio of the upper and lower torso areas. Sheldon observed this ratio remains constant even during weight gain or loss. Many other methods have been developed to estimate frame size (or somatotype) using similar methods (Carter and Heath 1990). Much of this work has been done by Christopher Ruff, PhD, who estimated body mass in elite athletes with minimal error (Ruff 2000); however, a simple literature search of somatotype will return several results and a review of each is outside of the scope of this chapter. As with any method using anthropometry, experience will increase the accuracy of the results. Individuals interested in using these methods should develop their own norms for the population, sports, or cohorts they work with to increase the accuracy of their estimations.

Using similar assumptions and anthropometric sites, we recently developed prediction equations to estimate the ideal weight and lean mass for an individual's frame size in a population of NFL football players using DXA. We measured 12 anatomical landmarks (e.g., shoulder width, hip width) and used multivariate linear regression to predict weight and lean mass adjusted for position and race. Our predicted weight and lean mass were strongly correlated with measured weight and lean mass (from DXA) at 0.93 and 0.90, respectively (unpublished data) (Figures 3.4 and 3.5). In

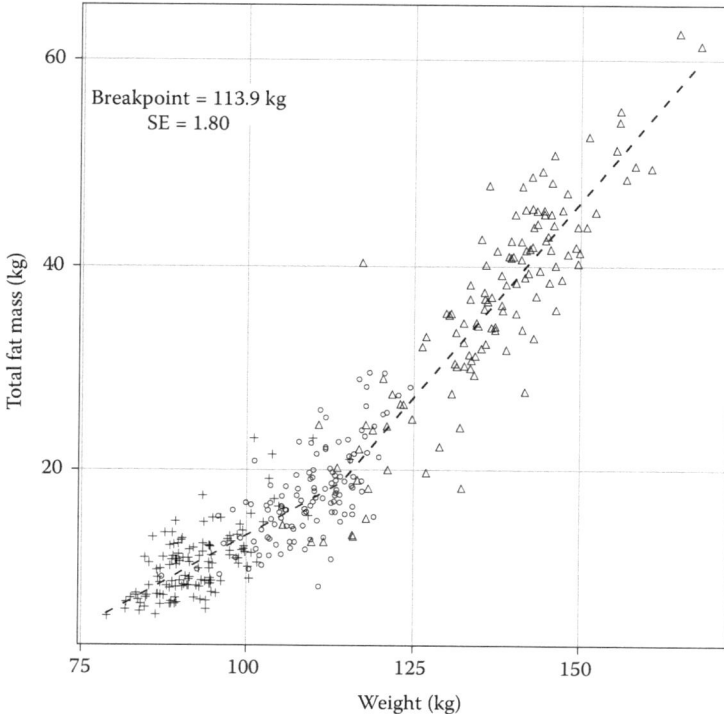

FIGURE 3.3 Total fat mass versus body weight with a change in slope at ~114 kg of body weight in linebackers, tight ends, running backs, quarterbacks, punters, and place kickers (open circles); offensive and defensive linemen (open triangles); wide receivers and defensive backs (plus symbol). (Adapted from Bosch, T. A. et al. 2014. *J Strength Cond Res* 28:3313–19).

simpler terms, our prediction equation explained 82% variance between an individual's lean mass. Currently, we are identifying the performance characteristics of individuals who are above, below, and on the regression line. This data will provide some evidence of whether having more or less lean mass than the ideal for an individual's frame is predictive of increased performance. Similar methods should be developed to predict change over time in less mature athletes (e.g., high school, college) to identify realistic changes in body weight or lean mass to maximize their performance. Doing so may improve projections of an athlete's capability of success in a particular task. As we observed, above 250 lbs., some individuals accumulate significantly more fat mass than lean mass. This could potentially be beneficial in some sports and positions, but may also decrease performance and increase injury risk.

3.6   BODY COMPOSITION CHARACTERISTICS OF ELITE ATHLETES: CURRENT AND FUTURE DIRECTIONS

We have described body composition characteristics of NFL football players, consistent with previous findings (Kraemer et al. 2005), position groups, and positions that mirror each other have similar body composition characteristics. Interestingly, searching the literature using "Body composition characteristics of elite" returns over 200 results ranging from fencers to basketball referees. Some of these reports are cross-sectional while some have measured longitudinal changes over time. In general, these typically use DXA to quantify percent body fat, fat mass, and lean mass.

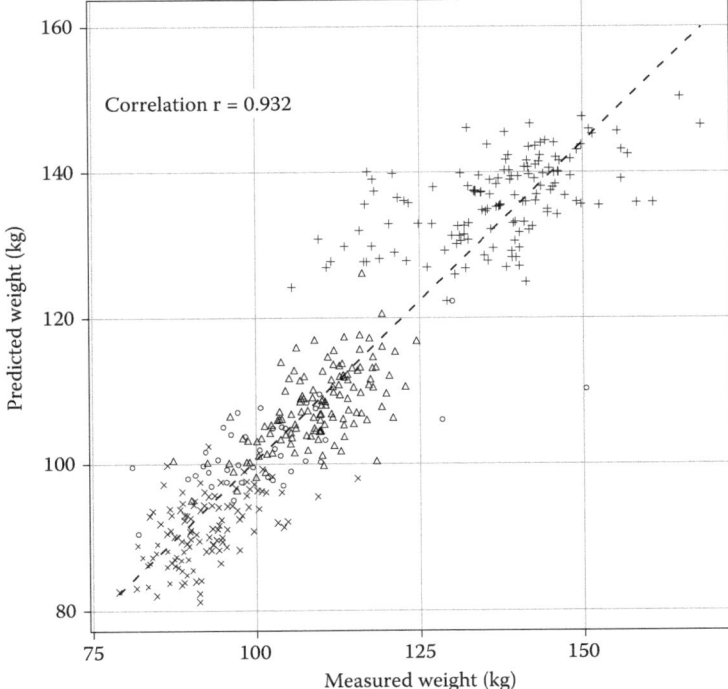

FIGURE 3.4 Predicted weight versus measured weight in linebackers, tight ends, and running backs (open circles); offensive and defensive linemen (open triangles); wide receivers and defensive backs (plus symbol); quarterbacks, punters, and place kickers (x symbol).

Over a given season, there is minimal change in these measures, ~1–2 kg on average. This is consistent with some of our yet unpublished data that measured changes in composition over several years of participation in the NFL. In our opinion, future studies need to examine regional changes as well as changes in the ratio of different tissues and body regions. Small changes in total mass do not mean significant changes have not occurred in different regions in the body. An individual that gains 4 kg of lean mass in his torso, but loses 4 kg of lean mass in his legs would have the same amount of total lean mass, but this shift could have a significant effect on their performance.

Similarly, total tissue mass will be different between individuals, particularly in sports with very different position groups (e.g., football, rugby, basketball). However, our data from NFL players (Dengel et al. 2014) suggests that the ratios of total mass (e.g., upper/lower body mass ratio or U/L ratio) are consistent across positions. Conversely, the ratio of total upper to lean leg mass was significantly different between positions. These data suggest that the proportion of mass may be more critical than the total mass. This would be consistent with biomechanical principles especially in sports that involve change in direction movements and contact. The legs are the primary movers through space, but the amount of mass in the upper body region will dramatically influence the amount of force necessary to change direction since the momentum of the upper body will need to be counteracted by the lower body force. Some anthropometric methods are capable of estimating these ratios, but the limitations discussed previously regarding the accuracy and assumptions of these methods will dramatically influence the precision error when calculating ratios. DXA provides accurate and reliable measures of body regions, but requires manual quantification of ratios. However, we feel ratio comparison is an important part of the future linking body composition characteristics to muscle function and athletic performance.

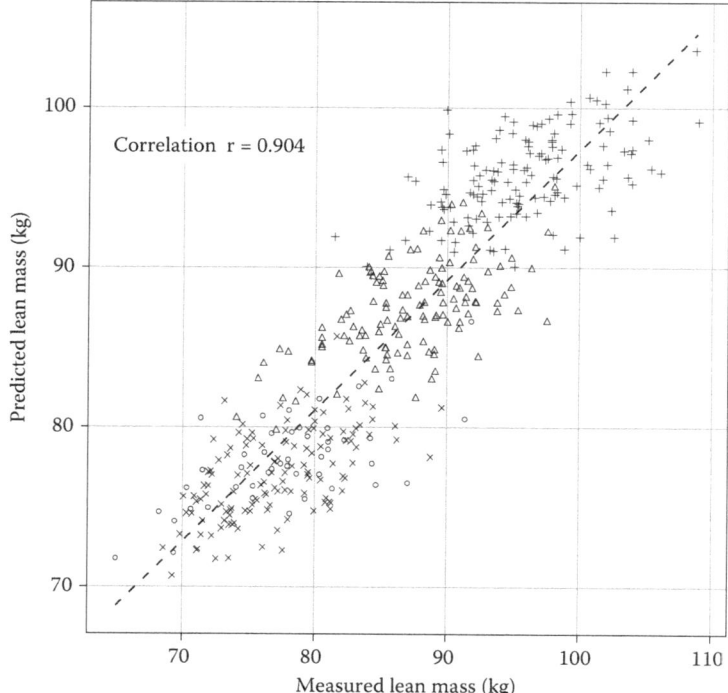

FIGURE 3.5 Predicted lean mass versus measured lean mass in linebackers, tight ends, and running backs (open circles); offensive and defensive linemen (open triangles); wide receivers and defensive backs (plus symbol); quarterbacks, punters, and place kickers (x symbol).

3.7 SKELETAL MUSCLE MASS AND SKELETAL MUSCLE FUNCTION

As we described above, several methods exist to measure skeletal muscle mass, although most actually measure lean tissue or fat-free mass. Most often in athletes these measures are correlated with muscle function (strength or power), athletic performance (e.g., measures of distance or time) or injury risk (e.g., relative risk differences in injury rates). Historically, one of the most common methods to measure muscle strength was isokinetic dynamometry (e.g., Biodex: Biodex Medical Systems, Shirley, New York, USA). This method measures the torque that a given limb places on an arm set to move at a specific speed (e.g., 60 degrees per second) in a given plane of motion (e.g., leg flexion/extension). This device measures peak torque for muscle groups muscles (e.g., quadriceps/hamstrings) as well as ipsilateral ratios to estimate muscle balance. This measurement is still collected at the NFL combine, and until recently was commonly used in rehabilitation from injury by physical therapists to compare involved and uninvolved legs. Although accurate and reliable, the use of this measurement has decreased because of the lack of functionality in measuring a specific range of motion compared to a movement (e.g., vertical jump). While true, unpublished data from a current study in our lab suggest a strong correlation between isokinetic dynamometer peak torque, force plate-derived peak power, and rate of force development (double and single leg). These relationships were consistent across sexes and sports (cross-country vs. football) suggesting dynamometry still provides relevant information about muscle function.

Recent innovations in force plate software have increased the availability and usability of force plate data. This information allows for immediate information about power output, rate of force development, and other characteristics of muscle function. These systems can be paired with motion analysis systems to identify biomechanical inefficiencies that may be limiting muscle function (i.e., power output). These methods allow for more accurate assessments of functional movements, compared to isokinetic dynamometry, that are more applicable to sports performance. The association between lean mass and power output during a countermovement jump is consistently strong across several populations (Bell et al. 2014). Using multiple force plates allows for the measurement of leg asymmetries. Bell et al. (2014) demonstrated that lean mass asymmetries in different segments of the leg were associated with power output asymmetries (explained 25% of the variance). This could provide important feedback for return to play following injury or injury prevention. However, 95% of their population had roughly 10% force and power asymmetry, thus more work is needed to identify significant asymmetry that may affect performance or increase risk of injury. More work is needed in this area to examine the relationship between lean mass asymmetries and power output.

3.8 SKELETAL MUSCLE MASS AND PERFORMANCE MEASURES

Skeletal muscle mass and cross-sectional areas are positively associated with strength and power measures; however, the translation to performance measures is more similar to the inverted U seen in the length–tension relationship of muscle. There is clearly an ideal total and lean mass for a given performance characteristic (e.g., jump height), but this does not equate to the ideal total and lean mass for sport performance. Addressing this, James L. Nuzzo (2015) questioned whether performance measures—in this case, NFL combine tests—need to be normalized to body mass. This study reported the percentile rankings of each test by position and compared absolute values, body mass adjusted values, and allometrically scaled values between positions. Not surprisingly, body mass and performance measures have strong associations (both positive and negative depending on the test). However, the need to normalize times, heights, and distances seems unwarranted, primarily because comparisons are rarely drawn across positions. Moreover, even in sports without such distinct size differences, these values are absolute measures that are important for sport. Regardless if an individual can run faster and jump farther when normalized or scaled relative to their mass, the absolute time and distance are most important. An argument can be made that when these values are used as surrogates for leg power, normalization or scaling provides an important marker to differentiate players, but again this depends on the sport or population being assessed. Nuzzo's work does build on the work of Robbins (2010, 2012) by providing position-specific criteria to normalize performance tests that may be useful when tracking an individual's change over time when there may also be changes in body mass.

In general, there remains a need to identify the ideal balance between skeletal muscle mass, performance measures, and sport-specific performance. Given the demands of each sport and other skills that contribute to sport-specific performance, there is likely a delicate balance between all three factors. As such, the training required to improve performance measures may not translate to improvements in sport-specific performance. The use of more sophisticated analysis techniques as well as more emphasis on body mass ratios and regional lean mass measurements may be critical to identifying this balance and shaping the future of training and development. The increased use of objective measures of force (force plates), velocity (movement tracking), and biomechanics (motion cameras) during training, paired with more accurate analysis of body composition (DXA) will be critical to the next step in sports performance.

3.9 CONCLUSION AND PERSPECTIVES

Over the last few decades, the ability to accurately measure skeletal muscle mass has evolved. This new-found accuracy has demonstrated the importance of a more detailed role for body composition than solely for height and weight measurements when examining overall health and disease risk (Prado and Heymsfield 2014). Newer imaging technology has allowed researchers to begin examining the quality of skeletal muscle mass, which in time may allow for more structural and functional information to be gathered regarding regional as well as total body skeletal muscle mass.

In addition, the role of body composition in sports performance, coupled with the lower cost of accurate body composition technology, has created a sports science market that continues to grow, giving professional and collegiate athletic teams access to more advanced body composition measurement methods. These new methods exceed simple measurements of total fat-free mass and have the ability to measure regional levels of lean body mass. This allows athletes and teams to look at asymmetry between left and right sides of the body or ratios of upper and lower skeletal muscle for the purpose of optimizing performance and preventing injury. Along these lines, research examining the ability of DXA to quantify, and longitudinally assess, ipsilateral, compartmental fat mass, and lean soft tissue may allow for a range of optimal ratios to be established. These ratios may ultimately be used to enhance sports performance, minimize injury risk, evaluate strength training and rehabilitation programs, and assess nutritional interventions.

As newer technologies of measuring total and regional skeletal muscle, the amount of information generated continues to grow. One of the new frontiers in using these new methods of body composition analysis in sports is the interpretation of the large amount of data gathered. It is therefore important to assess the new information gained from these advanced measures of skeletal muscle mass.

Finally, these newer, noninvasive methods of determining skeletal muscle mass now allow athletes, trainers, researchers, and health care providers to track changes in skeletal muscle mass over time. This information may therefore be used to examine a new training or diet regimen in an effort to help athletes perform at a higher level, to evaluate new medications to slow the advancement of sarcopenia in the elderly, or to examine individuals with rare diseases affecting skeletal muscle mass.

REFERENCES

Abate, N., D. Burns, R. M. Peshock, A. Garg, and S. M. Grundy. 1994. Estimation of adipose tissue mass by magnetic resonance imaging: Validation against dissection in human cadavers. *J Lipid Res* 35:1490–6.

Anderson, L. J., D. N. Erceg, and E. T. Schroeder. 2012. Utility of multifrequency bioelectrical impedance compared with dual-energy x-ray absorptiometry for assessment of total and regional body composition varies between men and women. *Nutr Res* 32:479–85.

Arif, H., S. B. Racette, D. T. Villareal, J. O. Holloszy, and E. P. Weiss. 2007. Comparison of methods for assessing abdominal adipose tissue from magnetic resonance images. *Obesity (Silver Spring)* 15:2240–4.

Baumgartner, R. N., S. B. Heymsfield, S. Lichtman, J. Wang, and R. N. Pierson Jr. 1991. Body composition in elderly people: Effect of criterion estimates on predictive equations. *Am J Clin Nutr* 53:1345–53.

Bell, D. R., J. L. Sanfilippo, N. Binkley, and B. C. Heiderscheit. 2014. Lean mass asymmetry influences force and power asymmetry during jumping in collegiate athletes. *J Strength Cond Res* 28:884–91.

Bellisari, A. and A. F. Roche. 2005. Anthropometry and ultrasound. In *Human Body Composition*, eds. S. B. Heymsfield, T. G. Lohman, Z. Wang, and S. B. Going, 109–28. Champaign, IL: Human Kinetics.

Bilsborough, J. C., K. Greenway, D. Opar, S. Livingstone, J. Cordy, and A. J. Coutts. 2014. The accuracy and precision of DXA for assessing body composition in team sport athletes. *J Sports Sci* 32:1821–8.

Blake, G. M. and I. Fogelman. 1997. Technical principles of dual energy x-ray absorptiometry. *Semin Nucl Med* 27:210–28.

Bosch, T. A., T. P. Burruss, N. L. Weir et al. 2014. Abdominal body composition differences in NFL football players. *J Strength Cond Res* 28:3313–9.

Brozek, J. F. Grande, J. T. Anderson, and A. Keys. 1963. Densitometric analysis of body composition: Revision of some quantitative assumptions. *Ann N Y Acad Sci* 110:113–40.

Buchholz, A. C., C. Bartok, and D. A. Schoeller. 2004. The validity of bioelectrical impedance models in clinical populations. *Nutr Clin Pract* 19:433–46.

Burkhart, T. A., K. L. Arthurs, and D. M. Andrews. 2009. Manual segmentation of DXA scan images result in reliable upper and lower extremity soft and rigid tissue mass estimates. *J Biomech* 27:197–206.

Carter, J. E. L. and B. H. Heath. 1990. *Somatotyping Development and Applications.* Cambridge: Cambridge University Press.

Cheek, D. B. 1968. *Human Growth.* Philadelphia: Lea and Febiger.

Delmonico, M. J., T. B. Harris, M. Visser et al. 2009. Longitudinal study of muscle strength, quality, and adipose tissue infiltration. *Am J Clin Nutr* 90:1579–85.

Dengel, D. R., T. A. Bosch, T. P. Burruss, K. A. Fielding, B. E. Engel, N. L. Weir, and T. D. Weston. 2014. Body composition of National Football League players. *J Strength Cond Res* 28:1–6.

Durnin, J. V. and J. Womersley. 1974. Body fat assessed from total body density and its estimation from skin-fold thickness: Measurements on 481 men and women aged from 16 to 72 years. *Br J Nutr* 32:77–97.

Edelman, R., J. R. Hesselink, M. B. Zlatkin, and J. V. Crues. 2006. *Clinical Magnetic Resonance Imaging* (Vol. 2), Philadelphia, PA: Saunders.

Engelke, K., J. E. Adams, G. Armbrecht et al. 2008. Clinical use of quantitative computed tomography and peripheral quantitative computed tomography in the management of osteoporosis in adults: The 2007 ISCD Official Positions. *J Clin Densitom* 11:123–62.

Erlandson, M. C., A. L. Lorbergs, S. Mathur, and A. M. Cheung. 2016. Muscle analysis using pQCT, DXA and MRI. *Eur J Radiol* 29:918–25. doi: 10.1016/j.ejrad.2016.03.001.

Esco, M. R., R. L. Snarr, M. D. Leatherwood et al. 2015. Comparison of total and segmental body composition using DXA and multifrequency bioimpedance in collegiate female athletes. *J Strength Cond Res* 29:918–25.

Fanelli, M. T. and R. J. Kuczmarski. 1984. Ultrasound as an approach to assessing body composition. *Am J Clin Nutr* 39:703–9.

Fosbøl, M. Ø. and B. Zerahn. 2015. Contemporary methods of body composition measurement. *Clin Physiol Funct Imaging* 35:81–97.

Fouladian, M., U. Korner, and I. Boasaeus. 2005. Body composition and time course changes in regional distribution of fat and lean tissue in unselected cancer patients on palliative care-correlations with food intake, metabolism, exercise capacity, and hormones. *Cancer* 103:189–98.

Fowler, P. A., M. F. Fuller, C. A. Glasbey et al. 1991. Total and subcutaneous adipose tissue in women: The measurement of distribution and accurate prediction of quantity by using magnetic resonance imaging. *Am J Clin Nutr* 54:18–25.

Frost, H. M. and E. Schoenau. 2000. The "muscle-bone unit" in children and adolescents: A 2000 overview. *J Pediatr Endocrinol Metab* 13:571–90.

Garby, L., O. Lammert, and E. Nielsen. 1990. Negligible effects of previous moderate physical activity and changes in environmental temperature on whole body electrical impedance. *Eur J Clin Nutr* 44:545–6.

Grant, J. P., P. B. Custer, and J. Thurlaw. 1981. Current techniques of nutritional assessment. *Surg Clin North Am* 61:437–63.

Gray, C., T. J. MacGillivray, C. Eeley et al. 2011. Magnetic resonance imaging with k-means clustering objectively measures whole muscle volume compartments in sarcopenia/cancer cachexia. *Clin Nutr* 30:106–11.

Hart, N. H., S. Nimphius, T. Spiteri, J. L. Cochrane, and R. U. Newton. 2015. Segmental musculoskeletal examinations using dual-energy x-ray absorptiometry (DXA): Positioning and analysis considerations. *J Sports Sci Med* 14:620–6.

Heymsfield, S. B., C. Arteaga, C. McManus, J. Smith, and S. Moffitt. 1983. Measurement of muscle mass in humans: Validity of the 24-h urinary creatinine method. *Am J Clin Nutr* 37:478–94.

Heymsfield, S. B., M. C. Gonzalez, J. Lu, G. Ja, and J. Zhreng. 2015. Skeletal muscle mass and quality: Evolution of modern measurement concepts in the context of sarcopenia. *Proc Nutr Soc* 74:355–66.

Jackson, A. S., and M. L. Pollock. 1978. Generalized equations for predicting body density of men. *Br J Nutr* 40:497–504.

Jackson, A. S., M. L. Pollock, and A. Ward. 1980. Generalized equations for predicting body density of women. *Med Sci Sports Exerc* 12:175–81.

Kraemer, W. J., J. C. Torine, R. Silvestre et al. 2005. Body size and composition of National Football League players. *J Strength Cond Res* 19:1061–2.

Lambrinoudaki, I., E. Georgiou, G. Douskas, G. Tsekes, M. Kyriakidis, and C. Proukakis. 1998. Body composition assessment by dual-energy x-ray absorptiometry: Comparison of prone and supine measurements. *Metabolism* 47:1379–82.

Latin, R. W. and R. O. Ruhling. 1986. Total lung capacity residual volume and predicted residual volume in a densitometric study of older men. *Br J Sports Med* 20:66–8.

Lee, M. K., M. Koh, A. C. Fang, S. N. Le, and G. Balasekaran. 2009. Estimation of body segment parameters using dual energy absorptiometry and 3-D exterior geometry. *13th International Conference on Biomedical Engineering: IFMBE Proc*, vol. 23, pp. 1777–80.

Lee, S. Y. and D. Gallagher. 2008. Assessment methods in human body composition. *Curr Opin Clin Nutr Metab Care* 11:566–72.

Lohman, M., K. Tallroth, J. A. Kettunen, and M. T. Marttinen. 2009. Reproducibility of dual-energy x-ray absorptiometry total and regional body composition measurements using different scanning positions and definitions of regions. *Metabolism* 58:1663–8.

Lohman, T. G. 1981. Skinfolds and body density and their relation to body fatness: A review. *Hum Biol* 53:181–225.

Lohman, T. G. and Z. Chen. 2005. Dual-energy x-ray absorptiometry. In *Human Body Composition: Methods and Findings*, eds. S. B. Heymsfield, T. G. Lohman, and Z. Wang, 63–77. Champaign, IL: Human Kinetics.

Lukaski, H. C. 1987. Methods for the assessment of human body composition: Traditional and new. *Am J Clin Nutr* 46:537–56.

Lukaski, H. C. 1989. Use of bioelectrical impedance analysis to assess human body composition: A review. In *Nutritional Status Assessment of the Individual*, ed. G. E. Livingston, 189–204. Trumbull, CT: Food and Nutrition Press.

Lykken, G. I., R. A. Jacob, P. M. Munoz, and H. H. Sandstead. 1980. A mathematical model of creatine metabolism in normal males—Comparison between theory and experiment. *The Am J Clin Nutr* 33:2674–85.

Mayans, D., M. S. Cartwright, and F. O. Walker. 2012. Neuromuscular ultrasonography: Quantifying muscle and nerve measurements. *Phys Med Rehabil Clin N Am* 23:133–48, xii.

Mitsiopoulos, N., R. N. Baumgartner, S. B. Heymsfield, W. Lyons, D. Gallagher, and R. Ross. 1998. Cadaver validation of skeletal muscle measurement by magnetic resonance imaging and computerized tomography. *J Appl Physiol* 85:115–22.

Modica, M. J., K. M. Kanal, and M. L. Gunn. 2011. The obese emergency patient: Imaging challenges and solutions. *Radiographics* 31:811–23.

Mourtzakis, M., C. M. M. Prado, J. R. Lieffers, T. Reiman, L. J. McCargar, and V. E. Baracos. 2008. A practical and precise approach to quantification of body composition in cancer patients using computed tomography images acquired during routine care. *Appl Physiol Nutr Metab* 33:997–1006.

Nuzzo, J. L. 2015. The National Football League scouting combine from 1999 to 2014: Normative reference values and an examination of body mass normalization techniques. *J Strength Cond Res* 29:279–89.

Pfeiffer, J. J., D. A. Galvao, Z. Gibbs et al. 2010. Strength and functional characteristics of men and women 65 years and older. *Rejuvenation Res* 13:75–82.

Prado, C. M. M. and S. B. Heymsfield. 2014. Lean tissue imaging: A new era for nutritional assessment and intervention. *JPEN J Parenter Enteral Nutr* 38:940–53.

Prevrhal, S., K. Engelke, and H. K. Genant. 2008. pQCT: Peripheral quantitative computed tomography. In *Radiology of Osteoporosis* (2nd Ed.), ed. S. Grampp, 143–62. Berlin, Heidelberg: Springer-Verlag.

Rauch, F., D. A. Bailey, A. Baxter-Jones, R. Mirwald, and R. Faulkner. 2004. The "muscle bone unit" during the pubertal growth spurt. *Bone* 34:771–5.

Robbins, D. W. 2010. The National Football League (NFL) combine: Does normalized data better predict performance in the NFL draft? *J Strength Cond Res* 24:2888–99.

Robbins, D. W. 2012. The normalization of explosive functional movements in a diverse population of elite American football players. *J Strength Cond Res* 26:995–1000.

Roche, A. F., S. B. Hemsfield, and T. G. Lohman. 1996. *Human Body Composition*. Champaign, IL: Human Kinetics.

Ross, R. and I. Janssen. 2005. Computed tomography and magnetic resonance imaging. In *Human Body Composition*, eds. S. B. Heymsfield, T. G. Lohman, Z. Wang, and S. B. Going, 89–108. Champaign, IL: Human Kinetics.

Ross, R., L. Leger, R. Guardo, G. J. De, and B. G. Pike. 1991. Adipose tissue volume measured by magnetic resonance imaging and computerized tomography in rats. *J Appl Physiol* 70:2164–72.

Roubenoff, R. and J. J. Kehayias. 1991. The meaning and measurement of lean body mass. *Nutr Rev* 49:163–75.

Roubenoff, R., J. J. Kehayias, B. Dawson-Hughes, and S. B. Heymsfield. 1993. Use of dual-energy x-ray absorptiometry in body-composition studies: Not yet a "gold standard". *Am J Clin Nutr* 58:589–91.

Ruff, C. B. 2000. Body mass prediction from skeletal frame size in elite athletes. *Am J Phys Anthropol* 113:507–17.

Schoenau, E., C. M. Neu, B. Beck, F. Manz, and F. Rauch. 2002. Bone mineral content per muscle cross-sectional areas as an index of the functional muscle-bone unit. *J Bone Miner Res* 17:1095–101.

Segal, K. R., M. Van Loan, P. I. Fitzgerald, J. A. Hodgdon, and T. B. Van Itallie. 1988. Lean body mass estimation by bioelectrical impedance analysis: A four-site cross-validation study. *Am J Clin Nutr* 47:7–14.

Sheldon, W. H., S. S. Stevens, and W. B. Tucker. 1940. *The Varieties of Human Physique*. New York: Harper and Brothers.

Shen, W. and J. Chen. 2008. Application of imaging and other noninvasive techniques in determining adipose tissue mass. *Methods Mol Biol* 456:39–54.

Shephard, R. J. 1991. *Body Composition in Biological Anthropology*. Cambridge, Great Britain: Cambridge University Press.

Sherk, V. D., M. G. Bemben, I. J. Palmer, and D. A. Beben. 2011. Effects of filtering methods on muscle and fat cross-sectional area measurement by pQCT: A technical note. *Physiol Meas* 32:N65–72.

Siervo, M. and S. A. Jebb. 2010. Body composition assessment: Theory into practice: Introduction of multi-compartment models. *IEEE Eng Med Biol Mag* 29:48–59.

Siri, W. E. 1956. The gross composition of the body. *Adv Biol Med Phys* 4:239–80.

Sjorstrom, L. 1991. A computer-tomography based multicompartment body composition technique and anthropometric predictions of lean body mass, total and subcutaneous adipose tissue. *Int J Obes* 15:19–30.

Sjorstrom, L., H. Kvist, A. Cederblad, and U. Tylen. 1986. Determination of total adipose tissue and body fat in women by computed tomography, ^{40}K, and tritium. *Am J Physiol Endocrinol Metab* 250:E736–45.

Stewart, A. D. 2001. Assessing body composition in athletes. *Nutrition* 17:694–5.

Wagner, D. R. 2013. Ultrasound as a tool to assess body fat. *J Obes* 2013:280713. doi: 10.1155/2013/280713.

Wang, J., J. C. Thornton, S. Kolesnik, and R. N. Pierson Jr. 2000. Anthropometry in body composition. An overview. *Ann N Y Acad Sci* 904:317–26.

Wang, Z. M., P. Deurenberg, S. S. Guo et al. 1998. Six-compartment body composition model: Inter-method comparisons of total body fat measurement. *Int J Obes Relat Metab Disord* 22:329–37.

Wang, Z., W. Shen, R. T. Withers, and S. B. Heymsfield. 2005. Multicomponent molecular-level models of body composition analysis. In *Human Body Composition* (2nd Ed.), eds. S. B. Heymsfield, T. G. Lohman, Z. Wang, and S. B. Going, 163–76. Champaign, IL: Human Kinetics.

Wells, J. C. and M. S. Fewtrell. 2006. Measuring body composition. *Arch Dis Child* 91:612–7.

Wilmore, J. H., P. A. Vodak, R. B. Parr, R. N. Girandola, and J. E. Billing. 1980. Further simplification of a method for determination of residual lung volume. *Med Sci Sports Exerc* 12:216–8.

4 Hydrometry, Hydration Status, and Performance

Ronald J. Maughan and Susan M. Shirreffs

CONTENTS

4.1 INTRODUCTION

Except in the very obese, water is the single largest component of the body, representing about 50%–70% of total body mass, and is present in variable amounts in all cells, tissues, and organs (Bender and Bender 1997). The total body water (TBW) content can be expressed in absolute terms (as a volume in mL or a mass in kg), or as a proportion of total body mass (TBW/body mass × 100%). Depending on how it is expressed, the body water content may change when TBW or body mass changes. Body water content is determined by the balance between the rates at which water is added to the body and the rate of water losses. It is tightly regulated to maintain a rather constant volume of water in the body and a constant tissue osmolality. Both the quantity of water in the body and hydration status are important in many different contexts, but unfortunately the two are often confused. The body's water content is quantified as a volume or mass of water, whereas hydration status takes account of tissue osmolality as well as water content. Body water content, and its measurement, is important for several reasons. As the fractional water content of tissues is relatively constant and the water content of lean tissue is much higher than that of adipose tissue, measurement of body water content can be used to estimate lean tissue mass and therefore body fat content. Body water content and hydration status affect all physiological functions, and if disturbances are sufficiently severe, both physical and cognitive functions are impaired. In extreme situations, death may result from both insufficient and excessive intake of water.

Lean tissue is normally about 70%–80% water, with an average value of 73.2% for the water content of the total fat-free mass being generally accepted, as originally proposed by Pace and Rathbun (1945). If the total body water content is known in absolute terms (in mL or kg), the total lean body mass may be estimated and, by difference from total body mass, the fat content can be estimated.

Those with a high body fat content will have a lower total body water content than their leaner counterparts of the same body mass. This assumes, of course, that the individual is euhydrated and it is usual to standardize premeasurement conditions to try to ensure that this is the case. From this it also follows, again assuming euhydration, that those individuals with a high body mass will have a greater total body water content than those with a lower body mass if body fat content is the same.

It is important to note, though, that the water content of lean tissue may vary substantially (from about 67% to 85%) between individuals (Moore and Boyden 1963; Sheng and Huggins 1979), leading to substantial errors in the estimation of lean tissue mass and therefore of fat mass. Application of a wide range of different methods to the assessment of body composition reveals poor agreement between them (Table 4.1). All of the methods used to produce the data in Table 4.1 estimate fat-free mass (FFM) and then calculate the percentage of fat from the difference between the total body mass (BM) and fat-free mass [(BM–FFM)/BM × 100%]. The methods rely on a two-component model to estimate FFM and assume a constant concentration of water or chemical composition of the fat-free body to estimate FFM. However, any interindividual variability in the assumed constant chemical composition of fat-free body leads to error that is propagated in calculation of the fat percentage. If the magnetic resonance imaging analyses are correct, then the data in Table 4.1 emphasize the weakness of the two-component model as related to technical (measurement) errors and biological variability errors of assumed constants (e.g., hydration and ^{40}K).

TABLE 4.1

Estimates of Body Fat Content (as % Body Mass) in a Sample of Lean and Overweight Women by Underwater Weighing (UWW), Body Water Dilution (BWD), Whole Body Counting (^{40}K), Skinfold Thickness (SFT), Bioelectrical Impedance (BEI), Magnetic Resonance Imaging (MRI), and a Combined Method (W+K: BWD and ^{40}K)

Subject	UWW	BWD	^{40}K	SFT	BEI	MRI	W+K	Range
Lean								
A	19.6	27.7	24.4	26.0	23.0	25.7	23.4	8.1
B	25.0	29.4	22.0	29.3	22.5	24.9	23.1	7.4
C	18.8	25.9	19.5	23.8	16.5	25.0	20.4	9.4
D	31.2	38.6	33.1	36.2	29.3	36.9	34.5	9.3
E	23.1	32.9	38.4	24.2	24.6	26.6	29.3	14.1
F	26.4	39.3	21.9	34.2	31.5	29.6	34.0	11.4
G	26.9	26.1	34.9	26.2	25.8	28.8	24.1	10.2
Mean	25.4	31.4	21.1	28.6	24.1	28.2	27.1	10.9
SD	6.1	5.7	1.5	4.9	4.9	4.2	5.6	3.7
Overweight								
H	39.6	46.7	41.5	38.4	36.1	43.8	44.3	10.8
I	35.8	39.1	32.3	34.2	35.2	36.3	36.6	6.8
J	43.5	51.4	52.3	41.1	43.4	41.3	50.1	10.3
K	41.4	50.5	45.1	41.2	35.1	44.1	41.7	15.4
L	38.2	36.5	45.3	43.3	31.6	43.8	37.4	8.8
M	50.0	53.0	42.9	40.6	48.5	48.9	50.6	12.4
N	42.1	38.5	39.0	39.6	40.4	44.4	39.2	5.9
Mean	42.4	45.1	43.5	39.8	39.6	44.1	43.1	10.1
SD	5.1	6.9	6.4	2.9	4.9	4.0	6.0	3.3

Source: Adapted from McNeill, G. et al. 1991. *Br J Nutr* 65:95–103.

TABLE 4.2

Solute Composition (mmol/L) of the Major Body Water Compartments and Normal Range of Sweat Composition

	Sweat	Plasma	Intracellular
Sodium	20–80	130–155	10
Potassium	4–8	3.2–5.5	150
Calcium	0–1	2.1–2.9	0
Magnesium	<0.2	0.7–1.5	15
Chloride	20–60	96–110	8
Bicarbonate	0–35	23–28	10
Phosphate	0.1–0.2	0.7–1.6	65
Sulfate	0.1–2.0	0.3–0.9	10

Note: Data from Maughan (1991) were compiled from various sources. The large variability in the composition of sweat and the relative constancy of the internal environment is striking.

The greater part (about two-thirds) of the total body water is contained within the intracellular space, with the remaining third found in the interstitial space and blood plasma. The distribution of water between these compartments has implications for cardiovascular and metabolic functions and is influenced by hydrostatic, oncotic, and osmotic pressures. The solute composition of these body water compartments is very different (Table 4.2). Changes in posture cause a redistribution of body water without affecting total body water content, though posture change may result in a change in the estimate of total body water when this is measured by bioimpedance analysis (Shirreffs and Maughan 1994). Likewise, short periods of intense exercise involving large muscle groups result in a large increase in the intracellular osmolality in the active muscles as a result of conversion of glycogen to small-molecule glycolytic intermediates and end products, resulting in a shift of water into the intramuscular space in response to the increased local osmolality (Maughan and Gleeson 2010): substantial reductions in blood volume may be observed without any change in total body water content. Assessment of total body water and of the volumes of the various compartments therefore requires careful standardization before and during the measurements.

Water is added to the body from food and fluid intake and is also generated by the oxidation of the macronutrients: fat, carbohydrate, protein, and alcohol. These inputs to the body water pool are matched by losses, which are normally accounted for mostly by urine but also include fecal, respiratory, and transcutaneous losses as well as sweat loss. Intake is episodic (though water of oxidation is produced continuously) but losses are continuous, so body water content is never constant: intake and output may not match over a period of hours, but are normally well matched over periods of 24 hours or more. Daily water turnover varies greatly between individuals but there can also be an enormous variability within individuals from day to day and at different times of year, depending primarily on temperature and humidity of the environment and on physical activity levels. In the sedentary individual living in a temperate climate, about 5% of total body water is typically lost and replaced on a daily basis, but when prolonged exercise is performed in a hot environment, 20%–40% of total body water can be turned over in a single day (Robinson and Robinson 1954). Voluntary control of intake can also override the physiological factors that regulate intake. For example, Flear et al. (1981) reported the case of a man who drank 9 L of beer, with a sodium content of 1.5 mmol/L, in the space of 20 min; his plasma sodium concentration fell from 143 mmol/L before to 127 mmol/L after drinking, but the man appeared unaffected.

Water intake (from food, beverages, and also water of oxidation generated during the catabolism of macronutrients) must match losses to maintain homeostasis, and the daily water intakes of various population groups have been reported in the literature. In the United States, the Adequate Intake (AI) for water for men aged 19–30 years of age is set at 3.7 L/day of total water (from foods and fluids), while the AI is set at 2.7 L/day for women in the same age group (Food and Nutrition Board 2005a). The European Food Standards Agency (EFSA; European Food Standards Agency 2010) has set adequate total water intakes for females of 2.0 L/day (95th percentile value 3.1 L) and for males 2.5 L/day (95th percentile value 4.0 L). In the case of both expert committee reports, the large interindividual variability was stressed as the reason for not defining a value for the estimated average requirement (EAR).

4.1.1 TERMINOLOGY

Hydration status is not the same as body water content as it also reflects the distribution of body water and the balance of the major electrolytes and other solutes. Hydration status, as indicated by plasma osmolality, is tightly regulated, and the body responds to even small changes in plasma osmolality: an increase stimulates thirst and reduces urinary losses, while a decrease promotes an increased water loss via the kidneys. Perturbations of water balance may be accompanied by, or may be caused by, alterations in the concentration of osmolytes in the various body water compartments, so euhydration usually includes a specified range of osmolality and/or sodium concentration, as sodium is the primary osmolyte of the extracellular space. Normal ranges for these variables will depend on the population of interest and on the laboratory methodologies used, but serum osmolality is normally within the range 281–297 mmol/kg and serum sodium concentration 134–143 mmol/L (Lentner 1984). Changes in electrolyte balance may occur independently of changes in water balance, further complicating both the definition and assessment of hydration status.

Euhydration occurs when body water content and the osmolality of the body water compartments are within the normal ranges. Dehydration is the process of water loss from the body and will lead to a state of hypohydration.

4.2 MEASUREMENT OF BODY WATER CONTENT

Various methods are available for the estimation of measurement of TBW content. The choice of method used is determined by a number of factors, including the precision required, the availability of the necessary facilities, the cost and the burden on the subject. Most involve dilution of a tracer in the body water space and measurement of the concentration of that tracer after a suitable equilibration period. It is assumed that complete equilibration with the total body water compartment occurs and that the tracer is not metabolized, excreted, or otherwise sequestered prior to sample collection (Heyward and Wagner 2004; Schoeller 2005).

4.2.1 ISOTOPE DILUTION

The water molecule consists of two atoms of hydrogen and one of oxygen: and isotopes of either of these components can be used as tracers to assess body water content. The stable isotopes deuterium (as deuterium oxide, ^2H_2O, or more correctly, ^2HHO) and ^{18}oxygen (as O), and the radioactive isotope tritium (as tritium oxide, ^3H_2O) appear to be appropriate tracers for water (Edelman 1952; Pinson 1952; Schoeller et al. 1980). Equilibration is achieved within about 3–4 hours and samples of body fluids may be obtained from blood, urine, saliva, or as a condensate from expired breath (Wong et al. 1988). Because of differences in the extent of isotope exchange with nonaqueous entities, the O dilution volume is about 3% smaller than the ^2HHO dilution volume and is closer to the true value of TBW (Schoeller et al. 1980). Based on several animal studies involving different species where total body water content of the whole body has been measured directly by desiccation, the use of hydrogen isotopes gives an overestimation difference of about 3.7% from the desiccation method with a standard deviation of 1.7%: for [18]oxygen, the corresponding overestimation values are 1.6% and 0.6% (Schoeller 2005).

The sensitivity and precision with which measurements can be made depend on several factors. Analytical variability, biological variability, and variations introduced by lack of standardization of conditions before and during measurements will all contribute. Because some of these factors will vary between laboratories, and even between individuals in the same laboratory, reported values for precision and sensitivity have limited relevance. Nevertheless, measurement of ^2H_2O by mass spectrometry has been reported to have a sensitivity of approximately 0.2 ppm (Halliday and Miller 1977) and a coefficient of variation (CV) of <2% (Leiper et al. 1988). Determination by infrared spectrometry can reliably detect differences of ≥ 10 ppm with a CV of 4.8% (Wemple et al. 1997). Tritium is radioactive and can be utilized in small doses for single measurements, but its use raises health issues, precluding frequent measurements in the same individual and even single measurements in some populations, such as pregnant women and children (Pinson 1952). Quantification of the tritium tracer concentration can be made using liquid scintillation counters, with assay sensitivity similar to that of mass spectrometry, and the radioactive dose received by subjects can be maintained within normal background radiation levels (Pinson 1952). The biological half-life of these tracers will depend on the rate of water turnover, but is typically about 7–14 days (Pinson 1952). [18]Oxygen is lost from the body in carbon dioxide as well as in water, so it cannot be used for estimates of water turnover. Either isotope may be used to measure the kinetic parameters of absorption and distribution of ingested water in the body water pool and of its subsequent disappearance from this pool (Peronnet et al. 2012).

4.2.2 Bioelectrical Impedance

Bioimpedance analysis (BIA) has been widely used to estimate both body water content and other aspects of body composition. The attractions of the method are based largely on its ease of use and its relatively low cost rather than on precision and validity. The principle of operation depends on the fact that the total volume of a conductor can be estimated from its length (L) and the resistance (R) to a single frequency electric current (L^2/R). The key assumption is that the conductor has a uniform shape and that the current is distributed throughout the conductor uniformly (Chumlea and Sun 2005). The National Institute of Health 1994 Technology Assessment Conference on Bioelectrical Impedance (National Institutes of Health 1994) concluded that "BIA provides a reliable estimate of total body water under most conditions." It carried on to state that "BIA values are affected by numerous variables including… hydration status" and that "Reliable BIA requires standardization and control of these variables." Much work in this area has generally highlighted the limitations of the technique. For example, Asselin et al. (1998) concluded that with acute dehydration and rehydration of 2%–3% of body mass, standard equations failed to predict changes in total body water as determined by changes in body mass. Shirreffs and Maughan (1994) found a progressive change in measured impedance over time when subjects went from an upright to a supine position, though there was clearly no change in total body water over this period. Berneis and Keller (2000), after inducing extracellular volume and tonicity alterations by infusion and drinking, concluded that BIA may not be reliable. Moon et al. (2010), however, found that some of the variability could be reduced by standardization of electrode placement, allowing smaller changes to be detected. Controlling other variables, such as posture, body temperature, prior food and fluid intake, and prior exercise may also help to reduce the variability, but the assumptions involved in the conversion of an impedance measurement to a body water content remain problematic.

Because of its low cost and ease of use, however, BIA has been used in many national surveys and large intervention studies as well as in laboratory investigations. Many equations have been reviewed and validated using a multicomponent model (Chumlea and Sun 2005). Though BIA can be used to estimate body composition, its accuracy is limited in estimating body water and body fatness. In a careful comparison between BIA and skinfolds among wrestlers, where several laboratories diligently followed the same measurement protocol, both methods were closely related to % body fat estimated from densitometry with a standard error of the estimate (SEE) of 3.5% (Lohman 1992). This indicates clearly the accuracy limits with these measurement techniques, and the SEE values are only obtainable only "within" specific groups, but not for mixed groups of athletes. When individual body composition is to be assessed, one should consider that, for example, 3% deviation from an assumed real value of 8% would result in % body fat values between 5% and 11%. This is far from the accuracy necessary for proper interpretation of health and performance optimization. A further limitation of the BIA method for athletes lies in the measurement prerequisites which include abstaining from exercise. However, a recently published pilot study (Gatterer et al. 2014) has concluded that after a bout of exercise-induced dehydration followed by a cold shower, the impedance results indicated that a fluid loss had occurred and that the impedance values obtained might be useful to evaluate fluid shifts between compartments. Thus, the use of bioelectrical impedance techniques for the assessment of body water volumes remains an area requiring significant research.

4.2.3 Measurement of Body Water Compartments

The total body water content includes both the intracellular water (ICW) and the extracellular water (ECW), and a number of markers have been used to estimate the ECW, with ICW being calculated by difference from TBW. The ICW can be estimated directly by measurement of total body potassium content, but few institutions have the facilities necessary for measurement of total body potassium.

Various tracers have been used to estimate the extracellular space but all have problems due to varying and uncertain distribution spaces, safety, or analytical difficulties. The most realistic tracer appears to be bromide, which tracks chloride, and is relatively easily measured using high-performance liquid chromatography (HPLC) (Schoeller 2005). Once again, the relatively long equilibration time (in the order of 4 h [Schoeller 2005]) that is necessary precludes the use of any of these tracer methods for repeated measures at short intervals.

4.3 WATER BALANCE

4.3.1 Estimates of Water Intake

The daily water requirement varies greatly between individuals because of differences in body size, dietary solute load from food consumed, environment (both indoors and outdoors), and physical activity level. Variations in intake are also introduced by conscious control of intake. As noted above, the U.S. AI for water for men aged 19–30 years of age is set at 3.7 L/day of total water (from foods and fluids), while the AI is set at 2.7 L/day for women in the same age group (Food and Nutrition Board 2005). The European Food Standards Agency (EFSA; European Food Standards Agency 2010) recently set adequate total water intakes for females of 2.0 L/day (95th percentile value 3.1 L) and for males 2.5 L/day (95th percentile value 4.0 L). The fact that these values are so different suggests some uncertainty in these values, and indeed there is an extremely large individual variability. In the case of both expert committee reports, the large interindividual variability was stressed as the reason for not defining an EAR value.

This variability arises in part from a true variability between individuals and between days within the same individual, but is also in part a consequence of the methods used to estimate intake. Intake can be estimated from dietary records, but these are often incomplete and therefore unreliable (Goris et al. 2000). A specific water balance questionnaire that was designed to evaluate water intake from fluid and solid foods and drinking water, and water loss from urine, feces, and sweat was reported to be both valid and reliable (Malisova et al. 2012). A median water balance of 27 mL/day was observed in a sample of 175 participants, and seems to support this. However, the variance was large, with 25% of the sample being in a negative balance of more than 1556 mL/day and 25% of the sample being in a positive water balance of more than 1200 mL/day. Cumulative daily water imbalances of such magnitude are clearly not sustainable, so the validity of the data is questionable.

4.3.2 WATER LOSSES

Water is lost from the lungs, through the skin, via the sweat glands, and in urine and feces (Table 4.3). Minerals and other solutes are lost in sweat, urine, and feces at varying concentrations. Water loss from the body is a continuous process, though the rate is constantly changing, but intake is episodic, so the body water content fluctuates over the course of the day. Water loss from the lungs and through the skin is determined largely by the temperature and humidity of the environment, while sweat loss is dictated by the need to adjust the rate of evaporative heat loss in order to maintain body temperature. Sweat rates may exceed 3 L/h in some individuals. There is a certain obligatory minimum urine output—about 500 mL per day—that is necessary to eliminate excess solute, mostly in the form of the end products of protein metabolism or dietary cations (sodium and potassium), from the body. This will be influenced by various factors, including especially body size and the composition of the diet. Fecal water loss is generally small—about 200 mL/day—but can reach 1 L/h in severe infectious diarrhea. Because water losses from the body depend largely on factors that are not under voluntary control, maintenance of water balance is achieved primarily by adjustment of intake. Change in body mass is often used as a proxy for water loss, with the assumption that 1 kg of mass loss represents 1 L of water loss. There are, however, a number of errors associated with this assumption, including loss of solid fecal matter for example, that may invalidate this assumption (Maughan et al. 2007). It is important to recognize too that water lost in urine and sweat is associated with electrolyte loss, while transcutaneous and respiratory water losses are not.

4.3.3 WATER TURNOVER

As highlighted above, there are formidable obstacles that tend to confound the results of measurements of the various components of water intake and water loss. Intake is usually estimated from

TABLE 4.3

Indicative Values (in mL/day) for the Main Components of 24-Hour Water Balance for a Typical 70 kg Sedentary Individual Living in a Temperate Environment and for the Same Individual Who Performs Hard Exercise in a Warm Environment

	Sedentary, Temperate	Active, Warm
	Intake	
Fluids	1250	4600
Food	800	1200
Metabolism	300	800
Total	2350	5600
	Loss	
Urine	1250	500
Feces	100	100
Respiratory	350	700
Transcutaneous	650	800
Sweat	0	3500
Total	2350	5600

weighed or measured food and fluid intake diaries, but the data are complicated by uncertainties in the water content of foodstuffs, and are subject to the usual reliability issues. Measurement of the various avenues of water loss is beset by similar problems.

These challenges can be avoided by the use of isotopic tracer methodologies that permit the noninvasive measurement of water turnover without any requirement for compliance by the subject. Deuterium is a nonradioactive isotope of hydrogen, and deuterium oxide can be used as a tracer for body water: [18]oxygen is a stable isotope of oxygen that accounts for about 0.2% of the oxygen in the atmosphere and can likewise be used as a tracer for water, but the isotope is lost from the body in carbon dioxide as well as in water, so it cannot be used for estimates of water turnover. The principle of the measurement and the practicalities are both relatively straightforward. Body water is labeled with the isotopic tracer and the water turnover is measured over a period of a few days from the rate of decrease in the tracer concentration in an accessible body water compartment. The measurement can be made conveniently on blood or urine samples, though saliva and the condensate from expired air can also be used. Collection of 24-hour urine output allows nonrenal losses (consisting mainly of sweat and transcutaneous losses, respiratory water loss, and fecal loss) to be calculated by difference.

The doubly labeled water method for assessment of energy expenditure (Roberts et al. 1995) allows calculation of whole body water turnover, but these data are seldom calculated or presented. Singh et al. (1989) published information on daily water turnover of Gambian women during periods of hard agricultural laboring work. These measurements were made as part of a study of energy balance in these women. A mean (SD) daily water turnover of 5.2 (1.4) L/day was observed for these women, who had a daily total energy expenditure of about 10.4 MJ/day: the water turnover ranged from 3.2 to 9.0 L/day. This value was compared with a mean value of 3.2 (0.8) L/day in sedentary women in Cambridge, England. The ambient temperature during the measurement period in the Gambia was 23–28°C, and in Cambridge it was 11–19°C. The water turnover values for the Gambian women are high, reflecting the strenuous labor carried out and the tropical climate.

Application of this method to two groups of subjects, one sedentary and one physically active, showed a higher rate of water turnover in the exercising group (Leiper et al. 1996). The active group were men with sedentary occupations who ran or jogged a mean distance of 103 (range 68–148) km during the week of the study: subjects in the sedentary group had a similar age, height, and weight, and were engaged in similar occupations, but undertook no physically demanding activities in their leisure time. Both groups had a similar total body water content. The median daily water turnover (averaged over 7 days) in the active group was 4673 (range: 4320–9609) mL/day, which was higher (P < 0.001) than that of the sedentary subjects (3256 [range: 2055–4185] mL/day). The average daily urine loss was greater (P < 0.001) in the exercising group (3021 [range: 2484–4225] mL) than in the sedentary group (1883 [range: 925–2226] mL). It might have been expected that the runners would have a greater daily sweat loss than the sedentary group, and that this would be reflected in a greater total nonrenal loss. There was, however, no significant difference between the groups in nonrenal water losses (runners: 1746 [range: 1241–5195]; sedentary: 1223 [range: 1021–1950] mL), although some tendency for there to be a difference (P < 0.08) was observed. These results seem surprising, but may reflect the relatively low total exercise load of the runners and the temperate climate (mean maximum daytime temperature of 14 (range: 7–21)°C at the time of the study. The results also suggest that the runners were habituated to drinking a volume of fluid in excess of that required to match the sweat loss incurred during exercise. The Cambridge women in the study of Singh et al. (1989) had a higher water turnover than the sedentary Aberdeen men, in spite of their smaller total body water content, and this presumably reflects the warmer weather conditions.

The same methodology has been applied to another physically active group, in this case cyclists covering an average daily distance of 50 km in training for competition, and another matched sedentary group (Leiper et al. 1995). Again, the median water turnover rate was higher (P < 0.001) in the active group (3.38 [range: 2.88–4.89] L/day) than in the sedentary individuals (2.22 [range: 2.06–3.40] L/day). In this study, however, there was no difference between the groups in the daily urine output (cyclists: 1.96 [range: 1.78–2.36] L; controls: 1.90 [range: 1.78–1.96] L), but the nonrenal losses were greater (P < 0.001) in the cyclists (1.46 [range: 1.06–3.04] L/day) than in the sedentary group (0.53 [range: 0.15–1.72] L/day). It was again rather cool during the measurement period, with maximum daily temperatures of 10 (4–18)°C, which might account for the rather low sweat rates in spite of the high physical activity level of the cyclists.

These two studies emphasize the variability in the normal pattern of fluid intake and loss in both sedentary and active individuals. In all cases, body mass remained rather constant throughout the measurement period, which suggests rather strongly that they were in energy balance and were maintaining normal hydration status. The variation between individuals was large: one subject (one of the more active members of the running group) had a daily urine output of 5786 mL, with a range of values from 2817–6290 mL: this is markedly different from the values obtained from most of the subjects, but this subject also had the greatest water turnover values, at an average of 9606 (SD 4328) mL/day (Leiper et al. 1996). This emphasizes the degree to which voluntary drive can override the physiological demand: this subject clearly ingested volumes of fluid greatly in excess of those necessary for maintenance of renal function.

In a study of groups of institutionalized and community-living elderly (69–93 years old) individuals, daily water turnover was higher in the community living group (2.1 [1.0–3.6] L/day; mean [SD]) than in the dependent group (1.5 [0.9–2.7] L/day), although there was no difference between the groups in total body water content (Leiper et al. 2005). The difference was entirely accounted for by a difference in urine output between the two groups, with no difference in nonrenal losses. The average daily water turnover values were lower than for the younger subjects, reflecting low urine outputs and also low nonrenal losses, a pattern that is not unexpected in these elderly individuals. This may reflect a decreased water requirement, a reduced sensitivity of the thirst mechanism, a decreased availability of fluids, or an impaired ability to respond to the dictates of thirst. There was also evidence in the subjects living in care that water turnover decreased as the degree of physical ability, as assessed by the Barthel scale, decreased, except in the group with the lowest level of independence. This is interpreted as reflecting the greater level of support offered to these individuals by the nursing staff.

An unpublished study of water turnover in a group of sedentary individuals living in Manila, in the Philippines, assessed whole body water balance before, during, and after the period of Ramadan, during which food and fluid are avoided during daylight hours. As might perhaps be expected, the whole body water turnover was lower during Ramadan (median 1.93 L/day, range: 0.58–5.08 L/day) than it was either before (2.24, 1.06–4.15) or afterward (2.19, 1.18–3.91 L/day): this difference was accounted for by a decrease in nonrenal losses, with urine output remaining rather constant throughout the measurement periods. Surprisingly, though, considering the prevailing weather, the water turnover was rather low. This seems to reflect the low level of physical activity of these subjects and the fact that they spent most of the day in an air-conditioned environment, with little exposure to outdoor conditions. It cannot be assumed, therefore that all individuals living in tropical regions are subjected to high heat stress: those who are not, and who are not physically active, may have low water requirements. During Ramadan, when access to food and water was restricted, subjects appeared to respond by further reducing their level of physical activity and/or exposure to the outdoor environment.

4.4 ASSESSMENT OF HUMAN HYDRATION STATUS

Assessment of hydration status—as opposed to body water content—is a topic of much controversy, and there have been many attempts over the years to assess hydration status in various different populations. Grant and Kubo (1975) classified the tests used in the clinical environment into three categories: laboratory tests, objective noninvasive measurements, and subjective observations. Laboratory tests included measures of serum parameters (osmolality and sodium concentration), blood urea nitrogen, hematocrit, and urine osmolality. Objective, noninvasive measurements included body mass, intake and output measurements, stool number and consistency, and vital signs, including temperature, heart rate, and respiratory rate. Subjective observations were skin turgor, thirst, and mucous membrane moisture. These authors concluded that, although the subjective measurements were least reliable in terms of consistency between measurers, they were the simplest, fastest, and most economical. Laboratory tests were deemed to be the most accurate means to assess a patient's hydration status.

Since this manuscript was published, a large body of research data has accumulated to further refine these observations. For laboratory investigations, a narrower range of indices of hydration status has been proposed, including body weight change, serum or plasma osmolality, and urine parameters (volume, frequency, color, specific gravity, and osmolality) and these markers and their limitations have been extensively reviewed (e.g., Kavouras 2002; Cheuvront et al. 2010; Cheuvront and Kenefick 2014). All methods, however, are subject to errors as a result of recent drinking behavior and other variables. Acute ingestion of a bolus of water can reduce plasma osmolality and result in relatively dilute urine even in a hypohydrated individual, while ingestion of solid food or strongly hypertonic drinks will result in temporary efflux of water into the gut, with a corresponding reduction in plasma volume and probably also in the volume of other body water compartments (Evans et al. 2009).

Currently, no "gold standard" hydration status marker exists, particularly for the transient and relatively modest levels of hypohydration or hyperhydration that frequently occur during the activities of daily living. The absence of such a criterion method makes it difficult to establish the accuracy of the various methods employed. The choice of marker for any particular situation will be influenced by the sensitivity and accuracy with which hydration status needs to be established and the level of subject compliance that can be ensured, together with the technical and time requirements and expense involved, but it does seem clear that the individual variability that exists precludes the use of any single biomarker to classify hydration status in all settings.

Cheuvront et al. (2004) reported a daily variability in body mass of less than 1% in soldiers exercising daily in a hot environment and concluded that "daily BM is a sufficiently stable physiological parameter for potential daily fluid balance monitoring". This, however, might be an optimistic interpretation as subjects in that study were military personnel living in a controlled environment and were required to ensure full replacement of fluid losses after each day's exercise. Lew et al. (2010) stated that Dore et al. (1975) and Grandjean et al. (2000) reported a daily variation on body mass within the range of ±1%, but some care needs to be taken with the interpretation of these results. While Grandjean et al. (2000) found a mean day-to-day variability of 0.30%, the range was from −1.52% to +0.90%. Similarly, Dore et al. (1975) found a mean daily weight change of 74 g in six subjects measured over three 6-day periods: the range was −800 g to +800 g in subjects with a body mass of 53–68 kg. While this level of variability may be acceptable in some situations, it would not detect a loss of body water sufficient to compromise both physical and mental performance.

4.4.1 BLOOD INDICES

The major components of blood are red cells (which contain intracellular fluid) and plasma (which is part of the extracellular fluid). Changes in blood volume and composition therefore reflect changes in hydration status. Given the ease with which blood can be sampled, it is not surprising that a range of blood markers of hydration status have been proposed.

Measurements of hemoglobin concentration and hematocrit have the potential to be used as markers of hydration status or change in hydration status provided a reliable baseline can be established. In this regard, standardization of posture for a time prior to blood collection is necessary to distinguish between postural changes in blood volume, and therefore in hemoglobin concentration and hematocrit, which occur (Harrison 1985) and changes due to water loss or gain. The volume of the red blood cells will also change if the plasma osmolality changes, tending to resist changes in plasma volume: this effect makes the use of automated cell counters, which rely on the dilution of blood in a medium of fixed tonicity, unreliable if the plasma osmolality differs markedly from that of the diluting medium (Watson and Maughan 2014).

The plasma concentration of most solutes will increase if there is a loss of volume from the vascular space. This has led to the use for assessment of hydration status on various markers that are routinely used in clinical practice, including urea, creatinine, albumin, and sodium (Vivanti et al. 2008). Plasma sodium concentration and osmolality will increase when the fluid loss inducing dehydration is hypotonic with respect to plasma. An increase in these values would be expected, therefore, in the majority of cases of hypohydration, including water loss by sweat secretion, urine production, or diarrhea. However, in subjects studied by Francesconi et al. (1987) who lost more than 3% of their body mass mainly through sweating, no change in hematocrit or serum osmolality was found, although some urine parameters did show changes. Similar findings to this were reported by Armstrong et al. (1994, 1998). This perhaps suggests that plasma volume is defended in an attempt to maintain cardiovascular stability, and so plasma variables may not be affected by hypohydration until substantial body water loss has occurred.

Cheuvront et al. (2010) explored the individual and population variability in the response of a variety of potential markers under standardized conditions and in response to dehydration. They reported that plasma osmolality, but not saliva osmolality, urine osmolality, or urine specific gravity, was a useful marker for the assessment of static dehydration. The range of morning, overnight-fasted plasma osmolality values on 18 subjects, each measured on three consecutive days was 284–298 mosmol/kg, revealing a large range even when an attempt was made to ensure euhydration by restricting physical activity on the previous day and by requiring subjects to drink 3 L of fluid in addition to their ad libitum intake from beverages and foods. They also induced dehydration of 2%–7% of body mass in their subjects by exercise on the previous day with limited fluid intake afterward. This revealed four separate values for plasma osmolality of between 290 and 295 mosmol/kg (i.e., within the euhydrated range) in individuals who were dehydrated by more than 2% of body mass, suggesting that plasma osmolality cannot always be relied upon to identify hypohydration.

Various circulation hormones have been proposed as markers of hydration status. Plasma testosterone, adrenaline, and cortisol concentrations were reported by Hoffman et al. (1994) not to be influenced by hypohydration to the extent of a body mass loss of up to 5.1% induced by exercise in the heat. Plasma noradrenaline concentration did respond to the hydration changes, but effects of stress and exercise on circulating noradrenaline concentrations preclude its use as a marker of hydration status, at least when changes are induced by exercise and/or heat stress. Secretion of arginine vasopressin (AVP) is sensitive to both blood volume and osmolality, but the response seems to be more sensitive to osmolality as AVP levels are suppressed by even small reductions in osmolality even in the presence of hypovolemia (Stricker and Verbalis 1986).

4.4.2 Urine Indices

Given a constant requirement for solute excretion, the kidneys respond to changes in hydration status by increasing or decreasing the volume of urine formed in an attempt to maintain the volume and osmolality of the vascular space. Collection of a urine sample for subsequent analysis has therefore been investigated and used as a hydration status marker. Possible urinary indices include osmolality, specific gravity, conductivity, color, volume, and frequency.

Measurement of urine osmolality has been extensively studied as a possible hydration status marker. Normal ranges will vary depending on the population of interest and on the sampling and analytical procedures (Bazari 2007), and the osmolality of random samples will vary greatly (from about 50 to 1400 mosmol/kg) depending on the recent history of fluid intake. The maximum values seen will decline with age due to loss of renal concentrating capacity (Kenney and Chiu 2001). For healthy adults, 24-hour urine osmolality should average between about 500 and 800 mosmol/kg, and the kidneys should concentrate the urine to an osmolality of more than 850 mosmol/kg after 12–14 hours of fluid restriction (Armstrong et al. 2013).

There has been some debate as to whether it is appropriate to collect the first sample of urine passed in the morning or whether this should be discarded and the second pass used, or indeed whether single readings have any value at all (Cheuvront et al. 2015). In a group of healthy young males, Shirreffs and Maughan (1998) observed first pass urine osmolality values of about 500–800 mosmol/kg in a group of healthy young males: when the same individuals performed exercise the evening before and did not fully replace sweat losses so that they were dehydrated by 1.9% of their body mass as determined by body mass changes, the corresponding values were about 850–1000 mosmol/kg, with most values in excess of 900 mosmol/kg.

In the study of Cheuvront et al. (2010) referred to above, urine osmolality was not deemed to be a sensitive or reliable marker of either static or dynamic hydration status. Some of the urine osmolality values in this study seem surprising, however: in subjects who were supposedly euhydrated and living under standardized conditions, the morning urine osmolality values ranged from 205 to 1091 mosmol/kg. Both the lower and higher values seem to lie outside of the range of values normally observed for morning samples (Shirreffs and Maughan 1998). This may be explained in part by uncertainties in the timing of these collections. According to the authors, subjects ingested 2 L of sports drink between 18.00 and 22.00 on the evening before and fasted from 22.00 to 06.00: they were then allowed 30 min for "personal hygiene" before reporting to the laboratory where a urine sample was provided. It is thus unclear if the sample provided at the laboratory was indeed the first of the day and it is also unclear whether food or fluid was allowed during the 30 min personal hygiene period if the fasting period did indeed end at 06.00.

Armstrong et al. (1994) have suggested that measures of urine osmolality can be used interchangeably with urine specific gravity. This was confirmed in a further study that compared these measures in both first pass samples and 24 h collections (Armstrong et al. 2010). Urine conductivity also gives results that follow closely the measured osmolality changes across a wide range of values (Shirreffs and Maughan 1998). It is important to recognize, however, that the apparently close statistical associations among these various markers also include a relatively wide scatter when individual samples are compared. Urine color is determined primarily by the amount of urochrome present (Diem 1962). When large volumes of urine are excreted, the urine is dilute and the solutes are excreted in a large volume. This generally gives the urine a very pale color. When small volumes of urine are excreted, the urine is concentrated and the solutes are excreted in a small volume. This generally gives the urine a dark color. Armstrong et al. (1998) investigated the relationship between urine color and specific gravity and conductivity. Using a scale of eight colors (Armstrong 2000), it was concluded that a linear relationship existed between urine color and both specific gravity and osmolality of the urine and that urine color could therefore be used in athletic or industrial settings to estimate hydration status when high precision may not be needed or where self-assessment may be required.

Urine indices of hydration status may be of limited value in identifying changes in hydration status during periods of rapid body water turnover. For example, Popowski et al. (2001) studied subjects who lost approximately 5% of their body mass during approximately 1 h of exercise in the heat and then rehydrated by replacing this lost fluid. In comparison to measures of plasma osmolality which increased and decreased in an almost linear fashion, urine osmolality and specific gravity were found to be less sensitive and demonstrated a delayed response, lagging behind the plasma osmolality changes.

4.4.3 Saliva Indices

Collection of saliva samples is noninvasive, making this an attractive option for a range of diagnostic purposes. Saliva flow rate, osmolality, and composition have all been identified as potential markers of hydration status. Of these, salivary osmolality has attracted the most attention (Walsh et al. 2004a,b; Oliver et al. 2008). Although some authors have concluded that saliva osmolality changes track urine (Walsh et al. 2004a) and plasma (Oliver et al. 2008) markers during periods of dehydration and rehydration, there are some practical difficulties in ensuring reliable collection of representative samples. Ely et al. (2011) confirmed that saliva osmolality was elevated by acute dehydration (4% loss of body mass) induced by exercise in the heat, but observed a large variability in the response: they also reported substantial decreases in saliva osmolality after a brief mouth rinse with water. These observations led them to cast doubt on the usefulness of this measure as a marker of hydration status.

While attempts to identify single markers that unequivocally establish hydration status seem doomed to failure, assessment of a change in hydration status of an individual can be made with greater certainty. Over a short timescale (of a few hours), changes in body mass reliably track changes in body water content, though variations in the electrolyte content of fluid losses will influence the plasma and urine composition (Maughan et al. 2007). Over a longer timescale of a few days, monitoring of morning urine concentration (whether by osmolality, specific gravity, or color), body mass, and subjective rating of thirst may give the best measure of hydration status. The method of choice will depend on many factors, including the precision required, the burden on the subject, equipment and resource availability, and cost.

4.5 HYDRATION, HEALTH, AND PERFORMANCE

It seems self-evident that hypohydration, if sufficiently severe, will result in impairment of all physiological and cognitive functions. Withdrawal of food and water intake typically results in death within a few (about 3–5) days, though this may be longer or shorter, depending on the environment and activity levels; paradoxically, intake of solid food, with its associated solute load, will generally shorten survival time by increasing the need for renal water loss, in spite of the associated water content and the water of oxidation that can be generated.

There is a strong body of experimental evidence to support the idea that a substantial reduction in body water content (of more than about 5% of body mass) will reduce performance in a range of exercise tasks involving strength, power, endurance, or skilled movement (Sawka et al. 2007). Equally, small fluctuations in body water content normally occur throughout the day with no perceptible effect on physical or mental performance. There is, however, considerable debate as to the effects of intermediate levels of body water loss, such as those that are likely to be incurred in daily living for some individuals, on exercise performance (Judelson et al 2007a,b; Goulet 2011). This debate arises in part because of

Confounding factors introduced by the various methods used to induce hypohydration. Methods used include fluid restriction, heat exposure, exercise and diuretic administration. Because of the variable composition of sweat, large sweat losses will have varying effects on the redistribution of water between the intracellular and extracellular spaces. Hypothermia, substrate depletion and electrolyte loss will all further complicate interpretation of results (Maughan and Shirreffs 2015).

Differences in the sensitivity of the measures of function or performance used and in the training and acclimation status of the participants (Maughan and Shirreffs 2015).

Different environmental conditions may affect the outcome. The effects of mild hypohydration are likely to be more apparent in the heat than in cool environments and at altitude rather than at sea level (Sawka et al. 2007).

Individual variability in the sensitivity to the effects of hypohydration and familiarity of the individual with both hypohydration and the test of function used (Fleming and James 2014).

Confounding effects introduced by preventing drinking when subjects wish to do so, requiring subjects to drink when they do not wish to do so, providing drinks that subjects like or do not like, providing familiar or unfamiliar drinks, and controlling effects other than those of hydration itself (carbohydrate content, temperature, etc.) (Maughan 2012). Because of these different factors, as well as the clear inter-individual variability in susceptibility to the effects of dehydration, it seems futile to attempt to define a precise point at which a water deficit will impair performance.

These considerations apply equally to physical and cognitive performance, and the evidence relating to hydration status and cognitive function is equally confusing. In a review of the evidence,

Benton and Young (2015) concluded that dehydration by more than 2% of body mass has been consistently shown to adversely affect mood, increase sensations of fatigue, and reduce levels of alertness. More recently, Muñoz et al. (2015) reported that, after accounting for other mood influencers, there was a positive association between total daily water intake and mood in a sample of 120 healthy young women.

There is also evidence that chronic mild hypohydration may be associated with a number of adverse health outcomes, but again there are inconsistencies and conflicts in the available evidence (El-Sharkawy et al. 2015a). Acute hypohydration may also be a precipitating factor in hospital admissions, especially in the elderly, and may have adverse implications for outcomes in terms of morbidity and mortality (El-Sharkawy et al. 2015b).

The resolution of these conflicts with regard to the effects of hydration on health and performance is important because of the implications for the advice that is appropriate. Though the thirst mechanism should ensure adequate hydration, assuming the availability of water or other drinks, it is apparent that this is not always sufficient (Stanhewicz and Kenney 2015). In mass participation marathon races, for example, the majority of finishers will be hypohydrated, but some will be hyperhydrated due to an intake of fluid greater than that lost in sweat. In a few cases, the hyperhydration is sufficient to result in hyponatremia: though benign in mild forms, this condition can be fatal (Hew-Butler et al. 2015).

REFERENCES

Armstrong, L. E. 2000. *Performing in Extreme Environments*. Champaign, IL: Human Kinetics.

Armstrong, L. E., C. M. Maresh, J. W. Castellani et al. 1994. Urinary indices of hydration status. *Int J Sport Nutr* 4:265–79.

Armstrong, L. E., J. A. Soto, F. T. HackerJr, D. J. Casa, S. A. Kavouras, and C. M. Maresh. 1998. Urinary indices during dehydration, exercise, and rehydration. *Int J Sport Nutr* 8:345–55.

Armstrong, L. E., A. C. Pumerantz, K. A. Fiala et al. 2010. Human hydration indices: Acute and longitudinal reference values. *Int J Sport Nutr Exerc Metab* 20:145–53.

Armstrong, L. E., E. C. Johnson, A. L. McKenzie, and C. X. Munoz. 2013. Interpreting common hydration biomarkers on the basis of solute and water excretion. *Eur J Clin Nutr* 67:249–53.

Asselin, M.-C., S. Kriemler, D. R. Chettle et al. 1998. Hydration status assessed by multi-frequency bioimpedance analysis. *Appl Radiat Isotop* 49:495–7.

Benton, D. and H. A. Young. 2015. Do small differences in hydration status affect mood and mental performance? *Nutr Rev* 70(Suppl. 2):S128–31.

Berneis, K. and U. Keller. 2000. Bioelectrical impedance analysis during acute changes of extracellular osmolality in man. *Clin Nutr* 19:361–6.

Bazari, H. 2007. Approach to the patient with renal disease. In *Cecil Medicine* (23rd Ed.), eds. L. Goldman and D. Ausiello, Philadelphia, PA: Saunders Elsevier. Chapter 115.

Bender, D. A. and A. E. Bender. 1997. *Nutrition a Reference Handbook*. Oxford, Oxford University Press.

Cheuvront, S. and R. Kenefick. 2014. Dehydration: Physiology, assessment, and performance effects. *Comp Physiol* 4:257–85.

Cheuvront, S. N., R. Carter, S. J. Montain, and M. Sawka. 2004. Daily body mass variability and stability in active men undergoing exercise-heat stress. *Int J Sport Nutr Exerc Metab* 14:532–40.

Cheuvront, S. N., B. R. Ely, R. W. Kenefick, and M. N. Sawka. 2010. Biological variation and diagnostic accuracy of dehydration assessment markers. *Am J Clin Nutr* 92:565–73.

Cheuvront, S. N., R. W. Kenefick, and E. J. Zambraski. 2015. Spot urine concentrations should not be used for hydration assessment: A methodology review. *Int J Sport Nutr Exerc Metab* 25:293–7.

Chumlea, W. C. and S. S. Sun. 2005. Bioelectrical impedance analysis. In *Human Body Composition* (2nd Ed.), eds. Heymsfield, S. B., T. G. Lohman, Z. M. Wang et al., 79–87. Champaign, IL: Human Kinetics.

Diem, K. 1962. *Documenta Geigy Scientific Tables*. Manchester: Geigy Pharmaceutical Company Limited, 538–9.

Dore, C., J. S. Weiner, E. F. Wheeler, and H. El-Neil. 1975. Water balance and body weight: Studies in a tropical climate. *Ann Hum Biol* 2:25–33.

Edelman, I. S. 1952. Exchange of water between blood and tissues. *Am J Physiol* 17:279–96.

El-Sharkawy, A. M., O. Sahota, and D. N. Lobo. 2015a. Acute and chronic effects of hydration status on health. *Nutr Rev* 73(S2):97–109.

El-Sharkawy, A. M., P. Watson, K. R. Neal et al. 2015b. Hydration and outcome in older patients admitted to hospital (The HOOP prospective cohort study). *Age Ageing* 44:943–7.

Ely, B. R., S. N. Cheuvront, R. W. Kenefick, and M. N. Sawka. 2011. Limitations of salivary osmolality as a marker of hydration status. *Med Sci Sports Exerc* 43:1080–4.

EFSA Panel on Dietetic Products, Nutrition, and Allergies (NDA). 2010. Scientific Opinion on Dietary reference values for water. *EFSA Journal* 8(3):1459 (48 pp). Doi:10.2903/j.efsa.2010.1459.

Evans, G. H., S. M. Shirreffs, and R. J. Maughan. 2009. Acute effects of ingesting glucose solutions on blood and plasma volume. *Br J Nutr* 101:1503–8.

Fleming, J. and L. J. James. 2014. Repeated familiarisation with hypohydration attenuates the performance decrement caused by hypohydration during treadmill running. *Appl Physiol Nutr Metab* 39:124–9.

Flear, C. T. G., C. V. Gill, and J. Burn. 1981. Beer drinking and hyponatraemia. *Lancet* 2:477.

Food and Nutrition Board. 2005. *Dietary Reference Intakes for Water, Potassium, Sodium, Chloride, and Sulfate*. Washington DC: The National Academies Press, 73–185.

Francesconi, R. P., R. W. Hubbard, P. C. Szlyk et al. 1987. Urinary and hematological indexes of hydration. *J Appl Physiol* 62:1271–6.

Gatterer, H., K. Schenk, L. Laninschegg et al. 2014. Bioimpedance identifies body fluid loss after exercise in the heat: A pilot study with body cooling. *PLoS ONE* 9(10):e109729. doi:10.1371/journal.pone.0109729.

Goris, A. H. C., M. S. Westerterp-Plantenga, and K. R. Westerterp. 2000. Undereating and under recording of habitual food intake in obese men: Selective underreporting of fat intake. *Am J Clin Nutr* 71:130–4.

Goulet, E. D. B. 2011. Effect of exercise-induced dehydration on time-trial exercise performance: A meta-analysis. *Br J Sports Med* 45:1149–56.

Grandjean, A. C., K. J. Reimers, K. E. Bannick, and M. C. Haven. 2000. The effect of caffeinated, non-caffeinated, caloric and non-caloric beverages on hydration. *J Am Coll Nutr* 19:591–600.

Grant, M. M. and W. M. Kubo. 1975. Assessing a patient's hydration status. *Am J Nurs* 75:1307–11.

Halliday, D. and A. G. Miller. 1977. Precise measurement of total body water using trace quantities of deuterium oxide. *Biomed Mass Spectrom* 4:82–7.

Harrison, M. H. 1985. Effects of thermal stress and exercise on blood volume in humans. *Physiol Rev* 65:149–209.

Hew-Butler, T., M. H. Rosner, S. Fowkes-Godek et al. 2015. Statement of the 3rd International exercise-associated hyponatremia consensus development conference, Carlsbad, California, 2015. *Clin J Sports Med* 25:303–20.

Heyward, V. H. and D. R. Wagner. 2004. *Applied Body Composition Assessment* (2nd Ed.), Champaign, IL: Human Kinetics.

Hoffman, J. R., C. M. Maresh, L. E. Armstrong et al. 1994. Effects of hydration state on plasma testosterone, cortisol, and catecholamine concentrations before and during mild exercise at elevated temperature. *Eur J Appl Physiol* 69:294–300.

Judelson, D. A., C. M. Maresh, J. M. Anderson et al. 2007a. Hydration and muscular performance—Does fluid balance affect strength, power and high-intensity endurance? *Sports Med* 37:907–21.

Judelson, D. A., C. M. Maresh, M. J. Farrell et al. 2007b. Effect of hydration state on strength, power, and resistance exercise performance. *Med Sci Sports Exerc* 39:1817–24.

Kavouras, S. A. 2002. Assessing hydration status. *Curr Opin Clin Nutr Metab Care* 5:519–24.

Kenney, W. L. and P. Chiu. 2001. Influence of age on thirst and fluid intake. *Med Sci Sports Exerc* 33:1524–32.

Leiper, J. B., A. Carnie, and R. J. Maughan. 1996. Water turnover rates in sedentary and exercising middle-aged men. *Br J Sports Med* 30:24–6.

Leiper, J. B., A. E. Fallick, and R. J. Maughan. 1988. Comparison of water absorption from an ingested glucose electrolyte solution (GES) and potable water using a tracer technique in healthy volunteers. *Clin Sci* 74(Suppl 18):68P.

Leiper, J. B., Y. P. Pitsiladis, and R. J. Maughan. 1995. Comparison of water turnover rates in en undertaking prolonged exercise and in sedentary men. *J Physiol* 483:123P.

Leiper, J. B., C. S. Primrose, W. R. Primrose, J. Phillimore, and R. J. Maughan. 2005. A comparison of water turnover in older people in community and institutional settings. *J Nutr Health Aging* 9:189–93.

Lentner, C. 1984. *Geigy Scientific Tables* (8th Ed.), Basle: Ciba-Geigy Limited.

Lew, C. H., G. Slater, G. Nair, and M. Miller. 2010. Relationship between changes in upon-waking urinary indices of hydration status and body mass in adolescent Singaporean athletes. *Int J Sport Nutr Exerc Metab* 20:330–5.

Lohman, T. G. 1992. *Advances in Human Body Composition*. Champaign, IL: Human Kinetics Publishers.

Malisova, O., V. Bountziouka, D. B. Panagiotakos, A. Zampelas, and M. Kapsokefalou. 2012. The water balance questionnaire: Design, reliability and validity of a questionnaire to evaluate water balance in the general population. *Int J Food Sci Nutr* 63:138–44.

Maughan, R. J. 1991. Fluid and electrolyte loss and replacement in exercise. *J Sports Sci* 9(Suppl 1):117–42.

Maughan, R. J. 2012. Investigating the associations between hydration and exercise performance: Methodology and limitations. *Nutr Rev* 11(Suppl 2):S128–31.

Maughan, R. and M. Gleeson, 2010. *The Biochemical Basis of Sports Performance* (2nd Ed.), Oxford: Oxford University Press.

Maughan, R. J. and S. M. Shirreffs. 2015. Water replacement before, during and after exercise: How much is enough? In *Fluid Balance, Hydration and Athletic Performance*, eds. F. Meyer, Z. Szygula, and B. Wilk, Boca Raton, FL: CRC Press.

Maughan, R. J., S. M. Shirreffs, and J. B. Leiper. 2007. Errors in the estimation of sweat loss and changes in hydration status from changes in body mass during exercise. *J Sports Sci* 25:797–804.

McNeill, G., P. A. Fowler, R. J. Maughan et al. 1991. Body fat in lean and overweight women estimated by six methods. *Br J Nutr* 65:95–103.

Moon, J. R., J. R. Stout, A. E. Smith et al. 2010. Reproducibility and validity of bioimpedance spectroscopy for tracking changes in total body water: Implications for repeated measurements. *Br J Nutr* 104:1384–94.

Moore, F. D. and Boyden, C. M. 1963. Body cell mass and limits of hydration on the fat-free body: Their relation to estimated skeletal weight. *Ann N Y Acad Sci* 110:62–71.

Muñoz, C. X., E. C. Johnson, A. L. McKenzie et al. 2015. Habitual total water intake and dimensions of mood in healthy young women. *Appetite* 92:81–6.

National Institutes of Health. 1994. Bioelectrical impedance analysis in body composition measurement. *NIH Technol Assess Statement*, Dec 12–14:1–35.

Oliver, S. J., S. J. Laing, S. Wilson, J. L. Bilzon, and N. P. Walsh. 2008. Saliva indices track hypohydration during 48 h of fluid restriction or combined fluid and energy restriction. *Arch Oral Biol* 53:975–80.

Pace, N. and E. N. Rathbun. 1945. Studies on body composition, III. The body water and chemically combined nitrogen content in relation to fat content. *J Biol Chem* 158:685–91.

Peronnet, F., D. Mignault, P. du Souich et al. 2012. Pharmacokinetic analysis of absorption, distribution and disappearance of ingested water labeled with D_2O in humans. *Eur J Appl Physiol* 112:2213–22.

Pinson, E. A. 1952. Water exchange and barriers as studied by the use of hydrogen isotopes. *Physiol Rev* 32:123–34.

Popowski, L. A., R. A. Oppliger, G. P. Lambert, R. F. Johnson, A. K. Johnson, and C. V. Gisolfi. 2001. Blood and urinary measures of hydration status during progressive acute dehydration. *Med Sci Sports Exerc* 33:747–53.

Roberts, S. B., W. Dietz, T. Sharp, G. E. Dallal, and J. O. Hill. 1995. Multiple laboratory comparison of the doubly labeled water technique. *Obesity Res* 3:3–13.

Robinson, S. and A. H. Robinson. 1954. Chemical composition of sweat. *Physiol Rev* 34:202–20.

Sawka, M. N., L. M. Burke, E. R. Eichner, R. J. Maughan, S. J. Montain, and N. S. Stachenfeld. 2007. Exercise and fluid replacement. *Med Sci Sports Exerc* 39:377–90.

Schoeller, D. A. 2005. Hydrometry. In *Human Body Composition* (2nd Ed.), eds. S. B. Heymsfield, T. G. Lohman, Z. Wang, and S. B. Going, 35–50. Champaign, IL: Human Kinetics.

Schoeller, D. A., E. van Santen, D. W. Peterson, W. Dietz, J. Jaspan, and P. D. Klein. 1980. Total body water measurement in humans with 18O and 2H labeled water. *Am J Clin Nutr* 33:2686–93.

Sheng, H. P. and R. A. Huggins. 1979. Review of body-composition studies with emphasis on total-body water and fat. *Am J Clin Nutr* 32:630–47.

Shirreffs, S. M. and R. J. Maughan. 1994. The effect of posture change on blood volume, serum potassium and whole body electrical impedance. *Eur J Appl Physiol* 69:461–3.

Shirreffs, S. M. and R. J. Maughan. 1998. Urine osmolality and conductivity as markers of hydration status. *Med Sci Sports Exerc* 30:1598–602.

Singh, J., A. M. Prentice, E. Diaz et al. 1989. Energy expenditure of Gambian women during peak agricultural activity measured by the doubly-labeled water method. *Br J Nutr* 62:315–29.

Stanhewicz, A. E. and W. L. Kenney. 2015. Determinants of water and sodium intake and output. *Nutr Rev* 73:73–82.

Stricker, E. M. and J. G. Verbalis. 1986. Interaction of osmotic and volume stimuli in regulation of neurohypophyseal secretion in rats. *Am J Physiol Regul Integr Comp Physiol* 250:R267–75.

Vivanti, A., K. Hervey, S. Ash, and D. Battistutta. 2008. Clinical assessment of dehydration in older people admitted to hospital. What are the strongest indicators? *Arch Gerontol Geriatr* 47:340–55.

Walsh, N. P., J. C. Montague, N. Callow, and A. V. Rowlands. 2004a. Saliva flow rate, total protein concentration and osmolarity as potential markers of whole body hydration status during progressive acute dehydration in humans. *Arch Oral Biol* 49:149–54.

Walsh, N. P., S. J. Laing, S. J. Oliver, J. C. Montague, R. Walters, and J. L. Bilzon. 2004b. Saliva parameters as potential indices of hydration status during acute dehydration. *Med Sci Sports Exerc* 36:1535–42.

Watson, P. and R. J. Maughan. 2014. Artifacts in plasma volume changes due to hematology analyzer derived hematocrit. *Med Sci Sports Exerc* 46:52–9.

Wemple, R. D., T. S. Morocco, and G. W. Mack. 1997. Influence of sodium replacement on fluid ingestion following exercise-induced dehydration. *Int J Sport Nutr* 7:104–16.

Wong, W. W., W. J. Cochran, W. J. Klish, E. O. Smith, L. S. Lee, and P. D. Klein. 1988. *In vivo* isotope-fractionation factors and the measurement of deuterium- and oxygen-18-dilution 6. *Am J Clin Nutr* 47(1):1–6.

Section II

Physical Activity and Body Composition

5 Physical Activity, Growth, and Maturation of Youth

Robert M. Malina and Manuel J. Coelho e Silva

CONTENTS

5.1 INTRODUCTION

Questions related to the potential influence of physical activity on the processes underlying growth have a long history. Studies span a spectrum from tissue level effects to the level of primary outcome variables in growth monitoring—height and weight. Studies dating to the late nineteenth century have highlighted the potentially positive and negative influences of regular physical activity on growth (Steinhaus 1933; Rarick 1960; Malina 1969, 1979). Current discussions, in contrast, are largely focused on potential health- and fitness-related benefits of regular physical activity and not on growth per se, while discussions of sport are often focused on potentially negative consequences of intensive training on growth and sexual maturation more so in females than in males.

This chapter briefly reviews several studies dating to the late nineteenth and early twentieth century through the 1960s, and then addresses issues related to evaluating potential effects of physical activity on growth and maturation of youth. The influence of physical activity on indicators of growth (height, weight), biological maturation (status, timing, tempo), and body composition (fat-free mass, adiposity, bone mineral) is then considered in the general population of youth and then in youth athletes.

5.2   HISTORICAL BACKGROUND

Several studies suggested beneficial effects of physical activity on the growth of adolescent and late adolescent boys. Short-term activity programs with youth 13–17 years (Schwartz et al. 1928) and with naval cadets 15–22 years (Beyer 1896) reported greater height gains in trained (largely gymnasium work) compared to untrained males. Greater heights of male gymnasts 14–18 years (Godin 1920) and 16–22 years (Matthias 1916) were attributed to the growth-enhancing effects of regular training. Sampling variation and lack of control for chronological age (CA) and individual differences in maturity status within and between groups were potential confounders. For example, in the study of boys 13–17 years, volunteers for the training program were of the same CA but shorter, lighter, and less mature (pubic hair, after Crampton 1908) than volunteers for the control group (Schwartz et al. 1928). To "adjust" for the difference, 16 boys were deleted by CA and height from the control group; all deleted boys were postpubertal.

A study of late adolescent/young adult American Black women 17–21 years compared the anthropometric characteristics of plantation workers and nonworkers. Workers were taller and heavier, on average, and had larger limb girths. The differences were attributed to physical work beginning at a relatively young age: "Hard labor apparently has a definite effect during youth as a stimulator of physical growth" (Adams 1938, p. 108).

The preceding emphasized physical activity as a stimulus for growth in height, but some questioned whether activity can stimulate or retard growth of long bones or height (Steinhaus 1933). Others cautioned about "…persons who claim that they can make your height increase by special exercises…" but "…I do not think it is worthwhile to exercise just for height increase" (Crampton 1936, p. 73).

With the emergence of school sport in the United States early last century, medical and educational authorities expressed concern for the potential downward extension of high school sport into junior high and elementary schools. The concern was noted in the proceedings of the 1930 White House Conference on Child Health and Protection (1932, p. 170):

> The marked expansion in recent years of organized athletic competition in the secondary schools, and the possibility in the future that it may also involve the grammar schools, makes it important to consider most seriously the question of whether the growth and development of the competitors is promoted or hindered by such athletic competition.

The discussion of sport, however, focused exclusively on adolescent boys.

The first study to suggest the potentially negative effects of participation in interscholastic sports on growth appeared shortly in the White House Conference proceedings. Heights and weights of interschool touch football participants and nonparticipants ~13–16 years were extracted from school records and gains over 3 years were compared (Rowe 1933). Initial comparisons were confounded by CA; players were older than nonplayers at the end of the third year, 16.7 and 15.7 years, respectively. To eliminate CA bias, data for players in the first 2 years were compared with nonplayers in the second and third years. After "equating" for CA, average height gain over 2 years was greater in nonplayers (7.8 cm) than players (3.2 cm), while weight gains did not differ, players (8.1 kg) and nonplayers (8.5 kg). The differences in height were not specifically attributed to sport, but the possibility was suggested. However, potential sampling bias was noted in a comment of T. Wingate Todd:

> …boys of athletic temperament mature earlier than do boys of non-athletic temperament …therefore… the athletic boy is not going to grow as much as the non-athletic boy over the period studied (Rowe 1933, p. 115, Note A).

In a similar study about 20 years later, 6-monthly gains in heights of 7th- and 8th-grade interschool football and basketball participants and nonparticipants were compared (Fait 1951). Estimated mean height gains over 6 months were less among sport participants in prepubertal, pubertal, and postpubertal groups (after Crampton 1908). Overall, the estimated mean height gain over 6 months was 0.9 cm less in sport participants, leading to the conclusion that "...growth of the long bones of the body is influenced negatively by strenuous activity" (Fait 1951, p. 49). CAs and heights were not reported, and CA was not controlled in the comparisons. Of interest, the author later noted that the results were "...far from conclusive" (Fait 1956).

Though limited in scope and analyses, the preceding (Rowe 1933; Fait 1951) were often cited as evidence that sport participation may negatively influence growth in stature (Rarick 1960; Pařizkova 1974; Lopez and Pruett 1982; Shephard 1982).

Surveys of the maturity status of participants in the 1955 and 1957 Little League World Series (baseball) brought attention to maturity-related selectivity in youth sport. The majority of players in each competition were, respectively, advanced in pubertal (pubic hair, Hale 1956) and skeletal (Krogman 1959) maturation. This selectivity along a maturity gradient has since been verified in male participants in many sports (Malina 2011).

Concern for potential risk associated with participation in competitive sports prompted the Medford Boys' Growth Study that was initiated at the University of Oregon in 1955 "...to investigate problems pertaining to interschool competitive athletics among elementary school boys" (Clarke 1971, p. 3). Athletes in four sports and nonathletes were compared in upper elementary, junior high, and senior high school grades. Athletes in football, basketball, and track were, on average, taller and heavier, and advanced in skeletal age (SA), especially between 12 and 15 years. At the other levels, differences in size and maturity between players and nonplayers were negligible. Baseball was not offered as a junior high sport.

The preceding discussion is limited to adolescent boys. Opportunities for organized sport among children of both sexes and adolescent girls were largely nonexistent in the first half of the twentieth century. Perhaps the first systematic study of girls in sport considered the growth, maturation, and functional capacity of elite teenage swimmers, who were taller and heavier than the Swedish reference at 7 (before systematic training) and 14 years, and attained menarche somewhat earlier than the reference (Åstrand et al. 1963). Training volumes varied from 5,000 to 65,000 meters per week, and swimmers from the club with the highest training volume attained menarche earlier than those with lesser volumes. This observation escaped the attention of later research attributing later recalled ages at menarche in athletes to training before menarche (Märker 1979; Warren 1980; Frisch et al. 1981).

Subsequent studies of female artistic gymnasts attributed their short stature and later maturation to intensive training (Ziemilska 1981; Jost-Relyveld and Sempé 1982; Jahreis et al. 1991; Theintz et al. 1993; Lindholm et al. 1994; Tofler et al. 1996; Daly et al. 2005). Males were not under the same scrutiny, although marked "deterioration of growth potential" was suggested in male more so than female gymnasts (Georgopoulos et al. 2010). These generalizations have contributed to concerns for potentially negative effects of intensive sport training on growth and maturation.

5.3 PHYSICAL ACTIVITY

Physical activity is a multidimensional behavior that occurs in many settings—play, physical education, sport, dance, deliberate exercise, chores, among others. It is also an important avenue for learning, enjoyment, social interactions, and self-understanding among youth. Motor skill (proficiency in a variety of movements) and fitness (performance- and health-related) are important correlates of activity that change with growth and maturation.

Methods for quantifying level of activity include direct observation, video, diary, questionnaire, interview, mechanical counters, and accelerometry. Each has limitations and advantages. Accelerometry is the preferred method at present, and provides estimates of time sedentary and time in activities of light, moderate, and vigorous intensity; specific contexts of activity are not provided. Moreover, equations to convert counts per minute to intensity levels are still a matter for debate. Videos and motion analysis are increasingly used to document activities during practice and matches in several sports.

Sport is a major context of activity for youth, and specialization in a single sport at relatively young ages has increased (Malina 2009, 2010a). It is important, however, to distinguish between participation and systematic training; the two are not equivalent.

Studies addressing activity and growth commonly classify youth as active and less active or as sport participants and nonparticipants. Hours per week or weeks per year spent in specific physical activities or training are also used. Time, however, is a limited indicator of the intensity of activity. Many activities of children and adolescents are intermittent and include intervals of "down time" (reduced activity). Practice and training for sport also include intervals of variable activity, for example, warm-up, stretching, instruction, drills, waiting between repetitions, and recovery. The intermittent nature of training is evident in observations of elite male gymnasts, 10.5 ± 0.9 years (Daly et al. 1998, 1999). About 63% of total training time was devoted to rest or recovery; work–rest ratios varied with context: strength and conditioning, 1:1.44, development of routines, 1:1.78; and precompetition, 1:1.94. Mean heart rate was 128 bpm, ~60% to ~65% of maximal values; peak rates were transient and varied with event: 158–184 bpm on the high bar and 171–184 bpm on the parallel bars.

Activity intensities during practice vary with sport. Estimates based on accelerometry contrast soccer (S) and baseball/softball (BSB) in boys and girls 7–14 years. Percentages of time in sedentary (S 28% vs. BSB 30%) and moderate (25% vs. 30%) activities were similar, but differed for light (S 19% vs. BSB 29%) and vigorous (28% vs. 11%) activities (Leek et al. 2011).

Activity intensities during competitions also vary. Intermittent activities are characteristic of gymnastics, diving, racket sports, and field events in athletics, while bouts of continuous activity occur more often in swimming and running events. Team sports such as soccer and field hockey involve reasonably continuous activities of variable intensity. Regular substitution in basketball and ice hockey provide rest intervals throughout a match, while baseball and American football involve intermittent activities among regular intervals of relative inactivity.

An observational study of boys 11–14 years participating in several sports highlights variability in intensity (Katzmarzyk et al. 2001). Sprinting (vigorous activity at great speed) and jogging (for ice hockey, steady skating at moderate intensity) accounted for 67% of game time in outdoor compared to 36% in indoor soccer, 31% in basketball, and 18% in ice hockey. Sitting accounted for 26% and 18% of game time in hockey and basketball, respectively, compared to <1% in soccer. Standing and walking (for hockey, coasting with few strides) accounted for 63% of game time in indoor soccer, 56% in hockey, 51% in basketball, and 33% in outdoor soccer.

Reported time in specific activities is thus a limited indicator of intensity. Estimated energy expenditure (metabolic equivalents [METs]) for different activities, games, and sports, and by intensity of effort among youth has been summarized (Ridley and Olds 2008; Ridley et al. 2008).

5.4   STUDIES OF YOUTH ATHLETES

Youth athletes have historically been used to highlight potential risks and benefits of physical activity for growth and maturation. It is often assumed that athletes have been regularly active in "training" and differences relative to nonathletes are attributed to training. Observations in this context have major limitations. First, sport is selective; the selection tends to follow a maturity gradient in many sports. Second, sport is characterized by differential persistence and drop-out, either voluntary or forced as in cutting. Third, successful young athletes of both sexes, especially the elite, tend to be different from nonathletes and also from drop-outs in size, maturation, and composition. Fourth and as already noted, time (hours per week, weeks per year) has limited utility as an indicator of the intensity sport-specific training. Except for sports that record distances covered in training (swimming, distance running), studies of young athletes ordinarily do not indicate specific training activities. Generalizations based on youth athletes are thus limited in applicability. In addition, the environments in which youth train have not been systematically evaluated in studies of growth and maturation. The environments, including coaching styles, demands, demeanors, etc., comprise the "culture" of a sport or of a particular gymnasium or club. These cultures require critical evaluation as potential influences on growth and maturation. The psychosocial environments of some sports, for example, may tacitly or explicitly foster behaviors which function to limit weight gain when accretion of mass is expected with growth.

5.5 PHYSICAL ACTIVITY, HEIGHT, WEIGHT

5.5.1 ACTIVITY AND HEIGHT AND WEIGHT IN THE GENERAL POPULATION

Longitudinal data on boys followed from childhood through adolescence, and girls followed during childhood indicate, on average, either no differences, or only small differences in height and weight between active and less active youth (Mirwald and Bailey 1986; Saris et al. 1986; Beunen et al. 1992). By inference, regular physical activity has no apparent effect on attained size and rates of growth in height and weight. Composition of body mass may be influenced by regular activity; this is discussed later in this chapter.

5.5.2 TRAINING FOR SPORT AND HEIGHT AND WEIGHT OF YOUTH ATHLETES

In order to evaluate the potential influence of training for a specific sport on the growth of young athletes, it is important to consider their status relative to the general population. Data on the growth and maturity characteristics of youth athletes in a variety of sports are reasonably comprehensive (Malina 1994a, 1998, 2002, 2006a, 2011; Beunen and Malina 2008; Malina et al. 2013a,b, 2015). With few exceptions, athletes of both sexes have, on average, statures that equal or exceed reference medians. Artistic gymnasts of both sexes have a profile of short stature; figure skaters of both sexes also present shorter statures though data are not extensive. Female ballet dancers tend to have shorter statures during childhood and early adolescence, but catch up with nondancers in late adolescence. Trends are similar for body weight, though more variable. Gymnasts, figure skaters, and ballet dancers of both sexes have lighter weights. Gymnasts and figure skaters have appropriate weight-for-height, while ballet dancers have low weight-for-height. Female distance runners have heights that approximate the reference, but present, on average, low weight-for-height.

Does training for sport affect growth in height and weight? Longitudinal studies, both short- and long-term, of athletes in several sports (Daniels and Oldridge 1971; Kotulan et al. 1980; Malina 1994b; Baxter-Jones et al. 1995; Malina et al. 1997c; Fogelholm et al. 2000; Eisenmann and Malina 2002; Kanehisa et al. 2006; Erlandson et al. 2008) indicate no influence of regular training on height and rate of growth in height. Body weight is more variable; changes with training are reflected in changes in body composition. Concern is often expressed for low weight-for-height among athletes in some sports (see Section 5.7.4).

In contrast and as noted earlier, the short statures of gymnasts, especially females, are often attributed to intensive sport-specific training. However, a consensus committee convened by the Scientific Commission of the International Gymnastics Federation concluded as follows:

> Adult height or near adult height of female and male artistic gymnasts is not compromised by intensive gymnastics training at a young age or during the pubertal growth spurt. …
> Gymnastics training does not attenuate growth of upper (sitting height) or lower (legs) body segment lengths (Malina et al. 2013a, p. 798).

Evidence is consistent in showing that artistic gymnasts are short before the start of training and have, on average, shorter parents. Though data are limited, gymnastics dropouts of both sexes tend to be, on average, taller, heavier, and advanced in maturity, whereas those who persist in the sport are shorter, lighter, and delayed in maturation (Malina 1999; Malina et al. 2013a).

5.6 PHYSICAL ACTIVITY AND BIOLOGICAL MATURATION

Biological maturation can be viewed in terms of status, timing, and tempo (Malina et al. 2004, 2015). Status refers to the state of maturation at observation. The two most commonly used indicators of status are SA and stage of puberty. SA has meaning relative to CA. SA is the only maturity indicator that spans childhood through late adolescence. Timing refers to the CA at which specific maturational events occur. The two events used most often are age at menarche and age at peak height velocity (PHV). Both require longitudinal data, though recalled ages at menarche are often used in epidemiological surveys of activity and studies of athletes. Tempo refers to the rate of maturation; data on tempo are very limited.

5.6.1 ACTIVITY AND MATURATION IN THE GENERAL POPULATION

Progress in SA relative to CA does not differ between active and nonactive boys followed from 11 to 15 years (Černý 1970) and from 13 to 18 years (Beunen et al. 1992). Longitudinal data on the sexual maturation of habitually active and nonactive boys and girls are not available. Some epidemiological data suggest an association between habitual activity and later recalled ages at menarche (Moisan et al. 1991; Merzenich et al. 1993), but other data do not (Moisan et al. 1990). The association is not strong and is confounded by other factors known to influence age at menarche (Malina 1998, 2010b).

Relatively small samples of boys classified as physically active and less active for the years prior to and during the growth spurt do not differ in estimated ages at PHV (Kobayashi et al. 1978; Mirwald and Bailey 1986; Šprynarova 1987; Beunen et al. 1992; Malina 1994b). Estimated peak velocities of growth in height also do not differ between active and less active boys. Corresponding data are not available for active and less active girls.

5.6.2 TRAINING FOR SPORT AND MATURATION OF YOUNG ATHLETES

Though data are limited, SAs of athletes span the spectrum from late through early maturation through about 11–12 years. Subsequently, male athletes in a variety of sports tend to be average (on time) or advanced in SA relative to CA; gymnasts present a profile delayed SA relative to CA. With increasing CA during adolescence, numbers of late-maturing boys decline while those of early-maturing boys increase; the opposite is true in gymnasts (Malina 2011). Nevertheless, some late-maturing boys are successful in sport in later adolescence (16–19 years), for example, track and basketball, which emphasizes catch-up in growth and maturation; adult size and maturity are attained by all boys albeit at different CAs. This highlights the reduced significance of maturity-associated variation in body size in the performances of boys in late adolescence.

SA data for female athletes are available primarily for artistic gymnasts and swimmers (Malina 2011). Late- and early-maturing girls are about equally represented among artistic gymnasts in late childhood. During adolescence, girls late and average in SA relative to CA dominate samples of elite gymnasts; early-maturing girls are a minority. The majority of swimmers <14 years are average in SA with several earlier than later-maturing girls. Among swimmers 14–15 years, equal numbers are average or mature, while most swimmers 16–17 years are skeletally mature.

Corresponding data for the pubertal status of youth athletes are relatively limited (Malina et al. 2015). Most discussions of sexual maturation focus on female athletes, specifically age at menarche, an indicator of timing that occurs late in the sequence of pubertal changes (Malina et al. 2004). Only prospectively collected and status quo data deal with youth athletes in the process of maturing; selective persistence and drop-out/exclusion from sport are major confounders. Prospective (longitudinal) data for individual athletes followed from prepuberty through puberty are commonly based on short-term studies and limited to small, select samples. Status quo data, in contrast, provide an estimated age at menarche for the sample. Given the selective nature of sport, samples in status quo surveys include athletes of different skill levels at younger ages and more select athletes at older ages. Most mean/median ages at menarche for prospective and status quo samples of youth athletes are within the range of normal variation and tend to approximate those for the general population; exceptions are later mean/median ages for artistic gymnasts, figure skaters, ballet dancers, and divers.

Most menarche data for athletes are retrospective, that is, based on recalled ages, in samples of postmenarcheal late adolescents and adults. Recalled ages are influenced by memory, recall bias (the shorter the interval, the more accurate the recall, and vice versa), and a tendency to report ages in whole years, typically age at the birthday before menarche. Mean ages based on the retrospective method are within the range of normal variation, and tend to be later in athletes in many, but not all sports (Malina 1983, 1998, 2006a; Malina et al. 2004). Mean ages based on recall vary among sports, within specific sports, and between "early" and "late" entry sports.

Estimated ages at PHV for samples of youth athletes are also limited (Malina et al. 2013a, 2015). Among athletes of European ancestry, studies that spanned most of adolescence indicate ages at PHV consistent with earlier maturation except for gymnasts. Most data for female athletes are available for artistic gymnasts; the limited data for athletes in other sports indicate ages at PHV, which approximate means for the general population. Ages at PHV of artistic gymnasts of both sexes are later. Ages at PHV of Japanese youth athletes on several nonselect school teams and a small sample of elite runners are generally consistent with those for the general population with the exception of a later age for school soccer players (elite academy soccer players in Japan are advanced in SA relative to CA, Malina 2011). Corresponding ages at PHV for regionally select Japanese female athletes in several sports are within the range of those of the general population.

A word of caution is warranted in the discussion of age at PHV. Studies of youth athletes are increasingly using predicted maturity offset (time before or after PHV) and age at PHV estimated as CA minus offset (Mirwald et al. 2002; Malina 2014). Validation studies in two longitudinal series of boys (8–18 years) and girls (8–16 years) indicate major limitations. Predicted offset and age at PHV are dependent upon CA at prediction, and as such intraindividual variation is considerable. Predicted ages at PHV have reduced ranges of variation within a CA group that will influence maturity status classifications. And predicted ages at PHV are affected by individual differences in observed (actual) ages at PHV. Among early-maturing boys and girls, predicted ages are consistently later than observed age at PHV, while among late-maturing youth of both sexes, predicted ages are earlier than observed age at PHV (Malina and Kozieł 2014a,b; Malina et al. 2016).

With the preceding as background, what is the influence of training for sport on the maturation of youth athletes? Short- and long-term longitudinal studies of youth athletes in several sports indicate no influence of regular training on indicators of maturity status, timing, and tempo (Kotulan et al. 1980; Novotný 1981; Eisenmann and Malina 2002; Malina 1994b; Baxter-Jones et al. 1995; Malina et al. 1997a,b; Geithner et al. 1998; Kanehisa et al. 2006; Erlandson et al. 2008). SA progresses, on average, in concert with CA; some athletes do in fact change in maturity status (SA relative to CA), but there is no clear pattern of acceleration or deceleration (Novotný 1981). Mean intervals for progression from one pubertal stage to the next or across two stages are similar to those for nonactive youth, and are within the range of normal variation in longitudinal studies of nonathletes. The interval between ages at PHV and menarche does not differ between girls active in sport and nonactive girls, and is similar to intervals in several samples of nonathletic girls, mean intervals of 1.2–1.5 years (Geithner et al. 1998). Overall, the results highlight sport-related variation in maturity status and timing, consistent with early maturation in males and on time maturation in females, except for artistic gymnasts who characteristically present later maturation which is often attributed intensive sport-specific training. The consensus committee convened by the Scientific Commission of the International Gymnastics Federation, however, arrived at the following conclusion:

> Gymnastics training does not appear to attenuate pubertal growth and maturation, including SA, secondary sex characteristics and age at menarche, and rate of growth and timing and tempo of the growth spurt (Malina et al. 2013a, p. 798).

Although SAs lag, on average, relative to CAs between 12 and 14 years in gymnasts of both sexes, both SA and CA show similar progress over the three observations (Keller and Fröhner 1989; Fröhner et al. 1990). The same trend is apparent in female gymnasts at 12 and 16 years over an interval of 4 years (Novotný 1981). Change in maturity status classification between 12 and 16 years occurred in 7 of 24 gymnasts but the pattern was variable: 1, early to average; 2, average to early; 1, late to average; and 3, average to late. Changes in status reflect individual variation, errors inherent in method of assessment, ceiling effect as skeletal maturity is attained, and variation among technicians. Given the preceding, the evidence indicates no influence of systematic gymnastics training on progress in skeletal maturation.

Variation in pubertal maturation of gymnasts of both sexes relative to athletes in other sports reflects differential timing; otherwise, gymnasts progress through puberty as expected (Baxter-Jones et al. 1995; Erlandson et al. 2008). The differential timing of pubertal maturation is consistent with later ages at PHV. Estimated ages at PHV and peak velocities of growth during the adolescent spurt for female and male gymnasts are similar, on average, to observations for short, normal, and late-maturing youth of both sexes (Malina et al. 2013a).

Menarche is a late event in pubertal maturation. It refers to the first menstrual flow. Early menstrual cycles are often irregular as normal regularity of cycles is gradually established with the continued maturation of the hypothalamic–pituitary–gonadal axis (Malina and Rogol 2011).

Later mean ages at menarche in athletes are often attributed to regular training for sport before menarche. Data underlying the inferred relationship are retrospective for ages at menarche and for ages at or years of training; moreover, details of training are not ordinarily specified. The conclusion is thus based on association and does not imply causality. The use of the term "delay" is misleading as it implies that regular training "causes" menarche to be later in athletes.

The association between years of training before menarche and later menarche may be an artifact (Stager et al. 1990). Assume two girls begin systematic training in a sport at 8 years of age. One girl is genetically an early maturer and attains menarche at 10 years and the other is genetically a late maturer and attains menarche at 15 years. The early-maturing girl has only 2 years while the late-maturing girl has 7 years of training before menarche.

A variety of factors are related to the timing of menarche—genotypic, dietary, nutritional, and ethnic among others (Malina et al. 2004). Age at menarche shows familial aggregation and is influenced by family size (Malina et al. 1994, 1997b) and home environments (Ellis 2004; Ellis and Essex 2007). Parental emotional and social investment in the careers of their child/children is substantial and affects the home environment. Coaches and the training environment may function to complement or disrupt the home lives of young athletes. The preceding factors are not ordinarily considered in discussions of menarche in athletes (Malina 2010b). They should also be viewed in the context of differential persistence and dropout in sport, the nonrandom nature of athlete samples, and athletes who change sports or take up sport after menarche. Nevertheless, discussions of the potential relationship between training before menarche and age at menarche have concluded with two observations: menarche occurs later in athletes in some sports, and the relationship between later menarche and training for sport is not causal (Loucks et al. 1992; Clapp and Little 1995). If training for sport is a factor, it interacts with or is confounded by a variety of other factors.

5.7 PHYSICAL ACTIVITY AND BODY COMPOSITION

The two-compartment model of body composition, that is, body weight = fat-free mass (FFM) + fat mass (FM), was used in many early studies of activity and body composition. Given advances in body composition technology, many studies partition FFM into lean tissue mass (LTM) and bone mineral content (BMC) or bone mineral density (BMD). Earlier studies of activity and body composition are largely limited to indirect indicators of FM, specifically, skinfolds, predicted percentage body fat (% FM), and the body mass index (BMI).

5.7.1 Activity and FFM in the General Population

It is often suggested that regular physical activity is associated with an increase in FFM and a decrease in FM. FFM is correlated with and has a similar growth pattern as height. FM increases from childhood through adolescence; % FM increases with CA during childhood but declines in males and increases in females during adolescence. The decline in % FM in males is a function of the adolescent spurt. Both sexes have a significant adolescent spurt in FFM, males more so than females (Malina et al. 2004).

It is difficult to partition potential effects of activity on FFM from expected changes with growth and maturation, specifically during adolescence. Peak velocity of growth in LTM (DXA) occurs, on average, after PHV in girls and boys (Iuliano-Burns et al. 2001). The use of multilevel modeling allowing for body size (height) and biological maturation (estimated years from PHV) in mixed-longitudinal observations for LTM (DXA) in boys and girls indicates several important observations (Baxter-Jones et al. 2008). Allowing for height and maturity, activity has an independent effect on growth in LTM in both sexes. At the same level of activity, the estimated effect on LTM is greater in boys than girls, especially for lean tissue accrual in the arms (boys 70 ± 27 g, girls 31 ± 15 g) and trunk (boys 249 ± 91 g, girls 120 ± 58 g) compared to the legs (boys 198 ± 60 g, girls 163 ± 40 g). Given relatively large gains in LTM and FFM during adolescence, the proportion attributed to activity is relatively small. The results highlight the need to consider interactions among body size per se, timing of maximal rate of growth during the adolescent spurt, growth in LTM, and sex in an effort to understand potential activity effects.

A study of 4 months of endurance activities designed to increase maximal aerobic power of boys provides insights into the difficulties in partitioning the effects of growth and training on FFM (Von Döbeln and Eriksson 1972). Height, weight, and ^{40}K were measured before and within 3 weeks after the program in nine boys. The interval between measurements was ~0.5–0.6 year. CAs ranged from 11.6 to 13.5 years at the second observation when testicular volume (pubertal status) was measured. Testicular volume (TV) was <9 mL in 6 boys (12.0 ± 0.6 years) and ≥9 mL in 3 boys (12.7 ± 0.7 years). Age-adjusted increments (mean±SE calculated from raw data in the paper) in ^{40}K, height, and weight in the two groups were as follows:

TV <9 mL, 11.2 ± 0.6 g, 2.7 ± 0.4 cm, and 0.3 ± 1.1 kg
TV ≥9 mL, 12.0 ± 0.9 g, 5.1 ± 0.7 cm, and 1.1 ± 1.8 kg

Although limited to small numbers, observed gains in height and ^{40}K were apparently influenced by age per se, sexual maturation, and perhaps the adolescent spurt, and not necessarily the aerobic activity program. Of note, endurance programs are not typically associated gains in FFM.

The results of resistance training programs designed to improve muscular strength are consistent with the preceding. Allowing for variable program durations and training protocols, changes in estimates of lean tissue (limb girths and areas, FFM) with resistance training in children and adolescents are variable and in most cases minimal (Malina 2006b).

A 10-month program of high-impact strength and aerobic activities among girls 9–10 years was associated with a larger mean increment in LTM and smaller increase in FM compared to girls following their normal pattern of activity (Morris et al. 1997). Changes in height, weight, and pubertal status were not controlled, and the groups overlapped considerably.

5.7.2 Training for Sport and FFM in Youth Athletes

A frequently cited study highlighting the influence of activity on growth in FFM (Pařizkova 1970, 1974) has relevance for youth athletes. Details of the study are reported in several papers and not always consistent. The project started in 1961 with 143 boys, mean CA 10.5 years (Pařizkova 1976); "boys with markedly accelerated or retarded somatic development were eliminated" (Pařizkova

1974, p. 235). Height, weight, and body composition (densitometry) of three groups of boys followed from 11 to 18 years were compared (Pařizkova 1974): active (n = 8, 6 h/week in "organized, intensive exercise" plus participation in "unorganized sports" and a 4-week summer camp in the first 5 years); moderately active (n = 18, 4 h/week in sport schools for 5 years, then continued training but not on a regular basis); least active (n = 13, <2.5 h/week in unsystematic sport activity, including physical education). Activity levels were described a bit differently in a related report (Šprynarova 1974): active (4 h/week 11–15 years, 6 h/week 15–18 years); moderate activity (2 h/week 11–15 years, 3 h/week 15–18 years); limited activity (1 h/week 11–15 years, no regular activity 15–18 years).

The groups differed slightly in body composition at 11–12 years, but the most active boys gained more FFM and less FM than the other groups between 11 and 18 years. The moderate and limited activity groups differed only slightly in FFM, but the least active boys had greater % FM. The larger gains in FFM among the most active boys were generally attributed to the effects of regular physical activity (Pařizkova 1974, 1977).

Subject selection and differential drop out over 8 years should be noted. Composition of the active group is relevant to this discussion; it included six or seven basketball players and two or one in athletics—running (Šprynarova 1974, 1987). The most active boys were likely youth athletes training for sport, primarily basketball; they were taller than the boys in the other groups throughout the study and heavier from 13 to 18 years.

Maturity status and timing were not considered in comparisons of body composition among activity groups. The initial report indicated no differences in SA (Pařizkova 1974). Data from the same research unit reported SA among three similarly labeled groups between 11 and 15 years (Černý 1970). Active boys (n = 14, described as training regularly in basketball and athletics, in addition to other sports) were, on average, advanced in SA at each CA compared to boys in the moderate (n = 32) and low (n = 24) activity groups; differences were most marked at 14 and 15 years. In a related report, advanced SA was reported in 12 active boys (labeled sportsmen—9 in basketball, 3 in light athletics) compared to 16 least active boys at each age from 11 to 17 years, but especially from 14 to 17 years (Ulbrich 1971). Estimated age at PHV was also described as not differing among the activity groups (Pařizkova 1974), but a subsequent report indicated an earlier estimated age at PHV (graphic interpolation) in active compared to moderately and least active boys (Šprynarova 1987). It is likely that the greater heights and FFM in active boys reflected advanced maturation and subject persistence/selectivity.

Other studies monitoring changes in body composition with sport-specific training and competition among youth athletes often focus on changes across a season, that is, pre- and postseason. As such, they provide limited insights into changes in FFM and FM associated with variation in training emphases and competitions during the season (Malina and Geithner 2011). A study of adolescent wrestlers is an exception. Among nine adolescent wrestlers (15.4 ± 0.3 years), body weight, FFM, and % FM (densitometry) declined from pre- to late-season, which likely reflected concern for "making weight" or maintaining weight, and then increased from late- to postseason (Roemmich and Sinning 1997). The seven nonathletes (15.0 ± 0.4 years) increased in weight and FFM but did not change in % FM. Across the interval of the season, gains in FFM and height, and changes in SA were the same in wrestlers and nonathletes. Overall changes in body composition were relatively small and sport-specific emphasis on body weight among the wrestlers contributed to variation in assessments during the season.

Similar trends were noted in 15 late adolescent/young adult collegiate female swimmers (19.1 ± 1.3 years). From October to December, FFM (densitometry) increased, while body weight, FM, and % FM decreased. This was an interval of dry land training, specifically weight training (high repetition, low resistance), which preceded swim training early in the season. The changes in weight and components of body composition were generally maintained from December to March, as swimmers tapered in preparation for the national championship (Meleski and Malina 1985). Unfortunately, the swimmers were not measured after the season.

5.7.3 Activity and Adiposity in the General Population

Longitudinal observations for boys and girls 6–12 years (Saris et al. 1986) and adolescent boys 13–18 years (Beunen et al. 1992) indicate negligible differences in skinfolds between active and less active youth, whereas higher physical activity is associated with lower FM in boys but not in girls after controlling for years from PHV and FFM in a mixed-longitudinal sample 8–15 years (Mundt et al. 2006). Activity prior to PHV may negatively influence the accumulation of FM in boys, consistent with a positive effect of activity prior to PHV on LTM (Baxter-Jones et al. 2008).

Correlation and regression analyses in youth of mixed weight status (normal, overweight, obese) generally indicate low and at best moderate relationships between habitual activity and indicators of adiposity (Strong et al. 2005; Malina et al. 2007a; Physical Activity Guidelines Committee 2008). Most of the variance in adiposity was not explained by activity; other factors need to be addressed. Variability in the measurement of skinfolds, both inter- and intraindividual, is well documented (Malina 1995), while skinfold-based equations for predicting % FM typically have an error range of 3%–5% (Lohman 1981, 1986). BMI, an indicator of weight-for-height, is about equally correlated with FFM and FM in normal-weight youth (Malina and Katzmarzyk 1999), and may be more closely correlated with lean tissue than with FM in relatively thin youth (Freedman et al. 2005). Growth and maturity status need to be considered. Individual skinfolds also behave differently with CA and relative to PHV (Beunen and Malina 1988; Malina et al. 1999).

Enhanced and experimental programs of variable duration in normal-weight youth show a minimal effect of activity on adiposity (Strong et al. 2005; Malina et al. 2007a). Activity volume needs further study; it is possible that normal-weight youth require a greater activity volume to modify adiposity. In contrast, activity interventions with overweight and obese youth are associated with reductions in overall and abdominal visceral adiposity. Programs included a variety of activities (largely aerobic) of moderate and vigorous intensity, 3–5 times per week, for 30–60 min duration. More consistent favorable effects are evident in studies using more direct estimates of adiposity, specifically DXA estimates of % FM and magnetic resonance imaging of visceral adiposity, in contrast to BMI, skinfolds, or predicted % FM (Strong et al. 2005; Malina et al. 2007a). Unfortunately, persistence of activity-related changes in adiposity is not ordinarily considered in experimental studies.

5.7.4 Training for Sport and Adiposity in Youth Athletes

Studies of the influence of activity/training on FFM in athletes also include estimates of FM and % FM. The three studies considered were based on densitometry. Athletes tended to have lower levels of FM and % FM, and the two studies evaluating changes across a season indicated a reduction in FM associated with training and weight control.

In contrast, most studies of body composition in youth athletes are cross-sectional and focus on % FM, given the generally negative influence of excess adiposity on performance. A variety of methods have been used to estimate % FM—densitometry, total body water, DXA, bioelectrical impedance, near-infrared interactance, and predictions from skinfolds using a variety of equations (Malina and Geithner 2011). Technical variation in measurement of skinfolds and errors inherent to prediction equations were noted earlier. Variation in body size and maturity status is not often considered in studies of relative fatness among youth athletes although some prediction equations are specific to the stage of pubertal status.

Estimates of % FM are somewhat more available for youth athletes in individual in contrast to team sports, especially for girls. On average, youth athletes tend to have a lower % FM than the reference, but there is considerable overlap between male athletes and the reference, while relatively few samples of female athletes have a % FM that approximates or exceeds the reference except for athletes in track and field throwing events and some team sports. The reference is an estimate based on densitometry compiled from samples of youth 9–19 years surveyed before the obesity epidemic

(Malina et al. 1988; Malina 1989). Estimates of % FM predicted from skinfolds show similar trends, but greater variability. Variation among athletes within the same sport and athletes in different sports is also considerable.

The low weight-for-height of female athletes in some sports is often viewed in terms of low levels of adiposity and attributed to intensive training and dietary restrictions. Relative to international criteria for mild, moderate, and severe thinness based on BMI (Cole et al. 2007), mild and moderate thinness occur among female youth athletes in several sports, but severe thinness is uncommon (Malina and Rogol 2011). Less weight-for-height is related in part to linearity of build, which is characteristic of later maturation in both sexes (Malina et al. 2004) and may not be the result of training or diet per se. Information on the BMI and menarcheal status (pre- or postmenarche) of athletes 10–16 years was available to the authors: U.S. Junior Olympic divers (n = 129, 8 with mild thinness, Malina and Geithner 1993), U.S. artistic gymnasts at a national training camp (n = 33, 4 with mild thinness, Malina unpublished), U.S. and Canadian figure skaters (n = 111, 11 with mild thinness, 3 with moderate thinness, Vadocz et al. 2002), and Polish distance runners (n = 23, 5 with mild thinness, 2 with moderate thinness, Malina et al. 2011). Of the 33 athletes with mild or moderate thinness, 23 were premenarcheal (mild 21, moderate 2). Data for elite female artistic gymnasts (Rotterdam World Championship in 1987, Claessens et al. 1992) were also available to the authors. Among gymnasts 13–16 years, 34 of 129 (26%) were mildly or moderately thin; 29 of the 34 were premenarcheal.

5.7.5 ACTIVITY AND BONE MINERAL IN THE GENERAL POPULATION

Advances in body composition technology have facilitated the measurement and evaluation of bone mineral status. Moreover, the benefits of regular activity on BMC have implications for longer-term skeletal health as bone mineral established during childhood and adolescence is a determinant of bone mineral status in adulthood.

Evidence from a variety of cross-sectional and longitudinal comparisons of active and less active youth indicate a beneficial effect of regular activity on BMC and/or BMD (Strong et al. 2005; Baptista and Janz 2012). Individual differences in the timing of the growth spurt influence observations in adolescents. Estimated peak velocity of total body BMC accrual occurs, on average, a bit more than one-half year after PHV. Peak velocities vary with maturity status in boys (early > average > late), and are similar in girls maturing early and on time but are less in girls maturing late (Iuliano-Burns et al. 2001). After adjusting for LTM and FM with multilevel modeling, BMC shows a maturity-related gradient in young adult females (early > average > late), but not males (Jackowski et al. 2011). The latter contrasts the gradient noted in males during adolescence and probably reflects the prolonged growth of late-maturing boys. Of interest, physical activity did not have a significant effect in the model. Nevertheless, active youth of both sexes gain more BMC than less active peers during the interval of rapid growth and also have greater BMC after peak velocity of growth in BMC (boys 9%, girls 17%) than less active peers (Bailey et al. 1999). Unfortunately, maturity status was not considered.

Physical activity interventions, 2 or 3 times per week of moderate-to-high-intensity activities, weight-bearing activities of a longer duration (45–60 min), and/or high-impact activities over a shorter duration (10 min) enhance BMC in youth (Strong et al. 2005). Changes in bone mineral are generally site-specific and reflect local mechanical strains. Activity programs in pre- and early pubertal youth of both sexes also influence bone geometry, which suggests enhanced bone strength (MacDonald et al. 2006). Results also suggest that short bouts of activity may have been as effective as sustained activity.

5.7.6 TRAINING FOR SPORT AND BONE MINERAL IN YOUTH ATHLETES

Studies of individuals participating in extreme unilateral activity of the arm have historically been used to address the potential influence activity on limb skeletal and muscle tissues (Malina 1979).

This is evident in the positive influence of racquet sports (tennis, squash) on BMC and bone strength of the dominant versus nondominant arms of female players grouped by recalled ages at which formal training began (Kannus et al. 1995, 1996; Kontulainen et al. 2001). Similar results are suggested for professional baseball players (Warden et al. 2014). Extreme unilateral activity during youth is associated with localized increases in bone mineral accretion.

An early study compared the throwing and nonthrowing arms of youth baseball players 8–19 years (Watson 1975). Differences in mineral and width measures at mid-humerus favored the throwing arm and increased with CA; corresponding comparisons of mineral and width at the distal third of the radius and ulna were inconsistent and showed no CA effect. Differences in mineral between humeri were not related to limb girths and grip strength after body weight was statistically controlled.

In contrast to baseball, effects of loading on bone variables (BMC, total and cortical areas, bending strength) in female tennis players 8–17 years were specific to region (mid and distal) and surface of the playing and nonplaying humeri, and varied among pre-, peri- (early), and postpubertal players (Bass et al. 2002). Muscle areas were larger in the dominant arms, but relative differences in bone variables and muscle area did not increase across maturity groups (Daly et al. 2004). Differences in muscle areas between playing and nonplaying arms explained only 12%–16% of the variance in BMC, cortical areas, and bending strength. Larger changes in the bone variables were also noted over a 1-year interval in the humerus of the dominant arm in pre/peripubertal and postmenarcheal tennis players 10–17 years, but the former experienced greater relative gains (Ducher et al. 2011).

Differences in muscle size (upper arm, forearm) and indicators of bone strength of the humerus, radius, and ulna favored the playing arms of elite female and male tennis players, 13.5 ± 1.9 years (Ireland et al. 2013). Although differences in bone and muscle size variables were related, a role for other factors that influence training-related side-to-side differences in bone strength was suggested.

In contrast to sports with dominant unilateral activities, studies of athletes in other sports have focused on high-impact (gymnastics, running) and low-impact (swimming, cycling) activities. Activity/training and BMC/BMD have received considerable attention in gymnasts as it is an early-entry sport. Mixed-longitudinal observations among girls 4–10 years showed greater accretion of BMC among gymnasts compared to dropouts and nongymnasts (Erlandson et al. 2011). Short-term studies of young female gymnasts indicated greater BMC and BMD especially at weight-bearing sites compared to controls (Bass et al. 1998; Courteix et al. 1999; Nickols-Richardson et al. 1999). Potential change in pubertal status was not considered, although SA, LTM, and FM were predictors of change in BMD (Courteix et al. 1999). After controlling for breast stage and estimated time from PHV, gymnasts accrued more BMC and BMD across puberty than nonathletes (Nurmi-Lawton et al. 2004). Training-related gains in BMD during youth also persisted into young adulthood in female gymnasts (Bass et al. 1998; Ducher et al. 2009). Corresponding data for males are not as extensive but are consistent with data for females. Cross-sectional data at 8 years (Zanker et al. 2003) and short-term observations of pre- and peripubertal male gymnasts indicate greater BMC/ BMD compared to nonathlete controls (Daly et al. 1999).

Reduced BMC in high school endurance runners was associated with training, menstrual function, reduced energy intake, and/or disordered eating across adolescence (Barrack et al. 2008, 2010a,b). The results highlight interactions between training and other factors to influence bone mineral accrual in adolescent female runners. Moreover, runners with low BMC at baseline (~15 years) were more likely to have low BMC 3 years later (Barrack et al. 2011).

Swimming, a non-weight-bearing sport, has also received attention. A systematic review of 14 studies of youth swimmers (7 of males, 7 of females, mean ages 8.7–16.1 years) indicated a BMD similar to sedentary controls and lower than athletes in weight-bearing sports (9 studies, 7 of females), primarily gymnasts and soccer players (Gomez-Bruton et al. 2016). Among age-matched males 9–18 years, swimmers had, on average, lower BMD and BMC than a combined sample in high-impact sports (gymnastics, handball, basketball). After controlling for pubertal status, height, and FFM, total body and lower limb BMD and BMC were significantly reduced in swimmers; corresponding comparisons of swimmers with nonathlete controls also indicated reduced total body and lower limb BMD and BMC in swimmers (Quiterio et al. 2011).

Cycling presents different demands from other sports. Overall BMC and BMD were less in 22 male road cyclists 15.5 ± 0.9 years and 18.4 ± 1.4 years than in 22 age-matched participants in recreational sports, but regional variation in BMC and BMD was substantial (Olmedillas et al. 2011). Among cyclists <17 years, BMC of the legs was lower and that of the hip was higher than in the controls, but among cyclists ≥17 years, BMC in the pelvis, femoral neck, and legs was lower compared to the controls. BMD was also lower at most sites in the two groups of cyclists. Allowing for small samples, the authors suggested that training in cycling "…may adversely affect bone mass during adolescence" (Olmedillas et al. 2011, p. 8).

The need for continued activity is suggested in a comparison of male ice hockey players and nonathlete controls observed at 16, 19, and 22 years (Gustavsson et al. 2003). Three BMD measures (total body, spine, and femoral neck) were slightly greater at 16 years, while total body and femoral neck BMD were significantly greater at 19 years in hockey players. Differences between active hockey players and controls were marked for the three BMD measures at 22 years; however, BMD measures of formerly active players were intermediate between the two groups, especially at the femoral neck. By inference, gains in BMD associated with active participation in ice hockey may not persist with the cessation of regular participation in the sport.

5.8 SUMMARY

Physical activity in the general population of youth and systematic training for sport among youth athletes have no effect on size attained and rate of growth in height and on maturity status and timing; however, data for ages at PHV and menarche for adolescent athletes are limited. Recalled ages at menarche are later in young adult athletes in some but not all sports, but the relationship between later menarche and training is not causal.

Physical activity and training may influence body weight and composition. Data for FFM/LTM are suggestive, but limited. Activity has a minimal effect on indicators of adiposity in normal-weight youth, but enhanced activity can have a favorable influence on adiposity in overweight and obese youth. Regular training for sport can positively influence adiposity in youth athletes. Activity and training have a beneficial influence on bone mineral, but variable effects are noted in some sports. The available data highlight the need to incorporate indicators of maturity status and timing in studies of activity and body composition during adolescence.

NOTE A

T. Wingate Todd was a professor of anatomy at Western Reserve University in Cleveland and a participant in the 1930 White House Conference on Child Health and Protection. He developed the atlas method for the assessment of skeletal maturation (Todd 1937). Wilton M. Krogman worked under the supervision of Todd before becoming a professor of anthropology in the Graduate School of Medicine at the University of Pennsylvania. In a comment to the Joint Committee on Athletic Competition for Children of Elementary and Junior High School age, Krogman referred to a comparison of SA in 1028 Cleveland high school boys classified as athletes and nonathletes; the former was biologically advanced in SA by about 2 years (American Association for Health, Physical Education, and Recreation 1952).

REFERENCES

Adams, E. H. 1938. A comparative anthropometric study of hard labor during youth as a stimulator of physical growth of young colored women. *Res Q* 9:102–8.

American Association for Health, Physical Education, and Recreation. 1952. *Desirable Athletic Competition for Children: Joint Committee Report*. Washington, D.C.: American Association for Health, Physical Education, and Recreation.

Åstrand, P. O., L. Engström, B. O. Eriksson et al. 1963. Girl swimmers. *Acta Paediatr* 147(Suppl):1–75.

Bailey, D. A., H. A. McKay, R. L. Mirwald, P. R. E. Crocker, and R. A. Faulkner. 1999. A six-year longitudinal study of the relationship of physical activity to bone mineral accrual in growing children: The University of Saskatchewan Bone Mineral Accrual Study. *J Bone Min Res* 14:1672–9.

Baptista, F. and K. F. Janz. 2012. Habitual physical activity and bone growth and development in children and adolescents: A public health perspective. In *Handbook of Growth and Growth Monitoring in Health and Disease*, ed. V. R. Preedy, 2395–411. New York: Springer.

Barrack, M. T., M. J. Rauh, H.-S. Barkai, and J. F. Nichols. 2008. Dietary restraint and low bone mass in female adolescent endurance runners. *Am J Clin Nutr* 87:36–43.

Barrack, M. T., M. J. Rauh, and J. F. Nichols. 2010a. Cross-sectional evidence of suppressed bone mineral accrual among female adolescent distance runners. *J Bone Min Res* 25:1850–7.

Barrack, M. T., M. D. Van Loan, M. J. Rauh, and J. F. Nichols. 2010b. Physiologic and behavioral indicators of energy deficiency in female adolescent runners with elevated bone turnover. *Am J Clin Nutr* 92:652–9.

Barrack, M. T., M. D. Van Loan, M. J. Rauh, and J. G. Nichols. 2011. Body mass, training, menses, and bone in adolescent runners: A 3-yr follow-up. *Med Sci Sports Exerc* 43:959–66.

Bass, S., G. Pearce, M. Bradney et al. 1998. Exercise before puberty may confer residual benefits in bone density in adulthood: Studies in active prepubertal and retired female gymnasts. *J Bone Min Res* 13:500–7.

Bass, S. L., L. Saxon, R. M. Daly et al. 2002. The effect of mechanical loading on the size and shape of bone in pre-, peri-, and post-pubertal girls: A study in tennis players. *J Bone Min Res* 17:2274–80.

Baxter-Jones, A. D. G., J. C. Eisenmann, R. L. Mirwald, R. A. Faulkner, and D. A. Bailey. 2008. The influence of physical activity on lean mass accrual during adolescence: A longitudinal analysis. *J Appl Physiol* 105:734–41.

Baxter-Jones, A. D. G., P. Helms, N. Maffulli, J. C. Baines-Preece, and M. Preece. 1995. Growth and development of male gymnasts, swimmers, soccer and tennis players: A longitudinal study. *Ann Hum Biol* 22:381–94.

Beunen, G. and R. M. Malina. 1988. Growth and physical performance relative to the timing of the adolescent spurt. *Exer Sports Sci Rev* 16:503–40.

Beunen, G. and R. M. Malina. 2008. Growth and biological maturation: Relevance to athletic performance. In *The Young Athlete*, eds. H. Hebestreit, and O. Bar-Or, 3–17. Malden: Blackwell.

Beunen, G. P., R. M. Malina, R. Renson, J. Simons, M. Ostyn, and J. Lefevre. 1992. Physical activity and growth, maturation and performance: A longitudinal study. *Med Sci Sports Exerc* 24:576–85.

Beyer, H. G. 1896. The influence of exercise on growth. *J Exp Med* 1:546–58.

Černý, L. 1970. The results of an evaluation of skeletal ages of boys 11–15 years old with different régime of physical activity. In *Physical Fitness and Its Laboratory Assessment*, eds. J. Kral and V. Novotný, 56–9. Prague: Charles University.

Claessens, A. L., R. M. Malina, J. Lefevrem et al. 1992. Growth and menarcheal status of elite female gymnasts. *Med Sci Sports Exerc* 24:755–63.

Clapp, J. F. and K. D. Little. 1995. The interaction between regular exercise and selected aspects of women's health. *Am J Obstet Gynecol* 173:2–9.

Clarke, H. H. 1971. *Physical and Motor Tests in the Medford Boy's Growth Study*. Englewood Cliffs: Prentice-Hall.

Cole, T. J., K. M. Flegal, D. Nicholls, and A. A. Jackson. 2007. Body mass index cut offs to define thinness in children and adolescents: International survey. *Br Med J* 335:194–201.

Courteix, D., E. Lespessailles, C. Jaffre, P. Obert, and C. L. Benhamou. 1999. Bone mineral acquisition and somatic development in highly trained girl gymnasts. *Acta Paediatr* 88:803–8.

Crampton, C. W. 1908. Physiological age: A fundamental principle. *Am Phys Educ Rev* 13:141–54.

Crampton, C. W. 1936. *Boy's Book of Strength*. New York: McGraw-Hill.

Daly, R. M., D. Caine, S. L. Bass et al. 2005. Growth of highly versus moderately trained competitive female artistic gymnasts. *Med Sci Sports Exerc* 37:1053–60.

Daly, R. M., P. A. Rich, and R. Klein. 1998. Hormonal responses to physical training in high-level peripubertal male gymnasts. *Eur J Appl Physiol* 79:74–81.

Daly, R. M., P. A. Rich, R. Klein, and S. Bass. 1999. Effects of high-impact exercise on ultrasonic and biochemical indices of skeletal status: A prospective study in young male gymnasts. *J Bone Min Res* 14:1222–30.

Daly, R. M., L. Saxon, C. H. Turner, A. G. Robling, and S. L. Bass. 2004. The relationship between muscle size and bone geometry during growth and in response to exercise. *Bone* 34:281–7.

Daniels, J. and N. Oldridge. 1971. Changes in oxygen consumption of young boys during growth and running training. *Med Sci Sports* 3:161–5.

Ducher, G., S. L. Bass, L. Saxon, and R. M. Daly. 2011. Effects of repetitive loading on the growth-induced changes in bone mass and cortical bone geometry: A 12-month study in pre/peri- and postmenarcheal tennis players. *J Bone Min Res* 26:1321–9.

Ducher, G., B. L. Hill, T. Angeli, S. L. Bass, and P. Eser. 2009. Comparison of pQCT parameters between ulna and radius in retired elite gymnasts: The skeletal benefits associated with long-term gymnastics are bone- and site-specific. *J Musculoskel Neuronal Interact* 9:247–55.

Eisenmann, J. C. and R. M. Malina. 2002. Growth status and estimated growth rate of young distance runners. *Int J Sports Med* 23:168–73.

Ellis, B. J. 2004. Timing of pubertal maturation in girls: An integrated life history approach. *Psychol Bull* 130:920–58.

Ellis, B. J. and M. J. Essex. 2007. Family environments, adrenarche, and sexual maturation: A longitudinal test of a life history model. *Child Develop* 78:1799–817.

Erlandson, M. C., S. A. Kontulainen, P. D. Chilibeck, C. A. Arnold, and A. D. G. Baxter-Jones. 2011. Bone mineral accrual in 4- to 10-year-old precompetitive, recreational gymnasts: A 4-year longitudinal study. *J Bone Min Res* 26:1313–20.

Erlandson, M. C., L. B. Sherar, R. L. Mirwald, N. Maffulli, and A. D. G. Baxter-Jones. 2008. Growth and maturation of adolescent female gymnasts, swimmers, and tennis players. *Med Sci Sports Exerc* 40:34–42.

Fait, H. F. 1951. An analytical study of the effects of competitive athletics upon junior high school boys. PhD dissertation, Iowa State University.

Fait, H. F. 1956. The physiological effects of strenuous activity upon the immature child. *FIEP-Bull* 26–7.

Fogelholm, M., R. Rankinen, M. Isokääntä, U. Kujala, and M. Uusitupa. 2000. Growth, dietary intake and trace element status in pubescent athletes and school children. *Med Sci Sports Exerc* 32:738–46.

Freedman, D. S., J. Wang, L. M. Maynard et al. 2005. Relation of BMI to fat and fat-free mass among children and adolescents. *Int J Obes* 29:1–8.

Frisch, R. E., A. V. Gotz-Welbergen, J. W. McArthur et al. 1981. Delayed menarche and amenorrhea of college athletes in relation to age of onset of training. *J Am Med Assoc* 246:1559–63.

Fröhner, G., E. Keller, and G. Schmidt. 1990. Wachstumsparameter von Sportlerinnen unter Bedingungen hoher Trainingsbelastungen. *Ärztl Jugend* 81:375–9.

Geithner, C. A., B. Woynarowska, and R. M. Malina. 1998. The adolescent spurt and sexual maturation in girls active and not active in sport. *Ann Hum Biol* 25:415–23.

Georgopoulos, N. A., N. D. Roupas, A. Theodoropoulou, A. Tsekouras, A. G. Vagenakis, and K. B. Markou. 2010. The influence of intensive physical training on growth and pubertal development in athletes. *Ann NY Acad Sci* 1205:39–44.

Godin, P. 1920. *Growth during School Age: Its Application to Education.* Boston: Gorham Press.

Gomez-Bruton, A., J. Montero-Marín, A. Gonzalez-Agüero et al. 2016. The effect of swimming during childhood and adolescence on bone mineral density: A systematic review and meta-analysis. *Sports Med* 46:335–79.

Gustavsson, A., T. Olsson, and P. Nordstrom. 2003. Rapid loss of bone mineral density of the femoral neck after cessation of ice hockey training: A 6-year longitudinal study in males. *J Bone Min Res* 18:1964–9.

Hale, C. J. 1956. Physiological maturity of Little League baseball players. *Res Q* 27:276–84.

Ireland, A., T. Maden-Wilkinson, J. McPhee et al. 2013. Upper limb muscle-bone asymmetries and bone adaptation in elite youth tennis players. *Med Sci Sports Exerc* 45:1749–58.

Iuliano-Burns, S., R. L. Mirwald, and D. A. Bailey. 2001. The timing and magnitude of peak height velocity and peak tissue velocities for early, average and late maturing boys and girls. *Am J Hum Biol* 13:1–8.

Jackowski, S. A., M. C. Erlandson, R. L. Mirwald et al. 2011. Effect of maturational timing on bone mineral content accrual from childhood to adulthood: Evidence from 15 years of longitudinal data. *Bone* 48:1178–85.

Jahreis, G., E. Kauf, G. Fröhner, and H. E. Schmidt. 1991. Influence of intensive exercise on insulin-like growth factor I, thyroid and steroid hormones in female gymnasts. *Growth Regulat* 1:95–9.

Jost-Relyveld, A. and M. Sempé. 1982. Analyse de la croissance et de la maturation squelettique de 80 jeunes gymnastes internationaux. *Pediatrie* 37:247–62.

Kanehisa, H., S. Kuno, S. Katsuta, and T. Fukunaga. 2006. A 2-year follow-up study on muscle size and dynamic strength in teenage tennis players. *Scand J Med Sci Sports* 16:93–101.

Kannus, P., H. Haapasalo, M. Sankelo et al. 1995. Effect of starting age of physical activity on bone mineral in the dominant arm of tennis and squash players. *Ann Intern Med* 123:27–31.

Kannus, P., H. Sievanen, and I. Vuori. 1996. Physical loading, exercise, and bone. *Bone* 18:S1–3.

Katzmarzyk, P. T., P. Walker, and R. M. Malina. 2001. A time-motion study of organized youth sports. *J Hum Move Stud* 40:325–34.

Keller, E. and G. Fröhner. 1989. Growth and development of boys with intensive training in gymnastics during puberty. In *Hormones and Sport*, eds. Z. Laron and A. D. Rogol, 11–20. New York: Raven Press.

Kobayashi, K., K. Kitamura, M. Miura et al. 1978. Aerobic power as related to body growth and training in Japanese boys: A longitudinal study. *J Appl Physiol* 44:666–72.

Kontulainen, S., P. Kannus, H. Haapasalo et al. 2001. Good maintenance of exercise-induced bone gain with decreased training of female tennis and squash players: A prospective 5-year follow-up study of young and old starters and controls. *J Bone Min Res* 17:195–201.

Kotulan, J., M. Řeznickova, and Z. Placheta. 1980. Exercise and growth. In *Youth and Physical Activity*, ed. Z. Placheta, 61–117. Brno: J.E. Purkyne University Medical Faculty.

Krogman, W. M. 1959. Maturation age of 55 boys in the Little League World Series, 1957. *Res Q* 30:54–6.

Leek, D., J. A. Carlson, K. L. Cain et al. 2011. Physical activity during youth sports participation. *Arch Pediatr Adol Med* 154:294–9.

Lindholm, C., K. Hagenfeldt, and B.-M. Ringertz. 1994. Pubertal development in elite juvenile gymnasts: Effects of physical training. *Acta Obstet Gynecol Scand* 73:269–73.

Lohman, T. G. 1981. Skinfolds and body density and their relationship to body fatness. *Hum Biol* 53:181–225.

Lohman, T. G. 1986. Applicability of body composition techniques and constants for children and youths. *Exerc Sport Sci Rev* 14:325–57.

Lopez, R. and D. M. Pruett. 1982. The child runner. *J Phys Educ Rec Dance* 53:78–81.

Loucks, A. B., J. Vaitukaitis, J. L. Cameron et al. 1992. The reproductive system and exercise in women. *Med Sci Sports Exerc* 24:S288–93.

MacDonald, H., S. Kontulainen, M. Petit, P. Janssen, and H. McKay. 2006. Bone strength and its determinants in pre- and early pubertal boys and girls. *Bone* 39:598–608.

Malina, R. M. 1969. Exercise as an influence upon growth: Review and critique of current concepts. *Clin Pediatr* 8:16–26.

Malina, R. M. 1979. The effects of exercise on specific tissues, dimensions and functions during growth. *Stud Phys Anthropol* 5:21–52.

Malina, R. M. 1983. Menarche in athletes: A synthesis and hypothesis. *Ann Hum Biol* 10:1–24.

Malina, R. M. 1989. Growth and maturation: Normal variation and the effects of training. In *Perspectives in Exercise Science and Sports Medicine, Vol. II, Youth, Exercise, and Sport*, eds. C. V. Gisolfi and D. R. Lamb, 223–65. Indianapolis: Benchmark Press.

Malina, R. M. 1994a. Physical growth and biological maturation of young athletes. *Exerc Sport Sci Rev* 22:389–433.

Malina, R. M. 1994b. Physical activity and training: Effects on stature and the adolescent growth spurt. *Med Sci Sports Exerc* 26:759–66.

Malina, R. M. 1995. Anthropometry. In *Physiological Assessment of Human Fitness*, eds. P. J. Maud and C. Foster, 205–19. Champaign, IL: Human Kinetics.

Malina, R. M. 1998. Growth and maturation of young athletes—Is training for sport a factor? In *Sports and Children*, eds. K.-M. Chan and L. J. Micheli, 133–61. Hong Kong: Williams and Wilkins.

Malina, R. M. 1999. Growth and maturation of elite female gymnasts: Is training a factor? In *Human Growth in Context*, eds. F. E. Johnston, B. Zemel, and P. B. Eveleth, 291–301. London: Smith-Gordon.

Malina, R. M. 2002. The young athlete: Biological growth and maturation in a biocultural context. In *Children and Youth in Sport: A Biopsychosocial Perspective* (2nd Ed.), eds. F. L. Smoll and R. E. Smith, 261–92. Dubuque: Kendall Hunt.

Malina, R. M. 2006a. *Crescita e maturazione di bambini ed adolescenti praticanti atletica leggera—Growth and Maturation of Child and Adolescent Track and Field Athletes* (in both Italian and English). Rome: Centro Studi e Ricerche, Federazine Italiana di Atletica Leggera.

Malina, R. M. 2006b. Weight training in youth—Growth, maturation, and safety: An evidence-based review. *Clin J Sports Med* 16:478–87.

Malina, R. M. 2009. Children and adolescents in the sport culture: The overwhelming majority to the select few. *J Exerc Sci Fit* 7:S1–10.

Malina, R. M. 2010a. Early sport specialization: Roots, effectiveness, risks. *Curr Sports Med Rep* 9:364–71.

Malina, R. M. 2010b. Growth and maturation: Interactions and sources of variation. In *Human Variation from the Laboratory to the Field*, eds. C. G. N. Mascie-Taylor, A. Yasukouchi, and S. Ulijaszek, 199–218. Boca Raton: CRC Press, Taylor & Francis Group.

Malina, R. M. 2011. Skeletal age and age verification in youth sport. *Sports Med* 41:925–47.

Malina, R. M. 2014. Top 10 research questions related to growth and maturation of relevance to physical activity, performance, and fitness. *Res Q Exerc Sport* 85:157–73.

Malina, R. M., A. D. G. Baxter-Jones, N. Armstrong et al. 2013a. Role of intensive training in the growth and maturation of artistic gymnastics. *Sports Med* 43:783–802.

Malina, R. M., C. Bouchard, and O. Bar-Or. 2004. *Growth, Maturation, and Physical Activity* (2nd Ed.), Champaign, IL: Human Kinetics.

Malina, R. M., Bouchard, C., and Beunen, G. 1988. Human growth: Selected aspects of current research on well-nourished children. *Ann Rev Anthropol* 17:187–219.

Malina, R. M., A. C. Chow, S. A. Czerwinski, and W. C. Chumlea. 2016. Validation of maturity offset in the Fels Longitudinal Study. *Pediate Exerc Sci* 28:433–55.

Malina, R. M., M. J. Coelho e Silva, and A. J. Figueiredo. 2013b. Growth and maturity status of youth players. In *Science and Soccer: Developing Elite Performers* (3rd Ed.), ed. A. M. Williams, 307–33. Abington: Routledge.

Malina, R. M. and C. A. Geithner. 1993. Background in sport, growth status, and growth rate of Junior Olympic Divers. In *U.S. Diving Sport Science Seminar 1993, Proceedings*, eds. R. M. Malina and J. L. Gabriel, 26–35. Indianapolis: United States Diving.

Malina, R. M. and C. A. Geithner. 2011. Body composition of young athletes. *Am J Lifestyle Med* 5:262–78.

Malina, R. M., E. Howley, and B. Gutin. 2007a. *Body mass and composition*. Report prepared for the Youth Health Subcommittee. Physical Activity Guidelines Advisory Committee.

Malina, R. M., Z. Ignasiak, K. Rożek et al. 2011. Growth, maturity and functional characteristics of female athletes 11–15 years of age. *Hum Move* 12:31–40.

Malina, R. M. and P. T. Katzmarzyk. 1999. Validity of the body mass index as an indicator of the risk and presence of overweight in adolescents. *Am J Clin Nutr* 70:131S–6S.

Malina, R. M., P. T. Katzmarzyk, C. M. Bonci, R. C. Ryan, and R. E. Wellens. 1997b. Family size and age at menarche in athletes. *Med Sci Sports Exerc* 29:99–106.

Malina, R. M. and S. M. Kozieł. 2014a. Validation of maturity offset in a longitudinal sample of Polish boys. *J Sports Sci* 32:424–37.

Malina, R. M. and S. M. Kozieł. 2014b. Validation of maturity offset in a longitudinal sample of Polish girls. *J Sports Sci* 32:1374–82.

Malina, R. M., S. Kozieł, and T. Bielicki. 1999. Variation in subcutaneous adipose tissue distribution associated with age, sex, and maturation. *Am J Hum Biol* 11:189–200.

Malina, R. M. and A. D. Rogol. 2011. Sport training and the growth and pubertal maturation of young athletes. *Pediatr Endoc Rev* 9:441–55.

Malina, R. M., A. D. Rogol, S. P. Cumming, M. J. Coelho e Silva, and A. J. Figueiredo. 2015. Biological maturation of youth athletes: Assessment and implications. *Br J Sports Med* 49:852–9.

Malina, R. M., R. C. Ryan, and C. M. Bonci. 1994. Age at menarche in athletes and their mothers and sisters. *Ann Hum Biol* 21:417–22.

Malina, R. M., B. Woynarowska, T. Bielicki et al. 1997c. Prospective and retrospective longitudinal studies of the growth, maturation, and fitness of Polish youth active in sport. *Int J Sports Med* 18(Suppl 3):S179–85.

Märker, K. 1979. Zur Menarche von Sportlerinnen nach merhrjährigem in Training in Kindersalter. *Med u Sport* 19:329–32.

Matthias, E. 1916. *Der Einfluss der Leibesübungen auf das Körperwachstum im Entwicklungsalter.* Zurich: Rascher.

Meleski, B. W. and R. M. Malina. 1985. Changes in body composition and physique of elite university-level swimmers during a competitive season. *J Sports Sci* 3:33–40.

Merzenich, H., H. Boeing, and J. Wahrendorf. 1993. Dietary fat and sports activity as determinants for age at menarche. *Am J Epidemiol* 138:217–24.

Mirwald, R. L. and D. A. Bailey. 1986. *Maximal Aerobic Power.* London, Ontario: Sports Dynamics.

Mirwald, R. L., A. D. G. Baxter-Jones, D. A. Bailey, and G. P. Beunen. 2002. An assessment of maturity from anthropometric measurements. *Med Sci Sports Exerc* 34:689–94.

Moisan, J., F. Meyer, and S. Gingras. 1990. A nested case-control study of the correlates of early menarche. *Am J Epidemiol* 132:953–61.

Moisan, J., F. Meyer, and S. Gingras. 1991. Leisure physical activity and age at menarche. *Med Sci Sports Exerc* 23:1170–5.

Morris, F. L., G. A. Naughton, J. L. Gibbs, J. S. Carlson, and J. D. Wark. 1997. Prospective ten-month exercise intervention in premenarcheal girls: Positive effects on bone and lean mass. *J Bone Min Res* 12:1453–62.

Mundt, C. A., A. D. G. Baxter-Jones, S. J. Whiting, D. A. Bailey, R. A. Faulkner, and R. L. Mirwald. 2006. Relationships of activity and sugar drink intake on fat mass development in youths. *Med Sci Sports Exerc* 38:1245–54.

Nickols-Richardson, S. M., P. J. O'Connor, S. A. Shapses, and R. D. Lewis. 1999. Longitudinal bone mineral density changes in female child artistic gymnasts. *J Bone Min Res* 14:994–1002.

Novotný, V. 1981. Veränderungen des Knochenalters im Verlauf einer mehrjährigen sportlichen Belastung. *Med u Sport* 21:44–7.

Nurmi-Lawton, J. A., A. D. Baxter-Jones, R. L. Mirwald et al. 2004. Evidence of sustained skeletal benefits from impact-loading exercise in young females: A 3-year longitudinal study. *J Bone Min Res* 19:314–22.

Olmedillas, H., A. González-Agüero, L. A. Moreno, J. A. Casajús, and G. Vicente-Rodriguez. 2011. Bone related health status in adolescent cyclists. *PLoS One* 6:e24841.

Pařizkova, J. 1970. Longitudinal study of the relationship between body composition and anthropometric characteristics in boys during growth and development. *Glasnik Antropoloskog Drustva Jugoslavije* 7:33–8.

Pařizkova, J. 1974. Particularities of lean body mass and fat development in growing boys as related to their motor activity. *Acta Paediatr Belg* 28(Suppl):233–44.

Pařizkova, J. 1976. Growth and growth velocity of lean body mass and fat in adolescent boys. *Pediatr Res* 10:647–50.

Pařizkova, J. 1977. *Body Fat and Physical Fitness*. The Hague: Martinus Nijhoff.

Physical Activity Guidelines Committee. 2008. *Physical Activity Guidelines Advisory Committee Report 2008, Part G, Section 9: Youth, G-1-G-9–33*. Washington, D.C.: Department of Health and Human Services.

Quiterio, A. L., E. A. Canero, F. M. Baptista, and L. B. Sardinha. 2011. Skeletal mass in adolescent male athletes and nonathletes: Relationships with high-impact sports. *J Str Cond Res* 25:3439–47.

Rarick, G. L. 1960. Exercise and growth. In *Science and Medicine of Exercise and Sports*, ed. W. R. Johnson, 440–65. New York: Harper.

Ridley, K., B. E. Ainsworth, and S. Olds. 2008. Development of a compendium of energy expenditures for youth. *Int J Beh Nutr Phys Act* 5:45–52.

Ridley, K. and T. S. Olds. 2008. Assigning energy costs to activities in children: A review and synthesis. *Med Sci Sports Exerc* 40:1439–46.

Roemmich, J. N. and W. E. Sinning. 1997. Weight loss and wrestling training: Effects on nutrition, growth, maturation, body composition, and strength. *J Appl Physiol* 82:1751–9.

Rowe, F. A. 1933. Growth comparison of athletes and non-athletes. *Res Q* 4:108–16.

Saris, W. H. M., J. W. H. Elvers, M. A. van't Hof, and R. A. Binkhorst. 1986. Changes in physical activity of children aged 6 to 12 years. In *Children and Exercise XII*, eds. J. Rutenfranz, R. Mocellin, and F. Klimt, 121–30. Champaign, IL: Human Kinetics.

Schwartz, L., R. H. Britten, and L. R. Thompson. 1928. *Studies in Physical Development and Posture*. Public Health Bulletin No. 179. Washington, D.C.: Government Printing Office.

Shephard, R. J. 1982. *Physical Activity and Growth*. St. Louis: Mosby.

Šprynarova, S. 1974. Longitudinal study of the influence of different physical activity programs on functional capacity of the boys from 11 to 18 years. *Acta Paediatr Belg* 28(Suppl):204–13.

Šprynarova, S. 1987. The influence of training on physical and functional growth before, during and after puberty. *Eur J Appl Physiol* 56:719–24.

Stager, J. M., J. K. Wigglesworth, and L. K. Hatler. 1990. Interpreting the relationship between age of menarche and prepubertal training. *Med Sci Sports Exerc* 22:54–8.

Steinhaus, A. H. 1933. Chronic effects of exercise. *Physiol Rev* 13:103–47.

Strong, W. B., R. M. Malina, C. J. R. Blimkie et al. 2005. Evidence based physical activity for school youth. *J Pediatr* 146:732–7.

Theintz, G. E., H. Howald, U. Weiss, and P. C. Sizonenko. 1993. Evidence for a reduction of growth potential in adolescent female gymnasts. *J Pediatr* 122:306–13.

Todd, T. W. 1937. *Atlas of Skeletal Maturation*. St. Louis: Mosby.

Tofler, I. R., B. K. Stryer, L. J. Micheli, and L. R. Herman. 1996. Physical and emotional problems of elite female gymnasts. *New Eng J Med* 335:281–3.

Ulbrich, J. 1971. Individual variants of physical fitness in boys from the age of 11 up to maturity and their selection for sports activities. *Medicina dello Sport* 24:118–36.

Vadocz, E. A., S. R. Siegel, and R. M. Malina. 2002. Age at menarche in competitive figure skaters: Variation by competency and discipline. *J Sports Sci* 20:93–100.

Von Döbeln, W. and B. O. Eriksson. 1972. Physical training, maximal oxygen uptake and dimensions of the oxygen transporting and metabolizing organs in boys 11–13 years of age. *Acta Paediatr Scand* 61:653–60.

Warden, S. J., S. M. Mantila Roosa, M. E. Kersh et al. 2014. Physical activity when young provides lifelong benefits to cortical bone size and strength in men. *Proc Nat Acad Sci* 111:5337–42.

Warren, M. P. 1980. The effect of exercise on pubertal progression and reproductive function in girls. *J Clin Endocrinol Metab* 51:1150–7.

Watson, R. C. 1975. Bone growth and physical activity in young males. In *International Conference on Bone Mineral Measurement*, ed. R. B. Mazess, 380–6. U.S. Department of Health, Education and Welfare, DHEW Publication No. (NIH) 75-683.

White House Conference on Child Health and Protection. 1932. *Growth and Development of the Child. Part I. General Considerations; Part IV. Appraisement of the Child.* New York: Century Company.

Zanker, C. L., L. Gannon, C. B. Cooke, K. L. Gee, B. Oldroyd, and J. G. Truscott. 2003. Differences in bone density, body composition, physical activity, and diet between child gymnasts and untrained children 7–8 years of age. *J Bone Min Res* 18:1043–50.

Ziemilska, A. 1981. *Wpływ intensywnego treningu gimnastycznego na rozwój somatyczny i dojrzewanie dzieci.* Warsaw: Akademia Wychowania Fizycznego.

6 Anthropometry in Physical Performance and Health

Arthur Stewart and Tim Ackland

CONTENTS

6.1 INTRODUCTION AND DEFINITIONS

Anthropometry is defined as "the scientific procedures and processes of acquiring surface anatomical dimensional measurements such as lengths, breadths, girths and skinfolds of the human body by means of specialist equipment" (Stewart 2010). This approach has altered little if at all over the last hundred years, and even in ancient Greece, we hear of systematic body measurement in order to produce statues that were appropriately sized to real individuals. Sculptors would have appreciated that this approach demands painstaking detail, adherence to best practice, and diligence in reducing errors, and few scientists would argue with this. Anthropometry sits within the field of kinanthropometry—"the academic discipline which involves the use of anthropometric measures in relation to other scientific parameters and/or thematic areas such as human movement, physiology or applied health sciences" (Stewart 2010). However, one of the issues for kinanthropometry, particularly in its applications for physical activity and sport, is that the tools have not advanced in parallel with those of other disciplines such as sports physiology and biomechanics. Researchers, therefore, may be persuaded to think that its relevance is reducing in a contemporary research context. Indeed, for publications in two main research journals, the prevalence of anthropometry as central to research (estimated from key word searches using similar terms) appears to have peaked a generation ago (Olds 2004). But perhaps kinanthropometry is on the verge of a renaissance for two reasons. First, the field has now largely embraced tightly defined standard procedures and error control, the lack of which previously diminished its ability to convince a research community becoming accustomed to more sophisticated methods. Second, recent advances in digital anthropometry, using three-dimensional (3D) body scanning, enable an unprecedented range of new measurement possibilities. These new measures can augment traditional anthropometry, and the combination of manual and digital anthropometry may allow new research questions to be addressed.

6.2 OVERVIEW OF THE PHYSICAL BASES OF MEASUREMENT

6.2.1 SKINFOLDS

The skinfold is a manually held, compressed layer of subcutaneous adipose tissue (SAT) plus skin. Most calipers seek to provide a constant compressive force of $10 \text{ g} \cdot \text{mm}^{-2}$ at all jaw opening distances. While validated against other measurements for fat quantity, several limitations have come to light from research evidence that are worthy of note. First, adipose tissue and the fat within it are compressible with a small applied force, and the compressibility curve of skinfolds varies both within and between individuals. This underscores the importance of rigor when locating skinfold sites (Hume and Marfell-Jones 2008), caliper orientation and other aspects of technique (Stewart et al. 2011a), and the time of compression (Himes et al. 1979). Different quantities of connective tissue structures embed the adipose tissue, meaning that skinfolds of a given magnitude represent a highly variable quantity of fat between individuals.

6.2.2 GIRTHS

Girths represent curvilinear distances around a body segment. As with skinfolds, their measured value will differ markedly if the measurement is made in a slightly different location (Daniell et al. 2010). Referred to as circumferences, they are not strictly circular but rather, irregular and at best elliptical, with the extent of noncircularity varying regionally and by overall body size. Empirical logic suggests girths may also be affected by hydration status, if significant water loss occurs from fluid compartments, and other circulatory responses do not compensate. In the case of thigh girth, for example, glycogen together with its bound water molecules can increase the girth value, if exercise or dietary intervention has perturbed levels prior to measurement. Metal tapes used to measure girths should not compress the skin surface, and close inspection of the girth should reveal no indentation of the skin (Stewart et al. 2011a). In practice, this is straightforward if the anthropometrist's fingers are used to pin the tape against the skin surface without compressing it. Girths should also span concavities—such as the lower back when measuring the waist. This does make girths measured by tape shorter than the equivalent surface distance—this may be an important distinction with 3D scanning, which generally identifies the surface distance. Tapes that are made of cloth may stretch and generally lack sufficient rigidity for easy measurement, and all tapes should have a stub beyond the zero value, which can be held by the measurer.

6.2.3 SEGMENT LENGTHS, SKELETAL BREADTHS, AND ANATOMICAL HEIGHTS

Linear distances between points on the body surface, or from the standing or sitting surface to key landmarks, provide valuable information of the body's proportions. The approach requires that landmarks can be located visually and in a systematic manner. The majority of landmarks are identified from the underlying skeletal structure, such as the anterior superior iliac spine (ASIS) and acromiale. Others are identified from soft tissue structures, such as the omphalion (midpoint of the naval) and tragion (the notch structure in the outer ear). Bony landmarks require palpation and it is paramount that these are marked once the skin has returned to its "resting orientation." In addition, tight clothing being moved to facilitate the marking may displace the skin surface by several centimeters, so care is required to ensure such marks are made appropriately. Segment lengths and heights are usually measured using a segmometer, large sliding caliper, or traditional rod anthropometer. Anatomical heights are best measured to an anthropometric box, rather than the floor, for ease of measurement. Care is required when placing the instrument on the landmarks to ensure correct alignment, to check for slippage, and to avoid compression of the skin. For skeletal breadths, compression of the overlying tissue is required, demanding a firm grip so the soft tissue contributes only minimally to the recorded measurements. This means traditional anthropometric measurements are not compatible with 3D scanning, in which breathing and postural artifacts can affect some measurements.

6.2.4 VOLUMES AND AREAS

Three-dimensional photonic scanning (3DPS) creates a digital shell of the body that can be interrogated for such measurements as surface distance, cross-sectional area, surface area, and segmental and total volumes. Certain mathematical assumptions are necessary with the different approaches to geometric calculations for body shape. Methods for acquiring scans vary, but typical "booth" scanners have footprints to guide participants when orienting themselves appropriately. With portable scanners, it is useful to capture a horizontal floor section that can be used to locate and rotate an "xyz positioning tool," which can then describe all landmarks and subsequent measurements in a standardized way. Identifying areas and segmental volumes vary by software options, with more primitive versions constraining subanalyses to orthogonal axes. More sophisticated software can depict the body at any angle by defining a slice plane based on a minimum of three points. So, for example, to replicate the waist girth or area, a landmark will be placed onto the torso and positioned to comply with the required waist protocol (Stewart et al. 2010). With more advanced software, tilting the waist plane is possible so that it could be made perpendicular to the torso, and thus comply with the minimum waist as identified by the International Society for the Advancement of Kinanthropometry (ISAK).

6.3 SEMINAL CONTRIBUTIONS TO THE FIELD OF KINANTHROPOMETRY

6.3.1 MATIEGKA'S ANATOMICAL PREDICTION OF BODY COMPOSITION

The first systematic body composition study was in 1921, when Jindrich Matiegka developed a validated method of quantifying bone, muscle, and adipose tissue, together with residual mass using a geometric anthropometric approach (Matiegka 1921). He applied this to quantify tissue components among different professional groups, including barbers, blacksmiths, hairdressers, and gymnastics instructors. Although his imperative was to examine the capacity of the body for physical work, which was an important consideration in the aftermath of World War I, Matiegka's approach spearheaded many other research efforts in body composition using anthropometry.

In the 1980s, our understanding of the anatomical model championed by Matiegka was considerably advanced with the advent of the Brussels Cadaver Study. This project involved the full anatomical dissection of 25 cadavers, with the separate tissue compartments fully dissected and weighed. The magnitude of this effort was enormous and perhaps only truly appreciated by those who have undertaken whole body dissections. The multiple anthropometric measurements made on the cadavers greatly enhanced our understanding of the nature of the skinfold (Clarys et al. 1987) and enabled the estimation of muscle mass (Martin et al. 1990) and skeletal mass (Drinkwater and Ross 1980).

6.3.2 LINDSAY CARTER: SOMATOTYPE, CRITICAL SKINFOLD ZONE, AND MORE

J.E. Lindsay Carter is perhaps best recognized as the protagonist of the Heath–Carter somatotype method in 1967. This method effectively brought the physique analysis schema, collectively referred to as "the somatotype," into a convincing and utilitarian process, which rated physique according to degrees of adiposity, musculoskeletal robustness, and linearity. This concept was to prove more popular than any before or since, partly because it enabled anthropometrists with a basic training in 10 measurements to become somatotype raters. Later, the somatotype concept was extended to provide reference ranges for a large number of different sporting groups, children, the elderly, and those of varying ethnicity (Carter and Heath 1990).

During the Olympic Games in Mexico City in 1968 and Montreal in 1976, Dr. Carter was instrumental in conducting systematic surveys of the Olympic athletes, reporting somatotypes and a range of other anatomical measurements. These landmark surveys would become some of the largest measurement endeavors ever undertaken, assessing nearly 2000 individuals in total. The breadth and depth of this athletic sample was unprecedented and is not likely to be repeated, due to greater logistical and security challenges facing measurers at public events. Dr. Carter's data led him to espouse a "critical skinfold zone," which identified the optimal and critical levels of skinfolds observed in athletes. This he related, subsequently, to a simple biomechanical model, first by suggesting that the human body comprises "productive mass," which contributes to movement (muscles, bone, nerve tissue, blood, and essential regulatory organs), and "ballast" (excess fat), which adds to the cost of movement (Carter 1985). Such an approach, while differing from contemporary understanding of adipose tissue as an endocrine organ (Kershaw and Flier 2004), was based on a very large number of observations that have been replicated by others since, and represents the biomechanical imperatives that continue to inform conditioning approaches in sport.

6.3.3 DEVELOPMENT OF VALIDATED PREDICTION EQUATIONS FOR BODY COMPOSITION

Over 100 prediction equations exist for adults, and specific subgroups by ethnicity, age, athletic status, or medical condition. These use skinfold values and are modeled (e.g., using linear, logarithmic, or quadratic equations) to predict fat as determined by another method, which has historically been underwater weighing. Some of the early generalized equations from the 1970s had very limited accuracy (standard error of the estimate ~5% fat, as determined by underwater weighing). In other words, if a person was measured at 15% fat, then the measurer could only be 68% confident of the true value falling between 10% and 20% fat, or 95% confident of the actual value falling between 5% and 25% fat. Furthermore, this fails to consider the possibility that the reference method itself may not be accurate, as Adams et al. (1982) demonstrated for underwater weighing in Canadian football players.

Sinning et al. (1985) revealed that the vast majority of generalized fat prediction equations were of very limited use for assessing athletes because they have less fat and distribute it differently from nonathletes. Furthermore, the reference methods often required unsupportable assumptions such as the constant density of the fat-free mass (Martin et al. 1986). Most equations in common use during the latter part of the twentieth century were of unacceptable accuracy for use with athletes, except for equations by Jackson and Pollock (1978) and Jackson et al. (1980). Crucially, these equations were validated as part of the original study, unlike those of Durnin and Womersley (1974), which by comparison, systematically overestimated fatness. This may be due, in part, to differences in the precise technique—descriptions of which left room for variable interpretation. In addition, Lohman (1992) observed that systematic differences of 3%–4% fat were obtained using different types of caliper.

Lohman had previously developed a robust procedure for cross-validation of equations (Lohman 1992). This outlined several key principles, including reporting standard errors of the estimate (SEE), total error (TE) = $[\Sigma(\text{reference method fat mass} - \text{predicted fat mass})^2/n]$, where n is the number of participants, and fitting curvilinear lines to data. Perhaps more than any other individual, Lohman shaped the progress of kinanthropometry by this approach, together with steps toward standardization of technique, which led to the *Anthropometric Standardization Reference Manual* (Lohman et al. 1988). He also recognized that too many researchers were developing new equations, many of which were no better than existing ones. As a result, Lohman recommended combining data from different studies, altering intercepts from existing equations, and only publishing new equations if they outperformed existing ones (Lohman 1992).

One study that did fulfil these criteria was that of Stewart and Hannan (2000) who predicted fat mass and fat-free mass from skinfolds in 106 male athletes from a wide variety of sports. The authors used dual x-ray absorptiometry (DXA) as the reference method and achieved a standard error of the estimate of 1.7 kg. This study utilized a stepwise regression method to select the optimal skinfolds from a total of 19 sites across different body regions, and concluded that appropriate skinfold selection is a crucial element in the accuracy of a prediction equation for a specific population. Using a random subsample of 82 to develop the equation and the remaining 24 to validate it, the following equation was produced:

$$\text{Fat mass (g)} = 331.5 \text{ (abdominal)} + 356.2 \text{ (thigh)} + 111.9M - 9108$$
$$(R^2 = 0.81; \text{SEE} = 1732 \text{ g}; \text{TE} = 2.9\%, P < 0.001),$$

where M is body mass in kg; skinfolds in mm.

With increased heterogeneity in a sample, there is greater scope for generalization of an equation, but this leads to poorer accuracy (i.e., a greater standard error). Researchers need to balance the capability for an equation to apply to other groups, with a low error. However, equations with a low SEE may still not be effective for fat prediction; it is also important to consider TE.

More recently, researchers have had access to four-compartment reference methods that separately divide the fat-free mass into bone mineral, water, and other tissue. These components represent the best-available criterion against which anthropometric predictions can be made, and contribute more valid equations for use in kinanthropometry. However, the costs for such investigations may limit the likelihood of them being repeated elsewhere. One example of excellent practice is the work of Evans et al. (2005) who studied collegiate athletes of both sexes and mixed ethnicity. Their resulting equation thus had separate gender and ethnicity terms in the regression, and yielded a prediction of body fat with a TE of 3.8%—which is lower than the equations from Jackson and Pollock (1978) and Jackson et al. (1980) developed using underwater weighing alone. Interestingly, the final regression that used only three skinfolds (abdominal, thigh, and triceps) had comparable accuracy as the one involving seven sites.

6.3.4 STANDARDIZATION OF ANTHROPOMETRY AND EMERGENCE OF INTERNATIONAL SOCIETY FOR THE ADVANCEMENT OF KINANTHROPOMETRY

Historically, routine anthropometric measurements have been employed in the fields of nutrition, medicine, sports, and ergonomics. Their use in diverse academic disciplines throughout multiple countries has led inevitably to different approaches, nomenclature, and practices, which represented a barrier to progress in the fields of application.

ISAK was founded in Glasgow, United Kingdom in 1986 at a conference of interested practitioners in the field, and members of the previous international working group in kinanthropometry, seeking to standardize practice. In the same year, a consensus conference in Virginia, USA sought to do the same. Both were motivated by the same drivers—the need for better standardization in measurement description, protocols and practice, and accuracy. Both were ultimately successful in achieving these aims, although their approaches differed. In the United States during the 1980s, the strong research base for clinical body composition covered a range of technologies, and anthropometry took its place alongside them. The standardization manual (Lohman et al. 1988) was a culmination of previous research and was, therefore, less didactic and constraining than the ISAK scheme, which was influenced more by the disciplines of sport, exercise science, and human biology. By contrast, ISAK's approach was to introduce a teaching and practice structure, which was subsequently manifest in a new qualifications scheme in 1996. It was heavily influenced by practitioners at the Australian Institute of Sport, with the first steps toward its definitive manual being Chapter 2 of the *Anthropometrica* book (Norton and Olds 1996), which systematically detailed protocols and applications of anthropometric measures in an accessible and unprecedented way. Comparing these two approaches reveals significant differences in perspective. The Lohman et al. (1988) manual provides a rich literature, strong evidence base, and relevant clinical detail, for instance, in the different contribution of various superficial fat depots to health risk (p. 55). However, it suggests that the location of skinfold sites need not be marked on the participant as a general rule, making exceptions for intercaliper differences, and the combination of skinfolds with girths to estimate limb cross-sectional areas. This contrasts with the strict adherence to the protocol for marking landmarks using the ISAK method for skinfolds, which considers it fundamental to anthropometric measurement. Moreover, the actual marking itself defines the orientation and precise alignment of the index finder prior to the fold being raised.

Perhaps the main reason for increased popularity of the ISAK approach is not its stance on landmarks, but the adoption of a four-level hierarchy of practitioner licencing, based on competence assessed by a practical exam. Crucially, ISAK requires that all measurers be licenced, even the examiners, who are required to examine one another's measurements. Such a comparison requires all measurers to pass error control targets in terms of reproducibility in a standardized setting. This includes intermeasurer as well as intrameasurer reliability, and represents a great advance for the methodology. While other schemes might be able to demonstrate reproducibility within a single laboratory, the ISAK protocols provide an indication of the comparability with others from various laboratory settings. Indeed, where technique, instruments, and protocols vary, there will inevitably be considerable interlaboratory variability, discussion of which has been conspicuously absent from the publication record. In contrast, adhering rigidly to the same protocol and quantifying error enables data to be pooled between laboratories with more confidence, and reference ranges to be constructed. ISAK has also championed the adoption of using raw data scores as opposed to conversion into % fat values, made possible only by strict protocol definitions and quality assurance of individual measures. In addition, the need for practitioners to have a measurement licence has fostered the automatic reskilling of practitioners, and enabled a forum for scrutiny and the practice of protocols and technique. Such scrutiny and feedback resulted in small but significant changes to the teaching manual, now in its third revision (Stewart et al. 2011a). This manual has been translated into several languages for use across the globe. Even in the United States where body composition research has been strongest, and the Lohman et al. (1988) manual has received widespread acclaim and usage, ISAK as a concept is being adopted, albeit more slowly than elsewhere in the world. The ISAK approach is not the only way of performing manual anthropometric measurements, but it continues to flourish, and is used more than any other protocol with elite athletes (Meyer et al. 2013).

6.3.5 Advent of Three-Dimensional Photonic Scanning

The advent of 3DPS has enriched the tools available for describing the body. Referred to in some circles as "digital anthropometry," 3DPS has made a vast contribution to body measurement. It has the capability for measurements, which include total volume, segmental volume, curved surface distances, direct distances, perpendicular planar distances, surface areas, and cross-sectional areas. Not only have these become valuable quantities in their own right, they have informed novel approaches to quantifying the body that are not possible with traditional anthropometry. The term "scanning" is used by medicine and industry to acquire a vast array of measurements. In humans, 3DPS involves approaches to acquiring the body shape, which most commonly include structured light, class 1 lasers, and more recently, depth cameras.

Structured light is projected onto the body to produce patterns distorted by the surface contour. Similarly, class 1 (eye-safe) lasers can project onto the body and for both, digital cameras placed around the body detect the deformed light stripe against a 3D reference grid, and individual points are calculated via triangulation. More complex approaches, such as stereo photogrammetry and others, are necessary when using handheld scanners that are not constrained to horizontal array beams.

Depth cameras, by contrast, acquire a single image and project an infrared speckle pattern onto the participant, while the sensor captures its deformation. This deformation, together with accurate distance sensing and RGB color, enables a 3D image to be acquired. For single depth cameras, software approaches include libraries of images to estimate the "blind side" data obscured from view. As yet, depth cameras lack the resolution and accuracy of structured light and laser scanners, although the technology is rapidly developing.

Once the primary measurement data are obtained in a point cloud, subsequent processing involving hole-filling and smoothing is done either manually or automatically via system software. In the case of handheld scanners, images require additional steps to register separate scan fragments, and then fuse them into a single object. Analysis can be performed either by the user identifying specific measurement locations, or from locations that are automatically detected from the shape itself. These "primary" landmarks frequently include the vertex, axilla, and crotch and may be used to generate secondary landmarks where specific measurements are made. Landmarks may also be applied via affixed reflective dots or triangles on the skin surface. Alternatively, landmarks may be created digitally once the 3D scan has been rendered into an object file. Increasingly, computing approaches can derive landmarks automatically from edge detection or shape curvature algorithms with minimum user involvement. Lastly, there is also a case for using visible landmarks, such as the Adam's apple, axillary fold, and navel, together with maxima and minima positions to describe the body. Some measurements are required to be made when posturally constrained, for example, in disabled participants, or for ergonomic applications. Maximum and minimum values can contribute to our knowledge of measurement variability in humans, for example, at the waist (Stewart et al. 2010).

Greater resolution of 3DPS systems means increasingly dense meshes to describe the body shape, at the expense of increasing file size. For example, early fixed-position industrial scanners developed for the clothing industry toward the end of the 1990s acquired about 200,000 points, and subsequent refinement of scanners increased this three- or fourfold. A typical adult scan from a Hamamatsu BLS 9036 (Hamamatsu Photonics, Hamamatsu, Japan) would have ~700,000 vertices and a file size of 13 MB. In contrast, a full body scan acquired by the portable Artec L scanner (Artec Group, Luxembourg) would have up to 20 million vertices with a corresponding file size of 500 MB.

In conventional anthropometry, there have been attempts to standardize practice for well over a century, illustrating a genealogy of protocols used in sports science, clothing, ergonomics, and health (Kupke and Olds 2008). Their work continues this process into the realm of 3D scanning, and identifies the need for generalized language, dimensional syntax, and the means to describe anthropometric functions. A project-specific landmarking manual (Olds et al. 2004) provides better definitions and more information than other standards (Robinette et al. 2002; BSI 2010), yet the disparity in what constitutes a standard definition underscores the diversity of approach in this new and expanding field. Efforts to standardize 3DPS are still limited by the relatively few scanning facilities for research, together with the rapid advancement of this technology. However, there is a burgeoning interest in professional meetings for 3DPS and, with the establishment of professional networks, the steps to formalize and standardize practice are imminent.

Total body volume enables the calculation of body density, and thus an estimate of % fat via the two-compartment method. Important validation work was carried out by Wang et al. (2006), with a C9036 laser scanner (Hamamatsu Photonics, Hamamatsu, Japan) compared to underwater weighing and anthropometry, using both a mannequin and human samples with a wide age range (6–83 years). Significantly larger body volumes with scanning were found compared with underwater weighing. This may be attributable to the difficulty in exhaling completely while standing upright in the scanning pose, the variable density of the fat-free mass in the sample, or the possibility that excess body hair causes the scanner to identify a false surface in some instances. The use of the mannequin to compare manual girths and those assessed by 3DPS revealed that manual anthropometry yielded mean values that were 0.87% greater at the waist and 0.55% greater at the hip, but 0.66% lower at the thigh. This difference is within the measurement error anticipated from experienced anthropometrists and may reflect minor orientation or positional differences in measurement. This should give confidence in the capability of 3DPS to extract valid measurements. However, like conventional anthropometry, hip girths and female chest girths will always be made over clothing, and the use of suitable form-fitting apparel is essential, provided it does not compress the body shape appreciably.

While 3D scanning will never be able to replace conventional skinfolds and skeletal breadths (due to the compression required to locate the bony landmarks), it offers a range of measurement possibilities that augment and enhance conventional anthropometry. First, there is the capability for retrospective measurement of a scan after a participant has left the laboratory, which can be subsequently interrogated for data—an approach used in telemedicine in remote regions of the world for medical data and investigations. Second, there is the opportunity for scan data to be sent elsewhere for analysis, using bespoke software for specialist purposes. Third, there is the opportunity to create a template-based approach for locating other measurements (e.g., skinfolds or ultrasound fat measurements) in xyz space in a composite model. Lastly, 3DPS allows the possibility of visualization, for instance, in body image assessment or somatotyping (Olds et al. 2013), which may extend to novel interfaces with interactive capabilities, rapid prototyping, and the construction of figurines to depict individuals or averaged shapes of groups. Such exciting new terrain will undoubtedly extend the applications of anthropometry into uncharted territory.

6.3.6 INTERNATIONAL OLYMPIC COMMITTEE AD HOC WORKING GROUP ON BODY COMPOSITION, HEALTH, AND PERFORMANCE

This working party met from 2010 to 2013 to address concerns related to the health and performance of athletes who attempt to modify their body composition using extreme and sometimes dangerous methods. This problem was of special concern for weight-sensitive sports, where athletes are required to make a weight category, or are judged on aesthetic criteria, or where body composition markedly affects performance. The group reviewed literature, conducted research, and surveyed scientists, coaches, and health professionals before disseminating their findings. Specifically, the aims and resulting outputs of this working party were as follows:

- To identify medical problems due to unhealthy practices in sport leading to extremes of underweight, weight reduction, and dehydration—see Sundgot-Borgen et al. (2013)
- To identify research needs in body composition, health, and performance—see Ackland et al. (2012); Meyer et al. (2013); Müller et al. (2013a,b, 2016)
- To identify current practice for body composition assessment globally—see Meyer et al. (2013)
- To develop suggestions for practical strategies capable of solving body composition and underweight problems in sports—see Müller et al. (2009)
- To establish, if practicable, an optimum body composition and/or minimum weight values for healthy competition in sports—see Sundgot-Borgen et al. (2013)

One of the important advances led by this group has been the development of an accurate and repeatable method for sampling the SAT layer using ultrasound (Müller et al. 2016). The standard methodology has been published, together with data on accuracy and repeatability, so now the group is completing a multicenter trial to assess inter- and intratester reliability and to compare ultrasound results with DXA, skinfolds, and a multicomponent model.

The ultrasound technique provides an accurate measure of the depth of the uncompressed SAT at several sites on the body surface. For several participants with extremely low fat content, measured during the multicenter trial, results were obtained that challenged conventional understanding relating to the fat content of skinfolds. One Caucasian athlete (soccer) with a skinfold total across the eight ISAK sites of 31.9 mm, had an uncompressed total fat depth of just 6.0 mm—only 19% of the skinfold total. One Afro-Caribbean athlete (track and field) whose skinfold total was 36.9 mm, had just 3.8 mm of total fat depth—only 10% of the skinfold total. Strikingly, significant connective tissue was apparent in the images of both, but more so in the track and field athlete. Both participants were apparently healthy and hydrated at the time of measurement. While these results require further replication in other centers, they challenge the concept of a minimum skinfold total for a certain amount of fatness in athletes, and cast doubt on the value of skinfolds to identify fat in extremely lean individuals.

6.4 ERROR CONTROL IN ANTHROPOMETRY

Error in anthropometric measurement is inevitable. It relates both to the acquisition of the measurement, where equipment calibration, site location, and technique are important, as well as the biological error, more correctly termed "biovariability," in which the true value changes over time. Biovariability relates to diurnal variation, hydration levels, temperature, and other metabolic processes. Errors associated with repeated measurements in anthropometry are quantified by the use of repeated measurements on the same testing occasion. Clearly, if measurements are made in rapid succession, the true value should not have changed. However, in the case of skinfolds, some residual compression may remain for up to 2 min, resulting from realignment of fat lobules in adipose tissue, so retesting within this time is discouraged. When measuring a parameter for the second time, it is important that the measurer is blinded to the first measurement scores. Quantification of the error is commonly achieved by the intraclass correlation coefficient and the technical error of measurement statistics.

The intraclass correlation coefficient is a correlation between successive measurements made on the same subject by a group of measurers. Although popular, it is sensitive to the sample mean and alternatively, the technical error of measurement (TEM) statistic, either as a raw score (absolute) or expressed as a percentage of the mean value (relative), may be preferable.

The absolute TEM is calculated by the expression

$$\text{TEM} = \sqrt{\frac{\Sigma d^2}{2n}}$$

where Σd^2 is the sum of squared differences between measurements and n is the number of participants measured. The absolute TEM is multiplied by 100 and divided by the "variable average value" (overall mean of the means between measurements of each participant for the same site) to provide the relative TEM (% TEM) for each site of measurement (Perini et al. 2005).

There exists a 1%–2% diurnal variation in stature as a consequence of gravitational forces acting on compressible structures within the spine when upright (Tyrrell et al. 1985). Coupled with the body's normal eating and bowel activity, this translates to the derived body mass index (BMI) varying by about 1 kg·m^{-2} per day for a typical adult, but considerably more where dehydration is also an issue, such as for athletes of certain sports. Gravity also influences fluid components of the body in other less rigid tissues, such that posture can influence body composition measurements. Carin-Levy et al. (2008) demonstrated such a difference in standing and supine skinfold measures. This may not come as a surprise, but should be considered in certain patient groups. Extending the logic of this finding, we know remarkably little about how the plasticity of tissues under their own weight affects the comparability of standing and supine measurements using medical imaging, as well as anthropometry.

6.5 APPLICATIONS IN HEALTH

The categorization of an individual's health risk based on simple anthropometric measurements has been a ubiquitous front line for health surveillance in medicine for over half a century. While this process assists in channeling resources to where they are most required, the candidate measures used to assess body size or relative weight also have the potential to mislead. This is a direct result not only of the variability in body composition and body proportions, but also the variable susceptibility for disease between different individuals. Increasing use of clinical guidelines and pathways has forced different measurements to be made, by different individuals, at different stages of diagnostic and care pathways. Simple anthropometric measures such as stature, mass, waist, and hip girth may engender a risk that the need for training and quality control is overlooked.

It is surprising, therefore, that the diagnosis of health risk could be based on measurements made by individuals whose error control may not have been properly appraised. As discussed in Section 6.4, precise anatomical location of the measurement site is pivotally important. Skinfolds show significant variation by distance at all eight standard sites, but the magnitude and direction of the differences varied by site location (Hume and Marfell-Jones 2008). Girths, while not appearing to be critical at the forearm and calf, demonstrate critical variation at the more commonly used waist and hip locations and show slightly greater variation in females than males (Daniell et al. 2010).

Anthropometric measurements are capable of providing a full fractionation of body mass using an anatomical model based on cadaver dissection (Drinkwater and Ross 1980). This expanded the original work by Matiegka (1921), including the prediction of skeletal, muscle, fat, and residual masses. The methodology of subtracting skinfolds multiplied by *pi* from body segment girths was applied as part of this to generate a theoretical lean girth, and this approach was applied to predict falling in the elderly using calf girth (Stewart et al. 2002). However, for most health purposes, such detailed measurement is not warranted. Nevertheless, some anthropometric measurements have a valuable role to play in health surveillance for appropriate weight and metabolic risk. In many cases, they may represent the first line of defense in flagging individuals for follow-up or specific treatment—either for undernourishment or excessive fatness. They represent convenient surrogates for health, at an appropriate level of technology and cost for screening initiatives.

The question of which measures are the most appropriate is a matter of heated debate between physicians, epidemiologists, and scientists. A large array of direct measures, derived indices, or composite indices are available from anthropometry, as illustrated in Figure 6.1.

Total body fatness might be the logical objective to address the obesity research agenda, not least because obesity is defined as an excess of bodily fat. However, there is neither clear linkage between fat levels and morbidity and mortality, nor recommended reference ranges of body fat that can be generalized with confidence (Gallagher et al. 2000). The metric for defining overweight and obesity—the BMI ($mass \cdot stature^{-2}$)—does have such reference ranges, but is at odds with the fundamental definition of obesity, assuming excess weight equates to excess fat. The BMI's critics point to the misclassification of muscular individuals as overweight or obese, and the challenges of applying different cut-off values to classify different groups, while its supporters will cite that at a population level, more individuals are likely to be heavy due to an excess of fat than muscle. If the body fat content can be measured, or predicted from skinfolds, the fat-free and fat masses can be used independently to calculate separate indices. Another improvement over BMI is the mass index (Ackland et al. 2012), which is based on the cormic index ($sitting\ height \cdot stature^{-1}$) and accounts for relative leg length in its scoring. This index is used in rule setting for ski length in Olympic ski jumping.

If the focus is on metabolic health, there is clear evidence that health risk relates more to centralized fat on the torso and abdomen, rather than total fat (Bjorntorp 1997). While logic would suggest the waist circumference should thus inform us more of health risk than would the BMI, it is unable to distinguish between SAT and visceral adipose tissue (VAT) compartments. Because visceral fat is an independent predictor of mortality (Kuk et al. 2006), for two individuals with a

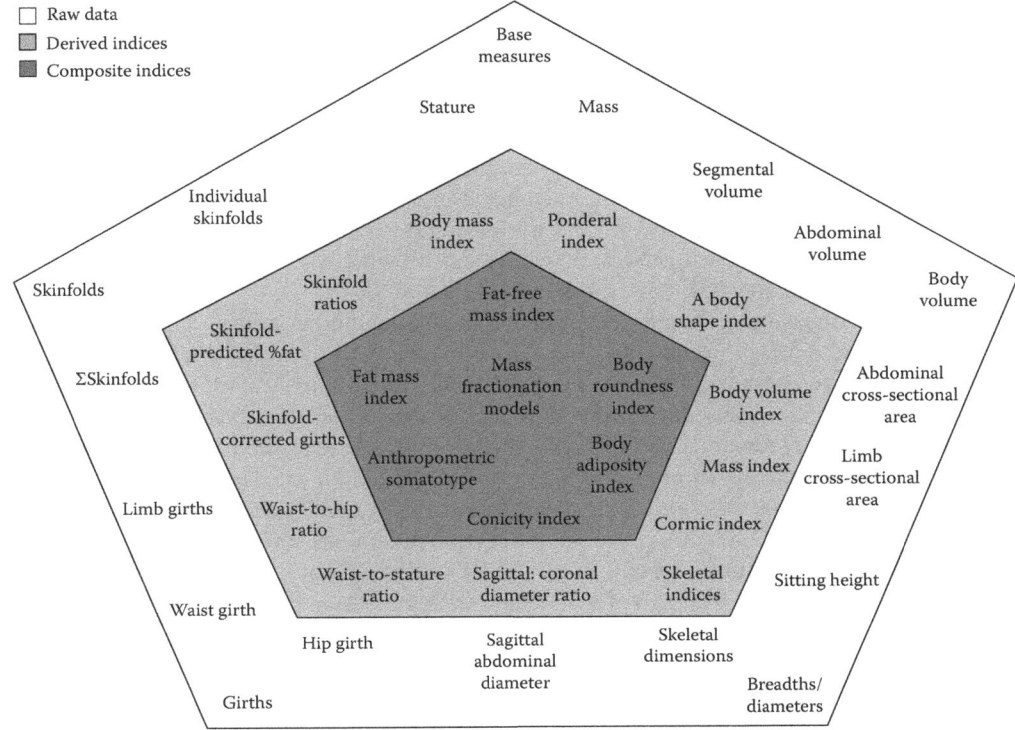

FIGURE 6.1 Schematic framework of anthropometric measurements, derived indices, and composite indices to describe anatomical factors.

similar waist girth, the one with greater visceral fat is likely to have an increased health risk relative to the other. The ratio of VAT to SAT has been well correlated to cardiometabolic risk (Kaess et al. 2012). However, expensive medical imaging technologies are required to identify visceral fat, usually involving equipment found only in hospital facilities. However, attempts to predict visceral fat using anthropometry are valuable because they have the potential to use a low-cost method to identify higher-risk individuals, who may be targeted with appropriate resources and treatment.

Relative girth (as opposed to relative weight) approaches include the well-established waist-to-hip ratio (de Koning et al. 2007) and also waist-to-stature ratio (Ho et al. 2003). While both can claim justification and are straightforward to measure, the question remains as to the likelihood of both numerator and denominator varying to a similar degree. The magnitude of the waist varies by much more than is generally appreciated even in healthy adults—approaching 12% variability in women, and 5% in men across the "waist zone" between the iliac crest and the tenth rib (Stewart et al. 2010). This not only influences the measurement value but also the accuracy of predicting visceral fat (Bosy-Westphal et al. 2009). This is due, in part, to protocol differences, but also because the shape of the visceral compartment itself varies axially and is prone to undersampling error (Thomas and Bell 2003). Waist girth has been shown to have a negative correlation with stature in a large UK sample (Wells et al. 2007), which is contrary to assumptions made in a range of anthropometric models that presume taller individuals have larger waists. The reality of using geometric models with girths is that the contained tissue is predicted using a circular model. In reality, the body is not circular in cross section, and the superficial fat depth is not uniform. Challenges to circular models have been leveled using elliptical approaches validated against MRI and have shown them to be superior to circular models (He et al. 2004). In this, both the total abdominal area and the visceral compartment area showed very strong predictions from anthropometric models.

Linear measures of skeletal dimensions have helped classify frame size and bodily proportions, but are of limited use in assessing health, because soft tissue is more influential. As such, the brachial, crural, and androgyny indices may be more valuable in identifying suitability for sports performance than health concerns. However, other linear dimensions are valuable in a health context. The sagittal abdominal diameter (SAD) at the waist section has received increasing attention over recent years. Several studies have demonstrated its association with visceral fat, and its utility in predicting an adverse metabolic profile (Valsamakis et al. 2004), and incident diabetes (Pajunen et al. 2013). While measurement standardization is essential to compare results in different studies (due to postural and breathing artifacts), as a single measure, the SAD has much in its favor, either on its own, or in combination with other measurements.

Other combined measurements have been used to derive composite indices. The conicity index (Valdez 1991) includes height, weight, and waist girth in a theoretical model of opposed truncated cones. The body adiposity index (Bergman et al. 2011) uses body height raised to the power of 1.5 and hip circumference, but subsequent work showed it was no better than BMI, waist or hip girth at predicting fatness (Freedman et al. 2012). The body roundness index considers the eccentricity of the body's height in relation to waist, and was successfully shown to relate to % fat and % VAT (Thomas et al. 2013). While this study appears very robust, its assumed circularity of the waist is a limitation, and the assumption that waist circumference should increase with stature is at odds with the aforementioned observations of Wells et al. (2007). Taken together, there are many anthropometric health indices to select from, all of which have their benefits and limitations. Although their applicability may be limited in some groups, especially athletes (Santos et al. 2015), the emergence of newer indices especially those that predict VAT is likely to supplant the overreliance on some of the more traditional indices that have been used ubiquitously in the past.

6.6 APPLICATIONS IN SPORT

Body composition is only one of many factors (physical, physiological, genetic, and psychological) that will determine athletic performance. And while the focus for many coaches and support staff is on adiposity of their athletes, it is important to remember other aspects of body composition, namely, the lean tissue components of muscle, bone, ligaments, and tendons, also affect sport performance. Many authors have noted that successful athletes in certain sports fit closely to an optimal body composition. While weight-sensitive sports (Ackland et al. 2012) compel the athlete to minimize body mass, other sports (e.g., contact sports) demand robust bodies in a musculoskeletal sense and can generally tolerate athletes with higher proportions of fat (e.g., American football linemen). Furthermore, some events (e.g., open water swimming) favor competitors with a degree of adiposity, providing a biomechanical advantage of buoyancy and a physiological benefit of insulation against heat loss.

Regardless of their sporting involvement, athletes appear to be in a perpetual state of body modification; this may be to gain mass, reduce fat, or make a weight category for competition. Therefore, it has become increasingly important to monitor the body composition status of athletes throughout the pre- and competition phases of the season. A variety of methods, involving both laboratory-based and field techniques, have been employed for this purpose. Ackland et al. (2012) summarize the current status of these techniques with commentary on the validity, repeatability, assumptions, advantages, and limitations of each method.

Meyer et al. (2013) used a 40-item instrument to survey the body composition methods used by sport scientists, and medical and health practitioners worldwide for the assessment of athletes. The data from 159 respondents were stratified according to demographics, sport type, and level of competition. While there were different methods favored in various parts of the world, it was clear that the majority relied upon skinfolds (though there was much variation in both technique standardization and postprocessing of data) as well as DXA. There was also support for bioelectrical impedance analysis (BIA) and air displacement plethysmography (ADP) methods. In terms of measurement frequency, a large cohort of respondents stated that this depended on the individual athlete and which sport they competed in, as well as the general goals of the intervention and phase of the training/competition season. Nevertheless, most athletes who were supported by these survey respondents appeared to be assessed between two to six times per year.

Body composition assessments have also formed an important component of large studies of elite performers at world and Olympic competitions. These studies have the dual purpose of providing contemporary normative data for athlete comparison, as well as to better understand the optimal morphology for a particular sport or event in terms of the athletes' physical and physiological characteristics. The first of these large-scale anthropometric surveys of elite performers began at the Rome Olympics with a study of 137 track and field athletes (Tanner 1964). Since this important work, anthropometic and other data have been published from the Mexico Olympics (deGaray et al. 1974), Montreal Olympics (Carter 1982), and Sydney Olympics (Kerr et al. 2007), as well as various World Championships covering many sports.

In one of the most comprehensive studies of aquatics athletes, a team of 33 anthropometrists measured full anthropometric profiles of 919 swimmers, divers, synchronized swimmers, and water polo players attending the 1991 World Aquatics Championships in Perth, Western Australia (Carter and Ackland 1994). For most of the swimming events, 70%–80% of all competitors were assessed, with a similarly high proportion of finalists measured. The data also included 82 divers (80% of the top 10 competitors), 137 synchronized swimmers (100% of the top 10 competitors), and 299 water polo players. Selected data for male competitors are shown in Table 6.1. According to Drinkwater and Mazza (1994), long-distance (open water) swimmers were significantly fatter (higher SUM6SF) than sprint and 1500 m swimmers—this additional adiposity was thought to aid buoyancy and thermal insulation during the open water events. Divers were shorter, lighter, and leaner than both swimmers and water polo players. There are significant biomechanical imperatives in the sport of diving that demand such characteristics from elite performers. With this body morphology, elite divers are able to minimize their rotational inertia and thereby, maximize somersault and twist velocity while in flight. The largest players in water polo are the center forwards and backs. In

TABLE 6.1

Body Composition of Male Aquatic Athletes Competing at the 1991 World Championships

Event	n	Stature (cm)	Body Mass (kg)	SUM6SF[a] (mm)	Muscle Mass[b] (kg)	Skeletal Mass[c] (kg)
			Freestyle Swimming			
50 and 100 m	47	186.4	79.8	44.0	57.8	13.3
200 and 400 m	34	185.2	79.1	50.4	57.0	13.0
1500 m	10	183.1	74.3	41.8	56.1	13.9
Long distance	13	179.6	78.1	60.3	56.3	13.0
Diving	43	170.9	66.7	45.9	58.6	12.9
			Water Polo			
Goalkeepers	30	189.1	86.2	60.9	56.6	13.1
Center backs	25	189.2	90.2	65.0	56.9	12.7
Center forwards	40	188.8	91.4	68.3	55.5	12.6
Others	95	184.0	82.7	59.9	55.8	12.8

[a] Sum of triceps, subscapular, abdominal, supraspinale, front thigh, and medial calf skinfolds.
[b] Estimated muscle mass calculated from anthropometry according to Martin et al. (1990).
[c] Estimated skeletal mass calculated from anthropometry according to Martin (1991).

TABLE 6.2

Factor B Weights and Regression Coefficients for Male and Female World Championship Triathletes

Dependent Variable (y)	B0	B1	B2	R²	F (* = sig p < 0.01)
Total time (s)	7434.9	324.8	−180.2	0.688	29.20*
Swim time (s)	1232.6	31.9	−44.3	0.549	17.10*
Cycle time (s)	3892.6	149.5	−99.9	0.659	24.88*
Run time (s)	2201.0	146.2	–	0.618	40.84*

Note: The general format for the multiple regression equation is y = B0 + (B1·x1) + (B2·x2) + Bn·xn), where x1 = adiposity; x2 = segmental lengths.

these positions, players are subjected to very heavy contact and body checking, and so demand very strong, robust, and buoyant bodies. In contrast, the other field position players need to be comparatively lighter and faster as they spend much of the time carrying the ball and setting up plays for the center forward.

Triathletes (n = 71) from 11 nations competing in the 1997 Triathlon World Championships were measured on a battery of 28 anthropometric dimensions. A factor analysis (Landers et al. 2000) reduced the number of variables to four (robustness, adiposity, segmental lengths, and skeletal mass) and these were used in a linear regression to determine which morphological characteristics were important to performance (Table 6.2). With respect to the total elapsed time for the event, and with male and female competitors combined, a regression equation using the adiposity and segmental length factors accounted for 47% of the variance in triathlon duration. The analysis illustrated the importance of low levels of adiposity and proportionally long limb segments for elite triathletes, especially in regard to total elapsed time, as well as swim time, cycle time, and run time treated separately. A higher level of adiposity hampers run times especially because it increases segmental inertia, diminishes running economy, and impairs heat loss. According to Landers et al. (2000) greater adiposity increases the energy demands for an athlete attempting to keep pace with a runner of equal body mass, but with reduced fat mass.

Both male and female lightweight rowers, as we might surmise, have significantly (p < 0.01) reduced stature, body mass, and adiposity compared to their open category counterparts (Table 6.3).

TABLE 6.3

Anthropometric Characteristics of Olympic Lightweight and Open-Class Rowers

Variable	Male Rowers		Female Rowers	
	Lightweight (n = 50)	Open-Class (n = 140)	Lightweight (n = 14)	Open-Class (n = 69)
Age (years)	27.1	26.4	26.0	27.8
Stature (m)	1.82	1.94	1.69	1.81
Sitting height (m)	0.95	0.99	0.89	0.94
Body mass (kg)	72.5	94.3	58.5	76.6
SUM8SF[a]	44.7	65.3	59.7	89.0

[a] Sum of triceps, biceps, iliac crest, subscapular, supraspinale, abdominal, front thigh, and medial calf.

These data were published for competitors at the Sydney Olympic Games in 2000 (Kerr et al. 2007), where 273 rowers were measured as part of the OZ2000 project. A further analysis compared the "best" crews (top 7 placings) to the "rest." The "best" open male crews were taller, heavier, and more robust than the "rest," but did not differ in terms of adiposity. For open women rowers, however, lower adiposity levels were characteristic of the "best" performers. Schranz et al. (2010) used 3D scanning to capture the morphology of elite rowers at two consecutive Australian national championships, and compared these to a control group of the general population. This insightful study was the first of its kind with body scanning, and was able to establish the effect size for a range of morphological variables, which differed between rowers and controls such as cross-sectional areas, surface areas, and segment volumes, which are not available using conventional anthropometry. As with the Olympic study, these data provide valuable information for coaches and support staff when selecting, developing, and monitoring elite-level crews.

While there are clear examples of absolute body size being advantageous, most obviously in basketball players and racing jockeys, there are subtler examples where the body's skeletal proportions may be influential. Short track speed skating favors the short limb length, low center of mass, and rapid power development. The dominance of Oriental nations such as Korea and Japan illustrate this point. Skeletal proportions are not "trainable," therefore athletes can be expected to self-select into sports in which they are likely to excel (Stewart et al. 2011b). For example, speed and endurance runners have greater crural indices (tibia:femur length ratio), which reduces inertial resistance. This concept extends to the identification of sporting talent, which has historically targeted exceptionally tall young rowers, with the potential to have long limbs and greater leverage. Onto this skeletal framework, soft tissues of muscle and fat respond to the training regimes and can be optimized for gaining and losing body weight, in a periodized training cycle.

The assessment and monitoring of body composition, using both anthropometric and other techniques, has become fundamental in the preparation of elite sporting competitors. As athletes strive to gain weight, lose weight, and make weight for competition, they are invariably subject to health risks due to some extreme practices. This is especially poignant for those competing in weight-sensitive sports—those sports in which high body weight restricts performance (gravitational sports), or where the athlete must meet a weight category restriction (weight-class sports), or in which the aesthetics of the performance contributes to the outcome (aesthetic sports). In a recent paper, Sundgot-Borgen et al. (2013) addressed some of the behaviors and health risks associated with these weight-sensitive sports and provided guidelines for athletes, coaches, support staff, and administrators for recognizing and preventing eating disorders. The authors also provide recommendations for sports administrators to consider rule modifications in their sport with a view to minimizing or eliminating some of the unhealthy behaviors and practices that these rules promote.

6.7 APPLICATIONS IN ERGONOMICS

Ergonomic applications of body dimensions relate the human shape and posture to function in working and living environments. The interface between human form and functional activity is at the very core of ergonomics, and influences a range of applications and agendas related to risk, safety, comfort, and productivity. The science of ergonomics encompasses a range of scientific disciplines—including physiology, biomechanics, human behavior, and others, all of which relate directly or indirectly to health and function. Many ergonomic challenges relate to such factors as vision, cognition, fatigue, and work capacity in complex ways, while others relate to body size in a more direct way.

Indigenous populations vary profoundly in their size and proportions, with the implication that size standards in one country may not be applicable in another. Genetic hybridization and secular trends for increase in stature (Cole 2002) have both influenced current, observed body size and bodily proportions, with implications for injury risk such as when operating machinery. The rising prevalence of global obesity (WHO 2000) has arguably had an additive effect, which has been more rapid and profound by affecting posture and locomotion (Wearing et al. 2006), and compromising movement and effective work in restricted space, with consequences for musculoskeletal health (Gallacher 2005).

Body size is also not the same between different professions within a country, and evidence exists that certain professions are associated with larger individuals, including truck drivers (Guan and Hsiao 2012) and firefighters (Hsaio et al. 2014). This has implication for extrapolating national size data to certain at-risk groups. As an example, consider the 67,000 UK offshore workers who are transported by helicopter to and from their work on installations in the North Sea. It was well established from a previous survey that UK offshore workers were heavier than UK norms (Light and Dingwall 1985), but this disparity in body weight has trebled since that time, during which the average male worker's weight increased by 19%. A subsequent study sought to quantify a large number of dimensions in relation to this trend for increased size (Ledingham et al. 2015).

In a recent safety review of helicopter operations, the UK Civil Aviation Authority altered seating rules to facilitate compatibility between passenger body size and the window diameter on the corresponding seat row. A recent study (Stewart et al. 2016), using a subsample of 404 offshore workers sampled across the entire weight spectrum, involved egressing through a window frame representing the minimum allowable size. Unsurprisingly, smaller individuals were more likely to succeed than their larger counterparts. Individual measurement dimensions obtained from 3D scanning were subjected to binary logistic regression to determine the optimal predictive test. Scrutiny of the effect size for the dimensional difference between those who passed and failed the egress task revealed any one of a number of candidate measurements (see Figure 6.2) could be used to inform an intelligent seating policy, although some of the measurements would not be practical to undertake for the industry. However, some false positives (large individuals succeeding) and false negatives (smaller individuals failing) suggest that body size is not the only predictive variable and that other factors such as flexibility and technique could also be influential.

6.8 CONCLUSION

What is the current state of anthropometry within the context of performance and health? Some would argue that the emergence of new techniques that are becoming increasingly affordable and portable, especially ultrasound and 3D scanning, could spell the end of the road for traditional anthropometry. Ethnic groups, children, and the elderly, together with participants from virtually every sport have already been characterized by anthropometry. While some studies of this nature may not be repeated, it is worth recognizing that very few studies with physical activity and performance or the wider realm of epidemiology do not involve *some* anthropometric measurements. Although it is hard to understand why the advances in standardization in traditional anthropometry were so long in coming, it is easy to recognize their benefits. The time is now ripe for equivalent standardization of 3D anthropometry (a young and rapidly evolving science by comparison), which will enable robust quality assurance of data, and an audit trail of competencies seen across other body composition disciplines. This will be essential if we are to create integrated composite models using a combination of methods, which could use a digital 3D template enriched by composition data located in xyz space. Such a "holy grail" could be expanded to include large data repositories and sharing arrangements, which would help us understand much finer morphological detail due to enhanced power to detect small differences, such as the intra- and interpersonal gradient in physique with sports performance standard, or shape change with disease progression with aging or muscle wasting.

However, we are not there yet, despite the aspiration of some, and the technological competence of many. First, as anthropometrists and practitioners of body composition, we need a more complete dialog and to agree to a common language on definitions, standards, and protocols. Second, we

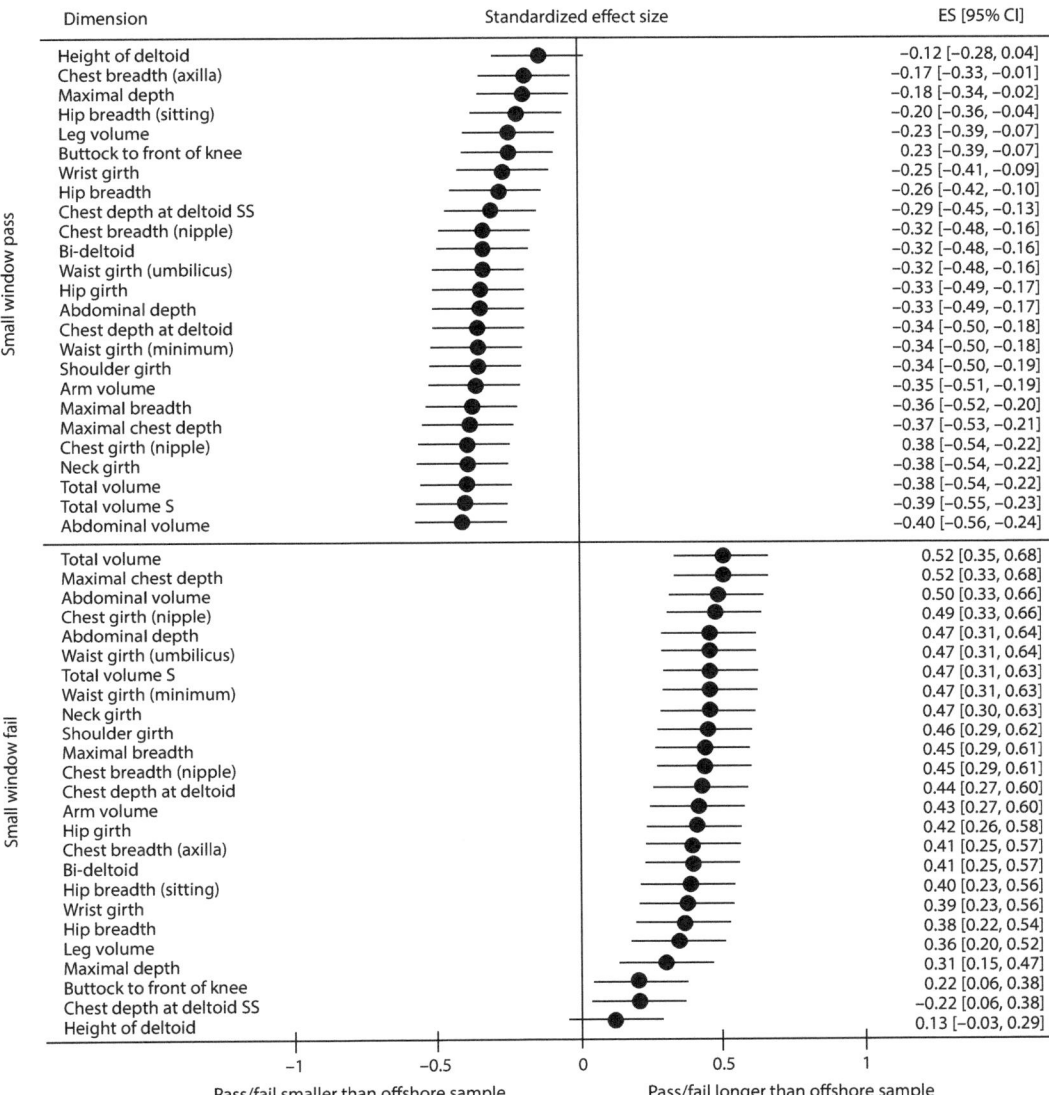

FIGURE 6.2 Comparison of the effect size of body dimensions between those passing and those failing a helicopter window egress test. (Reprinted from Stewart et al. 2015, with permission from Elsevier.)

need to define our aims collectively and build a path and structure that will help us toward achieving them. Neither of these tasks is straightforward, and both go well beyond the job descriptions of experts in the field. However, history will relate the pivotal role of key researchers who have defied the odds in encouraging entire disciplines to move in a certain direction. Individuals might need persuading that such efforts are worthwhile, because of the political hurdles in the path of international application and implementation. While there will always be differences on which path it is best to take, thanks to modern communication media, never before has such international dialog been as straightforward. The prominence of anthropometric measurement within the wider field of body composition throughout history will only be maintained or enhanced if such exchange of ideas embraces these new concepts. However, with the enthusiasm of its practitioners and the exciting developments anticipated, anthropometry may expect a promising future.

REFERENCES

Ackland, T. R., T. G. Lohman, J. Sundgot-Borgen et al. 2012. Current status of body composition assessment in sport. *Sports Med* 42:227–49.

Adams, J., M. Mottola, K. M. Bagnell, and K. D. McFadden. 1982. Total body fat content in a group of professional football players. *Can J App Sport Sci* 7:36–40.

Bergman, R. N., D. Stefanovski, T. A. Buchanan et al. 2011. A better index of body adiposity. *Obesity (Silver Spring)* 19:1083–9.

Bjorntorp, P. 1997. Body fat distribution, insulin resistance, and metabolic diseases. *Nutrition* 13:975–803.

Bosy-Westphal, A., C.-A. Booke, T. Blöcker et al. 2009. Measurement site for waist circumference affects its accuracy as an index of visceral and abdominal subcutaneous fat in a Caucasian population. *J Nutr* 140:954–61.

British Standards Institute. 2010. 3-D scanning methodologies for internationally compatible anthropometric databases. *BS EN ISO* 20685:2010.

Carin-Levy, G., C. A. Greig, S. J. Lewis, A. Stewart, A. Young, and G. E. Mead. 2008. The effect of different positions on anthropometric measurements and derived estimates of body composition. *Int J Body Comp Res* 6:17–20.

Carter, J. E. L. 1982. *Physical Structure of Olympic Athletes. Part 1. The Montreal Olympic Games Anthropological Study*. Basel, Switzerland: Karger.

Carter, J. E. L. 1985. Morphological factors limiting human performance. In *The Limits of Human Performance. The American Academy of Physical Education Papers, No. 18*. eds. H. M. Eckert and D. H. Clarke, 106–17. Champaign, IL: Human Kinetics.

Carter, J. E. L. and T. R. Ackland. 1994. *Kinanthropometry in Aquatic Sports*. Champaign, IL: Human Kinetics.

Carter, J. E. L. and B. H. Heath. 1990. *Somatotyping—Development and Applications*. Cambridge: Cambridge University Press.

Clarys, J. P., A. D. Martin, D. T. Drinkwater, and M. J. Marfell-Jones. 1987. The skinfold: Myth and reality. *J Sports Sci* 5:3–33.

Cole, T. 2002. The secular trend in human physical growth: A biological view. *Econ Hum Biol* 1:161–8.

Daniell, N., T. Olds, and G. Tomkinson. 2010. The importance of site location in girth measurements. *J Sports Sci* 28:751–7.

deGaray, A. L., L. Levine, and J. E. L. Carter. 1974. *Genetic and Anthropological Studies of Olympic Athletes*. New York: Academic Press.

de Koning, L., A. T. Merchant, J. Pogue, and S. S. Anand. 2007. Waist circumference and waist-to-hip ratio as predictors of cardiovascular events: Meta-regression analysis of prospective studies. *Eur Heart J* 28:850–6.

Drinkwater, D. T. and J. C. Mazza. 1994. Body composition. In *Kinanthropometry in Aquatic Sports*, eds. J. E. L. Carter and T. R. Ackland, 102–37. Champaign, IL: Human Kinetics.

Drinkwater, D. T. and W. D. Ross. 1980. Anthropometric fractionation of body mass. In *Kinanthropometry II*, eds. W. Ostyn, G. Beunen, and J. Simons, 177–88. Baltimore: University Park Press.

Durnin, J. V. G. A. and J. Womersley. 1974. Body fat assessed from total body density and its estimation from skinfold thickness: Measurements on 481 men and women aged from 16 to 72 years. *Brit J Nut* 32:77–97.

Evans, E. M., D. A. Rowe, M. M. Misic, B. M. Prior, and S. A. Arngrimsson. 2005. Skinfold prediction equation for athletes developed using a four-compartment model. *Med Sci Sports Exerc* 37:2006–11.

Freedman, D. S., J. Thornton, F. X. Pi-Sunyer et al. 2012. The body adiposity index (hip circumference/height(1.5)) is not a more accurate measure of adiposity than is BMI, waist circumference, or hip circumference. *Obesity (Silver Spring)* 20:2438–44.

Gallacher, S. 2005. Physical limitations and musculoskeletal complaints associated with work in unusual or restricted postures: A literature review. *J Safety Res* 35:51–61.

Gallagher, D., S. B. Heymsfield, M. Heo, S. A. Jebb, P. R. Murgatroyd, and Y. Sakamoto. 2000. Healthy percentage fat ranges: An approach for developing guidelines based on body mass index. *Am J Clin Nutr* 72:694–701.

Guan, J. and H. Hsiao. 2012. U.S. truck driver anthropometric study and multivariate anthropometric models for cab designs. *Hum Factors* 54:849–71.

He, Q., E. S. Engelson, J. Wang et al. 2004. Validation of an elliptical anthropometric model to estimate visceral compartment area. *Obes Res* 12:250–7.

Himes, J. H., A. F. Roche, and R. M. Siervogel. 1979. Compressibility of skinfolds and the measurement of subcutaneous fatness. *Am J Clin Nutr* 32:1734–40.

Ho, S-Y., T.-H. Lam, and E. D. Janus for the Hong Kong cardiovascular risk factor prevalence study steering committee. 2003. Waist to stature ratio is more strongly associated with cardiovascular risk factors than other simple anthropometric indices. *Ann Epidemiol* 13:683–91.

Hsaio, H., J. Whitestone, T. Kau, R. Whisler, G. Routley, and M. Wilbur. 2014. Sizing firefighters: Method and implications. *Hum Factors* 56:873–910.

Hume, P. and M. Marfell-Jones. 2008. The importance of accurate site location for skinfold measurement. *J Sports Sci* 26:1333–40.

Jackson, A. S. and M. L. Pollock. 1978. Generalized equations for predicting body density of men. *Brit J Nutr* 40:497–504.

Jackson, A. S., M. L. Pollock, and A. Ward. 1980. Generalized equations for predicting body density of women. *Med Sci Sports Exerc* 12:175–82.

Kaess, B. M., A. Pedley, J. M. Massaro, J. Murabito, U. Hoffman, and C. S. Fox. 2012. The ratio of visceral to subcutaneous fat, a metric of body fat distribution, is a unique correlate of cardiometabolic risk. *Diabetologia* 55:2622–30.

Kerr, D. A., T. R. Ackland, W. D. Ross, K. Norton, and P. Hume. 2007. Olympic lightweight and open rowers possess distinctive physical and proportionality characteristics. *J Sports Sci* 25:43–53.

Kershaw, E. E. and J. S. Flier. 2004. Adipose tissue as an endocrine organ. *J Clin Endocrinol Metab* 89:2548–56.

Kuk, J. L., P. T. Katzmarzyk, N. Z. Nichaman, T. S. Church, S. N. Blair, and R. Ross. 2006. Visceral fat is an independent predictor of all-cause mortality in men. *Obesity (Silver Spring)* 14:336–41.

Kupke, T. and T. Olds. 2008. Towards a generalised anthropometric language. In *Kinanthropometry IX. Proceedings of the 10th International Conference of the International Society for the Advancement of Kinanthropometry*, eds. M. Marfell-Jones and T. Olds, 213–30. London: Routledge.

Landers, G. J., B. A. Blanksby, T. R. Ackland, and D. Smith. 2000. Morphology and performance of world championship triathletes. *Ann Hum Biol* 27:387–400.

Ledingham, R., G. Alekandrova, M. Lamb, and A. Stewart. 2015. *Size and Shape of the UK Offshore Workforce 2014: A 3D Scanning Survey*. Aberdeen, UK: Robert Gordon University. ISBN 978-1-907349-10-2.

Light, I. M. and R. H. M. Dingwall. 1985. *Basic Anthropometry of 419 Offshore Workers (1984)*. Aberdeen, UK: Offshore Survival Centre, Robert Gordon's Institute of Technology.

Lohman, T. G. 1992. *Advances in Body Composition Assessment. Current Issues in Exercise Science Series Monograph No.3*. Champaign, IL: Human Kinetics.

Lohman, T. G., A. F. Roche, and R. Martorell. 1988. *Anthropometric Standardization Reference Manual*. Champaign, IL: Human Kinetics.

Martin, A. D. 1991. Anthropometric assessment of bone mineral. In *Anthropometric Assessment of Nutritional Status*, ed. J. Himes, 185–96. New York: Wiley-Liss.

Martin, A. D., D. T. Drinkwater, J. P. Clarys, and W. D. Ross. 1986. The inconstancy of the fat-free mass: A reappraisal with implications for densitometry. In *Kinanthropometry III*, eds. T. Reilly, J. Watkins, and J. Borms, 92–7. London: E. & F. N. Spon.

Martin, A. D., L. F. Spenst, D. T. Drinkwater, and J. P. Clarys. 1990. Anthropometric estimation of muscle mass in men. *Med Sci Sports Exerc* 22:729–33.

Matiegka, J. 1921. The testing of physical efficiency. *Am J Phys Anthropol* 4:223–30.

Meyer, N. L., J. Sundgot-Borgen, T. G. Lohman et al. 2013. Body composition for health and performance: A survey of the ad hoc research working group on body composition health and performance, under the auspices of the IOC Medical Commission. *Brit J Sports Med* 47:1044–53.

Müller, W. 2009. Towards research-based approaches for solving body composition problems in sports: Ski jumping as a heuristic example. *Brit J Sports Med* 43:1013–9.

Müller, W., M. Horn, A. Fürhapter-Rieger et al. 2013a. Body composition in sport: A comparison of novel ultrasound imaging technique to measure subcutaneous fat tissue compared with skinfold measurement. *Brit J Sports Med* 47:1028–35.

Müller, W., M. Horn, A. Fürhapter-Rieger et al. 2013b. Body composition in sport: Inter-observer reliability of a novel ultrasound measure of subcutaneous fat tissue. *Brit J Sports Med* 47:1036–43.

Müller, W., T. G. Lohman, A. D. Stewart et al. 2016. Subcutaneous fat patterning in athletes: Selection of appropriate sites and standardisation of a novel ultrasound measurement technique. *Brit J Sports Med* 50:45–54.

Norton, K. and T. Olds. 1996. *Anthropometrica*. Sydney: University of New South Wales Press.

Olds, T. 2004. The rise and fall of anthropometry. *J Sports Sci* 22:319–20.

Olds, T., N. Daniell, J. Petkov, and A. D. Stewart. 2013. Somatotyping using 3D anthropometry: A cluster analysis. *J Sports Sci* 31:936–44.

Olds, T., G. Tomkinson, M. Rogers, T. Kupke, L. Lowe, and N. Daniell. 2004. *3D Anthropometry ADAPT Landmarking Manual*. Adelaide, SA: University of South Australia.

Pajunen, P., M. Heliövaara, H. Rissanen, A. Reunanen, M. A. Laaksonen, and P. Knekt. 2013. Sagittal abdominal diameter as a new predictor if incident diabetes. *Diabetes Care* 6:283–8.

Perini, T. A., G. L. de Oliveira, J. S. Ornellas, and F. P. de Oliveira. 2005. Technical error of measurement in anthropometry. *Rev Bras Med Esporte* 11:86–90.

Robinette, K. M., S. Blackwell, M. Daanen et al. 2002. Civilian American and European surface anthropometry resource (CAESAR) Final Report, Vol 1: Summary. Ohio, USA: United States Air Force Research Laboratory, Wright-Patterson Air Force Base.

Santos, D. A., A. M. Silva, C. N. Matias et al. 2015. Utility of novel indices in predicting fat mass in elite athletes. *Nutrition* 31:948–54.

Schranz, N., G. Tomkinson, T. Olds, and N. Daniell. 2010. Three-dimensional anthropometric analysis: Differences between elite Australian rowers and the general population. *J Sports Sci* 28:459–69.

Sinning, W. E., D. G. Dolny, K. D. Little et al. 1985. Validity of "generalised" equations for body composition analysis in male athletes. *Med Sci Sports Exerc* 17:124–30.

Stewart, A., R. Ledingham, G. Furnace, N. Schranz, and A. Nevill. 2016. The ability of UK offshore workers of different body size and shape to egress through a restricted window space. *Appl Ergon* 55:226–33.

Stewart, A., M. Marfell-Jones, T. Olds, and H. de Ridder. 2011a. *International Standards for Anthropometric Assessment*. Lower Hutt, New Zealand: International Society for the Advancement of Kinanthropometry.

Stewart, A. D. 2010. Kinanthropometry and body composition: A natural home for 3D photonic scanning. *J Sports Sci* 28:455–7.

Stewart, A. D., P. J. Benson, T. Olds, M. Marfell-Jones, A. MacSween, and A. M. Nevill. 2011b. Self-selection of athletes into sports via skeletal ratios. *J Contemp Athletics* 5:153–67.

Stewart, A. D. and W. J. Hannan. 2000. Prediction of fat and fat-free mass in male athletes using dual x-ray absorptiometry as the reference method. *J Sports Sci* 18:263–74.

Stewart, A. D., A. M. Nevill, R. Stephen, and J. Young. 2010. Waist size and shape assessed by 3D photonic scanning. *Int J Body Comp Res* 8:123–30.

Stewart, A. D., A. Stewart, and D. Reid. 2002. Correcting calf circumference discriminates the incidence of falling but not bone quality by broadband ultrasound attenuation in elderly female subjects. *Bone* 31:195–8.

Sundgot-Borgen, J., N. L. Meyer, T. G. Lohman et al. 2013. How to minimize risks for athletes in weight-sensitive sports. *Brit J Sports Med* 47:1012–22.

Tanner, J. M. 1964. *The Physique of the Olympic Athlete*. London: George Allen & Unwin Ltd.

Thomas, D. M., C. Bredlau, A. Bosy-Westphal et al. 2013. Relationships between body roundness with body fat and visceral adipose tissue emerging from a new geometrical model. *Obesity (Silver Spring)* 21:2264–71.

Thomas, E. L. and J. D. Bell. 2003. Influence of undersampling on magnetic resonance imaging measurements of intra-abdominal adipose tissue. *Int J Obes* 27:211–8.

Tyrrell, A. R., T. Reilly, and J. D. G. Troup. 1985. Circadian variation in stature and the effects of spinal loading. *Spine* 10:161–4.

Valdez, R. 1991. A simple model-based index of abdominal adiposity. *J Clin Epidemiol* 9:955–6.

Valsamakis, G., R. Chetty, A. Anwar, A. K. Banerjee, A. Barnett, and S. Kumar. 2004. Association of simple anthropometric measures of obesity with visceral fat and the metabolic syndrome. *Diabet Med* 21:1339–448.

Wang, J., D. Gallagher, J. C. Thornton, W. Yu, M. Horlick, and F. X. Pi-Sunyer. 2006. Validation of a 3-dimensional photonic scanner for the measurement of body volumes, dimensions, and percentage body fat. *Am J Clin Nutr* 83:809–16.

Wearing, S. C., E. M. Henning, N. M. Byrne, J. R. Steele, and A. P. Hills. 2006. The biomechanics of restricted movement in adult obesity. *Obes Rev* 7:13–24.

Wells, J. C., P. Treleaven, and T. J. Cole. 2007. BMI compared with 3-dimensional body shape: The UK National Sizing Survey. *Am J Clin Nut* 85:419–25.

World Health Organization. 2000. *Obesity: Preventing and managing the global epidemic*. Report of a WHO Consultation. WHO Technical Report Series 894. Geneva: World Health Organization.

7 Exercise and Adipose Tissue Redistribution in Overweight and Obese Adults

Brittany P. Hammond, Andrea M. Brennan, and Robert Ross

CONTENTS

7.1 INTRODUCTION

Excess accumulation of adipose tissue (AT) in adults is positively associated with morbidity and mortality independent of age and gender (Poirier et al. 2006). Accumulation within the abdomen region, in particular, excess deposition of visceral adipose tissue (VAT), is the phenotype associated with the greatest health risk (Despres and Lemieux 2006). Chronic exercise combined with a healthful diet induces a substantial reduction in adiposity independent of age and gender. Whether regular exercise is associated with a redistribution of AT is unclear. Specifically, whether abdominal AT is preferentially reduced consequent to exercise remains a topic of debate.

Current knowledge regarding the dose–response relationships between exercise and total AT reduction depends in large measure upon a comparison of groups between studies that vary in exercise dose. In recent years, randomized controlled trials (RCTs) specifically designed to determine the effect of exercise dose on total and regional distribution of AT have emerged. The design of these trials employs multiple groups varying in exercise amount (exercise-induced energy expenditure; kcal) and/or intensity (% VO_2peak) permitting the isolation of these two components of exercise dose on AT distribution. The findings from these trials help resolve the following questions. For a fixed amount of exercise, does varying exercise intensity influence AT reduction? For a fixed exercise intensity, does varying exercise amount influence AT reduction?

In this chapter we address three main questions: "What are the separate effects of exercise amount and intensity on AT distribution?" "Is there preferential reduction of abdominal AT in response to exercise?" and "Is there a difference between exercise- and diet-induced reduction in total or abdominal AT?"

7.2 METHODOLOGY

7.2.1 SEARCH STRATEGY

A PubMed search was performed using the following keywords: (obesity OR overweight OR obese) AND (AT OR VAT OR subcutaneous adipose tissue [SAT] OR waist circumference [WC] OR body fat distribution OR abdominal AT) AND (exercise OR physical activity) AND (RCT OR random). The search strategy applied the following filters: publication date January 2000–April 2016, humans, English language, and adults >18 years old.

7.2.2 SELECTION CRITERIA

Search results were initially screened based upon the title and abstract. Identified studies were further reviewed using the following inclusion criteria:

1. Participants (male and female) were older than 18 years
2. Participants were overweight or obese (body mass index >25 kg/m²) and otherwise healthy (i.e., no diabetes)
3. Limited to primarily continuous aerobic exercise
4. The majority (90%) of exercise sessions were performed under direct supervision and/or monitored objectively
5. One of the following variables was provided: body weight or fat mass, WC, or abdominal fat mass

We restricted our search to randomized trials of 12 weeks' duration or more wherein the negative energy balance was induced by exercise alone; thus studies were excluded if a dietary intervention induced a negative energy balance. Studies meeting these inclusion criteria were deemed suitable and were examined for additional relevant references.

7.3 EXERCISE-INDUCED REDUCTION IN BODY WEIGHT OR TOTAL ADIPOSITY

A total of 10 RCTs met the inclusion criteria (Table 7.1). Inspection of Table 7.1 reveals that continuous aerobic exercise is associated with reductions in body weight and total adiposity independent of sex and age (Ross et al. 2000, 2004, 2015; Ross and Janssen 2001; Donnelly et al. 2003; Slentz et al. 2004; Davidson et al. 2009; Nordby et al. 2012). The majority of participants included in these studies are middle-aged white men and women. To date, there is limited evidence from RCTs that examine the effect of race on the relationship between exercise and total adiposity reduction in obese adults. One study within Table 7.1 reported no effect of race on exercise-induced reduction in body weight (Church et al. 2007).

7.3.1 SEPARATE EFFECTS OF EXERCISE AMOUNT AND INTENSITY ON BODY WEIGHT AND TOTAL ADIPOSITY REDUCTION

Current knowledge regarding the dose–response relationships between exercise and body weight or total AT reduction depends in large measure upon a comparison of groups between studies that vary in exercise dose.

TABLE 7.1
Randomized Controlled Trials Examining Exercise-Induced Changes in VAT, ASAT, and Total Adiposity

Study	Participants N (M/F)	Age (years)	Intervention Groups	Duration	Δ Weight (kg)	Δ WC (cm)	Δ VAT (Absolute)	Δ VAT (%)	Δ ASAT (Absolute)	Δ ASAT (%)	Δ Total Abdominal AT	Δ Total Fat Mass (kg)
Ross et al. (2000)	38 (38/0)	Control: 46.0 EWL: 45.0 EWW: 44.7	Control Exercise weight loss (EWL): 700 kcal/day Exercise without weight loss (EWW): 700 kcal/day and re-consume 700 kcal to maintain weight Intensity: <70% VO2peak (80% of max HR)	12 weeks	Control: +0.1 EWL: -7.5* EWW: -0.5 EWL sig. different from EWW	Control: -0.1 EWL: -6.5* EWW: -1.8 EWL sig. different from EWW	Control: 0.0 EWL: -1.1 kg* EWW: -0.4 kg* EWL sig. different from EWW	Control: 0.0 EWL: -28.2* EWW: -11.8* EWL sig. different from EWW	Control: N/A EWL: -0.8 kg EWW: not reported		Control: N/A EWL: -1.9 kg EWW: not reported EWL sig. different from EWW	Control: -0.6 EWL: -6.1* EWW: -1.5 EWL sig. different from EWW
Donnelly et al. (2003)	74 (31/43)	Control female: 21 Control male: 24 Exercise female: 24 Exercise male: 22	Control (C) Exercise (E): 55%–70% VO2max, 5 days/week, 400 kcal session (~2000 kcal per week)	64 weeks	C(M): -0.5 E(M): -5.2* C(F): +2.9 E(F): +0.6*		C(M): -6.3 cm² E(M): -22.4 cm² C(F): +3.1 cm² E(F): -3.2 cm²	C(M): -6.9 E(M): -22.9 C(F): +4.9 E(F): -5.3	C(M): -17.9 cm² E(M): -51.4 cm² C(F): +48.6 cm² E(F): -3.7 cm²	C(M): -5.8 E(M): -16.2 C(F): +12.5 E(F): -1.0*	C(M): -24.2 cm² E(M): -73.9 cm² C(F): +51.7 cm² E(F): -6.9 cm²	C(M): -0.7 E(M): -4.9* C(F): +2.2 E(F): -0.2*
Ross et al. (2004)	39 (0/39)	Control: 43.7 EWL: 43.2 EWW: 41.3	Control EWL: 500 kcal/day (0.45 kg per week) EWW: 500 kcal/day and re-consume 500 kcal to maintain weight Intensity: 80% of max HR	14 weeks	Control: +0.5 EWL: -5.9* EWW: -0.5	Control: +1.1 EWL: -6.5* EWW: -3.1* EWL sig. different from EWW	Control: -0.1 kg EWL: -0.7 kg* EWW: -0.4 kg*	Control: -4.3 EWL: -30.4* EWW: -18.2*	Control: +0.1 kg EWL: -1.1 kg* EWW: -0.3 kg*	Control: -1.7 EWL: -16.9* EWW: -4.9*	Control: no change EWL: -1.7 kg* EWW: -0.8 kg* EWL sig. different from EWW	Control: +0.8 EWL: -6.7* EWW: -2.7*

(Continued)

TABLE 7.1 (Continued)

Randomized Controlled Trials Examining Exercise-Induced Changes in VAT, ASAT, and Total Adiposity

Study	Participants N (M/F)	Age (years)	Intervention Groups	Duration	Δ Weight (kg)	Δ WC (cm)	Δ VAT (Absolute)	Δ VAT (%)	Δ ASAT (Absolute)	Δ ASAT (%)	Δ Total Abdominal AT	Δ Total Fat Mass (kg)
Slentz et al. (2004)	120 (65/55)	Control: 52.5 LAMI: 53.4 LAVI: 52.7 HAVI: 52.7	Control Low amount/ moderate intensity (LAMI): 12 miles/week at 40%–55% VO₂peak Low amount/ vigorous intensity (LAVI):12 miles/week at 65%–80% VO₂peak High amount/ vigorous intensity (HAVI): 20 miles/week at 65%–80% VO₂peak	32 weeks	Control: +1.1 LAMI: −1.3* LAVI: −1.1* HAVI: −3.5* HAVI sig. different from LAMI and LAVI	Control: +0.8 LAMI: −1.6* LAVI: −1.4* HAVI: −3.4*						
Slentz et al. (2005)	175 (91/84)	Control: 52.3 LAMI: 54.0 LAVI: 53.0 HAVI: 51.5	Control LAMI: 12 miles/week at 40%–55% VO₂peak LAVI:12 miles/week at 65%–80% VO₂peak HAVI: 20 miles/week at 65%–80% VO₂peak	32 weeks			Control: +14.2 cm² LAMI: +2.9 cm² LAVI: + 3.9 cm²* HAVI: −11.6 cm²*	Control: +8.6 LAMI: +1.7 LAVI: +2.5* HAVI: −6.9*	Control: + 3.4 cm² LAMI: −3.4 cm² LAVI: +9.0 cm² HAVI: −19.2 cm²* HAVI sig. different from LAMI, LAVI	Control: +1.1 LAMI: −1.2 LAVI: 3.1 HAVI: −7.0* HAVI sig. different from LAMI, LAVI		
Church et al. (2007)	464 (0/464)	57.3	Control 4 kcal/kg per week, 50% VO₂peak 8 kcal/kg per week, 50% VO₂peak 12 kcal/kg per week, 50% VO₂peak	24 weeks	Control: −2.2 4 kcal/kg: −0.4 8 kcal/kg: −2.2 12 kcal/kg: −0.6	Control: −1.4 4 kcal/kg: −1.9* 8 kcal/kg: −2.9* 12 kcal/kg: −1.4*						

(Continued)

TABLE 7.1 (Continued)
Randomized Controlled Trials Examining Exercise-Induced Changes in VAT, ASAT, and Total Adiposity

Study	Participants N (M/F)	Age (years)	Intervention Groups	Duration	Δ Weight (kg)	Δ WC (cm)	Δ VAT (Absolute)	Δ VAT (%)	Δ ASAT (Absolute)	Δ ASAT (%)	Δ Total Abdominal AT	Δ Total Fat Mass (kg)
Irving et al. (2008)	27 (0/27)	51	Control (NOET) LIET: 400 kcal/session, 5 days/week RPE 10–12 (at or below lactate threshold) HIET: 400 kcal/session, 5 days/week RPE 15–17 (above lactate threshold 3 days, less than lactate threshold 2 days)	16 weeks	NOET: −0.9 LIET: −2.1 HIET: −3.5	NOET: −0.7 LIET: −1.2 HIET: −5.6* HIET sig. different from LIET	NOET: −2 cm² LIET: −7 cm² HIET: −25 cm²	NOET: −1.0 LIET: −4.6 HIET: −14.5	NOET: −16 cm² LIET: −11 cm² HIET: −46 cm² HIET sig. different from LIET	NOET: −3.2 LIET: −2.3 HIET: −9.0	NOET: −28 cm² LIET: −11 cm² HIET: −58 cm² HIET sig. different from LIET	NOET: −0.3 LIET: −1.3 HIET: −2.8 HIET sig. different from LIET
Coker et al. (2009)	18 (9/9)	Control: 67 HI: 73 MI: 70	Control HI: 75% VO₂peak, 4–5 days/week (1000 kcal/week) MI: 50% VO₂peak, 4–5 days/week (1000 kcal/week)	12 weeks	Control: N/A HI: N/A MI: N/A		Control: N/A HI: −39 cm²* MI: N/A		Control: N/A HI: −12 cm² MI: −13 cm²			
Davidson et al. (2009)	136 (57/79)	Female: 67.5 Male: 67.7	Control Aerobic (AE): 30 min of moderate-intensity treadmill walking (60%–75% VO₂peak) 5 times per week	24 weeks	Control: +0.28 AE: −2.77*	Control: −0.28 AE: −5.08*	Control: +0.02 kg AE: −0.43 kg*		Control: −0.04 kg AE: −0.40 kg*		Control: −0.05 kg AE: −0.84 kg*	Control: −0.52 AE: −3.03*
Nordby et al. (2012)	36 (36/0)	Control: 28 Training: 32	Control Training (T): equivalent to 600 kcal/day, Combination of continuous exercise at ~65% HR-reserve and high intensity intervals for 5–6 bouts for 3–4 min at 85% HR-reserve Training and increased diet (T-iD): same training protocol with increased diet consumption of 600 kcal/day	12 weeks	Control: −0.2 T: −5.9* T-iD: −1.0 T sig. different from T-iD	Control: N/A T: −7* T-iD: −5*						Control: +0.1 T: −7.7* T-iD: −1.9 T sig. different from T-iD

(Continued)

TABLE 7.1 (Continued)

Randomized Controlled Trials Examining Exercise-Induced Changes in VAT, ASAT, and Total Adiposity

Study	Participants N (M/F)	Age (years)	Intervention Groups	Duration	Δ Weight (kg)	Δ WC (cm)	Δ VAT (Absolute)	Δ VAT (%)	Δ ASAT (Absolute)	Δ ASAT (%)	Δ Total Abdominal AT	Δ Total Fat Mass (kg)
Ross et al. (2015)	300 (104/196)	51.4	Control Low amount/low intensity (LALI; 180 and 300 kcal/session for women and men, respectively) High amount/low intensity (HALI; 360 and 600 kcal/session for women and men, , respectively) High amount/high intensity (HAHI; 360 and 600 kcal/session for women and men, respectively)	24 weeks	Control: N/A LALI: −3.8* HALI: −4.9* HAHI: −4.6*	Control: N/A LALI: −3.9* HALI: −4.6* HAHI: −4.6*						

Note: N, total number of participants; M, male participants; F, female participants; HR, heart rate; WC, waist circumference; VAT, visceral adipose tissue; ASAT, abdominal subcutaneous adipose tissue; AT, adipose tissue. *Significantly different from control, p < 0.05.

The findings of two prior reviews noted that upon comparison of groups across studies lasting <26 weeks, there was a positive dose–response relationship between exercise-induced energy expenditure (amount) and body weight or total adiposity (Ross and Janssen 2001; Shalev-Goldman et al. 2014). Body weight was reduced on average by 0.14 kg per week and total adiposity was reduced on average by 0.23 kg per week in both healthy and diabetic overweight adults (Shalev-Goldman et al. 2014). Subsequent to prior reviews five additional studies meeting the inclusion criteria were identified (Slentz et al. 2004, 2005; Church et al. 2007; Irving et al. 2008; Ross et al. 2015). Figure 7.1a depicts the relationship between energy expenditure and body weight reduction (n = 8), accounting

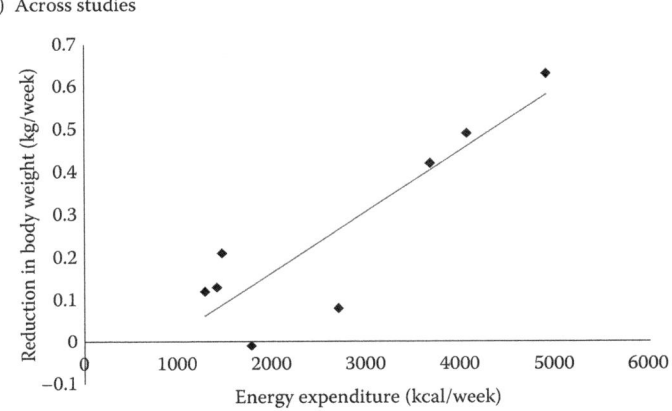

(a) Across studies

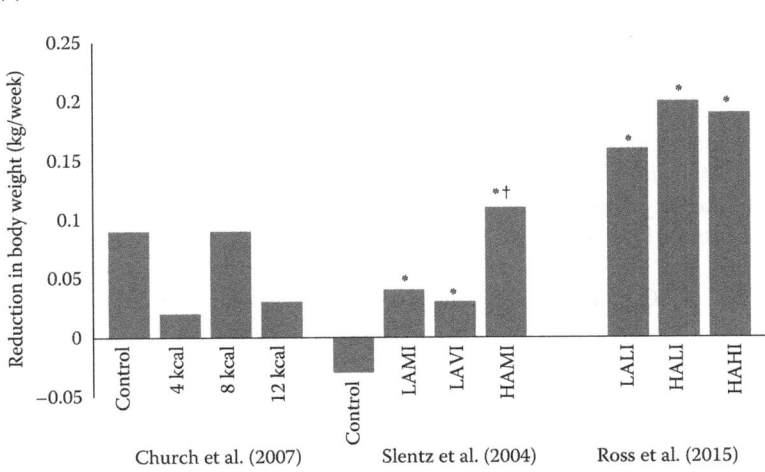

(b) Within studies

FIGURE 7.1 Relationship between energy expenditure and reduction in body weight (a) of groups across studies (N = 8, Table 7.1) and (b) groups within studies (N = 3, Table 7.1). Diamonds (♦) represent body weight reduction. Asterisks (*) represent significant reduction in body weight compared to control, p < 0.05. Crosses (†) represent significant reduction in body weight compared to low amount groups, p < 0.05. The data plotted in the figure are group means for the studies cited in Table 7.1. 4 kcal, 4 kcal/kg per week; 8 kcal, 8 kcal/kg per week; 12 kcal, 12 kcal/kg per week; LAMI, low amount moderate intensity (12 miles/week at 40%–55% VO₂peak, 14 kcal/kg per week); LAVI, low amount vigorous intensity (12 miles/week at 65%–80% VO₂peak,14 kcal/kg per week); HAMI, high amount moderate intensity (20 miles/week at 65%–80% VO₂peak, 23 kcal/kg per week); LALI, low amount low intensity (180 and 300 kcal/session for women and men, respectively); HALI, high amount low intensity (360 and 600 kcal/session for women and men, respectively); HAHI, high amount high intensity (360 and 600 kcal/session for women and men, respectively).

for differences in trial durations by representing change in units per week. The observations appear to be generally consistent with prior reviews that are indicative of a positive dose–response relationship, however, an evident gap in RCTs prescribing ~2000–4000 kcal per week precludes the ability to truly identify a linear dose–response relationship.

While comparison of exercise groups across studies is useful, limitations may confound interpretation. The majority of study groups included in Table 7.1 and the preceding reviews exercised at a similar intensity (~50%–70% VO_2peak); however, it is possible that the variation in exercise intensity plays a role in the observed dose–response relationship with exercise amount. The discrepancies in study design and methodology necessitate caution when comparing groups across studies. These limitations have been addressed by large RCTs specifically designed to determine the separate effects of exercise amount and intensity on adiposity reduction.

We have identified three studies depicted in Figure 7.1b (Slentz et al. 2004; Church et al. 2007; Ross et al. 2015) that have examined the separate effects of amount and intensity of aerobic exercise on body weight. Of these studies, one examined the dose–response relationship between exercise-induced energy expenditure (exercise amount) and reductions in body weight and total adiposity, as measured by skinfolds. Church et al. (2007) conducted a large RCT to examine the effect of 50%, 100%, and 150% of the consensus physical activity recommendations on change in cardiorespiratory fitness in women. A total of 464 hypertensive postmenopausal women were assigned to one of four groups: a no-exercise control group, 4, 8, and 12 kcal/kg body weight per week energy expenditure for the 6-month intervention period. All exercise groups performed activity at a fixed intensity of 50% VO_2peak. Despite the observation that improvements in cardiorespiratory fitness (VO_2peak) occurred in a dose–response manner—the greater the amount of exercise the greater the improvement in cardiorespiratory fitness—no change in body weight or percent body fat was observed. Though perplexing, this observation may be explained by the relatively low exercise-induced energy expenditure prescribed. Also, because the primary outcome of this trial was cardiorespiratory fitness and not weight loss, the participants were frequently encouraged to maintain other lifestyle habits including dietary intake throughout the study.

That increasing exercise amount at a fixed intensity is not associated with an increased reduction in weight loss has been confirmed by the findings of a large RCT that examined the separate effects of amount and intensity on changes in abdominal obesity and glucose tolerance over 24 weeks (Ross et al. 2015). Men and women (n = 300) were randomly assigned to one of four groups: control; low amount/low intensity (180 and 300 kcal/session for women and men, respectively, at 50% of VO_2peak); high amount/low intensity (360 and 600 kcal/session for women and men, respectively, at 50% of VO_2peak); and high amount/high intensity (360 and 600 kcal/session for women and men, respectively, at 75% of VO_2peak). Monitoring of dietary intake and physical activity (accelerometry) performed outside of the structured exercise regimen allowed for control of these potentially confounding variables. The authors observed that, unlike the observations of Church et al. (2007), all exercise groups experienced a substantial weight reduction (~5 kg) compared to control independent of sex and age. However, similar to findings from Church et al. (2007), at a fixed exercise intensity (50% of VO_2peak), a doubling of the exercise amount in the high compared to the low amount group did not result in greater weight loss (Ross et al. 2015). The authors noted that compensation in energy intake could have resulted in alterations in overall energy balance; however, this would mean the low amount group would have over reported their dietary intake which counters the dogma that obese persons generally underreport caloric intake (Livingstone and Black 2003).

Slentz et al. (2004) reported findings that contrast those of Ross et al. (2015). Men and women (n = 120) were randomly assigned to one of four conditions: control, low amount and moderate intensity (12 miles/week at 40%–55% VO_2peak), low amount and high intensity (12 miles/week at 65%–80% VO_2peak), or high amount vigorous intensity (20 miles/week at 65%–80% VO_2peak) (Slentz et al. 2004). After 32 weeks, despite the fact that participants were instructed to consume the equivalent number of calories expended in order to maintain weight, significant changes in weight were observed across both low and high amount exercise groups, with the high amount group observing greater reductions in weight compared to the low amount group (Slentz et al. 2004). Several factors may explain the discrepancy. First, Ross et al. (2015) used an intention-to-treat statistical analysis, which includes all participants originally randomized. Slentz et al. (2004) used a per protocol analysis, including only participants who completed both pre- and post-measurements. Second, in Slentz et al. (2004), participants were asked to increase their energy intake to compensate for the energy they expended in exercise so that they would not lose body weight. It is possible that those in the high amount group had difficulty consuming enough kilocalories (~23 kcal/kg) compared to the low amount group (~14 kcal/kg) for weight maintenance. This may have resulted in a greater negative energy balance, causing them to lose more weight and thus resulting in a greater difference between the high and low amount exercise groups.

From this review it is apparent that the effects of increasing exercise amount (kcal) on total adiposity depends on the literature reviewed. It appears upon comparison of groups across studies (Figure 7.1a), that a positive dose–response relationship exists between exercise amount and total adiposity reduction. However, this observation is based on a limited number of studies.

Furthermore, the findings illustrated in Figure 7.1b suggest that the effects of comparing increases in exercise amount between groups within the same study on total AT reduction are equally unclear. The findings from RCTs specifically designed to determine the effects of exercise amount on total adiposity are perplexing and, other than compensation in energy intake, are not readily explained.

The RCTs discussed above (Slentz et al. 2004; Church et al. 2007; Ross et al. 2015) offer additional insight into the independent effects of exercise intensity on body weight and total adiposity reduction. Both Slentz et al. (2004) and Ross et al. (2015) observed that, when the exercise amount is fixed, increasing exercise intensity does not result in greater reductions in body weight, independent of age and sex (Table 7.1). Taken together the observations reviewed here suggest that exercise amount is more important than exercise intensity, but these observations require confirmation.

7.4 EXERCISE-INDUCED REDUCTION IN WC AND ABDOMINAL ADIPOSITY

A total of 11 studies met the inclusion criteria and have examined the change in WC and/or abdominal adiposity in response to exercise (Table 7.1). Inspection of Table 7.1 reveals that regular aerobic exercise, ranging between 12 and 20 weeks at 50%–70% VO$_2$peak, is associated with reductions in WC (Ross et al. 2000, 2004; Slentz et al. 2004; Church et al. 2007; Irving et al. 2008; Davidson et al. 2009), VAT (Ross et al. 2000, 2004; Donnelly et al. 2003; Irving et al. 2008; Davidson et al. 2009), and abdominal SAT (ASAT) (Ross et al. 2000, 2004; Donnelly et al. 2003; Irving et al. 2008; Davidson et al. 2009). While the majority of studies include white middle-aged participants, Church et al. (2007) noted that exercise significantly reduced WC independent of race/ethnicity. This study included whites, blacks, and Hispanics. More studies are needed to determine the effect of ethnicity on the relationship between exercise and abdominal obesity reduction.

While exercise reduces abdominal obesity in both men and women, the magnitude of response may differ. A meta-analysis suggests that the effect size for reductions in VAT, in particular, was greater in men compared to women across studies including both healthy and diabetic participants (Vissers et al. 2013). The authors suggest this difference may be due in part to higher baseline VAT in men compared to women (Vissers et al. 2013). However, only absolute reduction in VAT was used in this review and it is unknown from this study whether women lost more VAT relatively (percent of VAT lost). Furthermore, studies included in this review examined men or women separately, or were not specifically designed to determine sex-specific responses.

7.4.1 SEPARATE EFFECTS OF EXERCISE AMOUNT AND INTENSITY ON WC AND ABDOMINAL OBESITY REDUCTION

Consistent with the observations previously described when considering the effects of exercise amount on total adiposity, current knowledge of dose–response relationships is based in large measure by comparison of exercise groups varying in exercise amount across studies. The findings of a prior review noted that upon comparison of groups across studies lasting <26 weeks, there was a positive dose–response relationship between exercise-induced energy expenditure (amount) and total abdominal adiposity (1.1% per week) (Ross and Janssen 2001; Shalev-Goldman et al. 2014). They reported that, on average, ASAT was reduced by 0.6%, VAT was reduced by 1.3%, and WC was reduced by 0.18% in healthy and diabetic overweight adults (Shalev-Goldman et al. 2014). Subsequent to this review, five additional studies meeting the criteria were identified (Slentz et al. 2004, 2005; Church et al. 2007; Irving et al. 2008; Ross et al. 2015). Inspection of Table 7.1 reveals a positive relationship between exercise amount and reduction in the components of abdominal obesity (Table 7.1). Specifically, Figure 7.2a depicts the relationship between energy expenditure

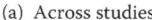
(a) Across studies

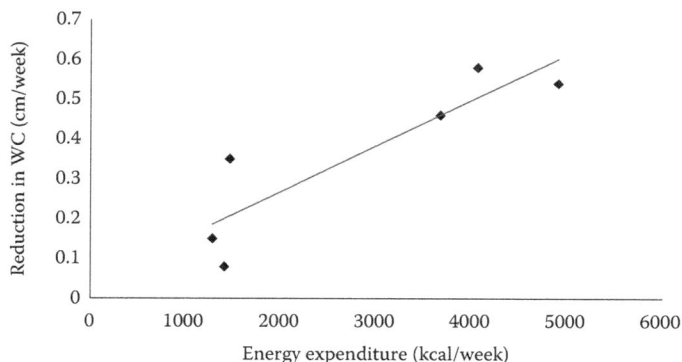

(b) Within studies

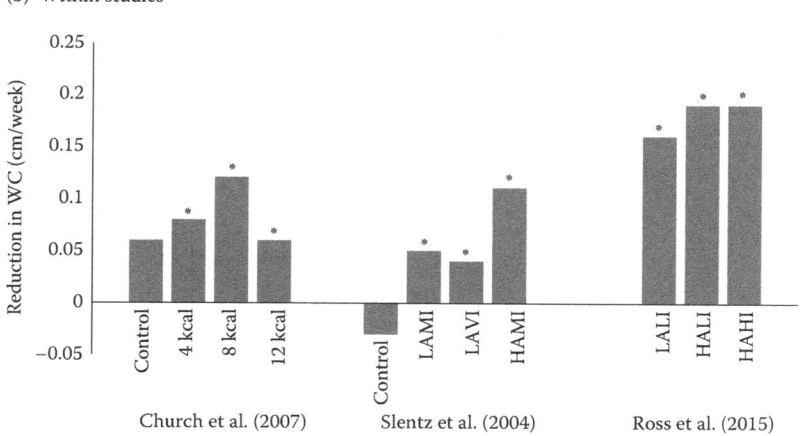

FIGURE 7.2 Relationship between energy expenditure and reduction in WC (a) of groups across groups (N = 6, Table 7.1) and (b) groups within studies (N = 3, Table 7.1). Diamonds (♦) represent WC reduction. Asterisks (*) represent significant reduction in WC compared to control, p < 0.05. Crosses (†) represent significant reduction in WC compared to low amount groups, p < 0.05. The data plotted in the figure are group means for the studies cited in Table 7.1. WC, WC; 4 kcal, 4 kcal/kg per week; 8 kcal, 8 kcal/kg per week; 12 kcal, 12 kcal/kg per week; LAMI, low amount moderate intensity (12 miles/week at 40%–55% VO$_2$peak, 14 kcal/kg per week); LAVI, low amount vigorous intensity (12 miles/week at 65%–80% VO$_2$peak, 14 kcal/kg per week); HAMI, high amount moderate intensity (20 miles/week at 65%–80% VO$_2$peak. 23 kcal/kg per week); LALI, low amount low intensity (180 and 300 kcal/session for women and men, respectively); HALI, high amount low intensity (360 and 600 kcal/session for women and men, respectively); HAHI, high amount high intensity (360 and 600 kcal/session for women and men, respectively).

and WC reduction, accounting for differences in trial durations by representing change in units per week. The observations appear to be indicative of a positive dose–response relationship, however due to the limited number of groups represented, this interpretation is not overly convincing.

Careful evaluation of RCTs specifically designed to examine the effect of increasing exercise amount on abdominal obesity reduction reveal conflicting findings. As illustrated in Figure 7.2b, three large RCTs previously described provide insight into the relationship between increasing exercise amount and WC reduction, for a given intensity (Slentz et al. 2004; Church et al. 2007; Ross et al. 2015). Church et al. (2007) found that, while all three groups significantly reduced WC compared to controls (−1.9, −2.9, and −1.4 cm for the 4, 8, and 12 kcal/kg per week, respectively), there were no between group differences despite the tripling of energy expenditure in the high amount compared to the low amount group (Church et al. 2007). As stated previously, participants were instructed that the primary outcome was not weight loss and they should maintain lifestyle habits throughout the intervention. This may have influenced the high amount group to compensate to a greater extent for the energy they expended in exercise, and thus may have attenuated the change in WC. These observations were confirmed by others. Ross et al. (2015) observed substantial reductions in WC (~5 cm) in all exercise groups compared to control, however, no differences between the low amount and high amount groups were noted despite the doubling in energy expenditure. Similarly, Slentz et al. (2004) observed significant reductions in WC ranging from 1.4 to 3.4 cm in all exercise groups compared to control, but again, no between group differences. These observations are not readily explained.

Only one study that fit the inclusion criteria examined the impact of increasing exercise amount at a fixed intensity on VAT and ASAT. Slentz et al. (2005) observed significant reductions in VAT in both the low and high amount groups, at a fixed intensity. However, there was no further reduction of VAT observed in the high amount compared to the low amount group. Only the high amount group showed significant reduction in ASAT compared to control (Slentz et al. 2005).

Albeit from a limited number of trials, the finding from RCTs that increasing exercise amount has modest effects on WC and no effect on VAT reduction is surprising and difficult to interpret, especially given the doubling of energy expenditure between some of the exercise conditions (Slentz et al. 2004, 2005; Church et al. 2007; Ross et al. 2015). As discussed above, it may be that individuals compensate for high amounts of exercise through increased energy intake. However, without exception the participants in these trials reported no increase in energy intake. Another possibility is that participants in the low amount groups overestimated their energy intake to disguise their attempts to achieve the same weight loss as those in the high amount groups. This contamination may be an unintended consequence of participants in various groups exercising together and sharing experiences.

Five studies examining the impact of exercise intensity on abdominal obesity reduction fit the inclusion criteria. With the exception of one study with a small sample size (Irving et al. 2008), for a given exercise amount (kilocalories), there was no effect of increasing exercise intensity on reduction in any of the components of abdominal obesity, including WC, VAT, and ASAT (Slentz et al. 2004, 2005; Coker et al. 2009; Ross et al. 2015). These findings suggest that adults can effectively reduce adiposity by choice of moderate intensity exercise for a longer duration (150 min at low intensity) or vigorous intensity exercise for a shorter duration (75 min at high intensity), of equivalent energy expenditure. However, it is important to note that while intensity does not appear to independently affect change in adiposity, it has been shown to have independent favorable effects on other cardiometabolic risk factors (Ross et al. 2015).

7.5 EXERCISE AND REGIONAL VARIATION IN AT REDUCTION

7.5.1 EXERCISE-INDUCED REDUCTION IN VAT VERSUS ASAT

It is established that VAT is the AT depot that conveys the greatest health risk (Despres and Lemieux 2006), thus there is great interest in determining whether there is preferential mobilization of this depot in response to exercise. Tchernof et al. (2006) examined whether regional differences in lipoprotein lipase (LPL) activity and lipolysis exist between VAT and ASAT in both women and men. The authors observed that in women, although visceral adipocytes were more responsive to lipolytic stimuli, abdominal SAT had larger adipocytes, higher lipolysis rates per cell, and higher LPL activity (Tchernof et al. 2006). In men, there were no differences in AT metabolism between the two AT depots (Boivin et al. 2007). This evidence supports the notion that VAT is not preferentially reduced compared to ASAT. These metabolic findings are confirmed by observations derived from RCTs (Table 7.1).

We identified seven studies that met the inclusion criteria that examined both VAT and ASAT reduction in response to exercise. Most adults have a greater quantity of ASAT compared to VAT (Schwartz et al. 1991). While none of the studies statistically compared VAT and ASAT response, the majority of studies revealed that for a given exercise-induced negative energy balance, the relative reduction in VAT is usually greater than ASAT (Table 7.1). Conversely, the absolute reduction in ASAT after exercise training is generally greater than VAT. Therefore, differences in AT responsiveness to exercise may well depend on whether the reduction in VAT or SAT is illustrated relative to its baseline (e.g., in percent), or as an absolute (e.g., in kilograms) reduction. This point is depicted in Figure 7.3, which shows both relative and absolute VAT and ASAT reduction measured by magnetic resonance imaging (MRI) in premenopausal women before and after 16 weeks of a continuous aerobic exercise intervention (Ross et al. 2000). While there are clear differences in abdominal AT distribution between men and women (Vague 1956; Kuk et al. 2005), wherein for a given WC premenopausal women typically have greater amounts of ASAT compared to men (Kuk et al. 2005) and vice versa for VAT (Kvist et al. 1988; Freedland 2004), whether there are sex-specific responses to exercise for abdominal AT reduction has not been reported. To address this question men and women would need to be matched for both VAT and ASAT pretreatment so that potential differences in regional abdominal AT response to exercise may be determined.

(a) 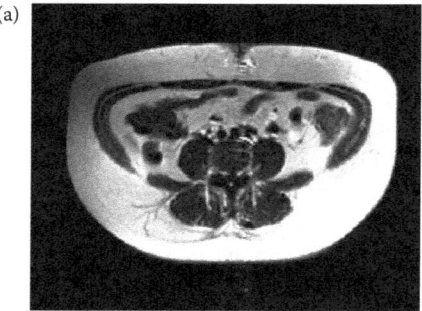 (b)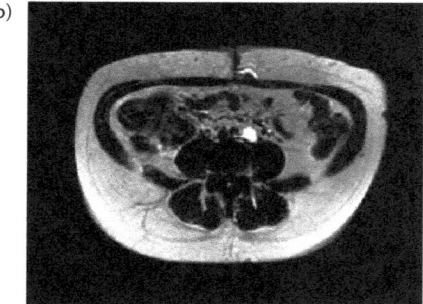

(c)

	Baseline	Post-intervention (7% weight loss)	
		Absolute change (cm²)	Relative change (%)
VAT (cm²)	124	−36	−29
ASAT (cm²)	430	−64	−15

FIGURE 7.3 Effects of 16 weeks of exercise-induced weight loss on VAT and ASAT in premenopausal women. (a) Abdominal AT distribution (MRI) at baseline (pre-exercise intervention); (b) Abdominal AT distribution (MRI) 16 weeks after exercise (60 min/session at 65% VO_2max) and (c) Absolute (cm²) and relative (%) changes in VAT and ASAT at baseline and post-exercise intervention. (Adapted from Ross, R., et al. 2004. *Obes Res* 12:789–98.)

It is established that the ratio of abdominal subcutaneous to VAT decreases with age, such that older adults have significantly greater amounts of VAT than their younger counterparts for a given WC, independent of sex (Zamboni et al. 1992; Kotani et al. 1994). Whether age influences the ratio of ASAT to VAT reduction consequent to exercise has not been studied. Concordant with previous observations in young adults, we would hypothesize that on an absolute basis, older adults will lose greater amounts of whichever AT depot is the largest.

Davidson et al. (2009) examined changes in adiposity in older adult men and women in response to exercise. Participants were randomized to one of four conditions lasting 6 months: control, aerobic exercise (30 min at 60%–75% VO$_2$peak, 5 days per week), resistance exercise (RE; 9 exercises, 3 days per week), or combined exercise (aerobic plus RE conditions). Using data from the aerobic exercise group only, at baseline older women had roughly two times the amount of ASAT compared to VAT (5.2 vs. 2.6 kg, respectively). However, counter to our hypothesis, on an absolute basis women lost relatively the same amount of ASAT (−0.2 kg) compared to VAT (−0.2 kg). Expressed relatively, the women lost double the amount of VAT (8%) compared to ASAT (4%). On the other hand, men presented with slightly similar amounts of VAT compared to ASAT at baseline (4.5 and 4.3 kg, respectively). In line with our hypothesis, they experienced similar absolute (0.7 vs. 0.6 kg for VAT and abdominal SAT, respectively) and relative (16% vs. 14% for VAT and ASAT, respectively). That women had such robust mobilization of VAT compared to ASAT for a given amount of AT differs from their middle-aged counterparts and is difficult to reconcile. It is possible that postmenopausal hormonal changes either enhanced responsiveness of visceral adipocytes or attenuated responsiveness of abdominal subcutaneous adipocytes in response to exercise, although this has yet to be identified and requires further investigation.

7.5.2 EXERCISE-INDUCED REDUCTION IN ABDOMINAL AT VERSUS LOWER BODY AT

While abdominal adiposity is recognized as a strong predictor of type 2 diabetes and cardiovascular disease risk, conversely there appears to be an inverse relationship between amount of lower-body SAT and cardiometabolic risk, wherein greater amounts of lower body SAT are considered protective against cardiometabolic risk (Ferreira et al. 2004; Lemieux 2004; Snijder et al. 2005).

It is clear that exercise is effective for abdominal obesity reduction (Section 7.4). Though few studies exist, available evidence suggests that exercise also reduces lower body adiposity (Slentz et al. 2004). Janiszewski et al. (2008) completed a secondary analysis using data from two RCTs that examined the effect of diet, exercise, and diet/exercise combinations on lower body SAT reduction. The authors observed significant reductions in lower body SAT in both men and women.

One study that examined changes in both lower body subcutaneous and abdominal AT was identified that met the inclusion criteria (Irving et al. 2008). The authors found that individuals in the high intensity exercise group lost a greater amount of abdominal AT on an absolute basis, but when expressed as relative to baseline AT amount, greater lower body SAT was lost. This finding is similar to the observations for ASAT versus VAT reduction, in that on an absolute basis, individuals typically lose more from whichever AT depot is the largest. It is important to note, however, that while participants experienced significant changes in both AT depots compared to baseline in the high intensity group, neither change was significantly different from control. Furthermore, the authors did not statistically compare changes in each AT depot relative to one another.

Though few studies that fit the inclusion criteria exist, two randomized studies without control groups have addressed this question. Carnero et al. (2014) investigated the effects of 20 weeks of aerobic exercise (AE; 60 min at 70% HR$_{max}$, 3 days per week), RE (10 exercises, 3 circuits, 3 days per week), and combination (AE/RE; 2, 12–20 min at 70% HR$_{max}$ + 8 exercises, 3 days per week) training on total and regional body composition in a small group of premenopausal women. While all exercise groups experienced significant reductions in total abdominal and lower body AT compared to baseline, there was greater mobilization of trunk AT compared to lower limb AT across all groups. After adjustment for baseline fat mass in each region, approximately twice the amount of fat mass was mobilized from the trunk compared to the lower limb across all groups (AE: −217.3 vs. −110.9, RE: −178.9 vs. −84.4, and AE/RE: −224.8 vs. −126.1 g/kg of fat mass, respectively). While limitations in sample size (n = 30) and absence of a control group necessitate caution of interpretation, these findings are supported by others who have previously observed greater mobilization of trunk AT in obese men with aerobic exercise (Despres et al. 1988).

The preceding findings are contrasted by those of Christiansen et al. (2009), who observed similar relative reductions in lower body SAT, VAT, and ASAT after 12 weeks of aerobic exercise in adult men and women (60–75 min at 70% HRreserve, 3 days per week). The discrepant findings could be explained by limitations in sample size (n = 19) that precludes the ability to detect differences in AT reduction, variation in regional AT measurement sites, and the inclusion of both men and women, as there is some evidence to suggest that response to exercise is affected by sex (Kuk and Ross 2009).

Differences in regional AT deposition between men and women should be considered when examining exercise-induced AT redistribution. It has long been established that premenopausal women typically display the "gynoid" phenotype, characterized by increased lower body SAT deposition, compared to men who exhibit an "android" phenotype characterized by increased abdominal AT deposition (Vague 1956). Thus, the question remains as to whether men and women respond differently to the same exercise stimulus beyond differences in baseline amounts of abdominal and lower body AT. Donges and Duffield (2012) recently addressed this question. Men and women (n = 67) were randomly assigned to control or aerobic exercise group where they participated in supervised exercise on a stationary cycle ergometer for 50 min at 75% of age-predicted HR_{max}, 3 days per week for 10 weeks. While both men and women experienced significant reductions in adiposity in response to exercise, men displayed greater (absolute and relative) reductions in both abdominal and lower body AT (hip and thigh) compared to women, after adjustment for age and BMI (Donges and Duffield 2012). While others have also suggested that women are resistant to exercise-induced reductions in AT compared to men (Despres et al. 1988; Donnelly et al. 2003), others have failed to observe any difference between the sexes (Irwin et al. 2003; Ross et al. 2004; Slentz et al. 2004). The discrepancies may be explained by how exercise is prescribed. For example, in Donges and Duffield (2012) men and women exercised for the same total number of minutes. It is known that for similar exercise intensity and duration, energy expenditure can vary significantly between men and women due to differences in baseline fat free mass and body size (Tooze et al. 2007). Consideration of studies in which men and women exercise for the same energy expenditure show that women lose similar relative amounts of AT as men (Ross et al. 2000, 2004).

7.6 DIET-INDUCED VERSUS EXERCISE-INDUCED WEIGHT LOSS AND AT DISTRIBUTION

In 1998 the National Institutes of Health in the United States sponsored a report on the clinical guidelines for the identification, evaluation, and treatment of overweight and obesity in adults (National Institutes of Health 1998). Among the primary findings of this report was the observation that diet-induced weight loss remained the cornerstone of obesity reduction programs and that exercise in the absence of caloric restriction was associated with only modest reductions in body weight (~2 kg) and WC (~2 cm). These observations were based upon a careful scrutiny of the existing literature and confirmed the findings of prior systematic reviews (Miller et al. 1997). However, upon inspection of the evidence it is clear that the negative energy balance induced within the diet (energy restriction) groups was substantially greater than the associated negative energy balance prescribed for the exercise (energy expenditure) groups (Miller et al. 1997). Given the gross difference in energy balance it comes as no surprise that diet-induced weight loss would be associated with substantially greater reductions in total and abdominal obesity compared to exercise-induced weight loss.

Ross et al. were the first to investigate whether differences in obesity reduction were observed in response to *equivalent* diet- versus exercise-induced weight loss in either men (Ross et al. 2000) or women (Ross et al. 2004). These RCTs were characterized by strict control of both energy expenditure (supervised exercise) and intake (self-reported intake every day), and change in AT distribution was measured using a whole body MRI protocol. The primary findings from these studies demonstrate that exercise-induced weight loss reduces total fat significantly more than equivalent diet-induced weight loss (Figure 7.4). In men, when the diet- and exercise-induced weight loss was carefully matched, reductions in abdominal obesity and visceral fat were similar. In women, the exercise-induced reduction in abdominal AT was greater compared to diet-induced weight loss. While these observations confirm that diet restriction is effective for reducing total and abdominal obesity, they also demonstrated that independent of gender, 12–14 weeks of approximately 60 minutes of daily exercise without caloric restriction was associated with substantial reductions in body weight, total fat, abdominal fat, and visceral fat (Figure 7.4). The discrepant findings with prior reports are likely explained by differences in study design. In the studies by Ross et al. the negative energy balance induced by exercise was substantial (~700 kcal/day) and was carefully matched with the negative energy balance induced by caloric restriction. Measured 24-hour energy expenditure values derived from doubly labeled water confirmed that participants did not perform substantial amounts of physical activity beyond the prescribed exercise (Ross et al. 2000). In previous studies, the exercise and diet groups were usually not well matched, 24-hour energy intake and expenditure values were not rigorously controlled or accurately measured, and the prescription of exercise programs did not induce a meaningful negative energy balance (Ballor and Poehlman 1994; Garrow and Summerbell 1995; Miller et al. 1997).

Weiss et al. (2006) performed a well-designed trial wherein previously sedentary men and women aged 50–60 year were randomly assigned to either exercise- or diet-induced weight loss interventions for 12 months. The negative energy balance prescribed for each group was similar. Consistent

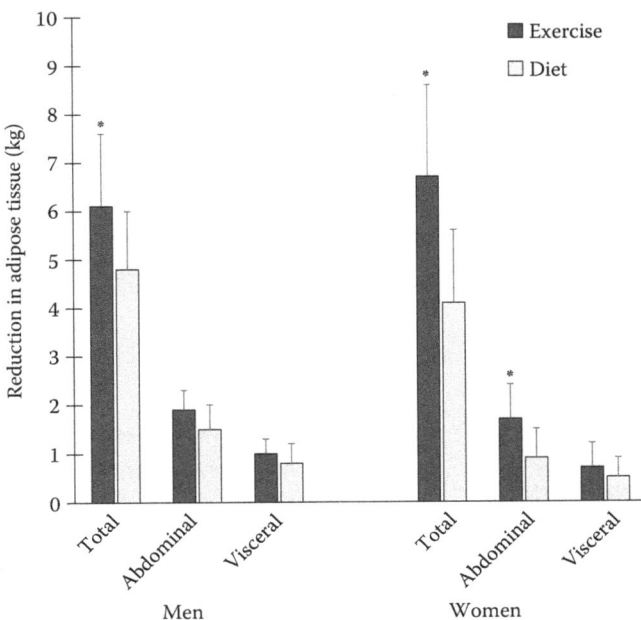

FIGURE 7.4 Comparisons of diet- and exercise-induced reductions in total, abdominal, and VAT in men (Ross et al. 2000) and women (Ross et al. 2004). Asterisks (*) represent significant differences in AT reduction between the exercise and diet groups, p < 0.05.

with the findings reported by Ross et al. (2000, 2004), Weiss et al. observed substantial reductions in total (exercise −5.6 kg vs. diet −6.3 kg) and abdominal (trunk fat measured by dual x-ray absorptiometry) fat (exercise −3.3 kg vs. diet −3.5 kg) within both groups over the 12 months which were not different from each other.

Together the findings from RCTs reviewed here counter the dogma that exercise (increasing energy expenditure) is inferior to diet (decreasing energy intake) as an effective strategy for reducing obesity in adults. This notion is underscored by Verheggen et al. (2016), who performed a systematic review and meta-analysis that compared exercise to diet as independent strategies for reducing body weight and VAT. Among the many informative conclusions emanating from this review, the author's analyses revealed that a 5% diet-induced reduction in body weight was associated with a 13% reduction in VAT whereas a 5% exercise-induced reduction in body weight was associated with a 21% reduction in VAT.

7.7   IS EXERCISE AN EFFECTIVE STRATEGY FOR REDUCING TOTAL AND REGIONAL ADIPOSITY?

The evidence reviewed here clearly suggests that chronic exercise without caloric restriction is associated with substantial reductions in total and abdominal obesity independent of age and gender. Why then, despite this evidence, do some scholars continue to question the utility of exercise alone as an effective strategy for reducing obesity (Luke and Cooper 2013)? The discrepant views may be explained by differences in the type of evidence used to support the contrasting opinion.

7.8   EFFICACY AND EFFECTIVENESS TRIALS

Intervention studies can be placed on a continuum, with a progression from efficacy trials to effectiveness trials. Efficacy can be defined as the performance of an intervention under ideal and controlled circumstances, whereas effectiveness refers to its performance under "real-world" conditions (Figure 7.5). Efficacy trials are characterized by having strong internal validity which in the context of this review implies intervention studies wherein all exercise sessions are supervised, the research

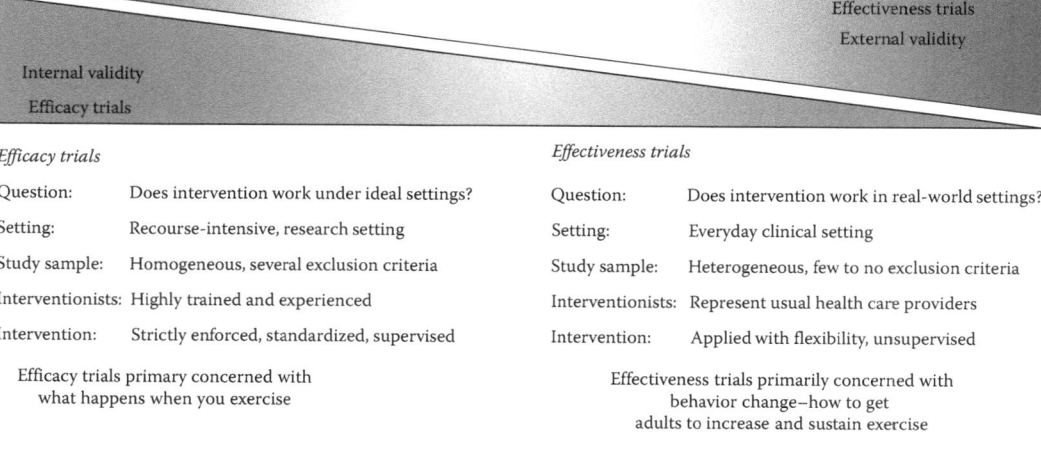

FIGURE 7.5   Intervention study continuum illustrating the major differences between efficacy and effectiveness study designs. (Adapted from Singal, A. G., P. D. Higgins, and A. K. Waljee. 2014. *Clin Transl Gastroenterol* 5:e45.)

takes place in research settings with highly qualified personnel who use criterion methods to measure all primary outcomes. The observations summarized in this review are derived from RCTs that by design are efficacy studies. Based on the evidence review it is clear that exercise is associated with substantial reductions in total and regional adiposity. However, a review of effectiveness outcome randomized trials wherein the participants are instructed or asked to adopt exercise combined with a healthful diet within a framework that incorporates cognitive behavioral techniques demonstrates very different results (Wadden et al. 2011). It is well established that trying to have adults adopt and sustain physical activity long-term in today's environment is extremely difficult for both men and women (Ross et al. 2012). What effectiveness trials demonstrate is the challenge inherent to getting people to adhere to the behavior, in this case exercise, *not* whether the behavior itself is efficacious. This distinction is largely ignored by those who criticize exercise as a meaningful strategy for reducing obesity. Indeed, sustaining healthy behaviors in today's environment whether it be increasing exercise and/or decreasing energy intake (diet), is extremely difficult for most adults and represents a major public health challenge.

7.9 CONCLUSIONS AND FUTURE DIRECTIONS

The findings of this review confirm and extend the observation that regular exercise (energy expenditure) in the absence of change in energy intake is associated with substantial reduction in both total and regional adiposity. Initial results from RCTs carefully designed to consider whether increasing exercise amount is associated with corresponding reductions in total or regional adiposity in a dose–response manner offer conflicting and perplexing results. While it is intuitive that increasing the amount of energy expended in response to exercise should be associated with further reductions in adiposity, current evidence suggests otherwise. No clear explanation for this observation exists. Further study that considers appetite regulation in combination with adipocyte metabolism will doubtless provide insight into this intriguing observation. While the effects of exercise amount of AT reduction remain to be clarified, initial evidence from well-controlled RCTs suggest that increasing exercise intensity does not influence AT reduction regardless of the AT depot considered. Further evidence from trials specifically designed to consider the independent effects of exercise intensity on AT metabolism are required to confirm these initial observations.

Whether a redistribution of AT occurs in response to exercise depends in large measure on the metric used to interpret the study findings. If one represents the results in relative terms (e.g., as a percent of baseline value), then the weighted evidence supports the view that, for example, VAT is preferentially mobilized and hence, a redistribution, or preferential reduction in abdominal AT, is the result. If, on the other hand, the absolute reduction for total SAT is compared to VAT, the redistribution reflects a preferential mobilization of SAT. Whether the differential mobilization of lipid from a given depot is clinically relevant is beyond the scope of this review. However, it is established that an exercise-induced reduction in adiposity conveys benefits across a wide range of health outcomes. The more important concern is how to encourage adults to sustain increased levels of exercise or physical activity in today's environment.

The evidence reviewed here suggests that exercise is associated with reductions in total adiposity that are comparable if not superior to diet-induced reductions. Systematic reviews comparing the two strategies suggest that exercise-induced weight loss is associated with greater reductions in visceral adiposity compared to equivalent diet-induced weight loss. The clinical relevance of the differences between the two strategies for reducing adiposity is unclear. More importantly, that increases in energy expenditure (exercise) or decreases in energy intake combined with a healthy diet are both associated with reductions in total and abdominal adiposity provide options to adults seeking to reduce adiposity. Allied health practitioners are encouraged to convey this positive message to the vast majority of adults in westernized society that seek treatment options to combat obesity.

REFERENCES

Ballor, D. L., and E. T. Poehlman. 1994. Exercise-training enhances fat-free mass preservation during diet-induced weight loss: A meta-analytical finding. *Int J Obes Relat Metab Disord* 18:35–40.

Boivin, A., G. Brochu, S. Marceau, P. Marceau, F. S. Hould, and A. Tchernof. 2007. Regional differences in adipose tissue metabolism in obese men. *Metabolism* 56:533–40.

Carnero, E. A., F. Amati, R. S. Pinto, M. J. Valamatos, P. Mil-Homens, and L. B. Sardinha. 2014. Regional fat mobilization and training type on sedentary, premenopausal overweight and obese women. *Obesity (Silver Spring)* 22:86–93.

Christiansen, T., S. K. Paulsen, and J. M. Bruun et al. 2009. Comparable reduction of the visceral adipose tissue depot after a diet-induced weight loss with or without aerobic exercise in obese subjects: A 12-week randomized intervention study. *Eur J Endocrinol* 160:759–67.

Church, T. S., C. P. Earnest, J. S. Skinner, and S. N. Blair. 2007. Effects of different doses of physical activity on cardiorespiratory fitness among sedentary, overweight or obese postmenopausal women with elevated blood pressure: A randomized controlled trial. *JAMA* 297:2081–91.

Coker, R. H., R. H. Williams, P. M. Kortebein, D. H. Sullivan, and W. J. Evans. 2009. Influence of exercise intensity on abdominal fat and adiponectin in elderly adults. *Metab Syndr Relat Disord* 7:363–8.

Davidson, L. E., R. Hudson, K. Kilpatrick et al. 2009. Effects of exercise modality on insulin resistance and functional limitation in older adults: A randomized controlled trial. *Arch Intern Med* 169:122–31.

Despres, J. P., and I. Lemieux. 2006. Abdominal obesity and metabolic syndrome. *Nature* 444:881–7.

Despres, J. P., A. Tremblay, A. Nadeau, and C. Bouchard. 1988. Physical training and changes in regional adipose tissue distribution. *Acta Med Scand Suppl* 723:205–12.

Donges, C. E., and R. Duffield. 2012. Effects of resistance or aerobic exercise training on total and regional body composition in sedentary overweight middle-aged adults. *Appl Physiol Nutr Metab* 37:499–509.

Donnelly, J. E., J. O. Hill, D. J. Jacobsen et al. 2003. Effects of a 16-month randomized controlled exercise trial on body weight and composition in young, overweight men and women: The midwest exercise trial. *Arch Int Med* 163:1343–50.

Ferreira, I., M. B. Snijder, J. W. Twisk et al. 2004. Central fat mass versus peripheral fat and lean mass: Opposite (adverse versus favorable) associations with arterial stiffness? The Amsterdam Growth and Health Longitudinal Study. *J Clin Endocrinol Metab* 89:2632–9.

Freedland, E. S. 2004. Role of a critical visceral adipose tissue threshold (CVATT) in metabolic syndrome: Implications for controlling dietary carbohydrates: A review. *Nutr Metab (Lond)* 1:12.

Garrow, J. S., and C. D. Summerbell. 1995. Meta-analysis: Effect of exercise, with or without dieting, on the body composition of overweight subjects. *Eur J Clin Nutr* 49:1–10.

Irving, B. A., C. K. Davis, D. W. Brock et al. 2008. Effect of exercise training intensity on abdominal visceral fat and body composition. *Med Sci Sports Exerc* 40(11):1863–72.

Irwin, M. L., Y. Yasui, C. M. Ulrich et al. 2003. Effect of exercise on total and intra-abdominal body fat in postmenopausal women: A randomized controlled trial. *JAMA* 289:323–30.

Janiszewski, P. M., J. L. Kuk, and R. Ross. 2008. Is the reduction of lower-body subcutaneous adipose tissue associated with elevations in risk factors for diabetes and cardiovascular disease? *Diabetologia* 51:1475–82.

Kotani, K., K. Tokunaga, S. Fujioka et al. 1994. Sexual dimorphism of age-related changes in whole-body fat distribution in the obese. *Int J Obes Relat Metab Disord* 18:207–12.

Kuk, J. L., S. Lee, S. B. Heymsfield, and R. Ross. 2005. Waist circumference and abdominal adipose tissue distribution: Influence of age and sex. *Am J Clin Nutr* 81:1330–4.

Kuk, J. L., and R. Ross. 2009. Influence of sex on total and regional fat loss in overweight and obese men and women. *Int J Obes (Lond)* 33:629–34.

Kvist, H., B. Chowdhury, U. Grangard, U. Tylen, and L. Sjostrom. 1988. Total and visceral adipose-tissue volumes derived from measurements with computed tomography in adult men and women: Predictive equations. *Am J Clin Nutr* 48:1351–61.

Lemieux, I. 2004. Energy partitioning in gluteal-femoral fat: Does the metabolic fate of triglycerides affect coronary heart disease risk? *Arterioscler Thromb Vasc Biol* 24:795–7.

Livingstone, M. B., and A. E. Black. 2003. Markers of the validity of reported energy intake. *J Nutr* 133(Suppl 3):895s–920s.

Luke, A., and R. S. Cooper. 2013. Physical activity does not influence obesity risk: Time to clarify the public health message. *Int J Epidemiol* 42:1831–6.

Miller, W. C., D. M. Koceja, and E. J. Hamilton. 1997. A meta-analysis of the past 25 years of weight loss research using diet, exercise or diet plus exercise intervention. *Int J Obes Relat Metab Disord* 21:941–7.

National Institutes of Health. 1998. Clinical guidelines on the identification, evaluation, and treatment of over-weight and obesity in adults: The evidence report. *Obes Res* 6(Suppl 2):51s–209s.

Nordby, P., P. L. Auerbach, M. Rosenkilde et al. 2012. Endurance training per se increases metabolic health in young, moderately overweight men. *Obesity (Silver Spring)* 20:2202–12.

Poirier, P., T. D. Giles, G. A. Bray et al. 2006. Obesity and cardiovascular disease: Pathophysiology, evaluation, and effect of weight loss. *Arterioscler Thromb Vasc Biol* 26:968–76.

Ross, R., D. Dagnone, P. J. Jones et al. 2000. Reduction in obesity and related comorbid conditions after diet-induced weight loss or exercise-induced weight loss in men. A randomized, controlled trial. *Ann Intern Med* 133:92–103.

Ross, R., R. Hudson, P. J. Stotz, and M. Lam. 2015. Effects of exercise amount and intensity on abdominal obesity and glucose tolerance in obese adults: A randomized trial. *Ann Intern Med* 162:325–34.

Ross, R., and I. Janssen. 2001. Physical activity, total and regional obesity: Dose-response considerations. *Med Sci Sports Exerc* 33:S521–7; discussion S528–9.

Ross, R., I. Janssen, J. Dawson et al. 2004. Exercise-induced reduction in obesity and insulin resistance in women: A randomized controlled trial. *Obes Res* 12:789–98.

Ross, R., M. Lam, S. N. Blair et al. 2012. Trial of prevention and reduction of obesity through active living in clinical settings: A randomized controlled trial. *Arch Intern Med* 172:414–24.

Schwartz, R. S., W. P. Shuman, V. Larson et al. 1991. The effect of intensive endurance exercise training on body fat distribution in young and older men. *Metabolism* 40:545–51.

Shalev-Goldman, E., T. O'Neill, and R. Ross. 2014. Energy cost of exercise, postexercise metabolic rates, and obesity. In Handbook of Obesity, Edited by Gary A. Bray and Claude Boucharde. Boca Raton: CRC Press, Taylor & Francis Group, pp. 1, 281–92.

Singal, A. G., P. D. Higgins, and A. K. Waljee. 2014. A primer on effectiveness and efficacy trials. *Clin Transl Gastroenterol* 5:e45.

Slentz, C. A., L. B. Aiken, J. A. Houmard et al. 2005. Inactivity, exercise, and visceral fat. STRRIDE: A randomized, controlled study of exercise intensity and amount. *J Appl Physiol (1985)* 99:1613–8.

Slentz, C. A., B. D. Duscha, J. L. Johnson et al. 2004. Effects of the amount of exercise on body weight, body composition, and measures of central obesity: STRRIDE—A randomized controlled study. *Arch Intern Med* 164:31–9.

Snijder, M. B., M. Visser, J. M. Dekker et al. 2005. Low subcutaneous thigh fat is a risk factor for unfavourable glucose and lipid levels, independently of high abdominal fat. The Health ABC Study. *Diabetologia* 48:301–8.

Tchernof, A., C. Belanger, A. S. Morisset et al. 2006. Regional differences in adipose tissue metabolism in women: Minor effect of obesity and body fat distribution. *Diabetes* 55:1353–60.

Tooze, J. A., D. A. Schoeller, A. F. Subar, V. Kipnis, A. Schatzkin, and R. P. Troiano. 2007. Total daily energy expenditure among middle-aged men and women: The OPEN Study. *Am J Clin Nutr* 86:382–7.

Vague, J. 1956. The degree of masculine differentiation of obesities: A factor determining predisposition to diabetes, atherosclerosis, gout, and uric calculous disease. *Am J Clin Nutr* 4:20–34.

Verheggen, R. J., M. F. Maessen, D. J. Green, A. R. Hermus, M. T. Hopman, and D. H. Thijssen. 2016. A systematic review and meta-analysis on the effects of exercise training versus hypocaloric diet: Distinct effects on body weight and visceral adipose tissue. *Obes Rev* 17:664–90.

Vissers, D., W. Hens, J. Taeymans, J. P. Baeyens, J. Poortmans, and L. Van Gaal. 2013. The effect of exercise on visceral adipose tissue in overweight adults: A systematic review and meta-analysis. *PLoS One* 8:e56415.

Wadden, T. A., S. Volger, D. B. Sarwer et al. 2011. A two-year randomized trial of obesity treatment in primary care practice. *N Engl J Med* 365:1969–79.

Weiss, E. P., S. B. Racette, D. T. Villareal et al. 2006. Improvements in glucose tolerance and insulin action induced by increasing energy expenditure or decreasing energy intake: A randomized controlled trial. *Am J Clin Nutr* 84:1033–42.

Zamboni, M., F. Armellini, M. P. Milani et al. 1992. Body fat distribution in pre- and post-menopausal women: Metabolic and anthropometric variables and their inter-relationships. *Int J Obes Relat Metab Disord* 16:495–504.

8 Changes in Body Composition with Exercise in Overweight and Obese Children

Scott Going, Joshua Farr, and Jennifer Bea

CONTENTS

8.1 INTRODUCTION AND BACKGROUND

Body composition refers to the amounts and proportions of the body constituents, the atoms, molecules, and tissues that comprise body mass (Going et al. 2012). Nothing is more fundamental to good health and function than optimal composition. Adequate intake of energy and nutrients are required for optimal development to occur. It is now clear that health and development are equally dependent on energy expenditure. When intake and expenditure are not balanced over the long-term malnutrition occurs, manifested as under or overweight, depending on the nature of the imbalance, with related comorbidities and changes in the relationships among the constituents of weight. Excess weight, especially adiposity, which is strongly associated with risk factors for cardiometabolic impairment even in childhood, has received a great deal of attention due to the health risks posed by obesity and its comorbidities. The usual approach to weight loss is to prescribe modest-to-moderate restriction of caloric intake depending on the severity of overweight and adiposity, with physical activity as a secondary component to boost energy expenditure. While caloric restriction is an effective strategy for acute weight loss, and is sometimes warranted in children and youth, there is risk, depending on the level of restriction, for impaired growth. In contrast, physical activity is critical for growth (Malina et al. 2004), and may be the most effective strategy for ultimately achieving optimal composition.

8.2 PHYSICAL ACTIVITY, EXERCISE, AND PARAMETERS AFFECTING DOSE AND ADAPTION

Physical activity is defined as all human movement; it is done at some rate of energy expenditure in all settings and for many different purposes. Exercise is a subcomponent of physical activity that is done for the purpose of increasing physical fitness. Body composition is one component of health-related fitness. Intensity (i.e., the rate of energy expenditure) is an important descriptor of physical activity, as well as the mode of activity, because different intensities have different physiologic effects, as do different modes of activity. It is critical to know the mode, intensity, and volume of exercise when evaluating the effects of exercise on body composition. Aerobic activities that engage large muscle groups and that require at least moderate levels of aerobic capacity are typically prescribed when the goal is to substantially increase levels of energy expenditure, often with the aim of reducing body weight and body fat. Moderate-intensity aerobic activities effectively increase cardiorespiratory capacity (Pate and Ward 1996) and generally improve cardiometabolic risk factors (Ho et al. 2013). In contrast, resistance exercise is typically prescribed when the goal is to promote lean mass and muscle strength. Whether resistance exercise improves cardiometabolic risk factors to the same degree as aerobic exercise has not been well tested, in part because energy expenditure is often not controlled or reported in studies of resistance training. When energy expenditure is equated, it may be that resistance exercise is equally beneficial for cardiometabolic risk with the added benefit of promoting musculoskeletal development. We focus primarily on controlled exercise studies in this chapter rather than the studies in which general physical activity is promoted, for example, studies with mixed mode aimed at increasing overall minutes of activity, since in those studies, adherence and dose of various modes of activity are difficult to discern. Gender, age, sexual maturation, and their interactions are other factors that can modify outcome and need to be controlled.

8.3 CROSS-TALK AND COUNTER-REGULATION AMONG TISSUES

Interventions designed to modify body composition often have a single aim, for example, to reduce weight and body fat or increase muscle or bone mass. Certainly an intervention can have effects on multiple tissues, directly or indirectly, depending on its design. For example, caloric restriction which effectively reduces body fat may also result in loss of lean tissue including muscle and bone. Although the interactions are complex and not completely understood, "cross-talk" among tissues plays a significant role in their regulation and in the regulation of energy expenditure. The views on regulation of composition and metabolism have changed markedly in recent years. Adipose tissue is now known to be considered an endocrine organ which secretes a number of adipokines with multiple effects on metabolically active tissue (Scherer 2006). Many adipokines are proinflammatory and have been implicated in the development of obesity-induced metabolic and cardiovascular disease. More recently, potential adverse effects for bone development have been noted (Rosen and Klibanski 2009). The associations between physical inactivity, obesity, and muscle and bone loss suggests skeletal muscle may mediate some of the established protective effects of exercise via secretion of proteins that could counteract harmful effects of proinflammatory adipokines. Indeed, muscle cells are now thought to produce hundreds of secreted factors (Bortoluzzi et al. 2006) and through these myokines, skeletal muscle plays a critical role in organ cross-talk, including muscle–adipose tissue and muscle–bone cross-talk during and/or after exercise (Hamrick 2011; Pedersen and Febbraio 2012; Bonewald et al. 2013). Given the cross-talk that occurs, interventions should be assessed for their effects on multiple components of composition.

Interventions in overweight and obese children and youth that promote musculoskeletal development while also improving body fat are needed. On this point Gutin (2011) has argued that exercise, rather than playing a supporting role to energy restriction, should be the primary approach for modifying body composition in overweight and obese youth. Based on observations that fatter youth (i) tend to ingest similar or less energy than their leaner peers, (ii) do not necessarily engage in less moderate-intensity physical activity, but (iii) do engage in less vigorous activity, Gutin (2011) suggests vigorous activity may encourage ingested energy to be partitioned into lean tissue rather than fat. In vitro, stem cells can differentiate into bone, cartilage, muscle, fat, and other connective tissues (Caplan 2009). Reciprocal relationships between fat and lean tissue exist, such that mechanisms that stimulate deposition of energy and nutrients in one direction tend to direct them away from the other (Muruganandan et al. 2009). In vitro studies have found that increasing concentrations of glucose and lipid can inhibit differentiation of mesenchymal stem cells into bone and direct these precursors toward the adipocyte lineage (Hamrick et al. 2009). In contrast, some data in rodents and a study in adolescent girls suggest mechanical signals induced by exercise inhibit development of fat mass while stimulating development of muscle and bone (Luu et al. 2009). Gutin posits that vigorous exercise may be most effective for directing energy and nutrients into lean tissue rather than fat mass. Because lean tissue has a relatively high metabolic rate, added lean mass may stimulate youth to ingest larger amounts of energy and nutrients needed for healthy growth, and explain why vigorously active youth with lower percent fat may ingest more energy than youth with a higher percent fat (Gutin 2011). Further investigation on these points is clearly needed.

8.4 EFFECTS OF EXERCISE ON BODY FAT

Concern for the obesity epidemic and the health risks associated with excess adiposity has motivated significant efforts to develop interventions for reducing body weight and body fat in overweight and obese children and youth. Weight loss requires an energy deficit, which can be easier to achieve with caloric restriction than exercise or a combination of decreased energy intake (caloric restriction) and greater expenditure (exercise). Consequently many studies include a diet component along with exercise (Ho et al. 2013), and surprisingly few studies have been designed to assess the independent contributions of diet and exercise (Watts et al. 2005) on body composition in overweight and obese youth.

8.4.1 Whole Body Fat

Recent reviews (Atlantis et al. 2006), including meta-analyses (Kelley and Kelley 2013) demonstrate a significant albeit small reduction in total body fat with exercise. Meta-analysis has the advantage of providing a quantitative summary of what is known on a topic while also examining the influence of relevant factors. Small-to-moderate standardized mean differences have been reported (Atlantis et al. 2006; Kelley and Kelley 2013), which translate into typical reductions on the order of 2%–4% fat units. Although the mode and duration of interventions are reported, adherence and energy expenditure are often unclear, and most interventions are of relatively short duration (<3 months). As might be expected, a recent analysis found that longer duration interventions had greater effects on body fat but the time-course of changes and dose–response relationships have not been delineated. In adults, initial levels of body fat influence fat loss (Going 1999). It seems reasonable to assume a similar relationship in youth but this supposition has not been carefully tested in studies with well-defined doses of exercise energy expenditure.

Whether different modes of exercise have similar effects on body fat is not clear. Most studies of the effects of exercise on body fat have employed aerobic exercise such as walking, swimming, and cycling, with the premise that aerobic activity elicits greater energy expenditure than other modes of activity. Few studies have compared aerobic exercise versus resistance exercise for fat loss (Watts et al. 2005) and comparative studies usually do not control energy expenditure. A meta-analysis showed greater effects of exercise on body fat when studies of resistance exercise were excluded from the analysis (Atlantis et al. 2006) possibly because studies of aerobic exercise achieved greater exercise energy expenditure. Study heterogeneity and failure to control energy expenditure are important limitations. It seems reasonable that resistance exercise would have similar effects on fat loss as aerobic activity when equal levels of energy expenditure and deficit are achieved. Given the greater muscle-building potential of resistance exercise it could have a greater overall effect on percentage body fat, although the effect would likely vary with maturation and gender and other factors that influence capacity for muscle hypertrophy.

8.4.2 Regional Body Fat

The notion that different fat depots confer different levels of risk for metabolic impairment and cardiometabolic disease is now accepted (Després 2012). Further, the risks associated with abdominal fat, especially intra-abdominal visceral fat, are well documented (Després 2006). Reduction of visceral fat in obese individuals is an important clinical goal. In adults, aerobic exercise reduces visceral fat, sometimes even with relatively small weight loss (Slentz et al. 2004; Ross and Janiszewski 2008). Available data suggest a similar effect in youth (Gutin et al. 2002; Atlantis et al. 2006), although results are conflicting, in part due to greater use of anthropometric indices of central adiposity (e.g., waist circumference and ratio of waist-to-hip circumference) than direct imaging techniques such as magnetic resonance imaging (MRI) or computed tomography (CT). Gutin et al. have done several studies in this area (Gutin and Owens 1999; Owens et al. 1999; Gutin et al. 2002). Using MRI to measure visceral adipose tissue, they showed both moderate-intensity (55%–60% peak oxygen uptake) and high-intensity (75%–80% peak oxygen uptake) aerobic exercise over 8 months improved visceral adiposity (Gutin et al. 2002) in obese youth. Treuth et al. (1998) examined the effects of 5 months of resistance exercise in obese pre-pubertal girls 7–10 years of age. Visceral adipose tissue measured by CT scan remained stable despite increases in body weight and fat mass. Unfortunately, this study was limited by small sample size (n = 11) and the lack of a control group.

Other fat depots expand as excess fat is gained, including pericardial, perirenal, hepatic, and intramuscular fat depots and these depots also confer risk (Going and Hingle 2010). These depots may respond to exercise similar to visceral fat. Farr et al. have shown a significant correlation between physical activity and thigh skeletal muscle density, a surrogate for skeletal muscle fat, in young girls across a range of fatness levels (Farr et al. 2012). To our knowledge the effects of exercise on intramuscular fat and other ectopic fat depots has not been investigated in controlled studies in overweight and obese children and youth.

Exercise dose–response studies are lacking and the optimal dose of exercise for reducing total body and regional fat is not known. In their analysis, Atlantis et al. (2006) found that moderate-to-high-intensity aerobic exercise significantly reduced body fat in obese boys and girls. Reductions in measures of central obesity were also reported that approached statistical significance. These investigators found larger effects after pooling studies which prescribed a higher versus lower dose of exercise (155–180 vs. 120–150 min/week). Current recommended doses (volumes) of exercise for treating overweight in children and adolescents (i.e., 210–360 min/week of moderate-to-vigorous physical activity) published by expert committees (Saris et al. 2003; Daniels et al. 2005; USDA 2005) are substantially higher than doses that have been tested in RCTs in young overweight and obese cohorts. Indeed, in their review, Atlantis et al. (2006) found no randomized controlled trial (RCT) that tested a dose of more than 200 min per week of exercise in overweight children. Although higher doses may in fact have greater benefits on body fat and central fat, this supposition must be tested in rigorous trials to demonstrate its feasibility and efficacy. Findings to date suggest a significant benefit of aerobic exercise at somewhat lower doses.

Gutin (2011) has made an interesting argument for the notion that vigorous exercise may have the most benefit for modifying body composition. Some studies that distinguish moderate from vigorous physical activity have shown that the amount of time spent in vigorous physical activity explains more of the variance in body fat than lower intensities of physical activity (Moliner-Urdiales et al. 2009; Steele et al. 2009). Gutin suggests there may be something about vigorous physical activity that encourages ingested energy and nutrients to be partitioned into lean rather than fat mass. Indeed, more vigorous, higher intensity activities (e.g., running, jumping, and resistance exercise) are typically recommended for musculoskeletal development. Studies of different modes and intensities of exercise controlling for energy expenditure in overweight and obese youth are lacking.

8.5 MUSCLE ADAPTATIONS TO EXERCISE

Skeletal muscle by weight is the largest soft-tissue component of body mass, increasing from ~40% in children to ~40%–45% in adults. Skeletal muscle is critical to energy expenditure, energy balance, and metabolic health. All bodily movement and its associated energy expenditure depend on muscle contraction. Resting energy expenditure, the single longest component of daily energy expenditure, is largely dependent on the skeletal muscle fraction of body weight. Skeletal muscle is also the largest site of glucose disposal. Low skeletal muscle mass (SMM) relative to height (Ralt 2007) may predispose children to obesity, given the interplay between lean muscle and more body fat. Ralt (2007) has suggested attempts to lessen the consequences of low muscle mass, which might be difficult in adulthood, could be more fruitful if initiated in childhood. Related to this point, Hanson and Gluckman (2011) suggest early intervention produces substantial disease risk intervention whereas the impact at adult intervention is small (Figure 8.1).

Whether early muscle adaptations confer advantages later in life is uncertain. It may be that early exercise ingrains a lifelong healthy behavior that maintains the benefit as long as participation continues. Early intervention, when muscle plasticity is high, may be important, as evidence that exercise promotes stem cell differentiation away from adipose tissue and toward muscle and bone suggests a long-term physiological as well as behavioral benefit.

8.5.1 EFFECTS OF EXERCISE ON SMM

In adults, resistance exercise more so than aerobic exercise is well accepted for enhancing muscle mass and strength. Results in children and adolescents are not as clear. Often, in studies of

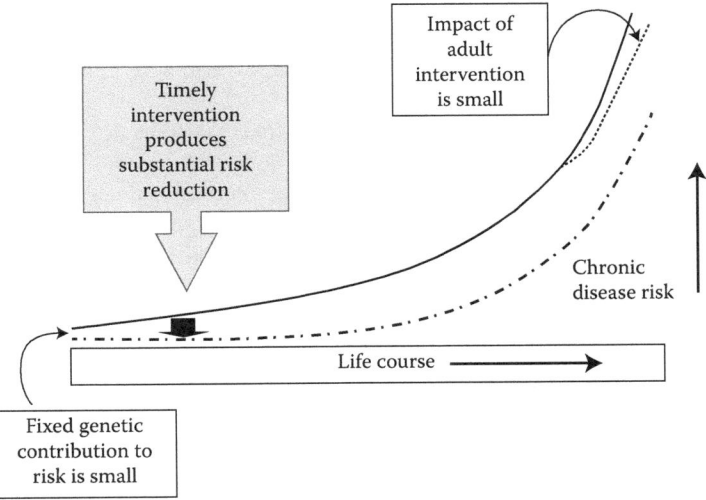

FIGURE 8.1 Early intervention has greater potential for optimizing body composition and reducing disease risk. (From Hanson, M., and P. Gluckman. 2011. Developmental origins of noncommunicable disease: Population and public health implications. *Am J Clin Nutr* 94(6, Suppl):1754S–58S. With permission.)

overweight and obese youth, the focus is more on body fat than muscle, and lean mass is often not reported unless the focus is on resistance training. Even then, strength is measured more often than lean mass. Interventions among overweight and obese youth are often multicomponent including caloric restriction and aerobic and resistance exercise, making it impossible to differentiate the effects of different modes of exercise and diet. The focus on adiposity rather than lean mass is evident in a recent systematic review of the effects of physical activity interventions on fitness and cardiovascular disease risk factors in overweight and obese adolescents in which lean mass was not systematically evaluated (Vasconcellos et al. 2014).

In multicomponent interventions with caloric restriction and aerobic and resistance training for weight loss among overweight and obese youth, short-term weight loss resulted in significant loss of lean tissue, whereas longer term programs appeared to protect lean tissue despite weight loss. An 8-week multicomponent inpatient program in 130 severely obese girls and boys, for example, resulted in significant losses of weight (girls 11.6 kg, boys 13.7 kg), fat (girls 7.0 kg, boys 9.4 kg), and fat free mass (girls 1.8 kg, boys 1.7 kg) (Knopfli et al. 2008). In contrast, in a similar but longer term (3–9 mo) program among extremely obese adolescents (N = 728), fat free mass increased despite greater weight loss (27.8 kg boys and 21.6 kg girls (Prado et al. 2009)). In the Malmö Pediatric Osteoporosis Prevention Study, one of the few long-term (5 year) multicomponent exercise RCTs without caloric restriction in younger children, there were no significant changes in lean mass despite improvements in strength, even after adjustments for Tanner stage and changes in body fat and weight (Lofgren et al. 2013; Detter et al. 2014; Fritz et al. 2016). These interventions were not designed to examine effects of aerobic versus resistance or power activities, nor is it possible to separate the effects of caloric restriction from exercise.

Several studies focused on resistance training have been conducted on youth. A meta-analysis including 40 RCTs, non-RCTs, and uncontrolled trials among overweight and obese children and adolescents found slight, nonsignificant increases in lean mass and fat free mass with resistance training and significant increases in strength. Resistance training alone compared to interventions that combined resistance training with diet education or behavior therapy (with or without caloric restriction) or aerobic training resulted in similar effects on body composition (Schranz et al. 2013). These studies demonstrate the ability for youth increasing strength without necessarily increasing lean mass, and reinforce the idea that neural adaptation may be more highly influenced with training than mass in children. The intervention duration, mode, and outcome assessment techniques varied widely, confounding comparisons. Subgroup analyses revealed no effect of sex, age, or training volume on lean mass for controlled trials, and only a small influence of those variables on change in body mass index (BMI) and body fat with resistance training (Schranz et al. 2013).

Understanding differences in the effects of aerobic versus resistance exercise on muscle adaptation to training remains an important area for research among overweight and obese youth. Whether aerobic and resistance exercise have similar benefit for increasing lean mass in youth remains unclear. One study that compared muscle adaptations to aerobic and resistance training versus control reported a significant increase in SMM in the resistance training group in obese boys (Lee et al. 2012) but not in the group undergoing aerobic training. Both aerobic and resistance training groups significantly and similarly reduced body fat and improved cardiorespiratory fitness (VO_2peak). Changes in lean mass in a similar study by the same group in obese girls were not significant in the exercise versus control groups (Lee et al. 2013). In the largest well-controlled RCT with resistance training, aerobic training, combination training, and control groups (N = 304) in obese male and female youth (or overweight youth with type 2 diabetes or cardiovascular risk factors), Sigal et al. reported significant increases in total body lean mass measured by MRI, ranging from 0.7 to 1.1 kg, and similar losses in fat mass (kg) for all training groups that were not different from control (Sigal et al. 2014). A significantly greater decrease in percent body fat was found for resistance training only group versus control, presumably as a result of a greater ratio of lean to fat after resistance training that did not occur with other types of training (Sigal et al. 2014).

Other, smaller studies comparing resistance training to aerobic training, typically with a dietary component across all groups, have found no significant differences between intervention groups for change in lean body mass in overweight and obese youth (Davis et al. 2009b; Suh et al. 2011; Damaso et al. 2014) while some have found significant increases in lean body mass for the intervention arms including resistance training compared to aerobic training, which lost lean mass (de Piano et al. 2012; Ackel-D'Elia et al. 2014). With its large sample size and comprehensive exercise regime, the Sigal study (2014) may provide the best comparison between aerobic and resistance training for changes in muscle. However, the intervention lasted only 6 months and findings from other multi-component interventions suggest that longer durations are needed to increase lean mass.

The wide variety of interventions reported in the literature and lack of dose–response studies make it difficult to determine the optimal mode, frequency, intensity, and duration of training to promote muscle in overweight and obese youth. The consistent findings of some fat loss with, at the very least, maintenance of lean mass suggests that when energy expenditure is similar and study duration is sufficient, resistance exercise may be as beneficial as aerobic exercise for improving cardiometabolic risk factors with the added benefit of protecting, if not promoting, muscle mass.

8.5.2 Quantity (Mass) versus Quality

Obesity is associated with functional limitations in muscle performance and increased likelihood of developing functional disability in adults (Tomlinson et al. 2016). Although obese individuals, regardless of age, have greater absolute maximum muscle strength in weight-bearing muscles of the lower limbs, when strength is normalized to body mass, they appear weaker than their normal weight counterparts. In adults, especially older adults, lower relative strength may partly be mediated via a higher state of systemic inflammation (Schrager et al. 2007; Tomlinson et al. 2014), due to obesity-related increases in proinflammatory cytokines (Schrager et al. 2007). These effects may be compounded by impaired skeletal muscle regeneration capacity in obese individuals due to compromised satellite cell function due to lipid overload (Akhmedov and Berdeaux 2013), but these notions have yet to be confirmed in human studies. Some evidence suggests that high levels of adiposity may impair against muscle activation in adolescents (Tomlinson et al. 2014), adding or perhaps lending to the functional limitation of low strength relative to body mass. Fatty infiltration accompanying obesity, leading to greater intramuscular fat and lower muscle quality, may also decrease relative force production through its effect on muscle mechanics (Rahemi et al. 2015). Muscle fiber type distribution is another feature of muscle quality that correlates with force production and potentially influences adaptions to exercise training, since Type II fibers may respond with greater hypertrophy to resistance exercise (Andersen and Aagaard 2010). Whether overweight and obese children and adolescents have a different fiber type distribution than their normal weight peers is not known. Similarly, whether muscle fibers convert between types because of exercise is uncertain. Certainly overweight and obese children and youth, like their normal weight peers, increase their force production per unit muscle cross-sectional (MCSA) area as a result of training. The extent to which the shift in force per unit MCSA is due to neural adaptations versus changes in muscle quality is uncertain since muscle quality is rarely investigated. Neural adaptations explain much of the adaptation in children whereas muscle mass explains a greater proportion of strength gains in adolescents, as the hormonal environment shifts in favor of accrual of muscle mass.

8.5.3 Muscle Adaptation Varies with Gender and Maturation

The effect of exercise on SMM is influenced by gender and maturation due to the hormonal differences that underlie muscle growth. Testosterone in boys, for example, promotes gains in SMM and strength during growth and in response to resistance exercise (Faigenbaum et al. 2003). Males tend to be stronger than females post puberty (Dodds et al. 2014) in large part due to their greater muscle mass. Studies examining force/MCSA, have shown its adaptation to exercise appears more dependent on duration and type of training rather than generalized differences between males and females (Jones et al. 2008). In a study of resistance exercise with nutrition education in overweight and obese Latino youth, for example, females demonstrated greater gains in bench press strength than males (5% vs. 3% gain) although lean mass was not improved (Davis et al. 2009a). Unfortunately, data are more often stratified by sex without directly comparing the adaptations in male to female to interventions. Alternatively, researchers use gender as a covariate or limit exercise training studies to one sex, making it difficult to understand the effects of gender on adaptation to training. The effect of adiposity, which is sexually dimorphic, on muscle strength and mass changes with training has not been well examined, likely due in part to limitation of subject selection to those who are obese or overweight.

8.5.4 Sarcopenia Prevention

SMM declines with aging (Lexell et al. 1988; Baumgartner et al. 1998b; Bailey 2000; Frost and Schonau 2000; Janssen et al. 2000) and contributes to important functional consequences (Baumgartner et al. 1998b; Baumgartner 2000; Melton et al. 2000; Janssen et al. 2002; Fisher 2004) and increased risk of morbidity and mortality (Roubenoff et al. 2003; Krakauer et al. 2004; Gale et al. 2007; Landi et al. 2010; Wijnhoven et al. 2012; Bea et al. 2015). While sarcopenia is not a concern among children, the potential for skeletal muscle optimization may be higher during growth (Frost and Schonau 2000; Aucouturier et al. 2011). When skeletal muscle accrual is most rapid, such as the period of peak height velocity in adolescence. Improving peak SMM during adolescence would be akin to increasing peak bone mineral density (BMD) and promoting adaptations in bone architecture that increase bone strength in youth, which is an accepted strategy for osteoporosis prevention (NIH 2012). The idea of prevention of sarcopenia in youth through exercise is further supported by the fact that there is a reduction in physical activity beginning in adolescence (Bailey 2000; Frost and Schonau 2000; Troiano et al. 2008) that may compromise muscle health across the life course (Ralt 2007; Hanson and Gluckman 2011). Some studies have related physical activity and muscle health in youth. Since females demonstrate lower peak SMM, more rapid SMM decline, and higher prevalence of sarcopenia than men (Baumgartner et al. 1998a; Garatachea and Lucia 2013), focusing on optimizing muscle in girls may be a priority.

Concern for the childhood obesity epidemic has resulted in weight management interventions among children and youth focused more on body weight and body fat than optimizing lean mass. Whether intentional weight loss during growth compromises muscle development is unclear and difficult to determine since BMI and body fat are far more often reported than lean mass in weight management studies. Loss of muscle mass, increasing the prevalence of sarcopenia, has been associated with weight loss interventions that do not include exercise in adult populations (Thomson et al. 2010; Weinheimer et al. 2010). Failure to optimize muscle mass during development could potentially lead to greater risk for sarcopenia later in life in overweight and obese children who seek weight loss through caloric restriction. Long-term maintenance of weight loss has not been good. The tendency to regain body fat, combined with lower muscle mass, may increase risk of sarcopenic-obesity and its functional and metabolic consequences. In adults who lose weight, exercise has been able to partially ameliorate loss of muscle mass (Weinheimer et al. 2010). Its role in weight management programs in children and youth needs to be thoroughly examined.

8.6 BONE ADAPTATIONS TO EXERCISE

Childhood is a period of rapid changes in stature, mass, and body composition which includes tremendous skeletal adaptations. Although skeletal morphology is largely determined genetically (Hopper et al. 1998) modifiable factors can also determine the final mass, architecture, and strength of the skeleton. Of all the modifiable lifestyle factors that can alter the skeleton, exercise may have the greatest potential to optimize bone strength during growth because of its ability to induce strains through gravitational loading and muscle contractions. Given the interdependence among adipose tissue, muscle, and bone, interventions such as exercise that can have beneficial effects on these tissues simultaneously have high potential to be successful in the prevention of metabolic and skeletal disorders.

The incidence of osteoporosis, a devastating skeletal fragility syndrome that increases fracture susceptibility, is projected to triple by the year 2040, reflecting expected population growth, prolonged life expectancy, and unhealthy lifestyles (Schneider and Guralnik 1990). It is now widely recognized that suboptimal peak bone strength early in life could be an important risk factor for osteoporosis later in life (Heaney et al. 2000). Appreciation of this fact underlies recent efforts to better understand how exercise effects bone adaptations during skeletal development and whether these adaptations during growth persist into later life. In addition to direct effects on the skeleton, exercise has the ability to modify soft-tissue composition, including adipose tissue and skeletal muscle, which both have direct and indirect effects on the skeleton (Rosen and Klibanski 2009; Kawai et al. 2012) even during childhood (Dimitri et al. 2012; Pollock 2015). Given the high prevalence of childhood obesity, there is considerable interest in how the skeleton adapts to exercise in overweight and obese children.

8.6.1 ADAPTIVE RESPONSE OF BONE TO MECHANICAL LOADING

In response to mechanical loading, bones adapt their mass, geometry, and material properties in order to keep typical strains within a safe physiological range and resist fractures. This basic concept has been known for many years (Wolff 1892). The mechanism controlling this feedback regulation, referred to as the "mechanostat" (Frost 1987), has been shown to be carried out at the cellular level by bone remodeling units (BMUs) comprised of osteoclasts that resorb bone and osteoblasts that lay down new bone. The activities of BMUs are coordinated by osteocytes, cells embedded in bone, which have the ability to respond to changes in mechanical loads and tailor the bone remodeling response by increasing the activity and/or number of osteoblasts relative to that of osteoclasts, resulting in net bone gain or loss.

8.6.2 CHARACTERISTICS OF EFFECTIVE SKELETAL LOADING

Because exercise is a critical part of building a healthy skeleton during growth, it is important to define the characteristics of mechanical stimuli that promote optimal skeletal adaptations so that these components can be incorporated into exercise prescriptions for promoting bone health. We know that dynamic loads are much more osteogenic than static loads (Rubin and Lanyon 1985), and that key features of osteogenic stimuli include high magnitude, high frequency, and abnormally distributed strains (Rubin and Lanyon 1985; Robling et al. 2001b). We also know that the osteogenic threshold is altered by an interaction between the amplitude of loading and the strain rate, such that activities involving high levels of both (e.g., jumping) will be more osteogenic than activities involving comparatively gentle strain (e.g., walking) or static loads (e.g., isometric strength exercises). There is substantial evidence demonstrating that the osteogenic response to loading saturates with relatively few loading cycles (Umemura et al. 1997), and is restored with rest (Robling et al. 2001a); thus, exercise prescriptions that involve relatively few high magnitude and frequency loading cycles separated by bouts of rest are thought to elicit the most adaptive skeletal responses (Turner and Robling 2003). Typical exercise recommendations aimed at cardiorespiratory endurance or weight maintenance alone may not be well suited for promoting skeletal adaptations. There is now considerable support for the view that (MacKelvie et al. 2002) the growing years are the most opportune period in life to optimize bone strength. Given the important interactions among tissues, it is important that interventions designed to prevent or treat obesity also consider the impact on bone.

8.6.3 Effects of Exercise on Skeletal Adaptations during Growth

The skeleton undergoes rapid changes during growth, and exercise has long been known to augment bone mineral accrual during childhood. This observation has been exemplified by studies of participants in unilateral racquet sports showing marked side-to-side differences in bone mass (10%–15%) of the playing versus the nonplaying arms in players who trained prior to skeletal maturity, whereas lesser differences were observed in age-matched controls (<5%), and in those who started playing in adulthood (Kannus et al. 1995; Bass et al. 2002). Beyond these changes in bone mineral mass, there is great interest in the underlying structural changes that occur in bone in response to exercise because, to improve fracture resistance, it is more beneficial to optimize the orientation of bone mineral than to increase bone mass per se. Because increasing the mass of the skeleton is not energetically cost efficient, adding bone to geometrically favorable surfaces translates into greater increases in bone strength and thus fracture resistance without unjustifiably increasing mass and metabolic costs. Exercise promotes the skeletal strength while maintaining lightness through adaptations in bone structure. Indeed, applications of 3D skeletal imaging techniques, such as quantitative computed tomography (QCT) and MRI, in unilateral racquet sport players have demonstrated that loading induces periosteal expansion (bone mineral accrued on the outer surface of long bones) during growth (Haapasalo et al. 2000; Bass et al. 2002), and this change in bone dimensions confers a dramatic increase in estimated bone strength (Figure 8.2).

8.6.4 Delivering Exercise Prescriptions during the Window of Opportunity

While the result of exercise on the adult skeleton is predominately maintenance, emerging evidence points to the prepubertal and early pubertal years as a unique period of life, coined "The Window of Opportunity" (MacKelvie et al. 2002), when the skeleton may be most sensitive to mechanical stimuli with consequent adaptations that promote strength. During this period, the convergence of

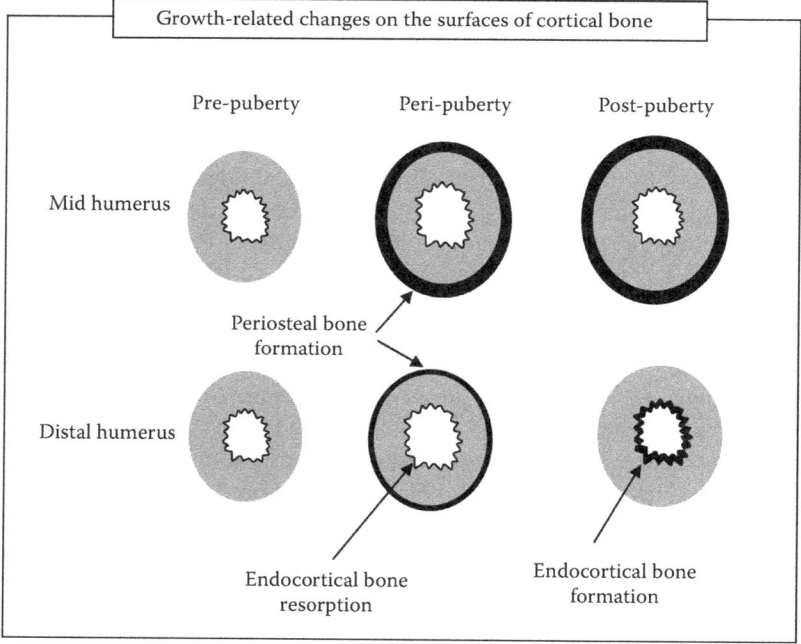

FIGURE 8.2 Growth-related changes on the surfaces of cortical bone. (From Bass, S. L. et al. The effect of mechanical loading on the size and shape of bone in pre-, peri-, and postpubertal girls: A study in tennis players. *J Bone Miner Res.* 2002. 17(12):2274–80. Copyright Wiley-VCH Verlag GmbH & Co. KGaA. Reproduced with permission.)

rapid skeletal changes (i.e., mineral mass accrual and structural adaptations) with skeletal loading through a combination of high-impact exercises and muscle forces generated during exercise can result in optimal skeletal adaptations. Thus, the delivery of effective skeletal loading prescriptions to prepubertal and early pubertal children could be an ideal strategy to elicit an increase in peak bone strength early in life that is reasonably sustained and that could offset the loss of bone strength that will inevitably occur with old age. Unlike general exercise recommendations, children may not need to participate in long periods of skeletal exercise prescriptions in order to achieve significant benefits, since the osteogenic loading effect saturates relatively quickly (Umemura et al. 1997) and exercise is more osteogenic if it is separated into shorter bouts with rest periods in between (Robling et al. 2001a).

Compelling evidence from exercise interventions and observational studies in children supports the central role for high-impact exercise to enhance bone strength during the prepubertal and early pubertal years in mixed samples of normal and overweight/obese children. Findings from these studies have been summarized in multiple reviews (MacKelvie et al. 2002; Hind and Burrows 2007; Behringer et al. 2014; Tan et al. 2014). One such review reported that 26/37 studies found a significant positive association between high-impact exercise and bone strength in both boys and girls (Tan et al. 2014). Studies that evaluated muscle *parameters* showed that muscle mass/size mediated the association between physical activity and bone strength. Despite the emerging evidence for the role that adipose tissue plays in skeletal development and perhaps in the bones' response to loading, very few studies examined the specific contribution of adiposity to bone strength, and no studies to date have delivered exercise interventions specifically to overweight and obese children.

8.6.5 RELATIONSHIPS BETWEEN ADIPOSE TISSUE AND BONE DURING GROWTH

Although osteoporosis and obesity have historically been considered independent disorders uncommonly diagnosed in the same individual, mounting evidence in recent years has unveiled an important interaction between adipose tissue and bone. Because peak bone strength early in life is a critical determinant of bone health and fracture risk later in life, understanding the influence of fat mass on skeletal changes during growth is critical for the development of exercise interventions aimed at improving peak bone strength. In adults, obesity has historically been considered protective against osteoporosis and fractures (Reid 2002, 2010). In contrast, obese children are overrepresented in fracture groups (Kessler et al. 2013), particularly those with distal forearm fractures (Goulding et al. 2000, 2005; Manias et al. 2006) suggesting excess adiposity may have detrimental effects on skeletal development (Dimitri et al. 2012; Pollock 2015).

Paradoxically, overweight and obese children tend to have higher bone mass, particularly at weight-bearing skeletal sites, which may result from the greater mechanical load on bone due to their higher body mass, their increased lean mass, or the hormones produced by their excess fat mass. Determining whether excess adiposity has beneficial or detrimental effects on other important determinants of bone strength, beyond bone mass, has been challenging due to methodological limitations. With the recent advent of technology with the ability to measure bone structure and aspects of bone quality, a number of studies have found that despite higher bone mass in overweight and obese children, other important determinants of bone strength may not be adapting appropriately during development, especially at non-weight-bearing skeletal sites. For example, a recent study using micro-finite element analysis (μFEA) of high-resolution peripheral QCT images in boys and girls (aged 8–15 years) found positive, albeit weak, associations between fat mass and μFEA-derived failure load (i.e., an index of bone strength that incorporates both the structure and quality of bone) at the distal tibia, but virtually nonexistent associations between fat mass and failure load of the distal radius (Farr et al. 2014). These observations suggest that the strength of the distal radius does not commensurately adapt to increases in fat mass during childhood, which may result in a mismatch between bone strength and the ability to resist the greater load experienced by the distal forearm during a fall in overweight and obese children (Farr et al. 2014). Thus, given the apparent skeletal site- and bone parameter-specific relationships between excess adiposity and skeletal development, the effects of fat mass on peak bone strength and whether exercise can improve skeletal adaptations in overweight and obese children are important clinical questions to address.

8.6.6 BONE ADAPTATIONS TO EXERCISE IN OVERWEIGHT AND OBESE CHILDREN

Given the prevalence of childhood overweight and obesity worldwide (Wang and Lobstein 2006) it is more urgent than ever to target this population for interventions to prevent downstream negative consequences, such as metabolic dysfunction and skeletal fractures. As a result of the interdependence among adipose tissue, muscle, and bone, interventions such as exercise that can target all of these tissues simultaneously are needed to prevent the dire consequences of childhood obesity. Aerobic endurance exercise regimens (e.g., walking, cycling, and swimming) that aim to improve cardiovascular fitness and energy expenditure and that are likely effective for improving cardio metabolic health outcomes, are less likely to improve the skeletal parameters that increase skeletal strength. This has certainly been the case in normal weight children, in whom high-impact exercise has repeatedly been shown to enhance bone strength during the prepubertal and early pubertal years, whereas general physical activity is less effective (MacKelvie et al. 2002; Hind and Burrows 2007; Behringer et al. 2014; Tan et al. 2014). While some studies have included small subsets of overweight and obese children, much less is known about the impact of exercise on the skeleton in these populations,

Given the higher forearm fracture risk in overweight and obese children (Goulding et al. 2000, 2005; Manias et al. 2006) interventions that safely target non-weight-bearing skeletal sites using osteogenic modes of exercise are needed. These skeletal sites may be particularly responsive to exercise prescriptions given the results from studies of normal weight children who participated in racquet sports during growth (Kannus et al. 1995; Bass et al. 2002). Similar studies are needed in overweight and obese children as well as longitudinal data from intervention studies. Whether beneficial exercise-induced effects on the skeleton during growth track into later life is an important question that must also be addressed.

8.7 METABOLIC OUTCOMES

The independent effects of exercise and changes in body composition on metabolic outcomes is important to understand, as the motivation underlying interventions aimed at modifying body composition is often to improve metabolic outcomes. Studies designed to address this question in adults suggest that cardiometabolic risk factors can be improved with exercise with little or no change in body weight and modest change in composition (Ross and Janiszewski 2008). Similar studies designed to estimate the independent effect of changes in weight and composition from exercise have not been conducted in children and youth. While numerous studies have examined metabolic outcomes in children and youth, few have examined the relationship between the changes in composition and the changes in metabolic outcomes. The results of recent reviews suggest a consistent effect of exercise on insulin and insulin resistance (Guinhouya et al. 2011; Fedewa et al. 2014; Vasconcellos et al. 2014). The results of studies that measured other cardiometabolic risk factors, including cholesterol and lipoproteins, markers of inflammation, and hemodynamic and hemostatic markers, were mixed. An important limitation in many studies is an inadequate assessment of exercise volume and energy expenditure. Direct comparisons between different modes of exercise without a diet component are infrequent and confounded by failure to control exercise energy expenditure. Aerobic exercise has been studied more frequently than resistance exercise, reflecting the notion that energy expenditure is more easily increased through aerobic activity. However, SMM is the major site for glucose disposal as well as critical to energy expenditure. Because sustained aerobic exercise may be difficult for obese youth, exercise aimed at increasing muscle strength may be advantageous in this population, either through effects on muscle mass and metabolic parameters or through improved muscle strength which could lead to greater physical activity and energy expenditure. That resistance exercise increases muscle strength in children and youth is clear, whereas its effect on lean tissue and cardiometabolic risk factors is less clear. In a recent review (Bea et al. 2017) of controlled trails on the effects of resistance exercise on cardio-metabolic risk factors in overweight and obese children and youth, only about half of the studies (9 of 18) demonstrated significant improvement in a metabolic outcome. It is difficult to determine to what degree changes in muscle mass, muscle quality, and body fat mediate changes in metabolic parameters, especially since many studies rely on indirect measures of body habitus and body composition. Even in studies with more direct measures of body fat (e.g., dual x-ray absorptiometry, bioelectrical impedance, and skinfolds), the results have been equivocal, with reports that improvements in cardiometabolic risk factors are independent of body fat, or attenuated or eliminated when body fat is controlled (Guinhouya et al. 2011). A common limitation is short-duration interventions. Given the variable nature of glucose and insulin levels during peak growth and maturation, including decreased insulin sensitivity (Moran et al. 1999), it is likely that longer duration interventions (>24 weeks) are necessary to show improvement in metabolic outcomes. Longer duration studies with direct measures of muscle and body fat and well-described training regimens (mode, exercise frequency, intensity, and duration) are needed to understand the contribution of changes in body composition versus exercise mode and dose to improvements in metabolic outcomes.

8.8 SUMMARY

Obesity, with its comorbidities, is a major public health issue. Excess adiposity tends to track. Without early intervention, adiposity often increases, contributing to cardiometabolic impairment and disease. Dietary interventions, with physical activity to increase energy expenditure as a secondary component, are often pursued. Long-term success has not been good. There is reason to believe that increased energy expenditure through increased physical activity should be the primary strategy. Caloric restriction may compromise nutrient intake and consequently, growth. Increased energy expenditure aids weight maintenance, and physical activity is vital to growth and optimal composition. The mechanisms whereby tissue compartments communicate, influence energy balance, and counter-regulate continue to be elucidated, although it is clear the effects of exercise on multiple compartments should be considered together. A fundamental role of exercise may be to influence stem cell differentiation and direct nutrients into lean tissue such as muscle and bone. In toto, studies in children and youth demonstrate significant reduction in body fat and a trend for reduction in abdominal visceral fat with aerobic exercise. Average reductions are modest, which is likely a consequence of short-term interventions which seek to increase energy expenditure by a modest amount. Whether resistance exercise has a similar effect is unclear. In contrast to aerobic exercise, resistance exercise may be more effective for promoting musculoskeletal development. The effect of resistance exercise on muscle is well described in adults. In children and youth, there are conflicting results, due, mostly, in our view, to the limitations of short-duration and moderate-intensity interventions, inadequate assessment methods and mixed samples (gender and maturation), and failure to adequately consider the effects of sexual maturation. Adolescents, more than children, and males more than females, due to the expected hormonal differences favoring accrual of lean tissue, are likely to benefit from resistance exercise. The results of longer duration multicomponent studies suggest an early effect on body fat and later effect on lean tissue but the nature of multi-component interventions precludes understanding the effects of different modes of activity. Higher intensity activities may be particularly beneficial for musculoskeletal development. Resistance exercise likely has advantages in obese youth who find other activities difficult to perform. Along with positive adaptations in body fat, muscle and bone, improvement in cardiometabolic risk factors occur, especially with aerobic exercise. The extent to which metabolic improvement with exercise is dependent on changes in body composition is not well described in youth although in adults significant improvement has been demonstrated with modest change in weight and composition. Dose–response studies in children and youth are lacking, as are well designed studies comparing modes of exercise. Early and sustained interventions are key to increase energy expenditure and partition nutrients to lean rather than adipose tissue. Emerging data suggest adaptations in bone architecture that promote bone strength in youth persist into adulthood. Whether adaptations in muscle early in life confer advantages in adulthood remains to be investigated.

8.9 FUTURE DIRECTIONS

Despite a growing body of literature, methodological limitations associated with many investigations have resulted in conflicting results; thus, the degree to which exercise and energy expenditure improve body composition in overweight and obese children, which mode and dose are best suited for improving a particular component of composition, and the associated health outcomes remain uncertain. Key questions, yet to be answered, include

1. What mode, intensity, and volume of exercise is optimal for improving various components of body composition in overweight and obese children and youth, and what are the associated cardiometabolic outcomes?
2. What are the time courses of adaptations to exercise by various components of composition and associated cardiometabolic outcomes?
3. Are acute adaptations maintained over the long-term and what volume of exercise is required to maintain adaptations?
4. How do sex, race, ethnicity, maturation, and initial body composition modify results?
5. To what degree are improvements in cardiometabolic outcomes dependent on changes in body composition?

Exercise interventions are expensive and challenging to deliver. As a result, most interventions test effects of one mode of exercise in one group over a short period of time. Dose–response designs are missing and long-term interventions are few in number, as are exercise interventions without a diet component in overweight and obese children and adolescents. Few studies compare the effects directly of different modes of exercise in different groups of children and adolescents. It is imperative that compliance, exercise dose, and energy expenditure be well described in order to understand the effects of the intervention on body composition and other outcomes.

REFERENCES

Ackel-D'Elia, C., J. Carnier, C. R. Bueno, Jr. et al. 2014. Effects of different physical exercises on leptin concentration in obese adolescents. *Int J Sports Med* 35(2):164–71.

Akhmedov, D., and R. Berdeaux. 2013. The effects of obesity on skeletal muscle regeneration. *Front Physiol* 4:371.

Andersen, J. L., and P. Aagaard. 2010. Effects of strength training on muscle fiber types and size; consequences for athletes training for high-intensity sport. *Scand J Med Sci Sports* 20(Suppl 2):32–8.

Atlantis, E., E. H. Barnes, and M. A. Singh. 2006. Efficacy of exercise for treating overweight in children and adolescents: A systematic review. *Int J Obes (Lond)* 30(7):1027–40.

Aucouturier, J., P. Duche, and B. W. Timmons. 2011. Metabolic flexibility and obesity in children and youth. *Obes Rev* 12(5):e44–53.

Bailey, D. 2000. Is anyone out there listening? *Quest* 52:344–50.

Bass, S. L., L. Saxon, R. M. Daly et al. 2002. The effect of mechanical loading on the size and shape of bone in pre-, peri-, and postpubertal girls: A study in tennis players. *J Bone Miner Res* 17(12):2274–80.

Baumgartner, R. N. 2000. Body composition in healthy aging. *Ann N Y Acad Sci* 904:437–48.

Baumgartner, R. N., K. M. Koehler, D. Gallagher et al. 1998a. Epidemiology of sarcopenia among the elderly in New Mexico. *Am J Epidemiol* 147(8):744–63.

Baumgartner, R. N., K. M. Koehler, D. Gallagher et al. 1998b. Epidemiology of sarcopenia among the elderly in New Mexico. [Erratum appears in *Am J Epidemiol* 1999 Jun 15;149 12:1161.] *Am J Epidemiol* 147(8):755–63.

Bea, J. W., C. A. Thomson, B. C. Wertheim et al. 2015. Risk of mortality according to body mass index and body composition among postmenopausal women. *Am J Epidemiol* 182(7):585–96.

Bea, J. W., R. M. Blew, C. How, M. Hetherington-Rauth, and S. B. Going. 2017. Resistance training effects on insulin resistance and metabolic syndrome among youth: A systematic review. PROSPERO registration number: CRD42015024433. *Pediatr Exer Sci.* doi: 10.1123/pes. 2016-0143. [E-pub ahead of print].

Behringer, M., S. Gruetzner, M. McCourt, and J. Mester. 2014. Effects of weight-bearing activities on bone mineral content and density in children and adolescents: A meta-analysis. *J Bone Miner Res* 29(2):467–78.

Bonewald, L. F., D. P. Kiel, T. L. Clemens et al. 2013. Forum on bone and skeletal muscle interactions: Summary of the proceedings of an ASBMR workshop. *J Bone Miner Res* 28(9):1857–65.

Bortoluzzi, S., P. Scannapieco, A. Cestaro, G. A. Danieli, and S. Schiaffino. 2006. Computational reconstruction of the human skeletal muscle secretome. *Proteins* 62(3):776–92.

Caplan, A. I. 2009. Why are MSCs therapeutic? New data: New insight. *J Pathol* 217(2):318–24.

Damaso, A. R., R. M. da Silveira Campos, D. A. Caranti et al. 2014. Aerobic plus resistance training was more effective in improving the visceral adiposity, metabolic profile and inflammatory markers than aerobic training in obese adolescents. *J Sports Sci* 32(15):1435–45.

Daniels, S. R., D. K. Arnett, R. H. Eckel et al. 2005. Overweight in children and adolescents: Pathophysiology, consequences, prevention, and treatment. *Circulation* 111(15):1999–2012.

Davis, J. N., L. A. Kelly, C. J. Lane et al. 2009a. Randomized control trial to improve adiposity and insulin resistance in overweight Latino adolescents. *Obesity (Silver Spring)* 17(8):1542–8.

Davis, J. N., A. Tung, S. S. Chak et al. 2009b. Aerobic and strength training reduces adiposity in overweight Latina adolescents. *Med Sci Sports Exerc* 41(7):1494–503.

de Piano, A., M. T. de Mello, L. Sanches Pde et al. 2012. Long-term effects of aerobic plus resistance training on the adipokines and neuropeptides in nonalcoholic fatty liver disease obese adolescents. *Eur J Gastroenterol Hepatol* 24(11):1313–24.

Després, J. P. 2006. Is visceral obesity the cause of the metabolic syndrome? *Ann Med* 38:52–63.

Després, J. P. 2012. Body fat distribution and risk of cardiovascular disease: An update. *Circulation* 126(10):1301–13.

Detter, F., J. A. Nilsson, C. Karlsson et al. 2014. A 3-year school-based exercise intervention improves muscle strength—A prospective controlled population-based study in 223 children. *BMC Musculoskelet Disord* 15:353.

Dimitri, P., N. Bishop, J. S. Walsh, and R. Eastell. 2012. Obesity is a risk factor for fracture in children but is protective against fracture in adults: A paradox. *Bone* 50(2):457–66.

Dodds, R. M., H. E. Syddall, R. Cooper et al. 2014. Grip strength across the life course: Normative data from twelve British studies. *PLoS One* 9(12):e113637.

Faigenbaum, A. D., L. A. Milliken, and W. L. Westcott. 2003. Maximal strength testing in healthy children. *J Strength Cond Res* 17(1):162–6.

Farr, J. N., S. Amin, N. K. LeBrasseur et al. 2014. Body composition during childhood and adolescence: Relations to bone strength and microstructure. *J Clin Endocrinol Metab* 99(12):4641–8.

Farr, J. N., M. D. Van Loan, T. G. Lohman, and S. B. Going. 2012. Lower physical activity is associated with skeletal muscle fat content in girls. *Med Sci Sports Exerc* 44(7):1375–81.

Fedewa, M. V., N. H. Gist, E. M. Evans, and R. K. Dishman. 2014. Exercise and insulin resistance in youth: A meta-analysis. *Pediatrics* 133(1):e163–74.

Fisher, A. L. 2004. Of worms and women: Sarcopenia and its role in disability and mortality. *J Am Geriatr Soc* 52(7):1185–90.

Fritz, J., M. E. Coster, S. Stenevi-Lundgren et al. 2016. A 5-year exercise program in children improves muscle strength without affecting fracture risk. *Eur J Appl Physiol* 116(4):707–15.

Frost, H. M. 1987. Bone "mass" and the "mechanostat": A proposal. *Anat Rec* 219(1):1–9.

Frost, H. M., and E. Schonau. 2000. The "muscle-bone unit" in children and adolescents: A 2000 overview. *J Pediatr Endocrinol Metab* 13(6):571–90.

Gale, C. R., C. N. Martyn, C. Cooper, and A. A. Sayer. 2007. Grip strength, body composition, and mortality. *Int J Epidemiol* 36(1):228–35.

Garatachea, N., and A. Lucia. 2013. Genes and the ageing muscle: A review on genetic association studies. *Age (Dordr)* 35(1):207–33.

Going, S. 1999. Body composition alterations with exercise. In *Lifestyle Medicine*. J. M. Rippe, ed. 1089–97. Malden, MA: Blackwell Science, Inc.

Going, S., and M. Hingle. 2010. Physical activity in diet-induced disease causation and prevention in women and men. In *Modern Dietary Fat Intakes in Disease Promotion* (1st Ed.), XXV. In *Nutrition and Health*, eds. R. R. De Meester, F. Watson, F. De Meester, and S. Zibadi, 443–54. New York: Humana Press (Springer Science + Business Media, LLC).

Going, S., M. Hingle, and J. Farr. 2012. Body composition. In *Modern Nutrition in Health and Disease* (11th Ed.), eds. B. Caballero, A. Catharine Ross, R. J. Cousins, K. L. Tucker, and T. R. Ziegler, 1648. Baltimore, MD: Lippincott, Williams & Wilkins.

Goulding, A., A. M. Grant, and S. M. Williams. 2005. Bone and body composition of children and adolescents with repeated forearm fractures. *J Bone Miner Res* 20(12):2090–6.

Goulding, A., L. Jones, R. W. Taylor, P. J. Manning, and S. M. Williams. 2000. More broken bones: A 4-year double cohort study of young girls with and without distal forearm fractures. *J Bone Miner Res* 15(10):2011–18.

Guinhouya, B. C., H. Samouda, D. Zitouni, C. Vilhelm, and H. Hubert. 2011. Evidence of the influence of physical activity on the metabolic syndrome and/or on insulin resistance in pediatric populations: A systematic review. *Int J Pediatr Obes* 6(5–6):361–88.

Gutin, B. 2011. The role of nutrient partitioning and stem cell differentiation in pediatric obesity: A new theory. *Int J Pediatr Obes* 6(Suppl 1):7–12.

Gutin, B., P. Barbeau, S. Owens et al. 2002. Effects of exercise intensity on cardiovascular fitness, total body composition, and visceral adiposity of obese adolescents. *Am J Clin Nutr* 75(5):818–26.

Gutin, B., and S. Owens. 1999. Rose of exercise intervention in improving body fat distribution and risk profile in children. *Am J Human Biol* 11(2):237–47.

Haapasalo, H., S. Kontulainen, H. Sievanen et al. 2000. Exercise-induced bone gain is due to enlargement in bone size without a change in volumetric bone density: A peripheral quantitative computed tomography study of the upper arms of male tennis players. *Bone* 27(3):351–7.

Hamrick, M. W. 2011. A role for myokines in muscle-bone interactions. *Exerc Sport Sci Rev* 39(1):43–7.

Hamrick, M. W., M. A. Della-Fera, C. A. Baile, N. K. Pollock, and R. D. Lewis. 2009. Body fat as a regulator of bone mass: Experimental evidence from animal models. *Clin Rev Bone Miner Metab* 7(3):224–9.

Hanson, M., and P. Gluckman. 2011. Developmental origins of noncommunicable disease: Population and public health implications. *Am J Clin Nutr* 94(6, Suppl):1754S–58S.

Heaney, R. P., S. Abrams, B. Dawson-Hughes et al. 2000. Peak bone mass. *Osteoporos Int* 11(12):985–1009.

Hind, K., and M. Burrows. 2007. Weight-bearing exercise and bone mineral accrual in children and adolescents: A review of controlled trials. *Bone* 40(1):14–27.

Ho, M., S. P. Garnett, L. A. Baur et al. 2013. Impact of dietary and exercise interventions on weight change and metabolic outcomes in obese children and adolescents: A systematic review and meta-analysis of randomized trials. *JAMA Pediatr* 167(8):759–68.

Hopper, J. L., R. M. Green, C. A. Nowson et al. 1998. Genetic, common environment, and individual specific components of variance for bone mineral density in 10- to 26-year-old females: A twin study. *Am J Epidemiol* 147(1):17–29.

Janssen, I., S. B. Heymsfield, and R. Ross. 2002. Low relative skeletal muscle mass (sarcopenia) in older persons is associated with functional impairment and physical disability. *J Am Geriatr Soc* 50(5):889–96.

Janssen, I., S. B. Heymsfield, Z. M. Wang, and R. Ross. 2000. Skeletal muscle mass and distribution in 468 men and women aged 18–88 yr. *J Appl Physiol* 89(1):81–8.

Jones, E. J., P. A. Bishop, A. K. Woods, and J. M. Green. 2008. Cross-sectional area and muscular strength: A brief review. *Sports Med* 38(12):987–94.

Kannus, P., H. Haapasalo, M. Sankelo et al. 1995. Effect of starting age of physical activity on bone mass in the dominant arm of tennis and squash players. *Ann Intern Med* 123(1):27–31.

Kawai, M., F. J. de Paula, and C. J. Rosen. 2012. New insights into osteoporosis: The bone-fat connection. *J Intern Med* 272(4):317–29.

Kelley, G. A., and K. S. Kelley. 2013. Effects of exercise in the treatment of overweight and obese children and adolescents: A systematic review of meta-analyses. *J Obes* 2013:783103.

Kessler, J., C. Koebnick, N. Smith, and A. Adams. 2013. Childhood obesity is associated with increased risk of most lower extremity fractures. *Clin Orthop Relat Res* 471(4):1199–207.

Knopfli, B. H., T. Radtke, M. Lehmann et al. 2008. Effects of a multidisciplinary inpatient intervention on body composition, aerobic fitness, and quality of life in severely obese girls and boys. *J Adolesc Health* 42 2:119–27.

Krakauer, J. C., B. Franklin, M. Kleerekoper, M. Karlsson, and J. A. Levine. 2004. Body composition profiles derived from dual-energy X-ray absorptiometry, total body scan, and mortality. *Prev Cardiol* 7 3:109–15.

Landi, F., A. Russo, R. Liperoti et al. 2010. Mid arm muscle circumference, physical performance and mortality: Results from the aging and longevity study in the Sirente geographic area (ilSIRENTE study). *Clin Nutr* 29(4):441–7.

Lee, S., F. Bacha, T. Hannon et al. 2012. Effects of aerobic versus resistance exercise without caloric restriction on abdominal fat, intrahepatic lipid, and insulin sensitivity in obese adolescent boys: A randomized, controlled trial. *Diabetes* 61(11):2787–95.

Lee, S., A. R. Deldin, D. White et al. 2013. Aerobic exercise but not resistance exercise reduces intrahepatic lipid content and visceral fat and improves insulin sensitivity in obese adolescent girls: A randomized controlled trial. *Am J Physiol Endocrinol Metab* 305(10):E1222–9.

Lexell, J., C. C. Taylor, and M. Sjostrom. 1988. What is the cause of the ageing atrophy? Total number, size and proportion of different fiber types studied in whole vastus lateralis muscle from 15- to 83-year-old men. *J Neurol Sci* 84(2–3):275–94.

Lofgren, B., R. M. Daly, J. A. Nilsson, M. Dencker, and M. K. Karlsson. 2013. An increase in school-based physical education increases muscle strength in children. *Med Sci Sports Exerc* 45(5):997–1003.

Luu, Y. K., E. Capilla, C. J. Rosen et al. 2009. Mechanical stimulation of mesenchymal stem cell proliferation and differentiation promotes osteogenesis while preventing dietary-induced obesity. *J Bone Miner Res* 24(1):50–61.

MacKelvie, K. J., K. M. Khan, and H. A. McKay. 2002. Is there a critical period for bone response to weight-bearing exercise in children and adolescents? A systematic review. *Br J Sports Med* 36:250–7.

Malina, R., C. Bouchard, and B. O. Oded. 2004. *Growth, Maturation, and Physical Activity* (2nd Ed.), Champaign, IL: Human Kinetics.

Manias, K., D. McCabe, and N. Bishop. 2006. Fractures and recurrent fractures in children; varying effects of environmental factors as well as bone size and mass. *Bone* 39(3):652–7.

Melton, L. J., 3rd, S. Khosla, and B. L. Riggs. 2000. Epidemiology of sarcopenia. *Mayo Clin Proc* 75(Suppl):S10–2; discussion S12–3.

Moliner-Urdiales, D., J. R. Ruiz, F. B. Ortega et al. 2009. Association of objectively assessed physical activity with total and central body fat in Spanish adolescents; the HELENA Study. *Int J Obes (Lond)* 33(10):1126–35.

Moran, A., D. R. Jacobs, Jr., J. Steinberger et al. 1999. Insulin resistance during puberty: Results from clamp studies in 357 children. *Diabetes* 48(10):2039–44.

Muruganandan, S., A. A. Roman, and C. J. Sinal. 2009. Adipocyte differentiation of bone marrow-derived mesenchymal stem cells: Cross talk with the osteoblastogenic program. *Cell Mol Life Sci* 66(2):236–53.

NIH. 2012. *Osteoporosis: Peak Bone Mass in Women.* NIH Osteoporosis and Related Bone Diseases National Resource Center. NIH Pub no. 15-7891.

Owens, S., B. Gutin, J. Allison et al. 1999. Effect of physical training on total and visceral fat in obese children. *Med Sci Sports Exerc* 31(1):143–8.

Pate, R. R., and D. S. Ward. 1996. Endurance trainability of children and youth. In *The Child and Adolescent Athlete. Volume 6 in Encyclopedia of Sports Medicine*, ed. O. Bar-Or. Oxford, England: Blackwell Science.

Pedersen, B. K., and M. A. Febbraio. 2012. Muscles, exercise and obesity: Skeletal muscle as a secretory organ. *Nat Rev Endocrinol* 8(8):457–65.

Pollock, N. K. 2015. Childhood obesity, bone development, and cardiometabolic risk factors. *Mol Cell Endocrinol* 410:52–63.

Prado, W. L., A. Siegfried, A. R. Damaso et al. 2009. Effects of long-term multidisciplinary inpatient therapy on body composition of severely obese adolescents. *J Pediatr (Rio J)* 85(3):243–8.

Rahemi, H., N. Nigam, and J. M. Wakeling. 2015. The effect of intramuscular fat on skeletal muscle mechanics: Implications for the elderly and obese. *J R Soc Interface* 12(109):20150365.

Ralt, D. 2007. Low muscle mass—Tall and obese children a special genre of obesity. *Med Hypotheses* 68(4):750–5.

Reid, I. R. 2002. Relationships among body mass, its components, and bone. *Bone* 31(5):547–55.

Reid, I. R. 2010. Fat and bone. *Arch Biochem Biophys* 503(1):20–7.

Robling, A. G., D. B. Burr, and C. H. Turner. 2001a. Recovery periods restore mechanosensitivity to dynamically loaded bone. *J Exp Biol* 204(Pt 19):3389–99.

Robling, A. G., K. M. Duijvelaar, J. V. Geevers, N. Ohashi, and C. H. Turner. 2001b. Modulation of appositional and longitudinal bone growth in the rat ulna by applied static and dynamic force. *Bone* 29(2):105–13.

Rosen, C. J., and A. Klibanski. 2009. Bone, fat, and body composition: Evolving concepts in the pathogenesis of osteoporosis. *Am J Med* 122(5):409–14.

Ross, R., and P. M. Janiszewski. 2008. Is weight loss the optimal target for obesity-related cardiovascular disease risk reduction? *Can J Cardiol* 24(Suppl D):25D–31D.

Roubenoff, R., H. Parise, H. A. Payette et al. 2003. Cytokines, insulin-like growth factor 1, sarcopenia, and mortality in very old community-dwelling men and women: The Framingham Heart Study. *Am J Med* 115(6):429–35.

Rubin, C. T., and L. E. Lanyon. 1985. Regulation of bone mass by mechanical strain magnitude. *Calcif Tissue Int* 37:411–7.

Saris, W. H., S. N. Blair, M. A. Van Baak et al. 2003. How much physical activity is enough to prevent unhealthy weight gain? Outcome of the IASO 1st Stock Conference and consensus statement. *Obes Rev* 4:101–14.

Scherer, P. E. 2006. Adipose tissue: From lipid storage compartment to endocrine organ. *Diabetes* 55(6):1537–45.

Schneider, E. L., and J. M. Guralnik. 1990. The aging of America: Impact on health care costs. *JAMA* 263(17):2335–2340.

Schrager, M. A., E. J. Metter, E. Simonsick et al. 2007. Sarcopenic obesity and inflammation in the InCHIANTI study. *J Appl Physiol (1985)* 102(3):919–25.

Schranz, N., G. Tomkinson, and T. Olds. 2013. What is the effect of resistance training on the strength, body composition and psychosocial status of overweight and obese children and adolescents? A Systematic review and meta-analysis. *Sports Med* 43(9):893–907.

Sigal, R. J., A. S. Alberga, G. S. Goldfield et al. 2014. Effects of aerobic training, resistance training, or both on percentage body fat and cardiometabolic risk markers in obese adolescents: The healthy eating aerobic and resistance training in youth randomized clinical trial. *JAMA Pediatr* 168(11):1006–14.

Slentz, C. A., B. D. Duscha, J. L. Johnson et al. 2004. Effects of the amount of exercise on body weight, body composition, and measures of central obesity: STRRIDE—A randomized controlled study. *Arch Intern Med* 164(1):31–9.

Steele, R. M., E. M. van Sluijs, A. Cassidy, S. J. Griffin, and U. Ekelund. 2009. Targeting sedentary time or moderate- and vigorous-intensity activity: Independent relations with adiposity in a population-based sample of 10-y-old British children. *Am J Clin Nutr* 90(5):1185–92.

Suh, S., I. K. Jeong, M. Y. Kim et al. 2011. Effects of resistance training and aerobic exercise on insulin sensitivity in overweight Korean adolescents: A controlled randomized trial. *Diabetes Metab J* 35(4):418–26.

Tan, V. P., H. M. Macdonald, S. Kim et al. 2014. Influence of physical activity on bone strength in children and adolescents: A systematic review and narrative synthesis. *J Bone Miner Res* 29(10):2161–81.

Thomson, C. A., A. T. Stopeck, J. W. Bea et al. 2010. Changes in body weight and metabolic indexes in overweight breast cancer survivors enrolled in a randomized trial of low-fat vs. reduced carbohydrate diets. *Nutr Cancer* 62(8):1142–52.

Tomlinson, D. J., R. M. Erskine, C. I. Morse, K. Winwood, and G. L. Onambele-Pearson. 2014. Combined effects of body composition and ageing on joint torque, muscle activation and co-contraction in sedentary women. *Age (Dordr)* 36(3):9652.

Tomlinson, D. J., R. M. Erskine, C. I. Morse, K. Winwood, and G. Onambele-Pearson. 2016. The impact of obesity on skeletal muscle strength and structure through adolescence to old age. *Biogerontology* 17:467–83.

Treuth, M. S., G. R. Hunter, R. Figueroa-Colon, and M. I. Goran. 1998. Effects of strength training on intra-abdominal adipose tissue in obese prepubertal girls. *Med Sci Sports Exerc* 30(12):1738–43.

Troiano, R. P., D. Berrigan, K. W. Dodd et al. 2008. Physical activity in the United States measured by accelerometer. *Med Sci Sports Exerc* 40(1):181–8.

Turner, C. H., and A. G. Robling. 2003. Designing exercise regimens to increase bone strength. *Exerc Sport Sci Rev* 31(1):45–50.

Umemura, Y., T. Ishiko, T. Yamauchi, M. Kurono, and S. Mashiko. 1997. Five jumps per day increase bone mass and breaking force in rats. *J Bone Miner Res* 12(9):1480–5.

USDA. 2005. USDA Dietary Guidelines for Americans. http://health.gov/dietaryguidelines/dga2005/document/. (Accessed April 5 2016).

Vasconcellos, F., A. Seabra, P. T. Katzmarzyk et al. 2014. Physical activity in overweight and obese adolescents: Systematic review of the effects on physical fitness components and cardiovascular risk factors. *Sports Med* 44(8):1139–52.

Wang, Y., and T. Lobstein. 2006. Worldwide trends in childhood overweight and obesity. *Int J Pediatr Obes* 1(1):11–25.

Watts, K., T. W. Jones, E. A. Davis, and D. Green. 2005. Exercise training in obese children and adolescents: Current concepts. *Sports Med* 35(5):375–92.

Weinheimer, E. M., L. P. Sands, and W. W. Campbell. 2010. A systematic review of the separate and combined effects of energy restriction and exercise on fat-free mass in middle-aged and older adults: Implications for sarcopenic obesity. *Nutr Rev* 68(7):375–88.

Wijnhoven, H. A., M. B. Snijder, M. A. van Bokhorst-de van der Schueren, D. J. Deeg, and M. Visser. 2012. Region-specific fat mass and muscle mass and mortality in community-dwelling older men and women. *Gerontology* 58(1):32–40.

Wolff, J. 1892. *The Law of Bone Transformation*. Berlin, Germany: A. Hirschwald.

Section III

Body Composition in Sports and Occupations

9 Body Composition Changes with Training
Methodological Implications

Luís B. Sardinha and Diana A. Santos

CONTENTS

9.1 OVERVIEW

Assessing body composition in the course of a sports season provides valuable information that can help sports professionals assess and monitor the success of training programs (Stapff 2000; Drinkwater et al. 2008) and also monitor the health status of athletes (Matzkin et al. 2015; Tenforde et al. 2016). Selecting a body composition method is frequently dependent on the intended purpose for which data are to be used and also on the availability of the techniques. Nonetheless, body composition estimates in athletes are diverse, in part because different assessment techniques of varying accuracy and precision are used to quantify exercise- and diet-related changes in body composition (Malina 2007). *In vivo* body composition methods rely on assumptions that may not be valid in athletes. Notwithstanding, laboratory methods can be time consuming, expensive, and may expose athletes to unnecessary radiation. Methodology and equipment to perform body composition assessment must be accessible and cost-effective. Not all of the methods meet these criteria. Furthermore, athletes and coaches should know that there are errors associated with all body composition techniques and that it is not appropriate to set a specific body composition profile for an individual athlete (Rodriguez et al. 2009). In this chapter, we will review some issues and concerns related to the precision and accuracy of most often used body composition methods that need to be taken into account when selecting a method.

9.2 WHY SHOULD WE TRACK BODY COMPOSITION IN SPORTS?

Numerous studies of athletic populations have reported that an enhanced body composition might have a positive impact on performance parameters such as maximal oxygen consumption (Hogstrom et al. 2012), the onset of blood lactate accumulation (Hogstrom et al. 2012), maximal strength (Granados et al. 2008; Silva et al. 2011, 2014), or muscle power (Granados et al. 2008; Silva et al. 2010, 2014; Santos et al. 2014). Accordingly, analyzing seasonal variation in body composition is extremely important, with studies commonly comparing the body composition of athletes during several critical periods of the season.

Another concern, particularly in weight-sensitive sports, is related to the health of the athletes (Matzkin et al. 2015; Tenforde et al. 2016). In weight-sensitive sports, there is a focus on leanness due to the possible negative impact of excessive weight on performance (Ackland et al. 2012; Sundgot-Borgen et al. 2013). In this regard, establishing a minimum weight and/or body composition for competition is becoming important to prevent unhealthy body composition profiles (Meyer et al. 2013).

Also in weight-sensitive sports, there are concerns related to energy availability (Loucks 2004; Loucks et al. 2011) and energy balance (Rodriguez et al. 2009). To accurately estimate energy availability (energy intake minus exercise energy expenditure per fat-free mass kg), it is necessary to have an accurate estimation of fat-free mass (FFM). To determine a given energy imbalance necessary to lose weight, considering the energy density of fat mass (FM) (Merril and Watt 1973) and FFM (Dulloo and Jacquet 1999) of 9.5 and 1.0 kcal/g/day, respectively, it is of the highest importance that body composition methods are able to accurately and precisely detect small but meaningful body composition changes.

Studies conducted over the course of a season reporting body composition changes have focused on the molecular and whole-body levels of body composition analysis. The majority of these studies used body composition techniques of limited accuracy.

9.3 WHAT BODY COMPOSITION METHODS ARE CURRENTLY BEING USED BY SPORTS PROFESSIONALS?

Numerous body composition methods are currently used in sports. Table 9.1 summarizes some methods that can be used to estimate body composition at the molecular, cellular, tissue, and whole-body level.

The variety of methods raises issues regarding research findings and precludes the possibility of comparisons between studies, sports, and seasonal variations.

The International Olympic Committee (IOC) established an *ad hoc* Research Working Group on Body Composition Health and Performance of Athletes (BCHP) in 2010. This group carried out (Meyer et al. 2013) a survey including demographic and content questions related to body composition assessment among sports dietitians, medical doctors, professors, sports scientists, coaches, athletic trainers, physical therapists, students, administrators, the self-employed, and competition judges (188 participants from 33 countries with 0.2–48 years of experience). The results showed a lack of standardization of the methods for body composition assessment. In Figure 9.1 are illustrated the most commonly reported body composition methods. Besides the methods described in Figure 9.1, other methods were reported, including ultrasound, MRI, CT, three-dimensional laser body scanner, lipometer, four-component (4C) model, assessment of extracellular fluids by bromide dilution, somatotype, five-way fractionation model and proportionality, and total body water (TBW) by deuterium dilution to estimate FFM.

The methods most commonly used by sports professional are skinfold (SKF) thickness, whether it is to convert to %FM or to use the sum of several sites. The use of dual x-ray absorptiometry (DXA) is more commonly reported for international-level athletes, and particularly in weight-sensitive sports; the other methods are equally used among different competitive levels. Bioimpedance

TABLE 9.1
Most Commonly Used Body Composition Methods at the Molecular and Whole-Body Level

	What Is Being Estimated	Setting
Molecular		
Four-component	FM	Laboratory
	FFM (water + mineral + protein/residual)	
Three-component	FM	Laboratory
	FFM (water + residual or mineral + residual)	
UWW/ADP	Body density ≫ FM	Laboratory
Hydrometry (D₂O)	TBW ≫ FFM	Laboratory
DXA	Total and regional BMC; FM; LST	Laboratory
BIA/BIS	R, Xc ≫ TBW ≫ FFM	Laboratory and field
SKF equations	Bd (%FM) or estimated %FM	Field
Whole Body		
BMI	Relative weight for height	Field
Mass Index	Relative weight for sitting height	Field
ΣSKF, SKF map, or SKF ratio	Subcutaneous adipose tissue thickness	Field
BIA/BIVA	R/H; Xc/H; Pha	Laboratory and field
Ultrasound	Uncompressed tissue layer thickness	Laboratory and field

Note: UWW, underwater weighting; ADP, air-displacement plethysmography; DXA, dual x-ray absorptiometry; BIA, bioimpedance analysis; BIS, bioimpedance spectroscopy; SKF, skinfold; BMI, body mass index; BIVA, bioimpedance vectorial analysis; FM, fat mass; FFM, fat-free mass; TBW, total body water; BMC, bone mineral content; LST, lean soft tissue; R, resistance; Xc, reactance; Bd, body density; H, height; Pha, phase angle.

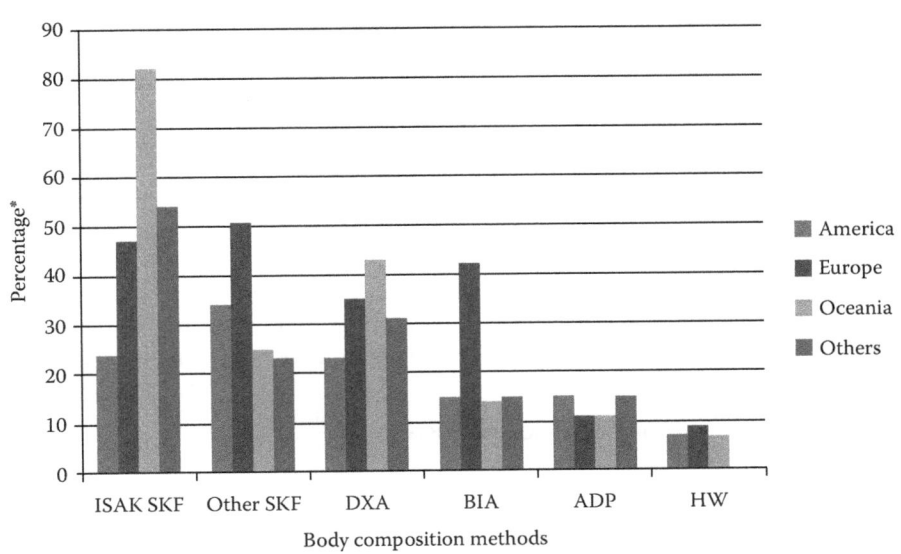

*More than one response was possible

FIGURE 9.1 **(See color insert.)** Most common body composition methods reported by Meyer et al. (2013).

analysis (BIA) is also often chosen by professionals, particularly in Europe. Air-displacement plethysmography and underwater weighting are also among the most frequently used body composition methods.

Additionally, some professionals choose to use more than one method; for example, the use of DXA is performed in specific time periods (e.g., 5 times/season) and SKFs can be taken on a monthly basis. Generally, dietitians and nutritionists most frequently assess athletes' body composition, particularly when it comes to weight-sensitive sports.

9.4 ACCURACY OR PRECISION?

When repeated measures of body composition are conducted, there are several aspects that need to be considered in the choice of the methodology. A method can be highly precise but gives inaccurate body composition measurements. Conversely, a method can be accurate but with a low degree of precision. Furthermore, it is important to be aware that there is currently no body composition method that is free of error. The selection of a method requires an understanding of error(s) associated with the basic assumptions of the method (biological error) and other errors associated with the technique and test administrator (technical error) (Lukaski 1987).

When a study reports the precision (reproducibility or repeatability) of the method, it refers to the degree to which the same method, under the same conditions, produces the same measurements. On the other hand, accuracy (or trueness) refers to the degree to which a method can estimate the true value.

Studies that determine the precision of a given method will conduct short-time interval assessments using the same equipment and under the same conditions and provide an estimate of the variability (e.g., coefficient of variation) of the measurement. However, the determination of accuracy requires a comparison of the measurement with the new or candidate method relative to an acknowledged reference method.

The precision of the method is particularly important when serial or multiple time-point assessments are performed. A survey of practices in body composition assessment (Meyer et al. 2013) demonstrated that the frequency of body composition assessment ranges from weekly to once per season. Key elements to increase the precision of the assessments include standardization of protocols, calibration of the equipment, or trained and certified technicians (Meyer et al. 2013).

9.5 BODY COMPOSITION CHANGES AND METHODOLOGICAL IMPLICATIONS

Body composition has been systematized into a five-level model in which body weight can be described as five distinct and separate but integrated levels of increasing complexity: atomic, molecular, cellular, tissue system, and whole body (Wang et al. 1992).

In the athletic field, the majority of the methods that are currently used by professionals are applied at the molecular and whole-body levels (Meyer et al. 2013); accordingly, this review will emphasize the main limitations of currently used methods at these body composition levels.

9.5.1 Molecular Models of Body Composition

The molecular level of body composition analysis consists of five major components: water, protein, carbohydrate (glycogen), mineral (bone and soft-tissue minerals), and lipid (Wang et al. 1992). The majority of the currently used body composition methods are based on the assumptions that acknowledge quantitative steady-state relations between molecular components. These associations are fundamental to the body composition methodology area, with the assumed physical density of the molecular components being of extreme importance for methodological advances (Table 9.2).

TABLE 9.2

Body Composition and Density (at 36°C) Based on Cadaver Analysis

Body Component	Fat-Free Mass (%)	Density (g/cm³)
Water	73.8	0.9937
Protein	19.4	1.34
Mineral	6.8	3.038
Osseous	5.6	2.982
Nonosseous	1.2	3.317
Fat-free mass	100	1.100
Fat		0.9007
Whole body		1.064

Source: Adapted from Brozek, J. et al. 1963. *Ann N Y Acad Sci* 110:113–40.

When using two-component (2C) models, body weight can be divided in FM and FFM, and the density and composition of the FFM are assumed to be constant (Table 9.2) (Behnke et al. 1942; Pace and Rathbun 1945; Siri 1961; Brozek et al. 1963). The physical density of the molecular components was of extreme importance for methodological advances. The calculated and assumed constant densities have allowed that, at the molecular level of analysis, body composition was traditionally investigated as the sum of two compartments, where the body mass equals the sum of FM and FFM (Behnke et al. 1942; Pace and Rathbun 1945; Siri 1961; Brozek et al. 1963). Equations 9.1 and 9.2 represent two commonly used 2C models that are based on the assumed FFM density (FFM_D) and composition. Using 2C models normally involves the determination of body density (densitometric models) or TBW (hydrometric models) (Withers et al. 1998).

$$\%FM = \left[\left(\frac{4.95}{Bd\ (g/cm^3)} \right) - 4.50 \right] \times 100 \qquad (9.1)$$

$$FM\ (kg) = BM\ (kg) - \frac{TBW\ (kg)}{0.732} \qquad (9.2)$$

In Equation 9.1 (Siri 1961), FFM_D is assumed to be 1.1 g/cm³, assuming constant proportions of water, protein, and mineral in FFM. In Equation 9.2 (Pace and Rathbun 1945), the hydration of FFM (TBW/FFM) is assumed to be constant (73.2%). Regardless, due to the wide variation of the FFM water compartment, even in healthy individuals, the use of a constant has been long stated as a limitation (Moore and Boyden 1963). The errors associated with 2C models exceed the relatively low technical accuracy of the measurements [TEM: underwater weighting = 0.4%FM, TBW = 0.6%FM (Withers et al. 1999)] and correspond to the inter-individual biological variability that can preclude the use of the assumed constants (Moore and Boyden 1963; Withers et al. 1999).

Figure 9.2 illustrates the differences in estimations of %FM when using densitometric and hydrometric 2C models versus using a 4C model, which controls for the variability of FFM density and composition.

As shown in Figure 9.2, it is possible to verify that using 2C models in athletes that deviate from assumed constants will lead to errors in the estimation of adiposity. When the water FFM compartment decreases, FFM density will increase, as the density of water is lower (0.9937 g/cm³) when

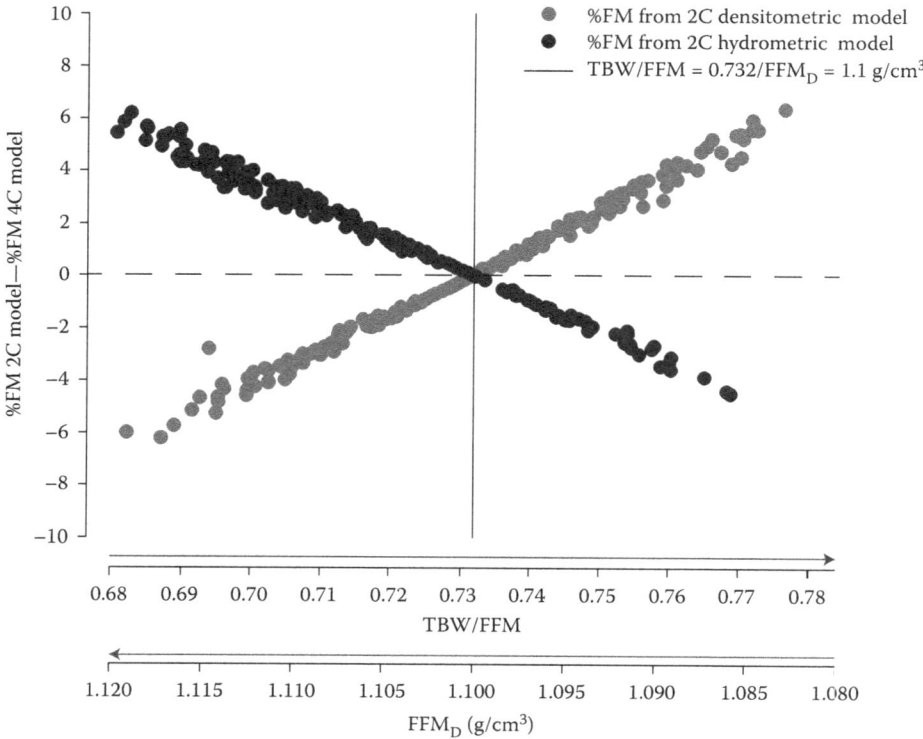

FIGURE 9.2 **(See color insert.)** Differences between percent fat mass estimated with 2C densitometric and hydrometric models versus a 4C model, accordingly to FFM density and hydration (data from 235 athletes, not published).

compared to the density of other FFM components (mineral = 3.038 g/cm³ and protein = 1.34 g/cm³). Accordingly, in an athlete that presents a lower FFM hydration, and consequently a higher FFM density, using 2C hydrometric models will lead to an overestimation of %FM whereas using a 2C densitometric model will result in underestimates of %FM.

Conversely, it has been demonstrated that athletes deviate (Modlesky et al. 1996; Prior et al. 2001; Silva et al. 2006, 2009; Santos et al. 2014) from these assumed constants that are based on the analysis of just three male cadavers (Brozek et al. 1963). Additionally, even for an individual athlete, seasonal variations may occur in the density and composition of FFM (van der Ploeg et al. 2001; Santos et al. 2014). Table 9.3 summarizes findings of changes in the density and composition of the FFM, by using a 4C model.

9.5.1.1 Two-Component Densitometric Models

The density of an object corresponds to its weight per unit volume. Accordingly, by measuring an athlete's body weight and density, we are able to calculate the body density. Using the Siri (1961) (Equation 9.1) or the Brozek et al. (1963) equation, it is possible to calculate %FM. The Siri (1961) equation lies on the premise that the density of FM at 37°C is 0.9 g/cm³ and that the density of FFM is 1.1 g/cm³. Despite the fact that body core temperature is close to 37°C, the average body temperature under basal conditions in a comfortable environment is 1–2°C lower (Withers et al. 1999); thus, Brozek et al. (1963) developed equations considering the density of body components at 36°C.

All 2C densitometric models will produce inaccurate values for the athlete's %FM whenever the density of the FFM is different from 1.1 g/cm³ (Withers et al. 1996). Santos et al. (2014) verified that, although, at a pre-season, female basketball players did not differ significantly from this

TABLE 9.3
FFM_D and Composition in Longitudinal Studies with Athletes

n/Sex/Sport/Level/Age range ($\bar{x}$ (sd) if range not available)	Time	FFM_D (g/cm³)	TBW/FFM	M/FFM	Prot/FFM	Body Density	Reference
12/male/basketball/national/16–17	Pre-season	1.101 (0.010)	71.3 (2.8)	5.6 (0.3)	23.1 (2.8)	Nr	Santos et al. (2014)
	Competitive period	1.103 (0.002)	70.6 (0.5)	5.6 (0.1)	23.8 (0.5)	Nr	
15/male/bodybuilding/≥3-year experience/19–44	Baseline	1.099 (0.004)	72.7 (1.1)	6.5 (0.6)	Nr	Nr	van Marken Lichtenbelt et al. (2004)
	8 weeks of strength training with AAS	1.099 (0.005)	72.4 (1.3)	6.2 (0.5)	Nr	Nr	
27/male/judo/top level/22.2 (2.8)	Weight maintenance	1.100 (0.007)	72 (2)	5.7 (0.3)	22 (2)	Nr	Santos et al. (2010)
	Prior to competition	1.102 (0.009)	71 (3)	5.7 (0.4)	23 (3)	Nr	
11/female/basketball/national/16–17	Pre-season	1.099 (0.005)	72.4 (1.6)	6.0 (0.5)	21.5 (1.7)	Nr	Santos et al. (2014)
	Competitive period	1.108 (0.007)	69.9 (1.7)	6.1 (0.5)	24.0 (1.7)	Nr	
5/female/bodybuilding/4-10-year experience/35.3 (5.7)	12 weeks prior to competition	1.0980 (0.0040)	73.9 (1.5)	4.98 (0.49)[a]	Nr	1.0560 (0.0103)	van der Ploeg et al. (2001)
	6 weeks prior to competition	1.0988 (0.0049)	73.8 (1.6)	5.07 (0.51)[a]	Nr	1.0605 (0.0109)	
	3–5 days prior to competition	1.1007 (0.0059)	73.3 (1.9)	5.12 (0.53)[a]	Nr	1.0706 (0.0104)	
8 + 8/male/bodybuilding/≥3-year experience/19–44	Baseline (placebo)	1.100 (0.004)	72.2 (0.8)	Nr	Nr	Nr	van Marken Lichtenbelt et al. (2004)
	After 8 weeks (placebo)	1.102 (0.003)	71.7 (0.7)	Nr	Nr	Nr	
	After 14 weeks (placebo)	1.100 (0.002)	72.1 (0.6)	Nr	Nr	Nr	
	Baseline (ND)	1.099 (0.004)	72.6 (1.2)	Nr	Nr	Nr	
	After 8 weeks (ND)	1.100 (0.004)	71.8 (1.0)	Nr	Nr	Nr	
	After 14 weeks[b] (ND)	1.1099 (0.003)	72.4 (0.7)	Nr	Nr	Nr	

Note: FFM_D, fat-free mass density; TBW, total body water; M, mineral; Prot, protein; AAS, androgenic-anabolic steroids; ND, nandrolone administration; Nr, not reported.

[a] BMM, bone mineral mass fraction.

[b] Assessments 7-weeks after the last nandrolone injection.

established value, at a competitive period, the FFM density was significantly higher compared to the established value that is based on cadaver analysis (Table 9.2). To understand the impact of deviations to these assumed constants in Table 9.4, we illustrate an example of the impact that deviations may have in estimating body composition. For this purpose, the Siri (1961) equation was derived (Table 9.4) using the assumed constants (left), the values of FFM density reported by the authors for the pre-season (middle), and the values reported for the competitive period (right), assuming that the body density and body weight were stable; the body density was 1.054 g/cm^3 and the body weight was 63.7 kg.

In the example, when using the original Siri (1961) equation (left), we will come up to a value with 19.6%FM. In the middle, we derived the equation taking into account the FFM density of the pre-season, which did not significantly differ from 1.100 g/cm^3, and the value was close to the one

---

TABLE 9.4

Derivation of the Siri (1961) Equation Using Data from Santos et al. (2014)

$$BW = FM + FFM \quad \text{and} \quad Bd = \frac{BW}{B\,Vol}$$

$$Bd = \frac{FM + FFM}{FM\,Vol + FFM\,Vol}$$

FM = 0.9 g/cm^3	FM = 0.9 g/cm^3	FM = 0.9 g/cm^3
dFFM = 1.100 g/cm^3	dFFM = 1.099 g/cm^3	dFFM = 1.108 g/cm^3
↓	↓	↓
$\frac{1}{Bd} = \frac{FM}{0.9} + \frac{FFM}{1.1}$	$\frac{1}{Bd} = \frac{FM}{0.9} + \frac{FFM}{1.099}$	$\frac{1}{Bd} = \frac{FM}{0.9} + \frac{FFM}{1.108}$
↓	↓	↓
$\frac{1}{Bd} = \frac{FM}{0.9} + \frac{1-FM}{1.1}$	$\frac{1}{Bd} = \frac{FM}{0.9} + \frac{1-FM}{1.099}$	$\frac{1}{Bd} = \frac{FM}{0.9} + \frac{1-FM}{1.108}$
$\frac{0.9}{Bd} = FM + \frac{0.9}{1.1} - \frac{0.9FM}{1.1}$	$\frac{0.9}{Bd} = FM + \frac{0.9}{1.099} - \frac{0.9FM}{1.099}$	$\frac{0.9}{Bd} = FM + \frac{0.9}{1.108} - \frac{0.9FM}{1.108}$
$\frac{0.9}{Bd} = FM + 0.8182 - 0.8182FM$	$\frac{0.9}{Bd} = FM + 0.8189 - 0.8189FM$	$\frac{0.9}{Bd} = FM + 0.8123 - 0.8123FM$
$\frac{0.9}{Bd} - 0.8182 = 1FM - 0.8182FM$	$\frac{0.9}{Bd} - 0.8189 = 1FM - 0.8189FM$	$\frac{0.9}{Bd} - 0.8123 = 1FM - 0.8123FM$
$\frac{0.9}{Bd} - 0.8182 = 0.1818FM$	$\frac{0.9}{Bd} - 0.8189 = 0.1811FM$	$\frac{0.9}{Bd} - 0.8123 = 0.1877FM$
↓	↓	↓
$FM = \frac{4.95}{Bd} - 4.50$	$FM = \frac{4.97}{Bd} - 4.52$	$FM = \frac{4.79}{Bd} - 4.33$

If Bd = 1.054 g/cm^3 and BW = 63.7 kg

$FM = \frac{4.95}{Bd\,(g/cm^3)} - 4.50$	$FM = \frac{4.97}{Bd\,(g/cm^3)} - 4.52$	$FM = \frac{4.79}{Bd\,(g/cm^3)} - 4.33$
↓	↓	↓
$FM = \frac{4.95}{1.054\,(g/cm^3)} - 4.50$	$FM = \frac{4.97}{1.054\,(g/cm^3)} - 4.52$	$FM = \frac{4.79}{1.054\,(g/cm^3)} - 4.33$
↓	↓	↓
FM = 19.6% (12.5 kg)	FM = 19.5% (12.4 kg)	FM = 21.5% (13.7 kg)

obtained with the Siri (1961) equation. On the other hand, when the FFM density was 1.108 g/cm³ (competitive period), the %FM was higher, for the same weight and body density (21.5%FM). This means that, when interpreting changes in body composition, changes in the density of FFM may affect the accuracy of our estimates, meaning that for the same body density, different %FM values may exist.

When using 2C densitometric models, it is necessary to estimate body density; there are two methods that allow the estimation of body density, namely, underwater weighting and air-displacement plethysmography. Furthermore, there are several anthropometric equations to estimate body density; the most commonly used is the Jackson and Pollock (1978) equation, although its use is inaccurate in detecting small changes in athlete's body composition (Tables 9.5 and 9.6) (Silva et al. 2009).

The use of underwater weighting and air-displacement plethysmography allows not only the estimation of FM using 2C models (Behnke et al. 1942; Siri 1961; Brozek et al. 1963) but also the estimations of body volume that are necessary for multicomponent models (Wang et al. 2005).

9.5.1.2 Two-Component Hydrometric Models

Calculating FFM from TBW is based on the assumption of a constant hydration of FFM (Schoeller 2005). Pace and Rathbun (1945) reviewed chemical composition data from several mammal species and concluded that the hydration of FFM corresponded to 73.2%. Considering a 2C model, where BM equals the sum of FM and FFM, it is possible to derive Equation 9.2, which is equivalent to FM = BM − (1.3661 × TBW). Infancy is a well-documented exception to this constant hydration of FFM, with children presenting higher FFM hydration compared to adults, and therefore a lower FFM density (Wells et al. 2010). Also in athletes, deviations from this constant value have been identified (Table 9.3). Accordingly, following the example given for densitometric models, in Table 9.7 we used data from a previous study that tracked body composition in female basketball players (Santos et al. 2014). The authors verified that both in the pre-season and at the competitive period, the FFM hydration was lower than 73.2% and, additionally, it decreased between assessments (34 weeks).

When using the assumed 73.2% FFM hydration (left panel), and assuming the mean body weight reported in the investigation (63.7 kg), it is verified that the %FM corresponds to 20.4%. With the pre-season FFM hydration (72.4%), the %FM would yield a value of 19.6% (middle panel), and when FFM hydration considerably decreased to 69.9%, the %FM was 16.6%. The only source of variation reported in Table 9.7 is the change that occurred in the FFM hydration in the course of the season. Accordingly, inaccurate measurements of body composition may arise when using 2C hydrometric models if changes in FFM hydration occur between assessments, with overestimation of %FM being expected whenever the FFM hydration is below 73.2%. van Marken Lichtenbelt et al. (2004) verified that, in male bodybuilders, similar accuracy was found between a 2C hydrometric and densitometric model, but when estimating %FM, the UWW provided a higher coefficient of determination and lower bias (Tables 9.5 and 9.6).

To use 2C hydrometric models, it is necessary to estimate TBW; for this purpose, deuterium dilution is the most commonly used tracer to estimate TBW (Schoeller 2005). Inherent in any tracer dilution technique are four basic assumptions: (1) the tracer is distributed only in the exchangeable pool; (2) it is equally distributed within this pool; (3) it is not metabolized during the equilibration time; and (4) tracer equilibration is achieved relatively rapid. Therefore, TBW can be measured by using a tracer dose of labeled water (tritium, deuterium, or 18-oxygen) (Ellis 2000; Schoeller 2005).

9.5.1.3 Multicomponent Models

FFM can be partitioned into several molecular components, including water, mineral, and protein (Wang et al. 1992). Multicomponent models are developed from equations that may include two or more unknown components; generally, for each unknown component that is estimated, there

TABLE 9.5
Validity of Body Composition Methods in Estimating %FM Changes in Athletic Populations Using 4C as the Reference Method

Alternative Method	%FM from 4C (T0) Mean (sd)	%FM from 4C (T1) Mean (sd)	Changes (%)	R^2	Bias (%)	95% LoA (%) (or error: 2sd)	Trend (R)	N/Sex/Sport/Level	Reference
Jackson and Pollock (1978), 7SKF	7.0 (3.3) (weight stability)	6.5 (3.4) (prior to competition)	−0.44 (2.17)	0.32	−0.1	−3.6; 3.5	−0.68	18/male/judo/top level	Silva et al. (2009)
Evans et al. (2005), 7SKF				0.34	0.0	−3.5; 3.6	−0.80		
Evans et al. (2005), 3SKF				0.36	0.1	−3.4; 3.6	−0.78		
DXA (fan beam)	9.2 (4.1) (weight stability)	8.0 (3.8) (prior to competition)	−1.22 (2.70)	0.29	0.81	−3.7; 5.3	−0.79	27/male/judo/top level	Santos et al. (2010)
Skinfolds	15.9 (4.4) (baseline)	14.4 (4.1) (after 8 weeks of strength training with AAS administration)	−1.6	0.31	0.29	3.04	ns	15/male/ bodybuilding/ ≥3-year experience	van Marken Lichtenbelt et al. (2004)
BIA				0.30	1.52	6.28	ns		
DXA (pencil beam)				0.27	−0.21	3.77	ns		
D_2O dilution				0.52	0.38	3.11	ns		
UWW (2C)				0.71	−0.09	2.39	ns		
3Cw				0.96	0.26	0.69	ns		
3Cb				0.42	−0.76	3.91	0.55		

Note: 3Cw, three-component model with body water; 3Cb, three-component model with body minerals; BIA, bioimpedance analysis; DXA, dual x-ray absorptiometry; D_2O dilution, dilution by deuterium; UWW, underwater weighing; AAS, androgenic-anabolic steroids; ns, nonsignificant.

TABLE 9.6
Validity of Body Composition Methods in Estimating FFM Changes in Athletic Populations Using 4C as the Reference Method

Alternative Method	FFM (kg) from 4C (T0) Mean (sd)	FFM (kg) from 4C (T1) Mean (sd)	Changes (kg)	R^2	Bias (kg)	95% LoA (kg) (or error: 2sd)	Trend (R)	n/Sex/Sport/Level	Reference
Jackson and Pollock (1978), 7SKF	68.3 (7.3) (weight stability)	67.9 (7.1) (prior to competition)	−0.41 (1.79)	0.52	0.1	−2.5;2.7	ns	18/male/judo/top-level	Silva et al. (2009)
Evans et al. (2005), 7SKF				0.53	0.0	−2.5;2.6	ns		
Evans et al. (2005), 3SKF				0.53	0.0	−2.5; 2.5	ns		
DXA (fan beam)	66.1 (6.4) (weight stability)	66.1 (6.0) (prior to competition)	0.07 (2.04)	0.38	−0.5	−3.7; 2.7	−0.33	27/male/judo/top-level	Santos et al. (2010)
BIS	66.1 (6.4) (weight stability)	66.1 (6.0) (prior to competition)	0.07 (2.04)	0.62	−0.5	−3.4; 2.6	ns	27/male/judo/top-level	Matias et al. (2012)
Skinfolds	65.2 (8.6) (baseline)	68.9 (8.9) (after 8 weeks of strength training with AAS administration)	3.7	0.77	0.29	2.27	ns	15/male/bodybuilding/≥3-year experience	van Marken Lichtenbelt et al. (2004)
BIA				ns	−1.14	5.16	ns		
DXA				0.59	0.22	3.11	ns		
D$_2$O dilution (2C)				0.81	−0.32	2.53	ns		
UWW (2C)				0.83	0.07	1.97	ns		
3Cw				0.98	−0.22	0.53	ns		
3Cb				0.66	0.69	3.11	ns		
Lean mass index[a]	81.6 (7.5)	81.4 (7.0)	−0.2 (3.0)	0.14	Na	Na	Na	12/male/rugby/elite	Slater et al. (2006)
Σ7SKF[a]				0.04	Na	Na	Na		
Forsyth and Sinning (1973)				0.07	Nr	Nr	Nr		
Thorland et al. (1984)				0.18	Nr	Nr	Nr		
Withers et al. (1996)				0.17	Nr	Nr	Nr		
2C (densitometric)				0.10	Nr	Nr	Nr		
3Cw				0.98	Nr	Nr	Nr		
TBW[a]				0.94	Na	Na	Na		

Note: 3Cw, three-component model with body water; 3Cb, three-component model with body minerals; BIA, bioimpedance analysis; DXA, dual x-ray absorptiometry; D$_2$O dilution, dilution by deuterium; UWW, underwater weighing; TBW, total body water; AAS, androgenic-anabolic steroids; SKF, skinfold; ns, nonsignificant; Nr, not reported; Na, not applicable.

[a] This method does not estimate kg of FM; only correlations are reported.

TABLE 9.7

Derivation of Hydrometric 2C Model Using Data from Santos et al. (2014)

$$FM\ (kg) = BM\ (kg) - \frac{TBW\ (kg)}{0.732}$$

If BW = 63.7 kg and TBW = 37.1 kg

$\frac{TBW}{FFM} = 0.732$	$\frac{TBW}{FFM} = 0.724$	$\frac{TBW}{FFM} = 0.699$
↓	↓	↓
$FM = 63.7 - \dfrac{37.1}{0.732}$	$FM = 63.7 - \dfrac{37.1}{0.724}$	$FM = 63.7 - \dfrac{37.1}{0.699}$
↓	↓	↓
FM = 13.0 kg (20.4%)	FM = 12.5 kg (19.6%)	FM = 10.6 kg (16.6%)

---

is one independent equation that includes the unknown component, the known component, and/or the measurable property. Measurable components include TBW or mineral, while measurable properties used in developing molecular-level multicomponent models include body mass and body volume (Heymsfield et al. 1997). The addition of an estimate of TBW by isotope dilution (Siri 1961; Withers et al. 1998) or mineral by DXA (Lohman 1986) to the 2C model (Equation 9.1) allows the development of three-component (3C) models. A 4C model can be derived by adding another component. The 4C models control for biological variability in TBW, bone mineral mass, and residual and can be generated using the same concept as the one previously described for 2C models (Figure 9.1), by knowing the density of the FFM components (Table 9.2).

Because multicomponent models control the biological variability in the FFM density and composition, it is often chosen as the reference method (Tables 9.5 and 9.6). Regardless, even 4C models are not error free. For example, assumptions for 4C models include that soft tissue minerals are a function of body weight (Selinger 1977), total body bone mineral (Heymsfield et al. 1990), or TBW (Wang et al. 2002). Another example is assuming different densities for the residual component. Friedl et al. (1992) and Withers et al. (1992) agree that the residual is composed of protein, soft minerals, and glycogen, but differ in the assumed densities, that is, 1.39 and 1.404 g/cm³ for Friedl et al. (1992) and Withers et al. (1992), respectively.

9.5.2 Dual X-ray Absorptiometry (Three-Component Model)

When using DXA to estimate body composition, it is assumed that the body consists of three components that are differentiated by their x-ray attenuation properties, namely, FM, bone mineral, and lean soft tissue (LST). Theoretically, knowing three unknown components would require measuring at three different photon energies. However, in practice, DXA can solve the fractional masses of only a 2C mixture. Accordingly, DXA initially divides pixels into those with soft tissue only (FM and LST) and those with soft tissue and bone mineral, based on the two different photon energies. Practically, this means that in pixels where there is bone mineral, soft tissue is not separately analyzed and the equipment will assume that the FM content of the adjacent area is analyzed (Pietrobelli et al. 1996). Between 40% and 45% of the scan contains bone in addition to soft tissue, and therefore a systematic individual error is introduced as there might be variations in body composition between measured and nonmeasured areas (Lohman and Chen 2005). For example, the influence of the arms and the thorax on the estimations can be underrepresented given the relatively large areas of bone in those regions (Roubenoff et al. 1993). Furthermore, this source of systematic error can be increased when tracking body composition compartments (Kiebzak et al. 2000).

For athletes, DXA measurements are appealing over other laboratory methods due to their good precision, large availability, and low radiation dose (Ackland et al. 2012; Toombs et al. 2012). The progressive replacement of the original pencil-beam densitometers by fan-beam devices in the early 1990 s allowed for better resolution and faster scan times, without compromising accuracy and without increasing radiation dose substantially, thus easing the burden of use for both athletes and technicians (Tothill et al. 2001; Toombs et al. 2012). Nevertheless, caution must be taken when using DXA on multiple occasions; Meyer et al. (2013) have suggested that DXA scans should not be performed more than twice during the season and preferably not close to competitions. The reasons to avoid multiple scans are not only related to the cumulative radiation dose (Ackland et al. 2012) but are also due to problems related to the accuracy and precision of the equipment (Toombs et al. 2012).

The precision of DXA depends on the tissue that we want to estimate; compared to FM, FFM provided more precise assessments. The coefficients of variation for FFM are about 1% whereas for FM and %FM range from 2.8% to 4.4% (Toombs et al. 2012). Also, considering one of the aspects that is most appealing for athletes' body composition assessment, which is the possibility of regional estimations (Ackland et al. 2012), there are concerns when it comes to precision of the equipment. Compared to whole-body estimations, regional body composition assessment provides poorer precision (Toombs et al. 2012).

Nana et al. (2013) have investigated this issues related to the precision of DXA in well-trained individuals (27 strength-trained male subjects, 14 female cyclists, and 14 male cyclists). The authors provide standardization tools to avoid errors that may lead to misinterpretations in body composition changes. Important standardization rules must include undertaking DXA scans in athletes who are in a fasting state and rested before assessment, and measurements should be conducted with a standardized positioning protocol by the same technician.

Tables 9.5 and 9.6 summarize the accuracy of DXA in tracking body composition. Santos et al. (2010) found that, when compared to a 4C model, DXA was not accurate in detecting small changes in body composition that occurred in judo athletes from a period of weight stability to prior to a competition, particularly for a given individual. The authors reported that DXA overestimated FM losses and underestimated FFM gains. Importantly, Santos et al. (2010) demonstrated that the accuracy of the DXA instrument to track body composition depended on the FFM hydration, with DXA overestimating FM with increases in FFM hydration and underestimating FFM with decreases in FFM hydration. van Marken Lichtenbelt et al. (2004) also reported that, when compared to a 4C model, DXA explained only 27% of %FM and 59% of FFM changes that occurred in 15 male bodybuilders after 8 weeks of strength training with androgenic-anabolic steroids administration.

There are other limitations that need to be pointed when using DXA to estimate body composition in athletes: the algorithms' calculations differ between manufacturers and are not published; pencil- and fan-beam densitometers differ in the accuracy of FM estimations and depend on the magnitude of FM that is being measured, with inaccuracies amplified in assessing very lean participants (Van Der Ploeg et al. 2003) (e.g., weight-sensitive sports athletes); and the assessment is limited to body regions within the scan area (Ackland et al. 2012). This last limitation particularly affects athletes involved in sports where height, which is a factor contributing to performance, such as basketball and volleyball, may exceed the length of the scan bed. Thus, Santos et al. (2013) suggested the use of the sum of two scans (head and trunk plus limbs) to assess body composition in athletes that are taller than the DXA scan area. Although the authors concluded that this procedure provided a valid approach to estimate body composition in athletes, it is important to verify its precision to conduct valid and accurate multiple time-point assessments during the sports season.

9.5.3 ANTHROPOMETRY

Anthropometric methods can be applied in both laboratory and sports field settings providing simple, inexpensive, and noninvasive body composition estimations (Bellisari and Roche 2005; Ackland et al. 2012). Commonly used anthropometric variables include lengths, breadths, circumferences,

SKF thicknesses, and body weight (Lohman et al. 1988; Stewart et al. 2011). To reduce errors associated with precision, standardized techniques have been developed (Jackson and Pollock 1985; Lohman et al. 1988; Stewart et al. 2011). The International Society for the Advancement of Kinanthropometry (ISAK) provides standardization (Stewart et al. 2011) and certification, ensuring that precision errors can be reduced. The ISAK accreditation scheme has a four-level hierarchy that requires that all levels have to meet initial technical error of measurement (TEM) criteria at the end of a course. To achieve certification, an anthropometrist must take a practical examination followed by the meeting of further TEM criteria on the measurement of 20 subjects to indicate satisfactory repeatability of measures. Reaccreditation is also necessary every 4 years by taking a practical exam in which inter-tester TEM targets (e.g., 10.0% for each SKF and 2.0% for each of the other measures) must be met in order to get certified (ISAK 2016).

The most commonly used anthropometric variable in the sports field is by far the SKF, which is a central anthropometric variable that allows approximations of adipose tissue patterning (Edwards 1951; Garn 1955), tissue mass fractionation (Martin et al. 1990), fat distribution (Clarys et al. 1987), and somatotyping (Carter and Heath 1990). To date, there are more than 100 equations that convert SKF values to body density (and posterior to FM by using the Siri (1961) or the Brozek et al. (1963) equation) or to FM. Nonetheless, it is important to consider that there are five assumptions implicit to convert SKF thickness total FM: (1) the constant compressibility of skin and subcutaneous fat, (2) the constancy of skin thickness, (3) the constancy of the fat fraction of adipose tissue, (4) the constancy of adipose tissue patterning, and (5) the constancy of internal to external fat ratio (Martin et al. 1985; Marfell-Jones 2001). Four of these assumptions have been shown not to be true while no validity has been recognized for the fifth. Accordingly, it seems unreasonable to bring additional errors by transforming anthropometric measurement values into %FM (Marfell-Jones 2001). The errors that are associated with transforming SKF thickness into %FM can be associated with violations in the assumptions of the FFM composition and density. Although anthropometric equations have been developed specifically for athletic populations (Forsyth and Sinning 1973; Thorland et al. 1984; Evans et al. 2005), these equations have been instigated not to be accurate in detecting %FM changes in athletes (van Marken Lichtenbelt et al. 2004; Slater et al. 2006; Silva et al. 2009).

To solve the limitations of converting the sum of SKFs into body density or %FM, Durnin (1995) has suggested that comparisons could be performed within and between individuals from the gross values of the SKFs. Accordingly, in athletic populations, the use of individual SKF map, SKF ratios, or the sum of SKFs has been suggested (Ackland et al. 2012; Meyer et al. 2013).

As an example, and using data from van der Ploeg et al. (2001), Figure 9.2 illustrates the changes that occurred in five female bodybuilders at 12 weeks, 6 weeks, and 3–5 days prior to a competition.

Use of the SKF map (Figure 9.3) enables evidence that not only whole subcutaneous fat decreased, which is consistent with the same tendency as 4C %FM (Van Der Ploeg et al. 2003), but also each individual SKF thickness decreased. Individual SKF thickness can, therefore, be used as an approximation for regional body composition; for example, by analyzing the SKF map, it is possible to characterize that adiposity is distributed mainly in the lower limbs (front thigh SKF). When using raw SKF values to track body composition, although we are limiting the inaccuracies associated with the conversion to %FM, we need to consider that the five assumptions that were mentioned above still exist (Martin et al. 1985; Marfell-Jones 2001). Also, it has been verified that, although summing SKF was cross-sectional associated with %FM from a 4C model, changes in this variable, though following the same trend, did not correlate with changes in %FM from the 4C model in the course of a season (Santos et al. 2014). Furthermore, the concerns associated with the precision of anthropometric measurements that were previously mentioned are still present.

9.5.4 BIA AND BIOIMPEDANCE SPECTROSCOPY

The ability of body tissues to conduct an electric current has been widely recognized (Ellis 2000). Due to their dissolved electrolytes, the aqueous tissues of the human body are the major

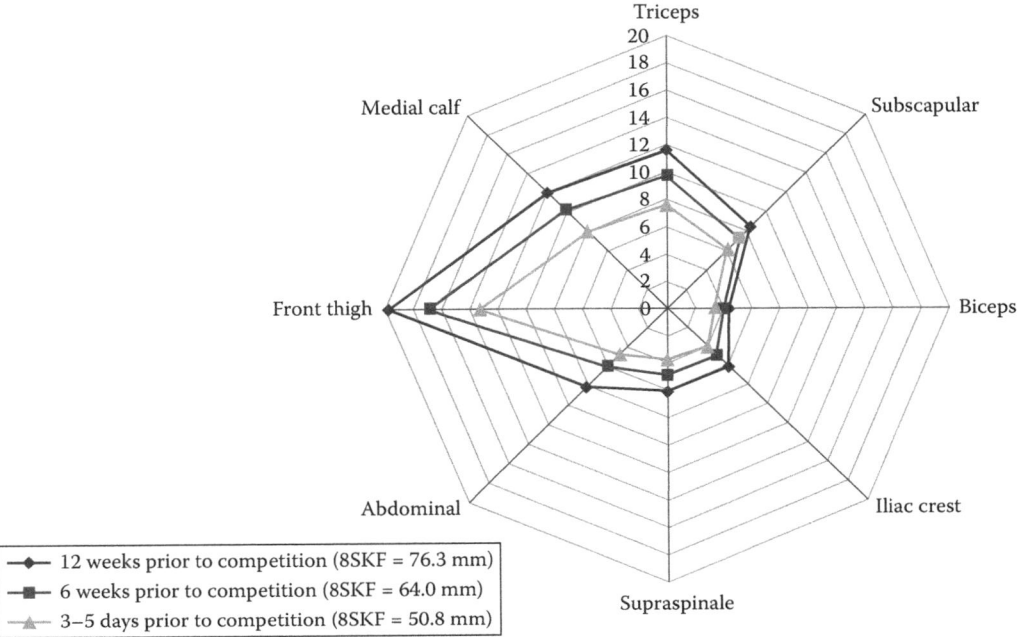

FIGURE 9.3 **(See color insert.)** An SKF map in five female bodybuilders at 12 weeks, 6 weeks, and 3–5 days prior to a competition. (Data from van der Ploeg, G. E. et al. 2001. *Eur J Clin Nutr* 55:268–77.)

conductors of an electric current whereas FM and bone present relatively poor conductance properties. Tissue conductivity is directly proportional to the amount of electrolyte-containing fluid present. Therefore, the main principle of the BIA method is that the resistance of a low-level electrical current applied to the body is inversely related to the TBW and electrolyte distribution (Ellis 2000; Jaffrin and Morel 2008). For single-frequency equipment, generally 50 kHz, an alternating current is passed through the outer pair of electrodes, while the voltage drop across the body is measured using the inner pair of electrodes from which the body's impedance is derived. The result of the current passage through the body gives a value of resistance and reactance. Impedance is a function of these two separate quantities and is also frequency dependent. The conductive characteristics of body fluids provide the resistive component, whereas the cell membranes, acting as imperfect capacitors, contribute to a frequency-dependent reactive component. Two assumptions are necessary to convert this information into volume of TBW. The first assumption is that the body can be modeled as an isotropic cylindrical conductor with length proportional to the participant's height. The other assumption is that the reactance term that contributes to the body's impedance is small, such that the resistance component can be considered equivalent to body impedance (Ellis 2000; Jaffrin and Morel 2008). Combining these assumptions, TBW can be estimated using equations. There are several equations that have been proposed to estimate TBW and FFM, but there is a lack of alternatives for athletic populations (Moon 2013; Matias et al. 2016). To solve this issue, Matias et al. (2016) have recently developed athlete specific prediction models, but this has not yet been validated to detect seasonal variations in TBW. In addition to the lack of validated equations, there is a wide variety of BIA equipment that considerably differs in accuracy and precision (Moon 2013).

The typical equipment works at a 50-kHz current, which does not penetrate completely into the cells, which can limit the accuracy in estimating TBW in participants with an abnormal ECW/TBW ratio (Jaffrin and Morel 2008). To solve this concern, bioimpedance spectroscopy (BIS) methods (with a large spectrum of frequencies) have been developed to assess water compartments. The use of BIS has been investigated to be accurate in detecting group changes in FFM in judo athletes; still, there are wide limits of agreement that may preclude its use to detect individual body composition changes (Matias et al. 2012).

Despite the fact that BIA or BIS outputs can be used to estimate TBW and FFM, similarly to other methods, the raw data of the equipment can be used. Cross-sectional and longitudinal studies with athletic populations reporting and analyzing bioelectrical impedance vectors and the phase angle (Nescolarde et al. 2011; Koury et al. 2014; Micheli et al. 2014; Matias et al. 2015) are emerging.

When using BIA or BIS to estimate body composition, concerns that are related to the hydration status exist. This is one of the sources of precision errors when estimating body composition, as dehydration in athletes is of concern (Ackland et al. 2012). Still, there are few sports professionals who assess the hydration status of the athlete before body composition assessments (Meyer et al. 2013).

9.5.5 ULTRASOUND

The ultrasound as an answer to estimate body composition has been recently suggested (Muller and Maughan 2013). The ultrasound technique allows measuring subcutaneous adipose tissue and embedded fibrous structures. Compared to anthropometry, the use of ultrasound avoids the compression of the tissues and the movement that may occur when using calipers to assess SKF thickness. An *ad hoc* working group on body composition, health, and performance under the auspices of the IOC Medical Commission has recently suggested a standardization of the ultra-sound technique for accurate and precise measurement of subcutaneous adipose tissue when using the ultrasound technique. The *ad hoc* group has suggested using eight site locations, which allows for inter-individual differences in the pattern of subcutaneous adipose tissue (Muller et al. 2016). Providing that the measurements are performed under standardized circumstances and that technicians are well trained, it is possible to have a high inter-observer reliability (Muller et al. 2013). Some cautions that need to be considered when applying this technique to estimate subcutaneous adipose tissue include the following: avoiding tissue compression by using a thick (3–5 mm) layer of ultrasound gel, the use of a semiautomatic image evaluation procedure, the orientation of the probe, or the use of standardized sites. In Figure 9.4 is illustrated an example of an ultrasound image that was captured for fat patterning analysis in the distal triceps site (Muller et al. 2016).

Similar to the anthropometry technique, the use of the sum of SKFs has been suggested for fat patterning in athletes (Muller et al. 2016). Despite the possible advantages of using ultrasound over anthropometry, due to its novelty, there are some concerns that need to be addressed: the use of ultrasound allows the quantification of only subcutaneous adipose tissue; the cost of the equipment is considerably higher when compared to the use of calipers; to date, there is no investigation to understand the accuracy of this technique to estimate athletes adiposity, and more particularly the changes that occur during the season; and there are no studies regarding athletes' health and performance in association with ultrasound measurements (Muller et al. 2016).

9.6   DETECTING MEANINGFUL BODY COMPOSITION CHANGES

When estimating the body composition of athletes, generally and when the health of the athlete is not at risk, professionals aim to track body composition changes that relate to the athletes' performance, which does not necessarily reflect accurate body composition estimations. At this regard, a meaningful body composition change will be related to an athlete's ability to perform (Colyer et al. 2016).

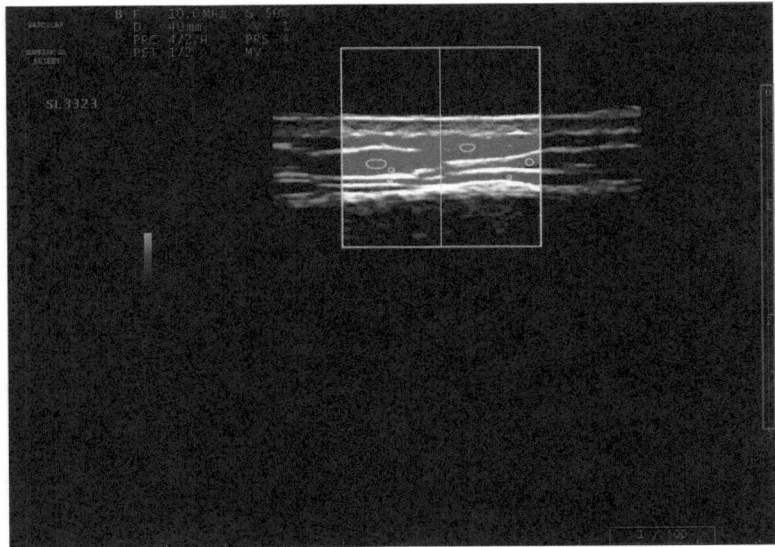

FIGURE 9.4 **(See color insert.)** Example of an ultrasound image that was captured in the distal triceps site (red represents subcutaneous adipose tissue).

Recently, Colyer et al. (2016) verified that, in bob skeleton athletes and elite rugby union players, changes in DXA body composition estimations were associated to lower limb strength-power indices. The author verified that increases in total and legs lean mass were related to improvements in jump performance. The author also verified that relative increases in total lean mass were associated with improvements in leg press and that a reduction in FM was associated with improvements in both leg press and jump performance. In top-level male judo athletes, Silva et al. (2010) observed that total and intracellular water decreases occurring from a period of weight stability to prior to a competition were associated with decreases in upper-body power.

Using anthropometric techniques, Legaz and Eston (2005) observed that in top-class runners, improvements in performance were associated with lower limbs SKF. Granados et al. (2008) and Gorostiaga et al. (2006) verified that changes in %FM, estimated by anthropometric techniques, correlated positively with changes in maximal strength and muscle power in male and female handball players, which means that those who developed larger decreases in %FM showed larger decreases in maximal strength (females) or muscle power (males and females) of the upper and lower extremities. Santos et al. (2014) reported that in male and female basketball players there was a positive association between seasonal variations in the countermovement jump with changes in calf muscle circumference, while negative associations were verified between the jump performance and the handgrip test changes with changes in the sum (Σ) of seven SKF (Σ7SKF: triceps, subscapular, biceps, suprailiac, abdominal, thigh, and medial calf). The authors also demonstrated that, when using a 4C model, there were associations between FM and FFM changes with alterations in jump performance, but not with the handgrip test. Appleby et al. (2012) showed that during a competitive season, increases in the lean mass index were related to squat 1 repetition maximum and bench press improvements. The lean mass index is a simple anthropometric variable that allows tracking body weight changes, adjusted for SKF thickness.

9.7 CONCLUSIONS AND NEW PERSPECTIVES

In this chapter, we reviewed the major limitations regarding the accuracy and precision of body composition methods that are most commonly used by sports professionals. All body composition methods present advantages and disadvantages; when choosing one method over another, it is important to be aware of the limitations of the method.

Currently, there are a variety of methods that are being used, precluding the possibility of comparisons between sports and establishing protocols. There is a need to establish protocols to standardize procedures across sports professionals.

To decrease the errors that are associated with precision, there are several aspects that professionals need to consider. Standardization of protocols, certification, and training of technicians, or maintenance and calibration of the equipment are among several easy steps that professionals can take to increase the precision of estimations; even a caliper needs to be calibrated.

The choice of a specific method over another is dependent on the purpose of what is being used; for example, if we need to establish a target body composition in weight-sensitive sports, care is necessary as errors associated with the assessment may have a negative impact on the health status of the athlete. Conversely, when performance is the goal, and if extreme leanness is not a concern, a method that estimates meaningful body composition changes should be preferred. Meaningful body composition changes do not necessarily relate to the most accurate method but are related to the performance of the athlete. If by detecting changes in the sum of SKFs one can predict changes in sports performance, that will be considered a meaningful body composition change, even though the sum of SKFs may not be associated to %FM from a reference method.

There are still issues and concerns in the field of body composition that currently available methods are not capable of responding. Athletes often deviate from assumed constants, which are the cornerstones of the methods, precluding accurate body composition estimates.

REFERENCES

Ackland, T. R., T. G. Lohman, J. Sundgot-Borgen et al. 2012. Current status of body composition assessment in sport: Review and position statement on behalf of the ad hoc research working group on body composition health and performance, under the auspices of the I.O.C. Medical Commission. *Sports Med* 42:227–49.

Appleby, B., R. U. Newton, and P. Cormie. 2012. Changes in strength over a 2-year period in professional rugby union players. *J Strength Cond Res* 26:2538–46.

Behnke, A. R., B. G. Feen, and W. C. Welham. 1942. The specific gravity of healthy men. Body weight divided by volume as an index of obesity. *J Am Med Assoc* 118:495–8.

Bellisari, A. and A. F. Roche. 2005. Anthropometry and ultrasound. In *Human Body Composition*, edited by S. B. Heymsfield, T. G. Lohman, Z. Wang, and S. B. Going, 109–28. Champaign, IL: Human Kinetics.

Brozek, J., F. Grande, J. T. Anderson, and A. Keys. 1963. Densitometric analysis of body composition: Revision of some quantitative assumptions. *Ann N Y Acad Sci* 110:113–40.

Carter, J. E. L. and B. H. Heath. 1990. *Somatotyping – Development and Applications*. New York: Cambridge University Press.

Clarys, J. P., A. D. Martin, D. T. Drinkwater, and M. J. Marfell-Jones. 1987. The skinfold: Myth and reality. *J Sports Sci* 5:3–33.

Colyer, S. L., S. P. Roberts, J. B. Robinson et al. 2016. Detecting meaningful body composition changes in athletes using dual-energy x-ray absorptiometry. *Physiol Meas* 37:596–609.

Drinkwater, E. J., D. B. Pyne, and M. J. McKenna. 2008. Design and interpretation of anthropometric and fitness testing of basketball players. *Sports Med* 38:565–78.

Dulloo, A. G. and J. Jacquet. 1999. The control of partitioning between protein and fat during human starvation: Its internal determinants and biological significance. *Br J Nutr* 82:339–56.

Durnin, J. V. G. A. 1995. Appropriate technology in body composition: A brief review. *Asia Pacific J Clin Nutr* 4:1–5.

Edwards, D. A. 1951. Differences in the distribution of subcutaneous fat with sex and maturity. *Clin Sci (Lond)* 10:305–15.

Ellis, K. J. 2000. Human body composition: *In vivo* methods. *Physiol Rev* 80:649–80.

Evans, E. M., D. A. Rowe, M. M. Misic, B. M. Prior, and S. A. Arngrimsson. 2005. Skinfold prediction equation for athletes developed using a four-component model. *Med Sci Sports Exerc* 37:2006–11.

Forsyth, H. L. and W. E. Sinning. 1973. The anthropometric estimation of body density and lean body weight of male athletes. *Med Sci Sports* 5:174–80.

Friedl, K. E., J. P. DeLuca, L. J. Marchitelli, and J. A. Vogel. 1992. Reliability of body-fat estimations from a four-compartment model by using density, body water, and bone mineral measurements. *Am J Clin Nutr* 55:764–70.

Garn, S. M. 1955. Relative fat patterning: An individual characteristic. *Hum Biol* 27:75–89.

Gorostiaga, E. M., C. Granados, J. Ibanez, J. J. Gonzalez-Badillo, and M. Izquierdo. 2006. Effects of an entire season on physical fitness changes in elite male handball players. *Med Sci Sports Exerc* 38:357–66.

Granados, C., M. Izquierdo, J. Ibanez, M. Ruesta, and E. M. Gorostiaga. 2008. Effects of an entire season on physical fitness in elite female handball players. *Med Sci Sports Exerc* 40:351–61.

Heymsfield, S. B., S. Lichtman, R. N. Baumgartner et al. 1990. Body composition of humans: Comparison of two improved four-compartment models that differ in expense, technical complexity, and radiation exposure. *Am J Clin Nutr* 52:52–8.

Heymsfield, S. B., Z. Wang, R. N. Baumgartner, and R. Ross. 1997. Human body composition: Advances in models and methods. *Annu Rev Nutr* 17:527–58.

Hogstrom, G. M., T. Pietila, P. Nordstrom, and A. Nordstrom. 2012. Body composition and performance: Influence of sport and gender among adolescents. *J Strength Cond Res* 26:1799–804.

ISAK. 2016. The ISAK Accreditation Scheme. Accessed April 4, 2016. http://www.isakonline.com/accreditation_scheme.

Jackson, A. S. and M. L. Pollock. 1978. Generalized equations for predicting body density of men. *Br J Nutr* 40:497–504.

Jackson, A. S. and M. L. Pollock. 1985. Practical assessment of body composition. *Phys Sportsmed* 13:76–90.

Jaffrin, M. Y. and H. Morel. 2008. Body fluid volumes measurements by impedance: A review of bioimpedance spectroscopy (BIS) and bioimpedance analysis (BIA) methods. *Med Eng Phys* 30:1257–69.

Kiebzak, G. M., L. J. Leamy, L. M. Pierson, R. H. Nord, and Z. Y. Zhang. 2000. Measurement precision of body composition variables using the lunar DPX-L densitometer. *J Clin Densitom* 3:35–41.

Koury, J. C., N. Mf Trugo, and A. G. Torres. 2014. Phase angle and bioelectrical impedance vectors in adolescent and adult male athletes. *Int J Sports Physiol Perform* 9:798–804.

Legaz, A. and R. Eston. 2005. Changes in performance, skinfold thicknesses, and fat patterning after three years of intense athletic conditioning in high level runners. *Br J Sports Med* 39:851–6.

Lohman, T. G. 1986. Applicability of body composition techniques and constants for children and youths. *Exerc Sport Sci Rev* 14:325–57.

Lohman, T. G. and Z. Chen. 2005. Dual-energy X-ray absorptiometry. In *Human Body Composition*, edited by S. B. Heymsfield, T. G. Lohman, Z. Wang, and S. B. Going, 63–77. Champaign, IL: Human Kinetics.

Lohman, T. G., A. F. Roche, and R. Martorell. 1988. *Anthropometric Standardization Reference Manual*. Champaign, IL: Human Kinetics Publishers.

Loucks, A. B. 2004. Energy balance and body composition in sports and exercise. *J Sports Sci* 22:1–14.

Loucks, A. B., B. Kiens, and H. H. Wright. 2011. Energy availability in athletes. *J Sports Sci* 29(Suppl. 1):S7–15.

Lukaski, H. C. 1987. Methods for the assessment of human body composition: Traditional and new. *Am J Clin Nutr* 46:537–56.

Malina, R. M. 2007. Body composition in athletes: Assessment and estimated fatness. *Clin Sports Med* 26:37–68.

Marfell-Jones, M. J. 2001. The value of the skinfold—Background, assumptions, cautions, and recommendations on taking and interpreting skinfold measurements. *Proceedings of the Seoul International Sport Science Congress*, Seoul, 313–23.

Martin, A. D., W. D. Ross, D. T. Drinkwater, and J. P. Clarys. 1985. Prediction of body fat by skinfold caliper: Assumptions and cadaver evidence. *Int J Obes* 9(Suppl. 1):31–9.

Martin, A. D., L. F. Spenst, D. T. Drinkwater, and J. P. Clarys. 1990. Anthropometric estimation of muscle mass in men. *Med Sci Sports Exerc* 22:729–33.

Matias, C. N., C. P. Monteiro, D. A. Santos, F. Martins, A. M. Silva, M. J. Laires, and L. B. Sardinha. 2015. Magnesium and phase angle: A prognostic tool for monitoring cellular integrity in judo athletes. *Magnes Res* 28:92–8.

Matias, C. N., D. A. Santos, D. A. Fields, L. B. Sardinha, and A. M. Silva. 2012. Is bioelectrical impedance spectroscopy accurate in estimating changes in fat-free mass in judo athletes? *J Sports Sci* 30:1225–33.

Matias, C. N., D. A. Santos, P. B. Judice et al. 2016. Estimation of total body water and extracellular water with bioimpedance in athletes: A need for athlete-specific prediction models. *Clin Nutr* 35:468–74.

Matzkin, E., E. J. Curry, and K. Whitlock. 2015. Female athlete triad: Past, present, and future. *J Am Acad Orthop Surg* 23:424–32.

Merril, A. L. and B. K. Watt. 1973. *Energy Value of Foods, Basis and Derivation.* Agriculture Handbook No. 74. Washington, DC: ARS United States Department of Agriculture.

Meyer, N. L., J. Sundgot-Borgen, T. G. Lohman et al. 2013. Body composition for health and performance: A survey of body composition assessment practice carried out by the *ad hoc* Research Working Group on Body Composition, Health and Performance under the auspices of the IOC Medical Commission. *Br J Sports Med* 47:1044–53.

Micheli, M. L., L. Pagani, M. Marella et al. 2014. Bioimpedance and impedance vector patterns as predictors of league level in male soccer players. *Int J Sports Physiol Perform* 9:532–39.

Modlesky, C. M., K. J. Cureton, R. D. Lewis, B. M. Prior, M. A. Sloniger, and D. A. Rowe. 1996. Density of the fat-free mass and estimates of body composition in male weight trainers. *J Appl Physiol* 80:2085–96.

Moon, J. R. 2013. Body composition in athletes and sports nutrition: An examination of the bioimpedance analysis technique. *Eur J Clin Nutr* 67(Suppl. 1):S54–9.

Moore, F. D. and C. M. Boyden. 1963. Body cell mass and limits of hydration of the fat-free body: Their relation to estimated skeletal weight. *Ann N Y Acad Sci* 110:62–71.

Muller, W., M. Horn, A. Furhapter-Rieger et al. 2013. Body composition in sport: Interobserver reliability of a novel ultrasound measure of subcutaneous fat tissue. *Br J Sports Med* 47:1036–43.

Muller, W., T. G. Lohman, A. D. Stewart et al. 2016. Subcutaneous fat patterning in athletes: Selection of appropriate sites and standardisation of a novel ultrasound measurement technique: Ad hoc working group on body composition, health and performance, under the auspices of the IOC Medical Commission. *Br J Sports Med* 50:45–54.

Muller, W. and R. J. Maughan. 2013. The need for a novel approach to measure body composition: Is ultrasound an answer? *Br J Sports Med* 47:1001–2.

Nana, A., G. J. Slater, W. G. Hopkins, and L. M. Burke. 2013. Effects of exercise sessions on DXA measurements of body composition in active people. *Med Sci Sports Exerc* 45:178–85.

Nescolarde, L., J. Yanguas, D. Medina, G. Rodas, and J. Rosell-Ferrer. 2011. Assessment and follow-up of muscle injuries in athletes by bioimpedance: Preliminary results. *Conf Proc IEEE Eng Med Biol Soc* 2011:1137–40.

Pace, N. and E. N. Rathbun. 1945. Studies on body composition—Body water and chemically combined nitrogen content in relation to fat content. *J Biol Chem* 158:685–91.

Pietrobelli, A., C. Formica, Z. Wang, and S. B. Heymsfield. 1996. Dual-energy x-ray absorptiometry body composition model: Review of physical concepts. *Am J Physiol* 271:E941–51.

Prior, B. M., C. M. Modlesky, E. M. Evans et al. 2001. Muscularity and the density of the fat-free mass in athletes. *J Appl Physiol* 90:1523–31.

Rodriguez, N. R., N. M. Di Marco, and S. Langley. 2009. American College of Sports Medicine position stand. Nutrition and athletic performance. *Med Sci Sports Exerc* 41:709–31.

Roubenoff, R., J. J. Kehayias, B. Dawson-Hughes, and S. B. Heymsfield. 1993. Use of dual-energy x-ray absorptiometry in body-composition studies: Not yet a "gold standard". *Am J Clin Nutr* 58:589–91.

Santos, D. A., L. A. Gobbo, C. N. Matias et al. 2013. Body composition in taller individuals using DXA: A validation study for athletic and non-athletic populations. *J Sports Sci* 31:405–13.

Santos, D. A., C. N. Matias, P. M. Rocha et al. 2014. Association of basketball season with body composition in elite junior players. *J Sports Med Phys Fitness* 54:162–73.

Santos, D. A., A. M. Silva, C. N. Matias, D. A. Fields, S. B. Heymsfield, and L. B. Sardinha. 2010. Accuracy of DXA in estimating body composition changes in elite athletes using a four compartment model as the reference method. *Nutr Metab (Lond)* 7:1–9.

Schoeller, D. A. 2005. Hydrometry. In *Human Body Composition*, edited by S. B. Heymsfield, T. G. Lohman, Z. Wang, and S. B. Going, 35–49. Champaign, IL: Human Kinetics.

Selinger, A. 1977. The body as a three component system. *Unpublished doctoral dissertation*, University of Ilinois.

Silva, A. M., D. A. Fields, S. B. Heymsfield, and L. B. Sardinha. 2010. Body composition and power changes in elite judo athletes. *Int J Sports Med* 31:737–41.

Silva, A. M., D. A. Fields, S. B. Heymsfield, and L. B. Sardinha. 2011. Relationship between changes in total-body water and fluid distribution with maximal forearm strength in elite judo athletes. *J Strength Cond Res* 25:2488–95.

Silva, A. M., D. A. Fields, A. L. Quiterio, and L. B. Sardinha. 2009. Are skinfold-based models accurate and suitable for assessing changes in body composition in highly trained athletes? *J Strength Cond Res* 23:1688–96.

Silva, A. M., C. N. Matias, D. A. Santos, P. M. Rocha, C. S. Minderico, and L. B. Sardinha. 2014. Increases in intracellular water explain strength and power improvements over a season. *Int J Sports Med* 35:1101–5.

Silva, A. M., C. S. Minderico, P. J. Teixeira, A. Pietrobelli, and L. B. Sardinha. 2006. Body fat measurement in adolescent athletes: Multicompartment molecular model comparison. *Eur J Clin Nutr* 60:955–64.

Siri, W. E. 1961. Body composition from fluid spaces and density: Analysis of methods. In *Techniques for Measuring Body Composition*, edited by J. Brozek and A. Henschel, 223–44. Washington, DC: National Academy of Sciences—National Research Council.

Slater, G. J., G. M. Duthie, D. B. Pyne, and W. G. Hopkins. 2006. Validation of a skinfold based index for tracking proportional changes in lean mass. *Br J Sports Med* 40:208–13.

Stapff, A. 2000. Protocols for the physiological assessment of Basketball players. In *Physiological Tests for Elite Athletes*, edited by C. J. Gore, 224–37. Champaign, IL: Human Kinetics.

Stewart, A. D., M. J. Marfell-Jones, T. Olds, and H. de Ridder. 2011. *International Standards for Anthropometric Assessment*. Lower Hutt, New Zealand: ISAK.

Sundgot-Borgen, J., N. L. Meyer, T. G. Lohman et al. 2013. How to minimise the health risks to athletes who compete in weight-sensitive sports review and position statement on behalf of the *ad hoc* Research Working Group on Body Composition, Health and Performance, under the auspices of the IOC Medical Commission. *Br J Sports Med* 47:1012–22.

Tenforde, A. S., M. T. Barrack, A. Nattiv, and M. Fredericson. 2016. Parallels with the female athlete triad in male athletes. *Sports Med* 46:171–82.

Thorland, W. G., G. O. Johnson, G. D. Tharp, T. J. Housh, and C. J. Cisar. 1984. Estimation of body density in adolescent athletes. *Hum Biol* 56:439–48.

Toombs, R. J., G. Ducher, J. A. Shepherd, and M. J. De Souza. 2012. The impact of recent technological advances on the trueness and precision of DXA to assess body composition. *Obesity (Silver Spring)* 20:30–9.

Tothill, P., W. J. Hannan, and S. Wilkinson. 2001. Comparisons between a pencil beam and two fan beam dual energy x-ray absorptiometers used for measuring total body bone and soft tissue. *Br J Radiol* 74:166–76.

van der Ploeg, G. E., A. G. Brooks, R. T. Withers, J. Dollman, F. Leaney, and B. E. Chatterton. 2001. Body composition changes in female bodybuilders during preparation for competition. *Eur J Clin Nutr* 55:268–77.

Van Der Ploeg, G. E., R. T. Withers, and J. Laforgia. 2003. Percent body fat via DEXA: Comparison with a four-compartment model. *J Appl Physiol* 94:499–506.

van Marken Lichtenbelt, W. D., F. Hartgens, N. B. Vollaard, S. Ebbing, and H. Kuipers. 2004. Body composition changes in bodybuilders: A method comparison. *Med Sci Sports Exerc* 36:490–7.

Wang, Z., R. N. Pierson Jr., and S. B. Heymsfield. 1992. The five-level model: A new approach to organizing body-composition research. *Am J Clin Nutr* 56:19–28.

Wang, Z., F. X. Pi-Sunyer, D. P. Kotler et al. 2002. Multicomponent methods: Evaluation of new and traditional soft tissue mineral models by *in vivo* neutron activation analysis. *Am J Clin Nutr* 76:968–74.

Wang, Z., W. Shen, R. T. Whithers, and S. B. Heymsfield. 2005. Multicomponent molecular level models of body composition analysis. In *Human Body Composition*, edited by S. B. Heymsfield, T. G. Lohman, Z. Wang, and S. B. Going, 163–75. Champaign, IL: Human Kinetics.

Wells, J. C., J. E. Williams, S. Chomtho et al. 2010. Pediatric reference data for lean tissue properties: Density and hydration from age 5–20 y. *Am J Clin Nutr* 91:610–8.

Withers, R. T., J. Laforgia, and S. B. Heymsfield. 1999. Critical appraisal of the estimation of body composition via two-, three-, and four-compartment models. *Am J Hum Biol* 11:175–85.

Withers, R. T., J. Laforgia, S. B. Heymsfield, Z. M. Wang, and R. K. Pillans. 1996. Two, three and four-compartment chemical models of body composition analysis. In *Anthropometrica*, edited by K. Norton and T. Olds, 199–231. Sydney, Australia: UNSW Press.

Withers, R. T., J. LaForgia, R. K. Pillans et al. 1998. Comparisons of two-, three-, and four-compartment models of body composition analysis in men and women. *J Appl Physiol* 85:238–45.

Withers, R. T., D. A. Smith, B. E. Chatterton, C. G. Schultz, and R. D. Gaffney. 1992. A comparison of four methods of estimating the body composition of male endurance athletes. *Eur J Clin Nutr* 46:773–84.

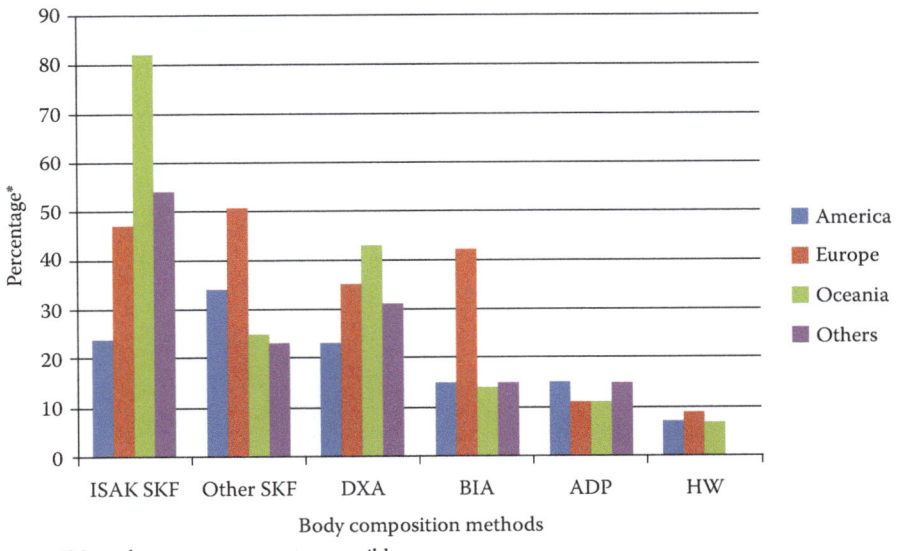

FIGURE 9.1 Most common body composition methods reported by Meyer et al. (2013).

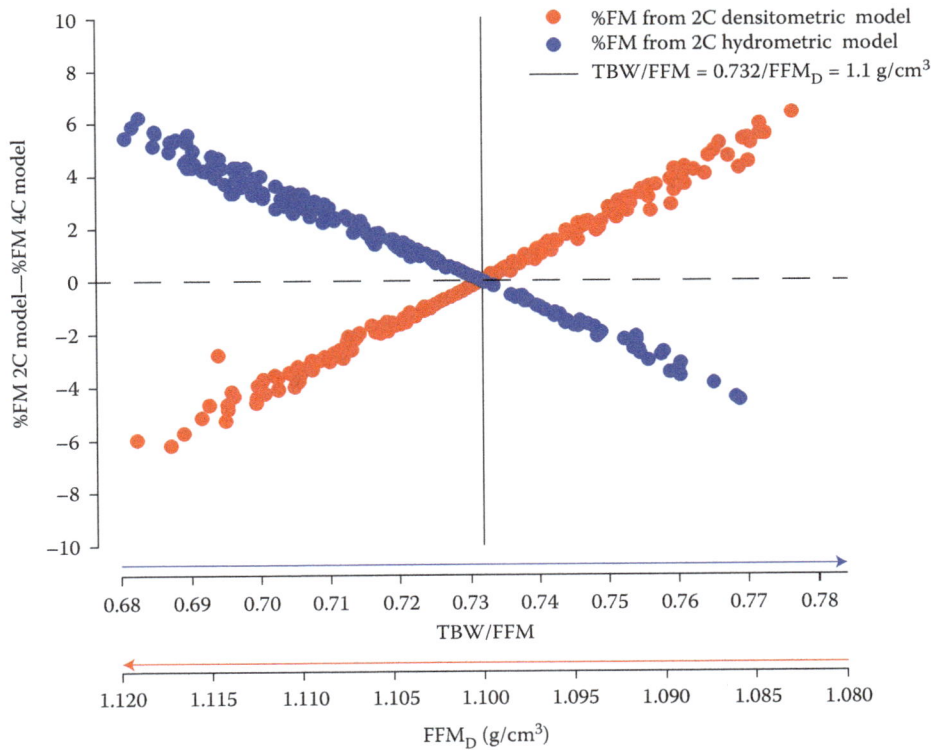

FIGURE 9.2 Differences between percent fat mass estimated with 2C densitometric and hydrometric models versus a 4C model, accordingly to FFM density and hydration (data from 235 athletes, not published).

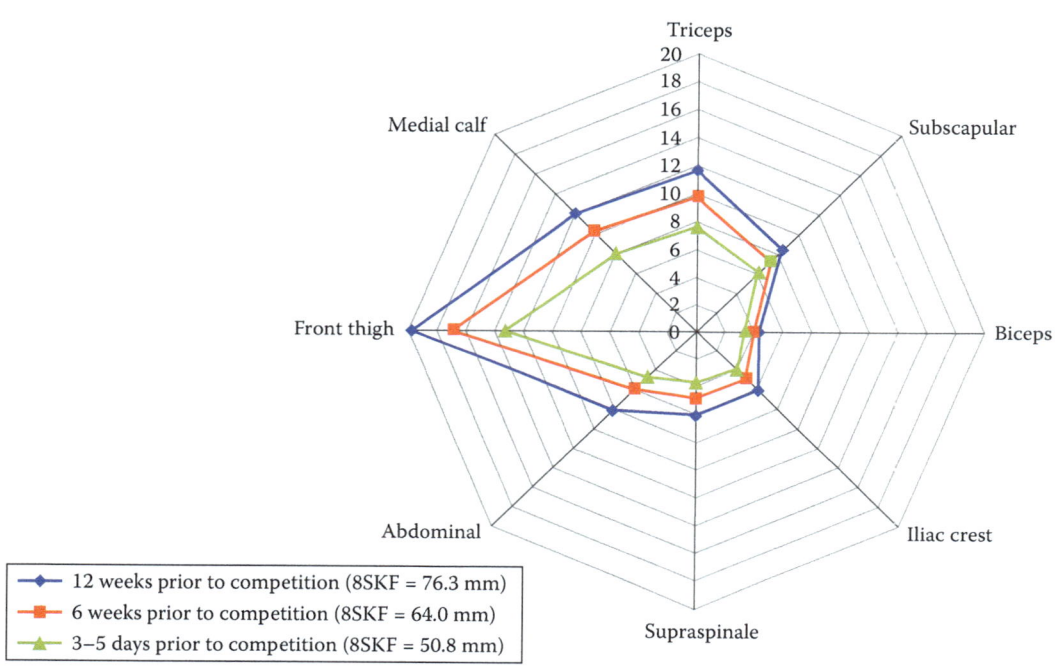

FIGURE 9.3 An SKF map in five female bodybuilders at 12 weeks, 6 weeks, and 3–5 days prior to a competition. (Data from van der Ploeg, G. E. et al. 2001. *Eur J Clin Nutr* 55:268–77.)

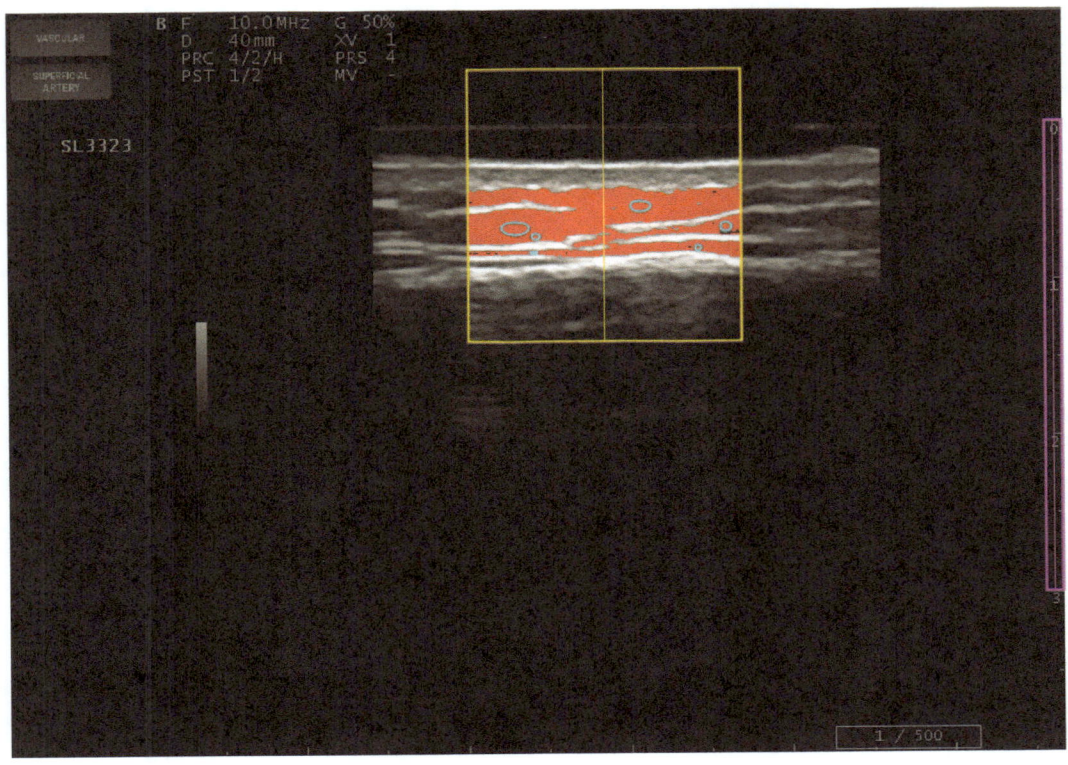

FIGURE 9.4 Example of an ultrasound image that was captured in the distal triceps site (red represents subcutaneous adipose tissue).

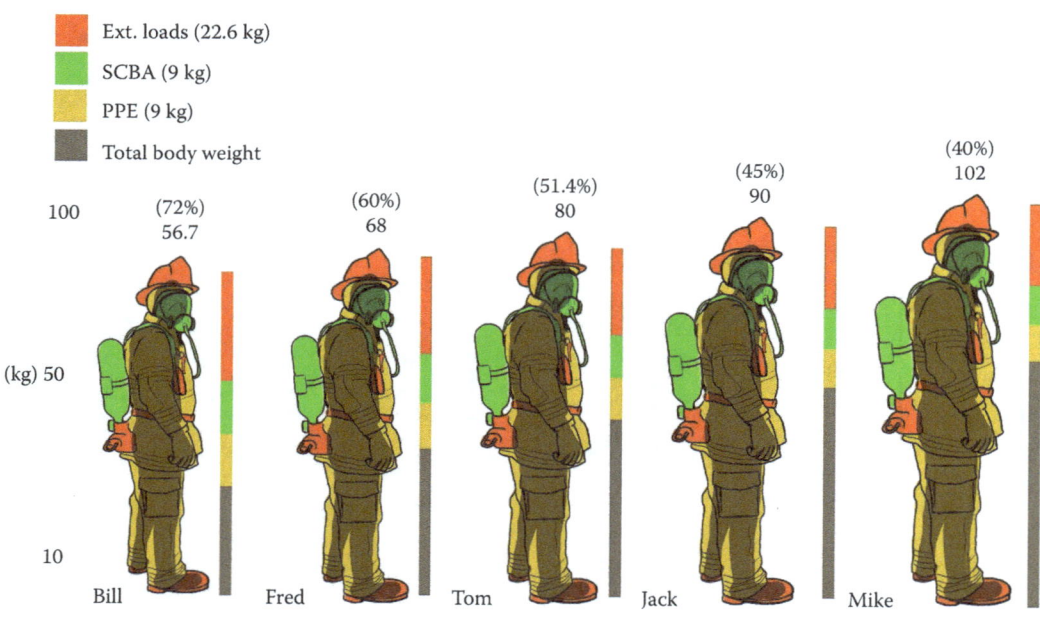

FIGURE 14.1 Body weight as a percentage of total load for firefighters. (Copyright 2016, Paul O. Davis.)

10 Endurance Athletes

Jordan R. Moon and Kristina L. Kendall

CONTENTS

10.1 INTRODUCTION

Several variables, including anthropometric and physiologic characteristics, can be used to differentiate endurance athletes from strength and power athletes. Athletes who compete in anaerobic sports tend to possess a large fat-free mass (FFM) to fat mass ratio and have a high proportion of Type II muscle fibers. This is not surprising as competition success is often based on rapid force production, maximal strength, and peak power output. Strength athletes are also more powerful and explosive compared to their endurance counterparts.

Endurance, compared to anaerobic (strength and power), athletes possess higher peak oxygen uptake (VO_{2max}) and anaerobic threshold levels, and have a predominance of Type I muscle fibers. They tend to be leaner and carry less body mass. Endurance training by definition is designed to enhance the overall aerobic capacity of not only muscle cells, but also of the body as a whole. Increased ability to take in and utilize oxygen is the most essential component for improving endurance performance regardless of the endurance sport. When comparing different levels (novice, trained, well trained, elite, etc.) of endurance athletes participating in the same sport, elite athletes have more Type I muscle fibers, greater capillary density, increased aerobic enzyme activity, higher absolute VO_{2max} values, improved economy, higher lactate thresholds, and overall superior endurance performance resulting in faster race times (Coyle 1995).

Despite these physiological differences and their fundamental role in determining overall endurance performance, endurance athletes also show variation in body types and composition within the same sport. While training status and age can also strongly influence endurance performance, differences in body size and shape (morphology) and composition can contribute to race speed and competition success. Specifically, when VO_{2max} and aerobic capacity are calculated relative to muscle mass, there appears to be no relationship with total body mass or body composition (Maciejczyk et al. 2014a,b). Therefore, increased amounts of muscle or fat mass can negatively impact endurance performance, and minimization of muscle mass and body fat of endurance athletes should enable optimal endurance performance.

This chapter examines the relationship between body composition and race performance in several different types of endurance athletes, including cross-country skiers, rowers, runners, cyclists, swimmers, and triathletes. In addition, it presents normative data from various endurance sports and identifies differences in body composition across multiple age groups and training status, performance, and event duration. These summary data can be used by athletes, coaches, trainers, and researchers to distinguish differences between endurance sports athletes to characterize body composition values for individual athletes (O'Connor et al. 2007). While changes in body composition and morphological characteristics are not discussed in this chapter, the data presented span across several decades with minimal changes observed in endurance athletes and body composition variables. Still, when using the data presented in this chapter, it is crucial to understand both the variability in the methods used to measure body composition as well as potential secular trends in the body composition of athletes across time. Finally, methodological considerations of various body composition techniques are discussed for use in endurance athletes.

10.2 CROSS-COUNTRY SKIERS

Cross-country skiing is considered one of the most demanding endurance sports. Compared to other endurance sports, cross-country skiing involves a variety of locomotion types (classical style, skate skiing, doubling poling, diagonal stride, etc.) on various terrains and different inclinations, highlighting the importance of both aerobic capacity and technique for optimal performance. Furthermore, cross-country skiing comprises different distances (0.8–50 km) and starting methods (interval and mass starts). Double pursuit with a mandatory ski change further adds to the complexity of the sport.

Because there are substantial differences in race distances, there are also differences in race times and energy contribution between the disciples. Sprint races generally last 2–4 min, with the majority of energy derived from aerobic processes (50%–70% aerobic, vs. 30%–50% anaerobic). Distance races, on the other hand, can range from 5 to 50 km, with skiing times from 13 min to more than 2 h. For distance cross-country skiers, aerobic processes account for 90%–99% of energy demands (Åstrand et al. 2003; Rusko 2003; Powers and Howley 2015). Maximal cardiac output has been shown to be in excess of 40 L/min, and stroke volumes over 200 mm have been measured in elite cross-country skiers, with relative maximal oxygen uptake values in the range of 80–90 mL/kg/min (Bergh and Forsberg 1992).

Successful ski racers have higher percentages of slow twitch muscle fibers and higher anaerobic thresholds than Alpine skiers, but lower anaerobic power scores. Cross-country skiers are also lean, comparable to distance runners. The absolute body mass of the ski racer, however, is much more variable than that of the distance runner. Lighter skiers may have an advantage on steep uphill courses, whereas heavier skiers will be favored on level, downhill, and less steep uphill courses (Eisenman et al. 1989).

10.2.1 Fat and FFM

The ideal body composition varies with each sport but, in general, the less fat mass, the greater the performance. When it comes to cross-country skiing, the success of an athlete depends heavily on body size, build, and body composition. Higher amounts of body fat can hinder performance by offering no strength advantages and potentially limiting endurance, speed, and movement.

The first likely study regarding the importance of body composition for performance in cross-country skiing was published by Niinimaa et al. (1978). They examined 10 intercollegiate skiers and found a strong, negative correlation between body fat percentage and performance in distance races. More recently, higher amounts of fat mass have been linked to slower race times and skiing speed. Larsson and Henriksson-Larsen (2008) found negative correlations between relative total fat mass and final race times, specifically in the uphill sections ($r = -0.661$ to -0.867). In addition, Stoggl et al. (2010) found that fat mass was negatively correlated with diagonal stride peak speed, whereas absolute and relative lean mass were positively correlated with stride speed ($r = 0.58$ and 0.76, respectively).

In cross-country skiing, the goal is to maintain as high a mean skiing speed as possible for the duration of the race. A high mean race speed is largely determined by the ability of the skeletal muscles to continuously generate high propelling forces throughout the race. Since the ability of a muscle to produce force is correlated with its cross-sectional area, theoretically, a skier with a large muscle mass has great potential to produce propelling forces and high race speeds (Hakkinen and Keskinen 1989; Alway et al. 1990; Akagi et al. 2008).

Larsson and Henriksson-Larsen (2008) reported significant associations between total body mass and total lean body mass and the lowest final race times ($r = -0.721$ and -0.830, respectively). Furthermore, body mass and lean body mass were both positive determinants of speed, with strong correlations observed in most sections of the course ($r = 0.636-0.867$). This supports the notion that the adverse effect on performance of a higher body weight is not of great importance in cross-country skiing compared to other weight-bearing sports like running.

Supporting this idea, Stoggl et al. (2010) found positive associations between body mass ($r = 0.57$) and total lean mass ($r = 0.69$) on double poling peak speed. The authors also found that a high absolute trunk mass in combination with a high lean mass appeared to be advantageous to race success. This finding confirmed results of previous studies of elite cross-country skiers that emphasized the importance of the trunk muscles in double pooling performance (Holmberg et al. 2005).

In addition to trunk mass, lean mass of the upper arms has been shown to be related to overall race performance, specifically in the uphill sections of a track. Larsson and Henriksson-Larsen (2008) found arm lean mass to be significantly related to final race time ($r = -0.648$) in college-aged elite male cross-country skiers; whereas, Carlsson et al. (2014) demonstrated a significant correlation between upper body lean mass and sprint performance in elite cross-country skiers of both sexes ($r = -0.66$ to -0.82).

10.2.2 Bone

Cross-sectional studies have shown that bone mineral density (BMD) is significantly higher in athletes compared with non-active controls (Risser et al. 1990; Heinonen et al. 1993, 1995; Slemenda and Johnston 1993). Furthermore, weight-bearing activities, like running and resistance training, seem to provide a more effective stimulus for bone growth than non-weight-bearing activity (like swimming). Swimmers and cyclists had BMD values not significantly different from non-active controls (Heinonen et al. 1993; Fehling et al. 1995; Taaffe et al. 1995).

Although cross-country skiing is a weight-bearing sport, most of the activity consists of gliding movements, with little impact and low ground reaction forces acting on the skeleton. During skiing, however, the femoral neck is subjected to ground reaction forces from the snow through the femur. Furthermore, off-season training for skiers includes impact loading exercises such as running and weight lifting. Not surprisingly, cross-country skiers have demonstrated significantly higher BMD of the femoral neck, femur diaphysis, and greater trochanter to non-active individuals (Pettersson et al. 2000).

As for the upper body, cross-country skiers are also subjected to higher levels of strain on the humerus due to the amount of arm work achieved during uphill skiing. Ground reaction forces in the poles have been shown to reach up to 50% of a skier's bodyweight (Komi 1987). As expected, cross-country skiers have significantly higher bone mass in the whole humerus in both arms (Pettersson et al. 2000). Both the primary activity (skiing) and off-season training likely contribute to the higher BMD observed in cross-country skiers as compared to non-active controls.

10.2.3 Summary

Upper body power and strength appear to be significantly related to cross-country skiing performance (Ng et al. 1988; Rundell and Bacharach 1995; Staib et al. 2000). The addition of greater muscle mass in both the upper and lower body seems to positively enhance performance with no negative side effects related to an increased body mass. Greater body fat can negatively impact performance and does not offer any strength advantages and may limit speed and movement. Coaches, trainers, and athletes should focus on developing lean mass and strength, specifically for the upper body, as these are important factors in race performance. Cross-country skiers are not at risk for having low BMD.

10.3 ROWERS

The sport of rowing demands a high level of both strength and endurance, as an elite male rower performs more than 200 strokes with a peak force of over 1000 N during a 2000 m race (Steinacker 1993). While maximal anaerobic and aerobic power are significantly correlated with rowing performance, body size and mass are undoubtedly performance-related factors (Jurimae et al. 1999).

Anthropometric data for both male and female rowers emphasize the importance of body mass and body size in determining successful rowing performance at an international level (Hebbelinck et al. 1980; Secher and Vaage 1983; DeRose et al. 1989). A typical heavyweight rower is tall, heavy, and lean, with a high percentage of slow twitch muscle fibers (Secher and Vaage 1983; Russell et al. 1998). Similarly, junior rowers also are taller, heavier, with greater length, breadth, and girth dimensions than the general population (Bourgois et al. 2000).

Due to the nature of the sport, both strength and endurance are needed for high-level rowing performance. Therefore, rowing-specific training programs combined with resistance training typically results in a large aerobic capacity and increased metabolic efficiency, a low percentage of body fat and increased muscle mass (Russell et al. 1998).

10.3.1 Fat and FFM

In rowing, an athlete's body mass is supported by a sliding seat in the boat or on a rowing ergometer, with heavier rowers possessing an advantage over lighter rowers (Secher 1983; Secher and Vaage 1983). Because body mass is supported, a higher body fat percentage in rowers does not put them at the same disadvantage that it would put a weight-bearing athlete (i.e., runners, triathletes, cross-country skiers, etc.). However, higher fat mass values have been reported to adversely affect 2000 m rowing ergometer performance (Secher and Vaage 1983; Ingham et al. 2002).

Amongst rowers, body fat, expressed as both fat mass and percent body fat was lower in junior rowers compared to both elite and sub-elite seniors (Mikulic and Ruzic 2008). One could argue that junior rowers tend to be leaner than senior rowers due to the fact that older, more experienced rowers tend to be heavier, and there is a positive correlation between rowing performance and body mass ($r = 0.41–0.85$, $p < 0.05$) (Russell et al. 1998; Yoshiga and Higuchi 2003b; Nevill et al. 2010; Akca 2014). Furthermore, it is difficult to combine high levels of muscularity with extreme leanness (Shephard 1998), although the percentage of body fat seems to decrease in recent years among elite rowers.

Although the measurement of body fat has been the prime focus of attention, many coaches working with elite athletes recognize that the amount and distribution of lean tissues like bone and muscle play an important role in determining sports performance. Yoshiga and Higuchi (2003b) found that the greater the FFM and maximal oxygen consumption (VO_{2max}) values in male and female rowers, the better the rowing performance, supporting the supposition that rowing demands high aerobic capacity and a large relative muscle mass.

The ability to maximize FFM at a given weight likely contributes to success through a greater power to body weight ratio (Yoshiga and Higuchi 2003b). Among both junior and senior heavy-weight rowers, FFM has been shown to be significantly correlated to both 2000 and 6000 m rowing performance ($r = 0.58–0.91$, $p < 0.05$) (Cosgrove et al.1999; Yoshiga and Higuchi 2003a,b; Mikulic 2009) and despite the weight limitations imposed on lightweight rowers, FFM remains a predictor of competitive success (Slater et al. 2005). Obtaining fast race times involves an element of dynamic strength and the ability to produce a large force during the stroke (Secher 1983). Rowers with a high lean body mass, and therefore a larger muscle mass, are potentially able to produce a greater force during each stroke compared to individuals with a lower lean body mass, ultimately leading to more successful rowing performances (Cosgrove et al. 1999).

Although the majority of body composition research in rowing has been conducted using sweepers (each rower only has one oar, typically held with both hands), it should be noted that scullers (each rower holds two oars, one in each hand), tend to be smaller, lighter, and have less muscle development compared to sweepers. However, FFM, specifically muscle mass and cross-sectional area of the thigh, have been shown to be significant predictors of 2000 m rowing ergometer performance in sculling (Jurimae et al. 2000). Furthermore, Purge et al. (2004) found that arm muscle mass was a strong predictor of sculling performance, indicating that the development of upper body musculature may have a high importance to race success in sculling.

It has been hypothesized that the correlation between rowing performance and FFM may be due to the direct relationship between skeletal muscle mass (a large component of FFM) and its capacity to consume oxygen for energy metabolism (Fleg and Lakatta 1988; Toth et al. 1994; Hunt et al. 1998). In addition, FFM may also be related to central circulatory factors known to influence maximal aerobic capacity (van Lieshout et al. 2001). Specifically, FFM is strongly related to blood volume and left ventricular hypertrophy, and may be a determinant of stroke volume (Coyle et al. 1986; Davy and Seals 1994).

10.3.2 Bone

Rowing is a sport that involves a unique loading pattern to the lumbar spine. Morris et al. (2000) conducted a biomechanical analysis of the force generated by the rowing stroke on the lumbar spine in rowing athletes. Their results indicated that the compressive force generated at the lumbar spine during the drive phase of the rowing stroke nearly reached five times the rower's body mass. This finding may help to explain the results of cross-sectional studies that have reported superior lumbar spine BMD in rowing athletes compared to their non-rowing counterparts (Wolman 1990; Morris et al. 2000).

Only a few longitudinal studies have reported lumbar spine BMD changes in rowing athletes over a competition season. The findings are somewhat conflicting, as some researchers reported no change in BMD (Lariviere et al. 2003; Jurimae et al. 2006), while others have reported significant increases (Cohen et al. 1995; Morris et al. 1999).

Cohen et al. (1995) showed that lumbar spine BMD significantly increased among male novice college rowers over a 7-month training period. Furthermore, mean bone mineral content increased by 4.2%. Lariviere et al. (2003) found that experienced rowers demonstrated a significant (2.5%) increase in BMD of the spine, compared to novice rowers, over a 6-month training season. The higher power output in the experienced rowers likely produced higher forces at the spine resulting in gains in BMD.

10.3.3 SPECIAL CONSIDERATIONS WITHIN THE SPORT OF ROWING

Body composition is a critical issue for the lightweight rower (e.g., male competitors weigh no more than 72.5 kg, with a boat average of 70.0 kg; and female competitors weigh no more than 59.0 kg, with a boat average of 56.7 kg). The goal of lightweight rowers is to maximize relative power output by increasing muscle mass while minimizing total body fat mass. It appears to be advantageous for the lightweight rower to lose body fat and increase muscle mass since muscle mass has been highly correlated to strength and power output (Mayhew et al. 1993), which is conducive to superior rowing performance (Secher 1983).

Slater et al. (2005) reported that lower body fat and higher levels of muscle mass were associated with faster heat times and better overall placing amongst lightweight rowers ($p < 0.01$). Using parameter estimates to predict 2000-m heat times, the authors concluded that for every 1-kg increase in fat mass, race time increases by 8.4 s. Conversely, for every 1-kg increase in muscle mass, race time decreases by 10.2 s. These findings confirm that lightweight rowers should prioritize the manipulation of not only fat mass, but also muscle mass, when they prepare to make weight for upcoming competition.

10.3.4 SUMMARY

A higher muscle mass and lower body fat percentage appear to be advantageous to both heavyweight and lightweight rowers. Because body mass is supported, a higher fat mass is less of a disadvantage in rowing compared to other endurance sports. However, lightweight rowers can benefit more than heavyweight rowers from having lower body fat percentage. Furthermore, rowers show a high level of BMD in the spine and should not be concerned with having low total body BMD.

10.4 RUNNERS

Since 1967 endurance runners have evolved to be taller, lighter, with increasingly lower amounts of body fat (Costill 1967) (Tables 10.1 and 10.2). Endurance running can include events as short as the 800 m run, which can demand as much as 50% of the required energy derived from aerobic sources, in comparison to a 10,000 m run or a marathon, which can require up to 100% energy coming from aerobic sources (Powers and Howley 2015). In addition to single long distance runs such as marathons, runners can compete in ultraendurance runs which can take several days and include distances of 338 km (>50 km a day) (Knechtle et al. 2009a).

Male endurance runners have demonstrated approximately 10% performance improvement when compared to females in the absence of body composition differences (Cheuvront et al. 2005). Specifically, males demonstrated a greater aerobic performance advantage in relation to VO_{2max} relative to lean/muscle mass. For every ounce of muscle, regardless of body fat and body mass, males appear to utilize more oxygen compared to females (Cheuvront et al. 2005). Regardless, body composition remains a major factor when it comes to racing performance for both sexes.

Compared to sprinters, endurance athletes have lower muscle cross-sectional area and fascicle length as well as smaller upper and lower body muscles (Abe et al. 2000). The smaller size of muscles in endurance athletes can be attributed to the greater dependence on Type I slow twitch muscle fibers which are smaller in size and diameter than fast twitch Type II muscle fibers (Coyle et al. 1991). Research has also demonstrated that VO_{2max}, percentage of Type I fibers, and lactate threshold are strong predictors of endurance running performance (Coyle 1995). However, researchers have evaluated the impact of body composition on performance with conflicting findings.

The literature appears to be in agreement regarding body size and running performance. Several studies have indicated that an increase in any mass, regardless of the composition, can negatively impact running performance (Costill 1972; Cureton et al. 1978; Hagan et al. 1987; Maciejczyk et al. 2014a,b). In 1972, Costill (1972) concluded that *"fat and massive skeletal structures serve as dead weight."* Later Cureton et al. (1978) stated that excess weight/fat lowers the *"oxidative energy available to move each kilogram of body weight"* and that for every 5% increase in body mass, a decrease in 89 m for a 12-min run, a 2.4 mL reduction in VO_2, and a 35-s reduction in maximal treadmill running time was observed. Recent studies confirm the findings from the 1970s and suggest that increasing muscle or fat mass for endurance runners can increase lactate production, reduce blood pH, and cause fatigue at a lower intensity than runners with less body mass with similar aerobic power (Maciejczyk et al. 2014a,b). Researchers have also suggested that larger body sizes can increase air resistance during running that can decrease running efficiency and ultimately race performance (Hagan et al. 1987). However, data also suggest that endurance runners with increased muscle size and quality tend to have improved performance and fewer stress fractures compared to those with lower body mass, higher fat mass, and lower vastus lateralis muscle cross-sectional area (Roelofs et al. 2015). Additional evidence reveals that small increases in body mass may reduce oxygen cost due to improved efficiency related to the stretch-shortening cycling and a greater return of elastic energy (O'Connor et al. 2007). The aforementioned findings challenge the idea that endurance runners should be as light as possible with only enough functional muscle mass to produce high aerobic power and running speed. Muscle quality along with size appears to benefit endurance athletes. The research is clear in that added body fat can lead to a reduction in performance and may increase the risk of injuries, even though it may slightly improve efficiency. However, the exact amount of muscle mass needed to optimize performance and reduce injuries remains unclear for various types of endurance runners participating in different events with varying distances.

Height and weight appear to be no different between elite runners (e.g., top 5% in the world) and high-level runners (Billat et al. 2001). However, elite males showed a significant increase in running speed and VO_{2peak}, while female elite runners were no different than high-level runners for VO_{2peak}, but were significantly faster, suggesting an improvement in running efficiency (Billat et al. 2001). In contrast, body mass index (BMI) was found to be highly variable between the top-five finishers of an ultramarathon, with a range of 22.4–24.7 for males and 17.3–21.1 for females (Hoffman 2008). There appear to be differences in the body composition values for both endurance runners at the same level, as well as endurance runners across different levels (elite, highly trained, trained, etc.).

10.4.1 Fat and FFM

Several studies looking at the relationships between various body composition variables and endurance running performance have produced conflicting findings. For recreational marathon runners, a greater body mass, BMI, thigh and calf circumferences, thigh and calf skinfolds, and percent fat (% fat) values were all significantly related to longer marathon race times (Rust et al. 2013). In male ultraendurance runners, upper arm circumferences were related to race performance, with greater circumferences being related to slower running times (decreased performance) (Knechtle et al. 2008). In ultraendurance athletes, only upper arm circumferences, BMI, and body mass were negatively related to performance (Knechtle et al. 2009a). In addition, past endurance runner research has shown that body mass, BMI, body fat, skinfold thicknesses, and circumferences of the upper arm and lower leg were related to endurance running performance (Knechtle et al. 2008). Thus, when using skinfolds to help predict running performance, it appears that individual skinfold site thicknesses are more valuable than just the sum of all skinfolds. Multiple skinfold locations have been shown to predict 1,500 m, 10,000 m, and marathon race times (Arrese and Ostariz 2006). In males, the thigh and calf skinfold thicknesses were significantly ($r > 0.56$) related to an increase in 1,500 and 10,000 m race times. In females, the suprailiac and abdominal skinfold thicknesses were significantly ($r > 0.60$) related to an increase in marathon race times (Arrese and Ostariz 2006). The exact reason why some skinfold sites may be related to running performance over other sites is unclear. Researchers have suggested that lower body skinfold sites may be better predictors over other sites because they relate to a higher lower body mass which could require more muscular effort to accelerate the legs compared to having more fat in the upper body which is relatively stationary while running (Arrese and Ostariz 2006). However, more research is needed to determine if individual skinfolds sites have a *"causal effect"* on endurance performance in runners (Arrese and Ostariz 2006).

In contrast, several studies have shown no relationships regarding anthropometric data and endurance running performance. In males who had completed at least nine marathons, there was no relationship between skinfold thicknesses, muscle mass, or body fat on performance during a 24-h run (Knechtle et al. 2009d). In nonprofessional male ultraendurance runners, anthropometric variables and % fat were not related to race performance (Knechtle et al. 2010f). Recently, researchers have questioned the use of anthropometric data alone to predict endurance performance and race time. Burtscher and Gatterer (2013) suggest that researchers should use both physiological and anthropometric data for predicting endurance performance, and that in the presence of physiological data such as VO_{2max} or peak power, the significant relationship between anthropometric data and race performance would disappear. In agreement, research conducted in male marathon runners demonstrated that while a lighter body mass and smaller skinfold thicknesses were related to faster running times, they were not major predictors of performance when physiological variables were included (Hagan et al. 1981). Specifically, less than 20% of the variation in endurance performance was attributed to skinfold thicknesses and body mass, while 71% was explained by VO_{2max}, average training speed, average distance per workout, and total workout distance. Still, the authors concluded there may be an added value when including physical characteristics such as body mass and skinfold thicknesses when predicting endurance race performance alongside physiological variables (Hagan et al. 1981).

For elite and world-ranked male and female runners, there appear to be no differences in skinfold thicknesses among runners who competed in the 100, 400, 800, 1,500, 3,000, 5,000, 10,000 m, and marathon races (Legaz Arrese et al. 2005). These findings suggest that subcutaneous fat does not differ significantly between different types of runners ranging from sprinters to endurance runners and that both types of athletes require low body fat values with sprint athletes requiring significantly more FFM. However, research has also shown that compared to elite male endurance runners, recreational male endurance runners have higher abdominal and total body fat, and elite female runners have less fat compared to moderate and good runners, and elite male runners have less fat, smaller skinfold thicknesses, and are lighter compared to average and good runners based on race speed (Bale et al. 1985, 1986; Hetland et al. 1998).

When looking at the combined percent body fat data for endurance athletes (Tables 10.1 and 10.2 and Figures 10.1 through 10.5), the largest differences can be seen between ultraendurance athletes and highly trained and elite distance runners. Ultraendurance athletes appear to have almost double the amount of relative body fat compared to non-ultraendurance runners. The added fat for ultraendurance athletes may be related to the sustained energy demands of the sport. Research has shown that ultraendurance runners (100 km) can lose a significant amount of both fat and muscle mass during a race (Knechtle et al. 2009c). Ultraendurance runners may have more fat compared to typical distance runners because of the relative importance of running speed, as ultraendurance athletes may be less worried about absolute speed and more focused on completing the race.

TABLE 10.1
Body Composition and Anthropometric Measurements of Male Endurance Athletes

Sports	Level	References		cm	kg			kg			DXA	Circumferences (cm)					Skinfold (mm)								
				Ht	Mass	BMI	%Fat	FM	FFM	SMM	%Fat	Waist	Hip	Biceps	Calf	Thigh	Chest	Triceps	Biceps	Subscap	Suprailiac	Calf	Axilla	Abd	Thigh
Cyclists	All adult	3,7,24,29	Mean	180.1	71.8	22.6	10.8	6.1	62.8	–	–	–	–	–	–	–	–	–	–	–	–	–	–	–	–
			SD BW	0.2	3.8	0.9	1.7	0.2	2.2	–	–	–	–	–	–	–	–	–	–	–	–	–	–	–	–
			SD WT	5.5	5.2	–	2.6	–	–	–	–	–	–	–	–	–	–	–	–	–	–	–	–	–	–
Cyclists	Youth	15	Mean	168.6	62.4	22.0	11.7	7.3	55.1	–	–	70.6	88.7	–	–	–	7.5	9.6	–	9.8	12.6	–	8.2	12.5	12.2
			SD BW	–	–	–	–	–	–	–	–	5.0	4.5	–	–	–	–	–	–	–	–	–	–	–	–
			SD WT	4.3	6.6	–	4.1	–	–	–	–	–	–	–	–	–	3.6	3.6	–	3.4	6.2	–	4.0	5.7	4.5
Rowers	Elite	31,43	Mean	187.6	88.9	25.2	13.3	12.0	76.9	–	–	–	–	34.9	40.3	63.2	–	–	–	–	–	–	–	–	–
			SD BW	9.1	11.7	0.9	3.7	4.9	6.9	–	–	–	–	–	–	–	–	–	–	–	–	–	–	–	–
			SD WT	3.8	4.2	–	3.4	–	–	–	–	–	–	0.7	2.0	2.2	–	–	–	–	–	–	–	–	–
Rowers	Highly trained	31	Mean	188.6	92.9	26.1	16.1	15.0	77.9	–	–	–	–	33.9	40.1	63.1	–	–	–	–	–	–	–	–	–
			SD BW	–	–	–	–	–	–	–	–	–	–	–	–	–	–	–	–	–	–	–	–	–	–
			SD WT	5.4	5.4	–	3.5	–	–	–	–	–	–	1.8	1.4	2.7	–	–	–	–	–	–	–	–	–
Rowers	Youth	31	Mean	188.9	86.1	24.1	12.9	11.1	75.0	–	–	–	–	31.4	39.4	60.2	–	–	–	–	–	–	–	–	–
			SD BW	–	–	–	–	–	–	–	–	–	–	–	–	–	–	–	–	–	–	–	–	–	–
			SD WT	3.6	4.1	–	2.1	–	–	–	–	–	–	1.4	2.0	2.2	–	–	–	–	–	–	–	–	–
Rowers	All adult	3,16,29,31,43	Mean	187.9	85.9	25.5	11.2	10.9	75.0	–	–	–	–	34.4	40.2	63.2	–	–	–	–	–	–	–	–	–
			SD BW	6.5	10.4	0.8	2.8	4.1	6.6	–	–	–	–	0.7	0.1	0.1	–	–	–	–	–	–	–	–	–
			SD WT	4.3	4.6	–	2.7	–	–	–	–	–	–	1.3	1.7	2.5	–	–	–	–	–	–	–	–	–
Runners	17–26 yrs	12	Mean	177.0	64.5	20.6	9.1	5.9	58.6	–	–	–	–	–	–	–	–	–	–	–	–	–	–	–	–
			SD BW	0.0	5.5	–	2.5	–	–	–	–	–	–	–	–	–	–	–	–	–	–	–	–	–	–
			SD WT	–	–	–	–	–	–	–	–	–	–	–	–	–	–	–	–	–	–	–	–	–	–
Runners	40–49 yrs	12	Mean	172.0	68.9	23.3	15.8	10.9	58.0	–	–	–	–	–	–	–	–	–	–	–	–	–	–	–	–
			SD BW	–	8.3	–	3.9	–	–	–	–	–	–	–	–	–	–	–	–	–	–	–	–	–	–
			SD WT	0.1	–	–	–	–	–	–	–	–	–	–	–	–	–	–	–	–	–	–	–	–	–
Runners	50–59 yrs	12	Mean	169.0	69.9	24.5	17.3	12.1	57.8	–	–	–	–	–	–	–	–	–	–	–	–	–	–	–	–
			SD BW	–	–	–	–	–	–	–	–	–	–	–	–	–	–	–	–	–	–	–	–	–	–
			SD WT	0.1	6.2	–	4.0	–	–	–	–	–	–	–	–	–	–	–	–	–	–	–	–	–	–
Runners	60–69 yrs	12	Mean	171.0	67.9	23.2	16.4	11.1	56.8	–	–	–	–	–	–	–	–	–	–	–	–	–	–	–	–
			SD BW	–	–	–	–	–	–	–	–	–	–	–	–	–	–	–	–	–	–	–	–	–	–
			SD WT	0.1	6.9	–	2.5	–	–	–	–	–	–	–	–	–	–	–	–	–	–	–	–	–	–

(Continued)

TABLE 10.1 (Continued)
Body Composition and Anthropometric Measurements of Male Endurance Athletes

Sports	Level	References		Ht (cm)	Mass (kg)	BMI	%Fat	FM (kg)	FFM (kg)	SMM (kg)	%Fat (DXA)	Waist	Hip	Biceps	Calf	Thigh	Chest	Triceps	Biceps	Subscap	Suprailiac	Calf	Axilla	Abd	Thigh
												Circumferences (cm)					Skinfold (mm)								
Runners	>70 yrs	12	Mean	166.0	67.3	24.4	20.0	13.5	53.8																
			SD BW																						
			SD WT	0.1	7.2		3.7																		
Runners	Elite	1,3,5,20,26	Mean	175.1	65.5	21.0	8.0	5.4	60.8		8.4			29.4	36.8		4.8	5.8	3.2	7.6	4.7	4.4	6.0	7.5	7.7
			SD BW		4.0		0.6	0.7	3.4								0.6	0.5	0.5	0.4	1.6	0.1		1.6	1.0
			SD WT	3.8	3.2		0.5				0.8						1.4	1.3		1.3	1.1	0.7	2.7	3.0	2.4
Runners	Highly trained	2,3,15	Mean	169.8	62.6	19.9	7.7	4.8	57.8			67.8	85.5				4.6	5.7		7.3	6.3		5.6	6.8	6.9
			SD BW		4.4		2.9	1.8	5.1																
			SD WT	3.7	4.3		2.8							1.2	2.5		1.2				2.8		1.7	2.4	2.5
Runners	Trained	3,5,7,20,36,37,47	Mean	178.5	72.7	22.5	12.1	9.7	63.0	38.1	10.6			29.0	36.3	54.8	8.1	8.5	4.1	9.6	9.5	5.4	9.5	14.7	11.9
			SD BW	3.0	8.5	2.3	5.0	5.2	3.8					0.2	1.4			1.0	0.5	1.1	7.9	0.7			
			SD WT	6.0	6.2		3.1			2.9	0.5			1.7	2.3	2.5	3.2	1.9	0.7	2.5	2.9		2.8	5.8	5.1
Runners	Youth	12,15	Mean	170.3	55.9	19.3	9.7	5.4	50.5			67.2	85.6				4.8	6.4		7.0	6.9		5.1	6.6	8.3
			SD BW									3.5	3.4				1.4								
			SD WT	4.4	5.3		2.2			2.9		3.4	2.7				1.8	2.0		1.2	1.9		1.4	1.9	2.7
Runners	All adult	1,2,3,5,7,15,16, 20,26,47	Mean	176.0	65.2	21.2	8.9	5.9	59.6	38.1	9.5	67.8	85.5	29.1	36.4	54.8	5.6	6.9	3.6	8.4	7.4	5.0	7.0	9.1	8.6
			SD BW	4.0	3.7	1.3	2.7	2.4	2.6	0.8	1.6			0.2	1.1		1.7	1.6	0.6	1.3	5.6	0.8	2.1	3.9	2.3
			SD WT	5.1	3.9		2.2			3.0	0.6	3.4	2.7	1.6	2.4	2.5	1.8	1.6	0.6	1.8	2.3	1.2	2.4	3.6	3.1
Ultra runners	All adult	30,34,38,41	Mean	177.5	72.9	23.1	15.0	10.9	61.9	37.2				28.8	36.9	53.2	5.5	7.5		8.8	10.6	6.7	6.8	14.1	9.7
			SD BW	1.0	1.6	0.4	1.5	1.3	0.7	0.8				1.0	2.6	1.4	0.5	0.6		0.1	1.0	0.6	0.3	2.2	1.6
			SD WT	6.0	7.9		3.9			3.0				2.1	2.3	3.0	2.5	2.1		2.3	4.9	2.9	1.6	7.9	4.5
Cross-country skiers	All adult	3,29	Mean		73.2		8.9	6.5	66.7																
			SD BW				2.3																		
			SD WT				1.5																		
Swimmers	Youth	15,29	Mean	163.6	52.9	19.4	11.6	6.1	48.1																
			SD BW	13.0	13.0	2.0	2.1	1.2	11.8																
			SD WT	2.9	5.2	3.1	3.1																		
Swimmers	All adult	3,7,16,23,29	Mean	181.3	75.8	23.0	9.7	8.0	67.8																
			SD BW				3.0																		
			SD WT	1.2	1.3		3.2																		

(Continued)

TABLE 10.1 (Continued)
Body Composition and Anthropometric Measurements of Male Endurance Athletes

Sports	Level	References		cm	kg			kg			DXA	Circumferences (cm)					Skinfold (mm)								
				Ht	Mass	BMI	%Fat	FM	FFM	SMM	%Fat	Waist	Hip	Biceps	Calf	Thigh	Chest	Triceps	Biceps	Subscap	Suprailiac	Calf	Axilla	Abd	Thigh
Distance swimmers	All adult	36,37,52	Mean	180.6	84.9	26.2	20.2	17.2	67.8	–	–	–	–	–	–	–	–	–	–	–	–	–	–	–	–
			SD BW	0.6	1.1	0.3	2.3	2.2	1.1	–	–	–	–	–	–	–	–	–	–	–	–	–	–	–	–
			SD WT	6.5	9.4	–	4.6	–	–	–	–	–	–	–	–	–	–	–	–	–	–	–	–	–	–
Triathletes	17–34 yrs	48	Mean	176.6	66.4	21.3	9.1	6.0	60.4	–	–	–	–	31.3	37.2	–	–	6.9	–	7.6	6.7	5.6	–	–	–
			SD BW	–	–	–	–	–	–	–	–	–	–	–	–	–	–	–	–	–	–	–	–	–	–
			SD WT	5.1	4.2	–	1.7	–	–	–	–	–	–	2.7	6.3	–	–	2.1	–	1.3	2.1	1.9	–	–	–
Triathletes	60–73 yrs	48	Mean	173.3	73.8	24.6	20.1	14.8	59.0	–	–	–	–	31.9	37.2	–	–	9.4	–	11.6	9.9	7.4	–	–	–
			SD BW	–	–	–	–	–	–	–	–	–	–	–	–	–	–	–	–	–	–	–	–	–	–
			SD WT	6.4	8.7	–	3.1	–	–	–	–	–	–	2.8	2.1	–	2.9	–	–	4.3	3.7	3.1	–	–	–
Triathletes	All adult	6,7,10,19,22,25, 39,40,42,44, 45,46,47,49	Mean	179.3	74.9	23.3	12.0	9.3	65.7	40.2	15.1	–	–	29.6	37.4	54.8	6.7	7.4	–	10.1	15.1	7.5	8.7	13.1	11.9
			SD BW	1.2	2.7	0.9	3.0	2.6	1.6	1.4	–	–	–	1.9	0.5	0.8	0.5	0.7	–	0.3	1.8	0.1	0.8	4.2	0.5
			SD WT	5.2	6.6	–	2.7	–	–	4.5	5.6	–	–	2.8	2.6	3.1	4.3	3.6	–	4.7	8.3	3.2	4.0	9.3	6.0
Triathletes	Elite	19,22	Mean	180.5	73.0	22.4	8.8	6.4	66.6	–	–	–	–	–	–	–	–	–	–	–	–	–	–	–	–
			SD BW	0.7	1.3	0.6	1.3	0.8	2.1	–	–	–	–	–	–	–	–	–	–	–	–	–	–	–	–
			SD WT	2.0	3.4	–	1.5	–	–	–	–	–	–	–	–	–	–	–	–	–	–	–	–	–	–
Triathletes	Trained	7,10,47	Mean	179.6	75.5	23.4	10.7	8.6	66.9	38.6	–	–	–	27.0	37.2	54.2	7.0	7.9	–	10.3	16.4	7.4	9.2	16.0	12.2
			SD BW	0.7	1.6	0.4	3.4	3.1	1.5	–	–	–	–	–	–	–	–	–	–	–	–	–	–	–	–
			SD WT	6.1	7.1	–	2.4	–	–	4.2	–	–	–	2.6	2.3	2.9	4.0	4.5	–	4.1	8.7	3.1	4.5	8.8	5.8
Ultra triathletes	All adult	27,28,32,33, 38,45	Mean	177.4	77.7	24.5	14.1	10.9	66.8	40.1	–	–	–	30.0	38.6	55.3	5.3	7.7	–	9.4	12.7	7.3	30.8	13.8	10.9
			SD BW	1.5	1.6	0.4	1.1	0.9	1.3	0.1	–	–	–	1.2	0.9	1.6	0.6	1.4	–	1.0	2.4	0.9	41.8	2.2	1.6
			SD WT	5.8	8.0	–	3.0	–	–	4.6	–	–	–	2.2	2.5	3.7	1.5	2.7	–	2.3	5.7	2.3	2.1	5.5	4.2

SD BW = standard deviations between studies, SD WT = average standard deviation within studies, Ht = height, Mass = body mass, %Fat = relative body fat measured using either densitometry-based methods or skinfold equations, FM = fat mass, FFM = fat-free mass, SMM = skeletal muscle mass, DXA = dual-energy x-ray absorptiometry, Abd = abdominal. Mean data reported was calculated by averaging the published means from multiple research studies (see table and figure references). Standard deviations (SD) were calculated by averaging the SDs published from the same research studies. When only ranges were provided, SDs were calculated using SD = range/4. Level of athlete included only adults unless identified as youth. References: [1]Costill et al. 1970, [2]Pipes 1977, [3]Fleck 1983, [3]Bale et al. 1986, [6]Holly et al. 1986, [7]O'Toole et al. 1987, [10]Dengel et al. 1989, [12]Grassi et al. 1991, [15]Tsunawake et al. 1994, [16]Krawczyk et al. 1995, [19]Rowbottom et al. 1997, [20]Hetland et al. 1998, [22]Schabort et al. 2000, [23]Prior et al. 2001, [24]Laursen et al. 2003, [25]Millet et al. 2003, [26]Legaz et al. 2005, [27]Knechtle et al. 2007a, [28]Knechtle et al. 2007b, [29]Malina 2007, [30]Knechtle et al. 2008, [31]Mikulic 2008, [32]Knechtle and Kohler 2009, [33]Knechtle et al. 2009b, [34]Knechtle et al. 2009d, [36]Knechtle et al. 2010a, [37]Knechtle et al. 2010b, [38]Knechtle et al. 2010c, [39]Knechtle et al. 2010d, [40]Knechtle et al. 2010e, [41]Knechtle et al. 2010f, [42]Knechtle et al. 2010g, [43]Arazi et al. 2011, [44]Knechtle et al. 2011a, [45]Knechtle et al. 2011b, [46]Knechtle et al. 2011c, [47]Gianoli et al. 2012, [48]Silva et al. 2012, [49]Mueller et al. 2013, [52]Diversi et al. 2016.

TABLE 10.2
Body Composition and Anthropometric Measurements of Female Endurance Athletes

Sports	Level	References		cm Ht	kg Mass	BMI	%Fat	Kg FM	Kg FFM	Kg SMM	DXA %Fat	Circ Waist	Circ Hip	Circ Biceps	Circ Calf	Circ Thigh	Chest	Triceps	Biceps	Subscap	Suprailiac	Calf	Axilla	Abd	Thigh
																					Skinfold (mm)				
Cyclists	All adult	3,7,8,13	Mean	169.3	61.5	21.5	13.8	8.7	55.0	–	–	–	–	–	–	–	–	–	–	–	–	–	–	–	–
			SD BW	6.2	5.5	1.1	2.8	1.3	5.5	–	–	–	–	–	–	–	–	–	–	–	–	–	–	–	–
			SD WT	3.2	4.3	–	2.4	–	–	–	–	–	–	–	–	–	–	–	–	–	–	–	–	–	–
Rowers	Elite	3,8,43	Mean	181.5	74.7	23.3	12.7	9.4	65.3	–	–	–	–	–	–	–	–	–	–	–	–	–	–	–	–
			SD BW	11.0	9.5	1.3	2.7	1.7	9.5	–	–	–	–	–	–	–	–	–	–	–	–	–	–	–	–
			SD WT	4.2	4.4	–	2.3	–	–	–	–	–	–	–	–	–	–	–	–	–	–	–	–	–	–
Rowers	Trained	29	Mean	–	–	–	20.6	–	–	–	21.9	–	–	–	–	–	–	–	–	–	–	–	–	–	–
			SD BW	–	–	–	2.6	–	–	–	–	–	–	–	–	–	–	–	–	–	–	–	–	–	–
			SD WT	–	–	–	3.5	–	–	–	2.3	–	–	–	–	–	–	–	–	–	–	–	–	–	–
Rowers	All adult	3,8,21,29,43	Mean	181.5	73.4	23.3	17.1	9.4	65.3	–	–	–	–	–	–	–	–	–	–	–	–	–	–	–	–
			SD BW	11.0	8.7	1.3	4.8	1.7	9.5	–	–	–	–	–	–	–	–	–	–	–	–	–	–	–	–
			SD WT	4.2	5.2	–	3.0	–	–	–	–	–	–	–	–	–	–	–	–	–	–	–	–	–	–
Runners	Elite	3,4,8,9,18,26	Mean	170.8	55.6	19.8	12.4	6.9	50.1	–	14.8	–	–	22.6	33.9	–	5.1	8.0	3.6	6.8	5.1	6.6	–	7.2	15.5
			SD BW	8.1	6.5	0.7	4.1	1.9	8.2	–	–	–	–	–	–	–	–	0.2	0.5	0.4	0.8	0.0	–	–	–
			SD WT	5.5	4.4	–	3.1	–	–	–	0.9	–	–	1.2	2.1	–	1.1	1.8	0.7	1.3	1.2	2.1	–	2.3	4.2
Runners	Highly trained	2,11,17,21	Mean	163.2	52.9	19.4	15.8	8.2	43.8	27.3	18.3	61.4	85.9	–	–	–	9.3	13.5	–	11.0	11.8	–	8.2	13.4	22.0
			SD BW	5.1	2.0	0.8	1.3	0.8	1.8	–	–	–	2.1	–	–	–	3.4	3.8	–	2.8	4.0	–	2.6	4.3	4.8
			SD WT	5.4	4.7	–	4.7	–	–	2.2	–	2.4	–	–	–	–	–	–	–	–	–	–	–	–	–
Runners	Trained	4,7,16,13,50	Mean	163.5	52.6	19.7	18.3	10.8	42.5	27.3	–	–	–	24.6	34.6	54.1	6.9	11.1	4.2	8.7	10.4	8.8	8.7	13.3	23.3
			SD BW	1.7	3.9	1.2	5.2	3.9	1.2	–	–	–	–	1.5	1.4	–	–	1.0	0.1	1.8	6.9	0.8	–	5.7	–
			SD WT	6.2	5.3	–	3.3	–	–	2.2	–	–	–	1.4	1.9	3.5	2.9	2.8	1.1	2.6	4.0	3.0	2.6	7.7	–
Runners	Youth	17	Mean	159.3	47.8	18.9	15.6	7.5	40.4	–	–	60.7	84.6	–	–	–	8.0	11.7	–	9.8	9.8	–	7.5	11.5	17.5
			SD BW	–	3.3	–	–	–	–	–	–	–	–	–	–	–	–	–	–	–	–	–	–	–	–
			SD WT	4.6	–	–	3.8	–	–	–	–	3.1	3.5	–	–	–	2.7	3.5	–	3.1	3.8	–	2.3	4.0	–
Runners	All adult	2,3,4,7,8,9,11,13,16,17,18,21,26,29,50	Mean	166.2	54.0	19.7	15.2	8.4	46.1	27.3	16.6	61.4	85.9	24.1	34.5	54.1	7.1	10.4	3.9	8.5	8.9	7.9	8.5	11.3	20.3
			SD BW	6.4	4.9	0.9	4.3	2.8	6.3	–	2.5	–	–	1.6	1.2	–	2.1	2.2	0.5	1.9	5.3	1.3	0.3	3.5	4.2
			SD WT	5.8	4.8	–	3.1	–	–	2.2	1.8	2.4	2.1	1.4	1.9	3.5	2.5	2.6	0.9	2.2	3.1	2.6	2.6	4.1	5.6

(Continued)

TABLE 10.2 (Continued)

Body Composition and Anthropometric Measurements of Female Endurance Athletes

Sports	Level	References		cm	kg			Kg			DXA	Circumferences (cm)					Skinfold (mm)								
				Ht	Mass	BMI	%Fat	FM	FFM	SMM	%Fat	Waist	Hip	Biceps	Calf	Thigh	Chest	Triceps	Biceps	Subscap	Suprailiac	Calf	Axilla	Abd	Thigh
Cross-country skiers	All adult	3,29	Mean	–	59.1	–	18.3	12.9	46.2	–	–	–	–	–	–	–	–	–	–	–	–	–	–	–	–
			SD BW	–	–	–	3.1	–	–	–	–	–	–	–	–	–	–	–	–	–	–	–	–	–	–
			SD WT	–	–	–	1.7	–	–	–	–	–	–	–	–	–	–	–	–	–	–	–	–	–	–
Swimmers	Youth	17,29	Mean	156.9	48.1	19.3	16.2	8.0	41.2	–	–	63.8	86.5	–	–	–	11.6	14.6	–	12.6	17.3	–	11.1	16.6	23.3
			SD BW	10.1	9.3	1.5	2.2	2.1	7.2	–	–	–	–	–	–	–	–	3.3	–	–	–	–	–	4.9	–
			SD WT	3.5	4.5	–	4.1	–	–	–	–	3.5	3.8	–	–	–	2.1	–	–	4.0	6.4	–	3.6	4.1	–
Swimmers	All adult	3,7,8,11,13,16,23,29,35,51	Mean	169.1	60.7	21.1	18.3	11.4	49.4	–	22.7	–	–	26.1	34.0	–	–	11.5	–	8.1	7.7	11.2	11.2	9.2	18.7
			SD BW	3.4	3.5	0.9	5.0	3.3	3.7	–	–	–	–	2.2	1.4	–	–	2.5	–	1.4	–	3.1	3.1	3.9	4.8
			SD WT	3.9	4.4	–	3.1	–	–	–	–	–	–	1.6	1.4	–	–	3.2	–	2.2	2.9	3.8	–	3.9	5.0
Distance swimmers	All adult	36,52	Mean	167.0	73.1	26.2	33.7	24.7	48.4	–	–	–	–	–	–	–	–	–	–	–	–	–	–	–	–
			SD BW	1.5	4.7	2.1	3.4	4.1	0.6	–	–	–	–	–	–	–	–	–	–	–	–	–	–	–	–
			SD WT	2.9	8.8	–	4.9	–	–	–	–	–	–	–	–	–	–	–	–	–	–	–	–	–	–
Triathletes	All adult	6,7,13,14,22,39,40,44,50	Mean	166.3	59.0	21.3	19.1	12.7	47.2	27.9	–	–	–	26.4	35.9	51.3	4.0	10.2	5.9	8.1	9.5	12.6	7.1	12.3	20.5
			SD BW	1.7	1.8	0.5	5.0	2.1	2.1	0.2	–	–	–	0.5	0.7	2.2	0.5	1.3	0.8	0.9	3.9	0.4	0.1	1.0	0.8
			SD WT	6.0	4.9	–	3.6	–	–	2.5	–	–	–	1.9	1.8	2.6	1.6	3.0	1.9	2.0	4.4	5.2	1.9	4.7	7.6

SD BW = standard deviations between studies, SD WT = average standard deviation within studies, Ht = height, Mass = body mass, %Fat = relative body fat measured using either densitometry-based methods or skinfold equations, FM = fat mass, FFM = fat-free mass, SMM = skeletal muscle mass, DXA = dual-energy x-ray absorptiometry, Abd = abdominal. Mean data reported was calculated by averaging the published means from multiple research studies (see table and figure references). Standard deviations (SD) were calculated by averaging the SDs published from the same research studies. When only ranges were provided, SDs were calculated using SD = range/4. Youth = 9-18 years, Adults ≥17 years. Level of athlete included only adults unless identified as youth. References: [2]Pipes 1977, [3]Fleck 1983, [4]Bale et al. 1985, [6]Holly et al. 1986, [7]O'Toole et al. 1987, [8]Withers et al. 1987b, [9]Withers et al. 1987a, [11]Johnson et al. 1989, [13]Leake and Carter 1991, [14]Laurenson et al. 1993, [16]Krawczyk et al. 1995, [17]Tsunawake et al. 1995, [18]Pichard et al. 1997, [21]Fornetti et al. 1999, [22]Schabort et al. 2000, [23]Prior et al. 2001, [26]Malina 2007, [29]Legaz et al. 2005, [35]Carbuhn et al. 2010, [36]Knechtle et al. 2010c, [39]Knechtle et al. 2010e, [40]Knechtle et al. 2010a, [43]Arazi et al. 2011, [44]Knechtle et al. 2011a, [50]Rust et al. 2013, [51]Stanforth et al. 2014, [52]Diversi et al. 2016.

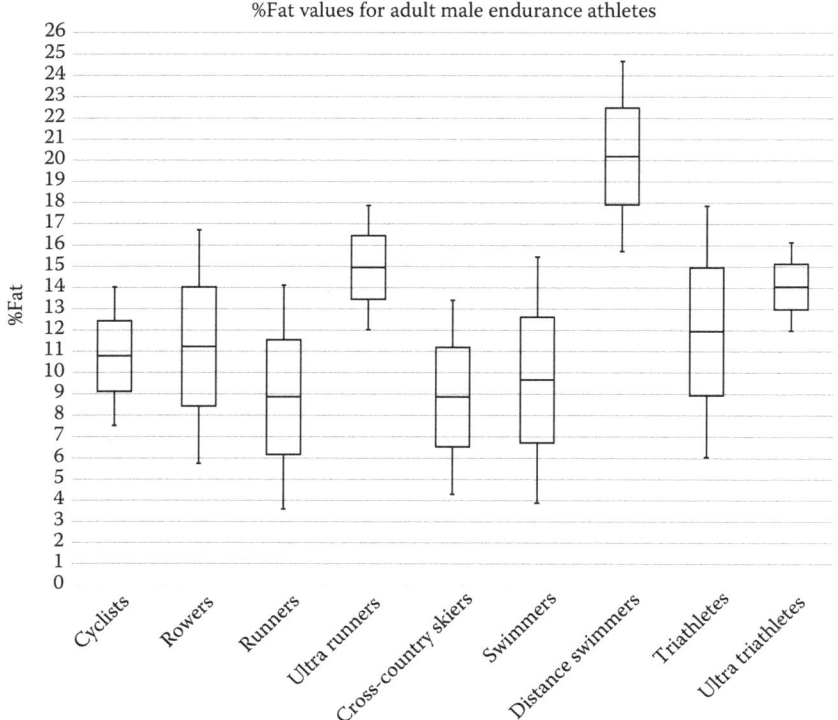

FIGURE 10.1 Mean data reported was calculated by averaging the published means from multiple research studies (see table and figure references). Standard deviations (SD) were calculated by averaging the SDs published from the same research studies. When only ranges were provided SDs were calculated using SD = range/4. Means are represented as the horizontal line inside each box. 68% confidence intervals from the SD are represented by each complete box. 95% confidence intervals from the SD are represented by the lines extending from the top and bottom of each box. Adult ≥17 years. References: Refer to Table 10.1.

Another simple explanation could be that ultraendurance athletes are less trained than elite and highly trained distance runners since their body fat values are similar to trained endurance runners.

Body fat also appears to change with age in endurance runners (Tables 10.1 and 10.2 and Figure 10.5). Percent fat values for male endurance runners under 18 and up to the age of 26 is 9%–10% with runners under 18 having less FFM than runners up to 26 years of age. Similar to males, females under 18 years of age have body fat values (19%–20%) similar to adult endurance runners but have less FFM. As youth runners develop into adults, they appear to maintain their % fat values while increasing FFM. In male endurance runners beyond the age of 26, body fat slightly increases by around 5%–6% and then remains the same up to the age of 70. In male endurance runners, FFM seems to be maintained until the age of 70. In male endurance athletes, FFM appears to be similar across different levels of runners with the largest lean mass associated with the lowest trained group. In contrast, female endurance runners in the highest performance group appear to have the highest FFM. Females in the highest training group are also taller and weigh more than the other levels with lower amounts of body fat.

10.4.2 BONE

Running is a highly weight-bearing activity which can enhance bone turnover and increase BMD (Maimoun and Sultan 2011). While endurance running is weight bearing, the body mass of endurance runners is very small and can limit the overall development of bone growth compared to

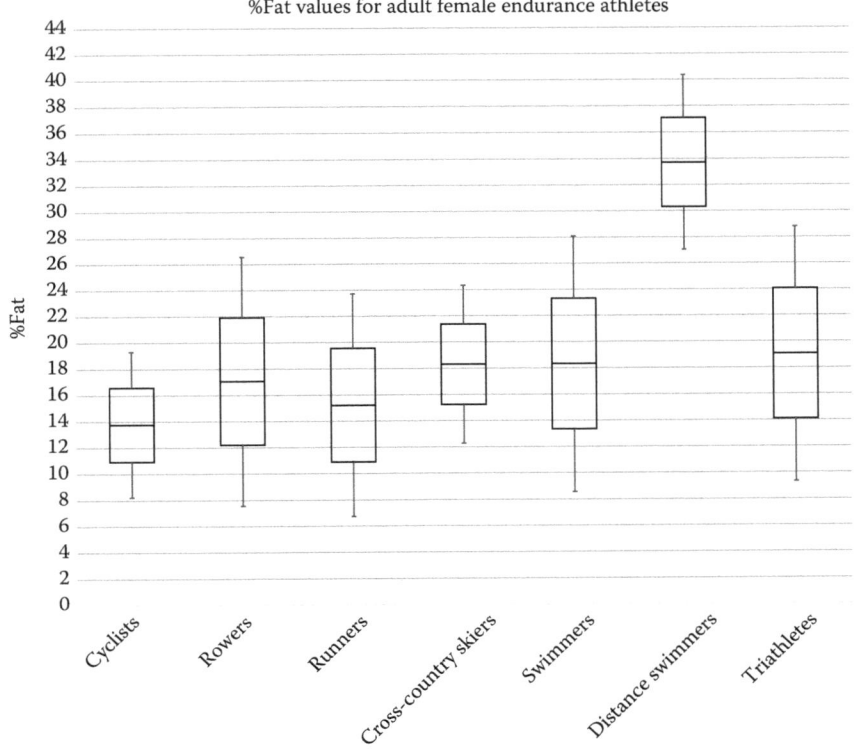

FIGURE 10.2 Mean data reported was calculated by averaging the published means from multiple research studies (see table and figure references). Standard deviations (SD) were calculated by averaging the SDs published from the same research studies. When only ranges were provided SDs were calculated using SD = range/4. Means are represented as the horizontal line inside each box. 68% confidence intervals from the SD are represented by each complete box. 95% confidence intervals from the SD are represented by the lines extending from the top and bottom of each box. Adult ≥17 years. References: Refer to Table 10.2.

strength and power athletes that are heavier and place a greater vertical load on the skeleton while training. Middle and long distance runners have demonstrated greater BMD compared to control subjects, but lower values compared to power athletes (Bennell et al. 1997). However, compared to other endurance athletes such as swimmers, cyclists, and triathletes, endurance runners appear to have significantly greater BMD (Rector et al. 2008; Scofield and Hecht 2012).

10.4.3 SUMMARY

While greater skinfold thicknesses and body fat may be related to an increase in endurance race time (slower finishing speed), there is no consensus on the usefulness of anthropometric and body composition data to predict individual performance when physiological variables are available such as VO_{2max}, lactate/ventilatory threshold, and training data. Anthropometric data alone should be used cautiously to predict endurance race performance for individual athletes but may be valuable when added to physiological variable-based endurance performance prediction equations.

Along these lines, the best use of individual skinfold thicknesses and body fat data appears to be to classify the level of an endurance runner and not to predict performance nor classify a runner into a specific distance or event. In addition, there seems to be a clear advantage for endurance runners to have low skinfold thicknesses, body fat, and body mass, but athletes, coaches, and trainers need to be aware of the possible health and injury risks associated with having too little body fat.

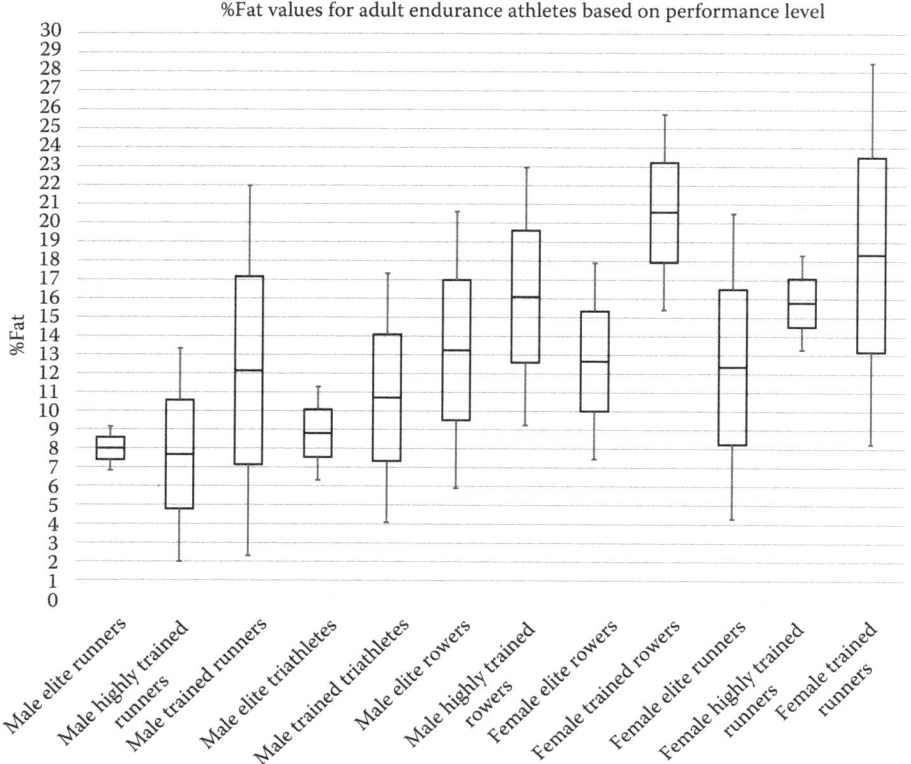

FIGURE 10.3 Mean data reported was calculated by averaging the published means from multiple research studies (see table and figure references). Standard deviations (SD) were calculated by averaging the SDs published from the same research studies. When only ranges were provided, SDs were calculated using SD = range/4. Means are represented as the horizontal line inside each box. 68% confidence intervals from the SD are represented by each complete box. 95% confidence intervals from the SD are represented by the lines extending from the top and bottom of each box. Adult ≥17 years. References: Refer to Tables 10.1 and 10.2.

FFM is a critical component for endurance runners and appears to initially change with age and then remain relatively consistent throughout a runner's career. Between fat and FFM, fat is the more dynamic component of body composition that a runner can manipulate to possibly enhance performance. When utilizing body composition data for adult runners, coaches, trainers, and athletes should consider pursuing maintenance in FFM while looking to modify % fat values. It appears that the lowest safe and healthy body fat percentage may produce the best performance for endurance runners, with ultraendurance runners possibly benefiting from having slightly more fat. Finally, runners are not at risk for low BMD due to the axial loading and weight-bearing nature of the sport.

10.5 CYCLISTS

Professional road cyclists perform in a great variety of terrains (i.e., level, uphill, and downhill roads) and competitive situations (i.e., individually or drafting behind other cyclists). In any of these situations, a cyclist's performance is largely determined by their anthropometric characteristics (Mujika and Padilla 2001). Body mass affects uphill cycling performance, as it determines gravity-dependent resistance. Uphill cyclists are generally shorter than flat terrain riders, but also lighter than all other riding specialists (all-terrain riders, time-trial specialists, and sprinters) (Swain et al. 1987). On the other hand, all-terrain and time-trial specialists appear to be taller and heavier.

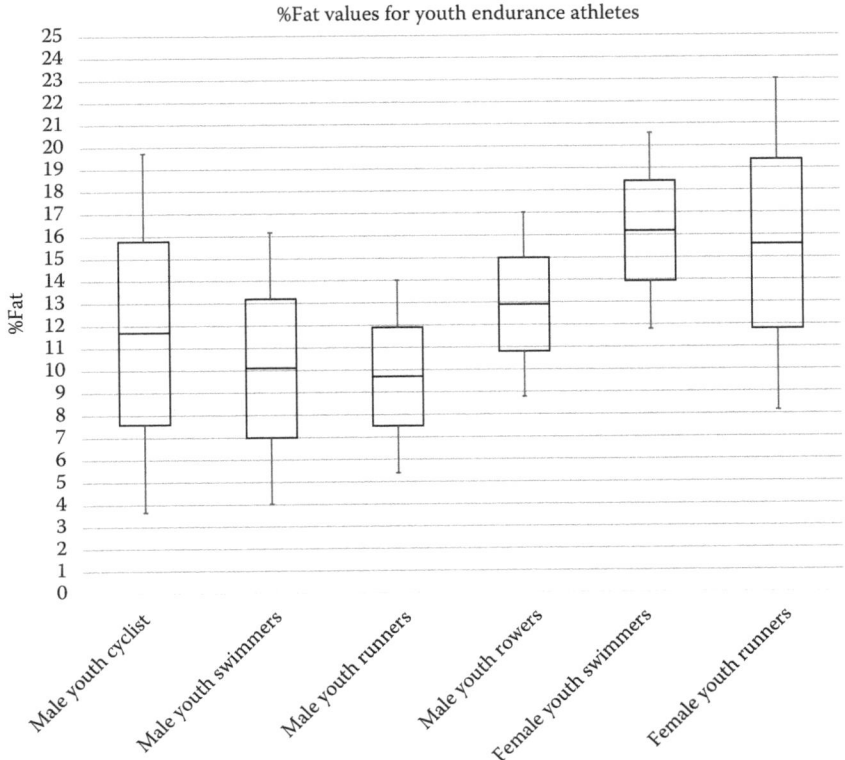

FIGURE 10.4 Mean data reported was calculated by averaging the published means from multiple research studies (see table and figure references). Standard deviations (SD) were calculated by averaging the SDs published from the same research studies. When only ranges were provided, SDs were calculated using SD = range/4. Means are represented as the horizontal line inside each box. 68% confidence intervals from the SD are represented by each complete box. 95% confidence intervals from the SD are represented by the lines extending from the top and bottom of each box. Youth = 9–18 years. References: Refer to Tables 10.1 and 10.2

Competitive cycling requires both aerobic and anaerobic power. Road and off-road races require the cyclist to possess the ability to generate a relatively high-power output of short duration during the mass start, steep climbing, and at the race finish (Faria et al. 2005). Typical road race and off-road cross-country events can range in duration from 1 to 5 h, while multistage races are characterized by several back-to-back days of racing consisting of mass-start stages and individual and team time trials. Professional cyclists are required to tolerate high workloads for long periods (3 weeks) during major tour races, like the Tour de France and the Giro d'Italia. Different by the nature of the setting, competitive track cycling demands acute bursts of high-power output followed by constant high-intensity sprinting (Faria et al. 2005).

There is a substantial evidence demonstrating that successful cyclists possess high VO_{2max} values ($\approx$74 mL/kg/min) and a lactate threshold around 90% of VO_{2max} (Faria et al. 1989; Coyle et al. 1991; Lucia et al. 1998; Fernandez-Garcia et al. 2000). Moreover, Pfeiffer et al. (1993) have demonstrated that VO_{2max} is a strong predictor ($r = -0.91$) of cycling performance during a multistage race. There is strong evidence that peak power output (W) obtained during a maximal incremental cycling test can be used as a predictor of cycling performance ($r = -0.91$; Hawley and Noakes 1992). These findings suggest that not only is a high aerobic capacity important for race success, but also a high amount of muscle mass and low % fat is important to maximize power out.

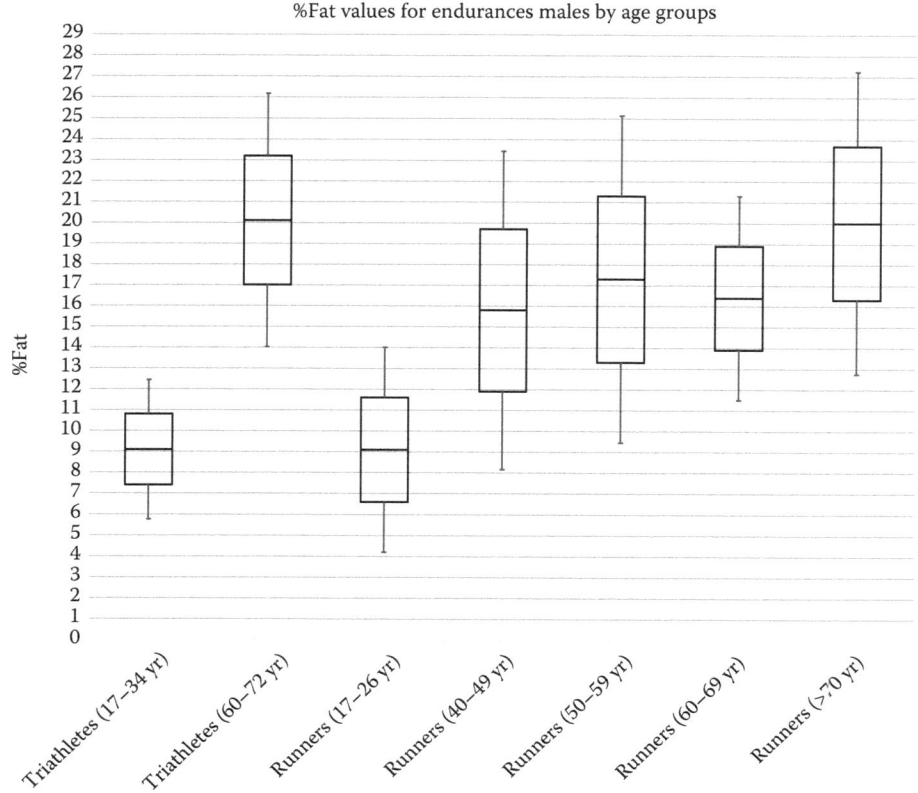

FIGURE 10.5 Mean data reported was calculated by averaging the published means from multiple research studies (see table and figure references). Standard deviations (SD) were calculated by averaging the SDs published from the same research studies. When only ranges were provided, SDs were calculated using SD = range/4. Means are represented as the horizontal line inside each box. 68% confidence intervals from the SD are represented by each complete box. 95% confidence intervals from the SD are represented by the lines extending from the top and bottom of each box. yr = years. References: Refer to Tables 10.1 and 10.2

10.5.1 FAT AND FFM

The physiological requirements for success in road cycling are unique for several reasons. Riders compete in mass start, multistage races characterized by stochastic shifts in work rate and/or speed that are largely dependent on terrain (Palmer et al. 1994; Padilla et al. 1999) and team tactics (Palmer et al. 1994; Padilla et al. 1999, 2000b; Mujika and Padilla 2001). In contrast, during individual (Padilla et al. 2000a,b) and team trials (Padilla et al. 2000b), a rider (or team) attempts to sustain the highest average power output possible for the duration of a race.

In contrast to other endurance sports, such as rowing and cross-country skiing, a slight increase in body mass significantly increases the energy requirement to overcome the resistive forces of gravity when cycling, especially during climbing and sprinting. Models of cycling performance have suggested that a 1-kg increase in body mass can increase cycling time up a 5% grade by 1% (Olds et al. 1995), which in international competition is significant.

A key performance indicator for both male and female cyclists is the maximal amount of power that can be generated for a given duration relative to body mass. A high power-to-weight ratio (>5.5 W/kg) is an important physiological characteristic for cyclists to be able to climb and accelerate quickly (Palmeri et al. 2007). Increasing lean mass, while reducing fat mass can help optimize relative power output, improving the performance of cyclists. It should also be noted that road cycling is characterized by many accelerations (Ebert et al. 2005), and that acceleration is inversely proportional to body weight. Because of these power–weight relationships, it is not uncommon to find low body fat values amongst elite cyclists.

Previous research has shown international competitive cyclists to be lighter and leaner than their lesser successful teammates (Martin et al. 2001). World-class female cyclists weigh less and have lower skinfolds (–5.0 mm) and % fat (–1.5%) compared to cyclists performing at lower levels (Haakonssen et al. 2015).

In general, elite off-road cyclists possess similar physiological profiles to those of elite road cyclists (Faria et al. 1989). In mountain bike races, body mass appears to be just as important for race success, as mountain bikers have been shown to be lighter and leaner compared to road cyclists (Lee et al. 2002). Contrary to previous findings of significant associations between % fat and running performance, Knechtle and Rosemann (2009) found no association ($r = 0.43$, $p > 0.05$) between % fat and race performance in male mountain bike ultramarathoners.

There appear to be noticeable differences in body composition between road and track cyclists. Compared to track endurance cyclists at the world-class level, female road cyclists have a significantly lower body mass (–6.04 kg; $p < 0.001$), significantly lower skinfold thicknesses (–11.5 mm; $p = 0.03$) and significantly lower % fat values (–2.7%; $p = 0.03$). Higher power output demands associated with track endurance events, such as the individual and team pursuit, may necessitate a higher body weight and greater functional lean mass, particularly at the world-class level. Absolute power may be more important for performance on the track compared to relative power (W/kg), given that track cyclists do not have to overcome gravity to the same extent as road cyclists, and there are fewer accelerations throughout the track races.

10.5.2 BONE

The prevalence of osteopenia and osteoporosis is alarmingly high in adult male road cyclists (Sabo et al. 1996; Stewart and Hannan 2000; Warner et al. 2002; Nichols et al. 2003), but not in distance runners (Stewart and Hannan 2000). The discrepancy in BMD between runners and cyclists has been attributed to the lack of ground reaction forces on the skeleton during cycling (Stewart and Hannan 2000; Warner et al. 2002; Nichols et al. 2003).

Despite similar stature, weight, and body composition, endurance runners have been shown to have significantly greater whole-body and lumbar spine BMD compared with cyclists (+10% and +4%, respectively) (Rector et al. 2008). Furthermore, 60% of the cyclists in the Rector et al. (2008) study were reported to have osteopenia of the spine compared to only 19% of runners exhibiting osteopenia. These results are consistent with previous studies documenting increased prevalence of osteopenia in adult male road cyclists (Sabo et al. 1996; Stewart and Hannan 2000; Warner et al. 2002), suggesting that non-weight-bearing exercise performed for long duration may be detrimental to the skeleton (Medelli et al. 2009; Smathers et al. 2009).

A 2010 study by Campion et al. (2010) found that professional cyclists had significantly lower total body BMD (–9.1%) and lumbar BMD (–16.0%) values compared to reference subjects. The results confirmed earlier findings by Sabo et al. (1996) who inferred that Tour de France riders had 10% lower BMD than controls. The findings of Campion et al. (2010) also supported earlier data that showed elite and professional road cyclists having lower total and regional BMD than a reference group (Medelli et al. 2009).

Results of these studies highlight the importance of sustaining skeletal loading to maintain bone mass. Cyclists are at an increased risk for traumatic injuries in the case of falls or collisions. The risk for traumatic fracture can be greatly increased by low bone strength, with low BMD being one of the best predictors of fractures in males (Gardsell et al. 1990; Melton et al. 1998). Bone loading activities such as running or jogging should be incorporated into training to help maintain bone mass in cyclists. Furthermore, the bone health and status of elite cyclists should be screened and monitored regularly since cycling may be a professional hazard for bone health.

10.5.3 Summary

The power to weight ratio (W/kg) is arguably the most important factor for cyclists. Higher amounts of muscle and lower body fat values are related to faster speed, more power, and better performance. Body fat amounts and the effects on performance can be related to the type of terrain with uphill riders needing to be lighter and have less body fat while track cyclists can have higher body fat values without an impact on performance due to a lack of change in elevation. Body fat can also impact a cyclist depending on the distance of the event. Cyclists who compete in longer events can benefit from having a lower body fat percentage compared to shorter distance cyclists who require more bursts of speed and require high-power outputs. Track cyclists can benefit from having more absolute power, while distance and road cyclists should focus on generating as much power per kilogram of body mass as possible. Low BMD, osteopenia, and osteoporosis are a concern in cyclists. Lack of ground contact reduces the ability to increase BMD and a cyclist may have much lower BMD in the lower body and spine compared to non-cyclists and other endurance athletes. Cyclists are at the highest risk for low BMD compared to all other endurance athletes referred to in this chapter.

10.6 SWIMMERS

The sport of swimming encompasses a wide range of anaerobic and aerobic energy demands. Events including 100 m distances and shorter may only require around 40% aerobic energy with a greater demand as distance increases (Powers and Howley 2015). Specifically, a 400 m swim nearly doubles the amount of aerobic energy demand to around 60%, an 800 m swim requires around 85% aerobic energy, and a marathon swim or longer demands nearly 100% aerobic energy (Powers and Howley 2015). In addition to distance variability, swimmers may also be subjected to various temperature conditions, ranging from the typical competitive indoor pool temperature of around 25–28°C (77–82°F) to much colder waters of 15–20°C (59–68°F) (Pendergast et al. 1977; Diversi et al. 2016). For distance swimmers, the ability to regulate core temperature in cold water can significantly impact both race speed and race completion (Pendergast et al. 1977; Diversi et al. 2016). Therefore, body composition plays a role in not only swimming speed but also body temperature regulation.

Several decades of research looking at marathon swimmers have shown females to have a significant advantage over males, with race times 12%–14% faster in females compared to males (Knechtle et al 2014). The advantage females have over males in distance swimming in both cold and comfortable water temperatures can be directly related to total fat, as well as fat distribution (Pendergast et al. 1977; McLean and Hinrichs 1998; Knechtle et al. 2014; Diversi et al. 2016).

While swimming distance and water temperature may vary across events, so may the strokes swimmers must perform. However, the effect of body composition on different swimming strokes is still unclear. Distance swimmers predominantly perform the freestyle stroke but may utilize multiple strokes throughout the race. The biomechanics may also vary between the freestyle stroke in open water distance events compared to shorter distances in a pool or in open water. Nevertheless, body composition plays an important role in all swimming strokes and events with significant differences between males and females and between shorter distance swimmers and longer distance swimmers. Most notably, the amount and location of body fat can impact a swimmer's drag and efficiency in the water, which can either hinder or enhance swimming speed (Pendergast et al. 1977; McLean and Hinrichs 1998; Knechtle et al. 2014; Diversi et al. 2016). The effects of body fat alone on drag and efficiency can influence speed in all events. Therefore, given the various aerobic demands ranging from 40% to 100% dependent on the distance and the impact body composition can have on swimming speed due to drag and efficiency, all types of swimmers should be considered when examining the impact of body composition and the sport of swimming.

10.6.1 FAT AND FFM

Fat mass and % fat values differ significantly when comparing distance swimmers to non-distance swimmers in both males and females (Tables 10.1 and 10.2 and Figures 10.1 and 10.2). Male distance swimmers (20.2% fat) appear to have nearly double the % fat compared to male non-distance swimmers (9.7% fat) (Table 10.1 and Figure 10.1). Female distance swimmers show a similar trend with distance swimmers having % fat values around 33.7% fat and non-distance swimmers having around 18.3% fat. The increase in % fat for distance swimmers appears to be directly related to an increase in swimming efficiency compared to lower % fat values. Specifically, an increase in % fat can significantly increase body buoyancy in the water, as well as reduce drag and increase efficiency (McLean and Hinrichs 1998; Knechtle et al. 2014). The increase in buoyancy due to fat is related to the density of the tissue. Body fat has a density of around 0.901 g/mL, and FFM has a density of around 1.100 g/mL. With 15.3% fat, a swimmer has a total body density (BD) of around 1.064 g/mL, while the density of water is around 1.000 g/mL (Brozek et al. 1963). Anything less than the density of water will float, and anything greater will sink. Therefore, fat will float in water and muscle will sink. The more body fat a swimmer has, the more buoyant he/she will be and the closer the total BD will be to that of the surrounding water. It should also be noted that swimmers who compete in salt and/or cold water have an advantage over swimmers who compete in warm fresh water because salt water and cold water have a greater density which allows the human body to be more buoyant. The density of water should impact all athletes competing in a single event equally, but should be noted when comparing distance swimming times performed in different types of water as the efficiency of a swimming stroke can be improved by swimming in cold salty water.

When comparing males to females, as noted earlier, females have a significant advantage over males in distance swimming. Research has suggested males will never overtake females in distance swimming events when comparing race times between the top female and male athletes. The advantage females have in distance swimming is both related to the total amount of body fat and distribution of the fat. Female swimmers compared to males have a significantly greater distribution of body fat in the lower body (hips, thighs, and legs) which results in a greater mechanical efficiency when swimming (Pendergast et al. 1977). The distribution of body fat in the lower body for females allows the center of buoyancy to be closer to the center of mass when swimming horizontally (all competitive swimming strokes) (Pendergast et al. 1977; McLean and Hinrichs 1998; Knechtle et al. 2014). With a center of buoyancy closer to the center of mass, most noticeably increases the buoyancy of the legs. With greater fat distributions in the lower body, females use significantly less energy per kick compared to males to produce the same linear force (Pendergast et al. 1977).

The additional body fat found in distance swimmers compared to non-distance swimmers is clearly a function of efficiency. However, having an additional body fat can increase body surface area and drag which can slow a swimmer down when swimming at full speed. Having greater buoyancy allows for a more efficient use of energy, but it appears to hinder maximum speed due to the associated increase in mass and surface area. The differences in body fat between non-distance and distance swimmers demonstrate this finding. When swimming at submaximal speeds an efficient (buoyant) body mass and fat distribution is ideal, but when swimming at near-max and at maximal speed a reduction in body fat and body mass is warranted. Both male and female distance swimmers have not only a greater amount of body fat, but also greater body mass around 9.1 and 12.4 kg compared to non-distance swimmers, respectively. The added body mass is almost completely in the fat compartment with FFM being no different between types of swimmers (Tables 10.1 and 10.2).

Young male swimmers tend to have a slightly higher percent body fat and lower body mass compared to non-distance adult male swimmers, and lower percent body fat and body mass compared to adult male distance swimmers. As male youth swimmers develop into adult swimmers, there appears to be an increase in total mass and FFM, with a decrease in % fat (Table 10.1). However, female youth swimmers tend to have less fat, FFM, and body mass compared to both non-distance and distance adult female swimmers. As female youth swimmers develop into adult swimmers, there appears to be an increase in total mass, FFM, and % fat (Table 10.2). Depending on the type of swimmer (non-distance vs. distance), youth swimmers should look to achieve a body composition similar to those of their adult counterparts if looking to achieve optimal performance.

Unlike fat mass and percent body fat, FFM does not differ much between distance and non-distance swimmers (Tables 10.1 and 10.2). Swimmers have a greater amount of FFM than runners and triathletes, with cyclists and rowers having a greater amount of FFM than both male and female swimmers. A large FFM does not appear to be beneficial for either distance swimming or non-distance swimming, as any increase in muscle mass can decrease buoyancy since muscle is denser than water. However, if a swimmer can increase power along with muscle mass and has the body size (arm and leg length) to support a greater total mass and muscle mass, he or she could significantly increase his/her maximal sprint performance with an unchanged body fat percentage. Thus, a non-distance swimmer could improve performance by increasing muscle mass and power that overcomes the loss due to increased body size and drag. However, over long distances, this extra muscle mass does not provide any benefit to the swimmer as the athlete needs to exert more energy and use more oxygen to swim through the water at a submaximal speed.

10.6.2 BONE

In a recent systematic review looking at swimmers and bone, researchers concluded that "swimming does not produce enough power to stimulate bone growth above the regular pattern, with most studies showing similar bone mineral density or bone mineral content to control groups" (Gomez-Bruton et al. 2013). The authors further concluded that swimming may help reduce bone loss related to aging but that the reduction in bone loss may not be directly related to swimming and could be related to an overall more active lifestyle (Gomez-Bruton et al. 2013). When bone density values of female Division I collegiate swimmers were compared to softball, volleyball, basketball, and track and field athletes, swimmers had significantly lower values for their total body, arms, legs, pelvis, and the spine (Carbuhn et al. 2010). The differences between swimmers and other athletes can be attributed to the lack of weight bearing in swimming. While weight-bearing sports and activities can significantly increase BMD, swimming appears to have little effect. However, research has shown that unlike cyclists, swimming does not negatively impact bone density, and swimmers are not at a greater risk for osteoporosis or osteopenia (Carbuhn et al. 2010; Gomez-Bruton et al. 2013). However, swimmers who regularly participate in strength training outside the pool may be able to increase BMD beyond inactive control or reference subjects.

10.6.3 SUMMARY

Guidelines for body fatness of swimmers range significantly more in females compared to males with % fat values between 4.3% and 13.4% for non-distance males and 8.6%–28.1% for non-distance females and 15.7%–24.7% fat for distance males and 27.1%–40.4% fat for distance females. In swimming, unlike other endurance sports, having the lowest possible % fat and body mass does not appear to be beneficial. While the relationship between % fat, subcutaneous fat, intramuscular fat, and distance swimming performance warrants further investigation, some researchers have speculated that increasing subcutaneous fat can increase cold water distance performance by helping regulate body temperature, as females can swim longer in cold water compared to males in the same conditions (Knechtle et al. 2014). For endurance (long distance) swimmers, there appears to be no added benefit to increasing muscle mass due to the submaximal nature of the sport. The ideal amount of FFM and muscle mass will depend on the amount of muscle needed to produce optimal aerobic performance without a loss in swimming efficiency, which can vary depending on the individual swimmer's body size and structure. Swimmers tend not to have an increased BMD above normal values but are not at an increased risk for low BMD.

10.7 TRIATHLETES

Triathletes must be proficient in endurance running, swimming, and cycling. Although events such as a super sprint triathlon can be as a short as a 250 m swim, 5 km cycle, and a 1.5 km run, sprint triathlons require a great deal of endurance. Each single event demands more than 50% energy from aerobic sources, and each successive event can have a compounding effect on aerobic demand (Powers and Howley 2015). However, most triathlon events are much longer than a super sprint triathlon. The distance for an Olympic triathlon is a 1.5 km swim, 40 km cycle, and a 10 km run. Ironman triathlons require triathletes to swim 3.86 km, cycle 180.25 km, and run 42.2 km (Knechtle and Kohler 2009). Finally, there are ultraendurance triathletes who compete in an event called a triple iron triathlon which requires participants to run three Ironman triathlons over a 3-day period, which in total comprises an 11.6 km swim, 540 km cycle, and a 126.6 km run (Knechtle and Kohler 2009).

Although many triathletes have body types more similar to swimmers than runners (Leake and Carter 1991), research has shown that triathletes who have a physique like runners, but do not have a running background, may have the best performance potential in the sport. Specifically, athletes with a history in marathon running do not appear to be ideal Ironman triathletes (Gianoli et al. 2012). Research also supports that triathletes have greater variability in body fat, muscle mass, and skinfold thicknesses compared to other endurance athletes (Knechtle and Kohler 2009). Ultraendurance triathletes also appear to have body types more similar to ultraendurance cyclists than ultraendurance runners (Knechtle et al. 2007b, 2010c). Thus, there are several different body types of triathletes, and each athlete typically has one event (swim, cycle, and run) in which he or she excels, suggesting that body type and composition are related to the performance of not only a single event, but also possibly all events. Understanding the body composition of triathletes and how they compare to endurance swimmers, cyclists, and runners can be useful in determining performance and race time for triathletes.

10.7.1 Fat and FFM

Conflicting findings exist in the relationship between body fat and subcutaneous fat on race performance in triathletes, with several studies showing a relationship (Landers et al. 2000; Knechtle et al. 2009b, 2010d, 2011c; Gianoli et al. 2012) and many more showing no relationship (Leake and Carter 1991; Laurenson et al. 1993; Schabort et al. 2000; Knechtle et al. 2007a,b, 2010g; Knechtle and Kohler 2009; Rust et al. 2013). In addition, other reports identify a relationship for male triathletes, but not females (Knechtle et al. 2010e, 2011a).

Studies that reported significant relationships between triathlon performance and body composition have concluded that fat mass, % fat, skinfold thicknesses, upper arm and thigh circumferences, BMI, and body mass are related to overall race time and split times in cycling, swimming, and running (Landers et al. 2000; Knechtle et al. 2009b, 2011c; Gianoli et al. 2012; Rust et al. 2013). These findings suggest that an increase in any of the aforementioned variables could make a triathlete slower and a decrease in these variables may reduce running time and improve overall performance.

Comparing less-trained and experienced male and female triathletes, fat mass, % fat, BMI, skinfold thicknesses, and muscle mass were only related to performance in males, while training volume was related to performance in females. Thus, it appears that experience is the most important factor for predicting race success in female triathletes, while body composition may be a more important predictor for success in males (Knechtle et al. 2010d,e, 2011a).

Compared to Ironman triathletes, ultraendurance triathletes appear to be smaller and have more body fat, shorter limbs, and larger limb circumferences (Knechtle et al. 2011b) (Table 10.1).

Training variables appear to be more important than anthropometric variables for determining race performance in ultraendurance triathletes than in Ironman triathletes (Knechtle et al. 2011a). These findings come as no surprise as ultraendurance athletes are often more focused on finishing the race rather than finishing the fastest. Specifically, the impact of the differences in body composition and anthropometric variables and race time appears to be irrelevant in races that exceed an Ironman distance, and training for such long events is the most important aspect related to race time in ultraendurance triathletes. Training for the physical and mental demand of ultraendurance triathlons clearly supersedes any minor differences in body composition.

However, there is still a clear body type and relatively ideal body composition for ultraendurance triathletes compared to Ironman triathletes, which is most likely related to increased energy demand spanning across multiple days. Being smaller with more body fat may provide an added benefit during ultraendurance events. Although swimming and cycling training speed does not appear to be any different between ultraendurance and Ironman triathletes, ultraendurance triathletes train at a slower running speed (−0.6 km/h) compared to Ironman triathletes (Knechtle et al. 2011a). While racing, however, ultraendurance triathletes swim, cycle, and run significantly slower than Ironman triathletes, suggesting a conservation of energy in order to complete the longer race.

10.7.2 Bone

Typically, triathletes train for swimming, cycling, and running equally (Gulbin and Gaffney 1999). Thus, any changes in bone should be related to all three types of training. Triathletes should not experience the same risks of osteopenia and osteoporosis as endurance cyclists due to the running component of their training. The addition of running and skeletal loading is the most important component for triathletes and bone density. The swimming component does not appear to enhance bone density beyond non-active control subjects (Gomez-Bruton et al. 2013). However, due to the combined training and less running frequency compared to endurance runners, triathletes do tend to have lower BMD compared to runners (Rector et al. 2008; Scofield and Hecht 2012). If a triathlete is running with similar frequency to that of swimming and cycling, there should not be a concern for low BMD, although he or she may not have bone density values much different from active males and females. As is the case of cyclists and swimmers, triathletes may benefit from incorporating strength training and load-bearing exercises into their routines to enhance bone density. A study of over 240 triathletes found that 42% reported never strength training, with 22% strength trained regularly (Gulbin and Gaffney 1999). Most likely the 22% who participated in regular strength training had higher BMD than the 42% who never strength trained, and may have been at a lower risk for fractures, osteopenia, and osteoporosis.

10.7.3 Summary

Not surprisingly, triathletes have body composition values similar to runners, swimmers, and cyclists. Female triathletes appear to have % fat values similar to swimmers and FFM values similar to cross-country skiers, swimmers, and less-trained runners. Similar to runners, highly trained male triathletes tend to have lower % fat values compared to less-trained triathletes. Percent fat values for triathletes also appear to be similar to cyclists, rowers, runners, and cross-country skiers. FFM values for all levels of male triathletes seem to be about the same, with similar values to cross-country skiers, swimmers, and distance swimmers. Thus, while triathletes have similar body composition values to other endurance athletes, they have greater variability as a whole possibly due to being more dominant in a certain stage of their race (running, swimming, and cycling). Triathletes may benefit by slightly modifying their body composition to be more successful at their weaker stages, but this may decrease the performance in their best stage. Nonetheless, triathletes, like runners, cyclists, and swimmers, can benefit from having a low % fat with similar benefits to those seen in each sport independently.

Much like with runners, most research does not support the use of anthropometric data alone to predict triathlon performance and race time in the presence of physiological variables (Leake and Carter 1991; Laurenson et al 1993; Schabort et al. 2000; Knechtle and Kohler 2009; Knechtle et al 2010g). Similarly, researchers, athletes, coaches, and trainers should use both physiological and anthropometric data when predicting endurance performance and in the presence of physiological data such as VO_{2max} or peak power, the significant relationship between anthropometric data and race performance may disappear. Triathletes have greater BMD compared to swimmers and cyclists, and due to the running component are not typically at risk for low BMD.

10.8 METHODOLOGICAL CONSIDERATIONS

The exact amount of essential fat for males and females is controversial. The standard lower levels for male and female athletes have been reported to be 5% and 12%–16%, respectively (Heyward and Wagner 2004). However, researchers (Fleck 1983; Heyward and Wagner 2004) have recommended these cutoff values in part based on factors such as averages of percent body fat values measured from skinfold equations from sports with lean athletes (Tcheng and Tipton 1973) and from the lowest reported values of athletes measured using a water-based two-component model (Novak et al. 1968).

Novak et al. (1968) used the Pace and Rathbun (1945) two-component model along with deuterium oxide to test a small ($n = 16$) sample of Division I male athletes and reported body composition values which have been used to set the standard of 5% as the lower end for essential fat in males. While the Pace and Rathbun (1945) equation has been shown to be as accurate as the Siri (1961) three-component model, both the water-based two-component and three-component model have been shown to have an individual error of over 0.5% fat (Wang et al. 1998; Moon et al. 2009a). Furthermore, two-component models using density, such as hydrostatic weighing (HW) and air displacement plethysmography (BOD POD®), as well as skinfold prediction equations have produced individual errors of around ±3%–6% fat with skinfold equations typically resulting in larger individual variability when compared to a five- or six-component model in athletes and non-athletes (Wang et al. 1998; Silva et al. 2006; Moon et al. 2009a). Female essential fat values have been determined the same way as the males, but with some focus on amenorrhea. Data suggest the need for a minimal amount of fat for ovulation and menstrual cycles in females as high as 22% body fat (Fleck 1983; Frisch and McArthur 1974).

A majority of the aforementioned studies are over 40 years old and may not represent the athletes of today. Furthermore, with newer technology allowing for easier deployment of multicomponent models along with computerized tomography (CT) and magnetic resonance imaging (MRI) techniques, it is only a matter of time before new essential fat values are recommended for athletes that may better represent specific sports, ages, and athletic levels. However, until then the best recommendation based on the methods used to establish essential fat values and their known variability and lack of current more-advanced measurement data in this area, the following essential fat ranges are proposed when using any method other than a water-based multicomponent model:

Males: 5±4% fat (1%–9% fat)
Females: 14±4% fat (10%–18% fat)

While the suggested ranges are appropriate for skinfold-based methods along with densitometry-based two-component models, without proper technique and testing guidelines the individual errors may be larger than ±4% fat. Larger errors of over ±4%–6% fat can be caused by using estimated lung volumes for BOD POD® and HW, uncontrolled test conditions (diet and hydration) and testing protocols, inaccurate skinfold equations and uncalibrated skinfold calipers, and inadequately trained personnel to make accurate and reliable measurements. Even in ideal conditions, individual variability for skinfold-based methods and densitometry-based two-component models makes determining valid assessments of body fatness useful for an individual. One recommendation for athletes with borderline low % fat is to use multiple measurements and track over time if a loss of body fat is taking place, since a single measurement of fat or lean mass does not reflect health status.

Dual x-ray absorptiometry (DXA) is another tool that may be useful for determining body composition in athletes. However, when compared to densitometry-based two-component models, as well as skinfold equations based on HW, DXA appears to produce significantly higher values by as much as 3%–6% fat female athletes (Silva et al. 2006; Moon et al. 2009a). However, in male athletes, the difference between DXA and densitometry-based two-component models is much lower with differences around −4% to 2% fat (Arngrimsson et al. 2000; Silva et al. 2006). Therefore, when working with female endurance athletes, be aware that DXA values may be higher than skinfold equations or HW or BOD POD®, but in males, the values may be more interchangeable. One benefit of using DXA for assessing body composition in endurance athletes is that DXA can look at specifics segments like the arms and the legs together or independently. DXA can also be used to look at BMD. While MRI and CT scans are considered the "*most accurate methods for in vivo quantification of body composition on the tissue level*," they are less readily available for athletes to use and are more expensive compared to DXA scans (Ross and Janssen 2005). DXA instruments are being purchased and used by the National Football League (NFL) and other professional sports programs, in addition to more college athletic departments purchasing and using DXA for assessing and monitoring their athletes. DXA manufacturers claim more than 100 machines are being used in professional sports and at the college level. Growing research is being published with DXA normative data for athletes including recent studies looking at NFL and college football players (Bosch et al. 2014; Dengel et al. 2014; Melvin et al. 2014). Having total body, segmental, and site-specific normative data can help coaches, trainers, and athletes compare specific body sections of elite athletes beyond subcutaneous fat measurements available with skinfold calipers and ultrasounds. Also, DXA allows for the analysis of muscle symmetry between limbs, which could be used to help prevent injuries by identifying muscle imbalances (Dengel et al. 2014).

Bioelectrical impedance (BIA) is another method that has been used in endurance and various other athletes, but normative data is hard to interpret due to the use of various machines and methods, in addition to several studies not using ideal pretesting protocols to ensure proper hydration. Researchers are in agreement that BIA is a faster technique than skinfolds, DXA, HW, and BOD POD®, but when electrolyte and hydration balances are abnormal, the measurement errors for BIA become almost too large to be of practical value (Williams and Bale 1998; Berneis and Keller 2000; Ostojic 2006; O'Connor et al. 2007; Moon 2013; Hew-Butler et al. 2015).

Researchers have also cautioned against using BIA devices in athletes due to these aforementioned issues along with a lack of validated devices and equations in the athletic population (Moon 2013). Still, BIA techniques and devices may provide valuable data in endurance athletes as a complement to other techniques such as skinfolds, circumferences, DXA, HW, or BOD POD® (Ostojic 2006). Newer stand-alone multi-frequency BIA machines may also provide more valid and reliable data for endurance athletes compared to single frequency devices, but more research is needed before these devices can be used in place of trusted methods such as skinfolds, circumferences, and densitometry-based two-component models that have been used in the literature for decades.

A relatively new method for measuring endurance and strength athletes that provides a segmental analysis with great detail involves the use of brightness mode (B-Mode) ultrasound, which can provide muscle cross-sectional area as well as muscle quality in addition to lean and fat mass (Roelofs et al. 2015; Hirsch et al. 2016). This method can provide additional data that could be useful to athletes, but the availability of ultrasound machines and training may be a limiting factor for athletes, coaches, and trainers due to high cost and detailed protocols. Amplitude mode (A-Mode) ultrasound devices may provide more information than skinfold calipers, with the additional ability to look at both muscle and fat thicknesses. Research has shown that in rowers A-Mode ultrasound provides similar measurements to densitometry (BOD POD®) and skinfold equations for % fat and could be useful for endurance athletes in the place of skinfold calipers, HW, or BOD POD®

(Kendall et al. 2017). However, similarly with skinfold techniques, training is required, and testers may significantly influence the outcome of the measurements by not following proper guidelines.

Another relatively new method to measure body composition and collect anthropometric data in athletes involves three-dimensional (3D) whole-body scanning devices. Some examples of the use of 3D scanners in athletes include comparing elite rowers to a general population as well predicting performance in junior rowers (Schranz et al. 2010, 2012). 3D scanners can increase the number of anthropometric measurements compared to using tape-based circumference measurements, but there are limitations to the technology. While comparison data may be valuable from 3D scanners, there is a lack of validity when it comes to specific site measurements compared to tape-based circumference measurements in addition to validity issues when attempting to predict % fat. Furthermore, there are numerous 3D scanners from different manufacturers with limited research comparing machines and calculations. These scanners also only measure circumferences, necessitating the use of either an ultrasound device or skinfold calipers to determine subcutaneous fat. The high cost, questionable validity across all devices, lack of portability, and limited additional data compared to skinfold/ultrasound and tape-based circumference measurements, limit the application of 3D scanners for use in endurance athletes.

Anthropometric measurements such as skinfold and circumference measurements are the most used methods in the endurance athlete literature. The plethora of anthropometric data in the published literature allows for normative data to be established for multiple types of endurance athletes (Tables 10.1 and 10.2), although secular trends may reduce the utility of this data over time. Not all researchers have used the same skinfold equations to predict % fat, and many used different calipers as well as slightly different measurement sites. Still, the majority of the research has used standard skinfold sites such as those suggested by pioneers in the field of body composition as well as the standards suggested by the International Olympic Committee and taught by the International Society for the Advancement of Kinanthropometry (ISAK) (Jackson and Pollock 1985; Stewart and Marfell-Jones 2006). While there is little research on the differences in skinfold thicknesses, most locations are similar, and using either of the two suggested protocols should provide sound data for comparison using Figures 10.1 and 10.2. There is, however, a good deal of research looking at differences between skinfold calipers. In female college athletes, the differences between Lange and Harpenden calipers resulted in an average % fat of around 2.82% fat higher for the Lange caliper, which provides a slightly higher compression rate (Lohman et al. 1984). Another study reported that the Lange caliper produced skinfold sums across seven sites to be 10.6 mm higher in females and 9.9 mm higher for males, which resulted in a higher % fat of around 1.5% fat for males and 1.5%–2% fat for females (Gruber et al. 1990). It has been suggested that equations using either a Lange or Harpenden caliper can be adjusted based on these constant differences (Moon et al. 2009b). Specifically, if a Lange caliper is used for an equation that was developed using a Harpenden caliper, simply subtracting 1.5% for males or females may provide a more accurate % fat value that more precisely estimates the criterion method used to develop the skinfold equation.

Research supports the use of the Brozek et al. (1963) equation (Equation 10.5) to convert BD to % fat, as endurance and strength and power athletes appear to have a similar FFM density ($\approx$1.100 g/mL) and FFM water content ($\approx$73%) to the reference body used in Brozek et al. study (Arngrimsson et al. 2000; Moon et al. 2009a). However, the Siri (1961) equation has been proven to be just as valid as the Brozek equation in athletes and could also be used (Silva et al. 2006; Moon et al. 2009a).

When tracking changes in body composition, regardless of the method, errors will be present. Some researchers have recommended avoiding converting skinfold thicknesses to % fat altogether (O'Connor et al. 2007), and many coaches, athletes, trainers, and researchers have opted to measure anthropometric data and interpret the raw data without converting it to % fat. By using raw skinfolds and circumferences, one can determine both changes in subcutaneous fat and location, and this raw data can also be used with circumference measurements to calculate changes in muscle mass. While some researchers suggest that more-advanced techniques for measuring and tracking body composition do not offer any additional information beyond skinfold and circumference measurements, more-advanced methods may still serve as valuables tools for endurance athletes. An alternative to using skinfold measurements is DXA, as research has shown DXA to be a reliable body composition tool. A loss of as little 300 g of appendicular lean tissue has been shown to increase health risks in older adults, suggesting good reliability and sensitivity when measuring muscle in the arms and legs of an athlete (Szulc et al. 2010). However, there appears to be a lack of research using DXA, skinfold-based equations, and densitometry-based two-component models to track both large and small changes in lean and fat masses of all athletes compared to criterion water-based multicomponent models. On the other hand, there is research suggesting the aforementioned methods are valid and reliable when tracking both lean and fat masses in various other populations (Minderico et al. 2006, 2008; Moon et al. 2013). Therefore, both total body and segmental DXA measurements along with skinfold and circumference measurements in addition to HW and BOD POD® (with measured lung volumes) may be used together or independently as valuable tools when assessing the body composition of endurance athletes. Currently, there is not enough evidence to support using predicted lung volumes for HW and BOD POD® when tracking changes or for a single measurement in endurance athletes, and this may result in errors too large to be of practical value. Research has shown that predicted lung volumes for densitometry-based, two-component models can increase errors from ±0.5% fat to ±5% fat with the majority of the data suggesting around a ±2.5% fat increased error (Withers et al. 1990).

Other factors to consider for endurance athletes that can impact body composition measurements include acute changes in diet and hydration. Low carbohydrate diets could impact glycogen stores and may reduce body water, giving invalid body composition measurements for techniques that assume a constant hydration status of FFM. Being dehydrated or over-hydrated from not drinking enough water or drinking large amounts of water could also impact the accuracy of body composition methods that rely on a constant hydration status of FFM. This applies to any method that directly includes a body water estimation including skinfold equations, HW, BOD POD®, and DXA. When abnormal hydration is known, one should consider using methods that measure body water, such as the Pace and Rathbun two-component model, the Siri three-component model, and all four-component models that include a total body water measurement (Pace and Rathbun 1945; Siri 1961). Also, given the known acute changes in hydration within individuals and with training and diet interventions, body composition methods that include a body water measurement should be used when tracking small changes in individuals. Larger changes in body composition may be needed before methods that do not measure total body water can detect true changes. It has been suggested that methods that do not measure body water may require a change to be greater than 4–5 kg in FFM or fat mass before an individual change can be determined with confidence (Moon 2013; Moon et al. 2013). This limitation supports the idea of using skinfold and circumference measurements in addition to other methods for tracking changes in individual endurance athletes. Changes in skinfold (also ultrasound) and circumference measurements may detect smaller changes in muscle and fat compared to methods like HW, BOD POD®, and DXA. Using skinfold and circumference-based equations that do not rely on body mass to predict muscle mass and % fat will be less susceptible to errors related to changes in hydration status and should detect small changes accurately when performed under ideal conditions by a trained individual.

Both seven- and three-site skinfold equations have produced similar results compared to criterion methods, and it has been suggested that three-site equations are just as accurate as seven-site equations for athletes (Moon et al. 2008, 2009b). However, for athletes, it may be beneficial to measure as many skinfold sites as possible to identify site-specific changes in subcutaneous fat. This is even more important when attempting to track small changes in an athlete.

Suggested equations for use in endurance athletes are provided below. Included are the Jackson and Pollock equations (Equations 10.1 through 10.4) (Jackson and Pollock 1978; Jackson et al. 1980) that predict HW BD and have been validated in multiple athletic populations including endurance athletes (Thorland et al. 1984; Silva et al. 2006; Moon et al. 2008, 2009b). The Jackson and Pollock (1978) and Jackson et al. (1980) equations have also been used in multiple research studies to establish normative data for endurance athletes (Tables 10.1 and 10.2), making them ideal for comparing data of individual athletes to other athletes within the same sport and level. Also suggested are Equations 10.6 and 10.7 used to estimate DXA percent body fat that have been used in several endurance athlete studies (Ball et al. 2004a,b). The final % fat equations (Equations 10.8 and 10.9) suggested were developed using a four-component model to estimate % fat and have also been validated in various athletic populations (Evans et al. 2005; Moon et al. 2009b). Each equation suggested has advantages and disadvantages, but all can be used in endurance athletes as long as the variances are understood. The Jackson and Pollock equations are probably the best option since these equations have been used for several decades to determine normative data and have been validated more than any other skinfold equation. They should also produce similar results to HW or BOD POD® which are also the most common methods used over the last few decades to measure the body composition of endurance athletes. If one does not have access to HW or a BOD POD®, the Jackson and Pollock skinfold equations can be used as a substitute. If one is trying to predict DXA percent body fat values, the Ball equations are more appropriate, but they may produce slightly higher values than some of the normative data that is based on HW. Table 10.3 includes a comparison of the Ball equations (Ball et al. 2004a,b) and indicates a higher % fat of around 3% for females and 4% for males compared to the Jackson and Pollock equations. The final Evans et al. percent body fat equation has been used the least to determine % fat normative data in endurance athletes, but as one can see in Table 10.3 the values should be similar to the average of the Jackson and Pollock and Ball equations, and the equation is easier to use. However, Table 10.3 is only an example for a single male or female, and this may not be the case in all athletes. Thus, when looking to compare an athlete to the data in Tables 10.1 and 10.2, using all three equations would likely provide the most comprehensive analysis. Also, it should be noted that the Evans et al. equation was created using a Harpenden skinfold caliper, and when corrected for a Lange caliper, the values will be closer to the Jackson and Pollock equations. Nevertheless, the same measurements were used for all equations in Table 10.3, so regardless of the caliper, the results should be similar to this table in various endurance athletes. There is also an anthropometric equation to predict skeletal muscle mass that was developed using MRI as the criterion method and was used exclusively to determine normative data in Tables 10.1 and 10.2 (Lee et al. 2000). This equation requires both skinfold and

TABLE 10.3
%Fat Equation Comparisons

Equation	Equation No.	Men %Fat	Women %Fat
Ball	10.6, 10.7	10.7	20.3
Evans 7	10.9	8.9	20.7
Evans 3	10.8	8.7	19.4
Jackson 3	10.1, 10.3	6.7	16.5
Jackson 7	10.2, 10.4	7.1	17.4

Source: Jackson, A. S., M. L. Pollock, and A. Ward. 1980. *Med Sci Sports Exerc* 12:175–81; Jackson, A. S. and M. L. Pollock. 1985. *Phys Sport Med* 13:76–90; Ball, S. D., T. S. Altena, and P. D. Swan. 2004a. *Eur J Clin Nutr* 58:1525–31; Ball, S., P. D. Swan, and R. DeSimone. 2004b. *Res Q Exerc Sport* 75:248–58; Evans, E. M. et al. 2005. *Med Sci Sports Exerc* 37:2006–11.

Note: Comparison between equations for a 20-year-old male and female runner using all adult means for height, body mass, with anthropometric data from Tables 10.1 and 10.2.

circumference measurements and should provide valid estimations of muscle mass in endurance athletes in addition to being used to compare an athlete to the data in Tables 10.1 and 10.2.

The suggested equations in this chapter were selected for their previous use in all types of athletes, contributions to Tables 10.1 and 10.2, unique criterion method to predict % fat (HW, DXA, four-component, MRI muscle mass), as well as their reported low standard error of the estimate (SEE) values. The SEE value is regarded as one of the single most important statistics for determining the "relative worth of a prediction equation" (Heyward and Wagner 2004). All % fat equations suggested have produced SEE values from 2% to 3% fat which is considered "ideal" to "very good" using the subjective rating of Heyward and Wagner (2004) (Thorland et al. 1984; Ball et al. 2004a,b; Silva et al. 2006; Moon et al. 2008, 2009b). The Lee et al. (2000) MRI prediction equation for skeletal muscle mass has a reported SEE value of 2.2 kg, which is also considered "ideal" to "very good" using the subjective rating of Heyward and Wagner (2004) for FFM, which is similar to muscle mass in tissue mass. When contemplating the use of other skinfold prediction equations not suggested in this chapter, one should look for SEE values under 3% fat in addition to the equation being specific and/or cross-validated in the population being tested.

When comparing a group of athletes or a single athlete to Tables 10.1 or 10.2 or Figures 10.1 through 10.5, the standard deviations and confidence intervals must be considered. Tables 10.1 and 10.2 report both the average standard deviations within a study (SD WT) as well as between studies (SD BW). Figures 10.1 through 10.5 report only the SD BW, and include both the 68% and 95% confidence intervals, which means that 95% of the data from all the studies used for that type of athlete fall within the highest and lowest points on the lines and that 68% of the athletes were within the box for each type of athlete and level. These tables and figures should only be used as a general guide for comparison, as each athlete is unique and may not compare exactly to the research subjects used to create the tables and figures. However, it is suggested when using these tables and figures that one considers the relatively large standard deviations for each type of endurance athlete and also considers both the range of healthy minimum % fat values as well as the errors associated with the method one is using to estimate body composition. This also applies to the other values in Tables 10.1 and 10.2 such as skinfold thicknesses and circumferences. It may not be best to strive to be exactly within one standard deviation of the mean, but rather to look at all the data from an athlete together to determine if he or she has an ideal body composition for his or her sport and level. Again, these tables and figures are guides to compare different athletes and to show the range within the same type of athlete, and caution should be used when using these tables and figures as grounds to modify an athlete's body composition through diet and training.

The ethnicity of an athlete is another methodological consideration for testing body composition in endurance athletes. The Evans and Lee equations (Equations 10.8 through 10.10) have an ethnicity component incorporated to help improve % fat estimations. However, limited data are available regarding the effect of ethnicity and body composition on endurance performance. One study compared female white and black college middle distance runners and found % fat values calculated using skinfold equations were nearly identical for both ethnicities. The largest impact of ethnicity in endurance athletes is most likely related to the measurement tools being used and not the effects of body composition, in particular, % fat and performance. More research is needed to determine the effects of anthropometric skinfold equations on various ethnicities of endurance athletes. Also, more research is needed to determine the differences in various ethnic groups and body composition values and to establish normative data for different ethnicities. When measuring non-Caucasian endurance athletes, the Evans and Lee equations (Equations 10.8 through 10.10) may provide more accurate predictions compared to the Jackson and Pollock and the Ball equations (Equations 10.1 through 10.4, 10.6, and 10.7), but the data in Tables 10.1 and 10.2 and Figures 10.1 through 10.5 may not apply to all ethnicities. Still, the limited research that is available does suggest that body composition may not differ significantly between endurance athletes of different ethnicities.

Finally, when working with athletes regardless of their % fat values, there may be an underlying concern that an athlete may become obsessed or too focused on the percent body fat numbers and risk developing emotional and psychological issues which could result in health issues. For this reason, it is recommended that coaches, trainers, and researchers who work with athletes be cautious when interpreting and sharing results with their athletes (O'Connor et al. 2007). There is a burden placed on the coach, trainer, or researcher considering the known individual variability with most body composition methods and the fact that a single measurement of FFM or fat mass cannot determine true health status, along with the errors associated with every repeated measurement. It is crucial that anyone interpreting body composition data and administering body composition tests on not only endurance athletes, but also all athletes, be well educated in the errors of their chosen methods and the proper testing protocols, in addition to understanding the ranges for minimum essential and healthy % fat among different endurance athletes. Endurance athletes are at a higher risk of having % fat values that are too low because of the direct relationship between low % fat and increased performance. It may not always be best to have a % fat value as low as possible, especially in female athletes. It has been suggested that anthropometric measures be performed on athletes regularly and as often as every few weeks (O'Connor et al. 2007). At-risk endurance athletes may benefit from having more frequent measurements using methods sensitive enough to detect small changes and trends in body fat.

10.9 SUGGESTED EQUATIONS

$$\text{Females BD} = 1.0994921 - 0.0009929(\text{SUM3.1}) + 0.0000023(\text{SUM3.1})^2 - 0.0001392(\text{Age}) \quad (10.1)$$

$$\text{Females BD} = 1.097 - 0.00046971(\text{SUM7}) + 0.00000056(\text{SUM7})^2 - 0.00012828(\text{Age}) \quad (10.2)$$

BD = Body density
SUM3.1 = Triceps + suprailiac + thigh skinfold thicknesses in mm
SUM7 = Chest + axilla + triceps + abdomen + suprailiac + subscapular + thigh skinfold
    thicknesses in mm
Age = Age in years
Calipers used in original study: Lange
(Jackson et al. 1980)

$$\text{Males BD} = 1.10938 - 0.0008267(\text{SUM3.2}) + 0.0000016(\text{SUM3.2})^2 - 0.0002574(\text{Age}) \quad (10.3)$$

$$\text{Males BD} = 1.112 - 0.00043499(\text{SUM7}) + 0.00000055(\text{SUM7})^2 - 0.00028826(\text{Age}) \quad (10.4)$$

BD = Body density
SUM3.2 = Chest + abdominal + thigh skinfold thicknesses in mm
SUM7 = Chest + axilla + triceps + abdomen + suprailiac + subscapular + thigh skinfold
    thicknesses in mm
Age = Age in years
Calipers used in original study: Lange
(Jackson and Pollock 1985)

$$\%\text{Fat from BD} = ([4.57 / \text{BD}] - 4.142) \times 100 \quad (10.5)$$

BD = Body density
(Brozek et al. 1963)

$$\text{Males DXA } \%\text{Fat} = 0.465 + 0.180(\text{SUM7}) - 0.0002406(\text{SUM7})^2 + 0.06619(\text{Age}) \quad (10.6)$$

SUM7 = Chest + axilla + triceps + abdomen + suprailiac + subscapular + thigh skinfold
thicknesses in mm
Age = Age in years
Calipers used in original study: Lange
(Ball et al. 2004a)

$$\text{Females DXA \%Fat} = -6.40665 + 0.41946(\text{SUM3.1}) - 0.00126(\text{SUM3.1})^2$$
$$+ 0.12515(\text{Hip}) + 0.06473(\text{age}) \tag{10.7}$$

SUM3.1 = Triceps + suprailiac + thigh skinfold thicknesses in mm
Hip = Circumference of the hip at the level of the trochanter in cm
Age = Age in years
Calipers used in original study: Lange
(Ball et al. 2004b)

$$\text{E3\%Fat} = 8.997 + 0.24658(\text{SUM3.3}) - 6.343(\text{Sex}) - 1.998(\text{Race}) \tag{10.8}$$

$$\text{E7\%Fat} = 10.566 + 0.12077(\text{SUM7}) - 8.057(\text{Sex}) - 2.545(\text{Race}) \tag{10.9}$$

SUM3.3 = Triceps + abdomen + thigh skinfold thicknesses in mm
SUM7 = Chest + axilla + triceps + abdomen + suprailiac + subscapular + thigh skinfold
thicknesses in mm
Sex = 1 for male, 0 for female
Race = 1 for black, 0 for white
Calipers used in original study: Harpenden
(Evans et al. 2005)

$$\text{MRI Skeletal Muscle Mass} = \text{Ht} \times (0.00744 \times \text{CAG}^2 + 0.00088 \times \text{CTG}^2 + 0.00441 \times \text{CCG}^2)$$
$$+ 2.4 \times \text{Sex} - 0.048 \times \text{Age} + \text{Race} + 7.8 \tag{10.10}$$

Ht = Body height in m
CAG = skinfold-corrected upper arm girth
CTG = skinfold-corrected thigh girth
CCG = skinfold-corrected calf girth
Corrected girth = Limb circumference (cm) $- \pi \times$ skinfold thickness (cm)
Sex = 1 for male, 0 for female
Age = Age in years
Race = 0 for whites and Hispanics, 1.1 for blacks, −2.0 for Asians
Calipers used in original study: Lange
(Lee et al. 2000)

ACKNOWLEDGMENT

We would like to thank Patty Wilson for her tireless efforts in locating all of the full text articles for this chapter.

REFERENCES

Abe, T., K. Kumagai, and W. F. Brechue. 2000. Fascicle length of leg muscles is greater in sprinters than distance runners. *Med Sci Sports Exerc* 32:1125–9.

Akagi, R., H. Kanehisa, Y. Kawakami, and T. Fukunaga. 2008. Establishing a new index of muscle cross-sectional area and its relationship with isometric muscle strength. *J Strength Cond Res* 22:82–7.

Akca, F. 2014. Prediction of rowing ergometer performance from functional anaerobic power, strength and anthropometric components. *J Hum Kinet* 41:133–42.

Alway, S. E., J. Stray-Gundersen, W. H. Grumbt, and W. J. Gonyea. 1990. Muscle cross-sectional area and torque in resistance-trained subjects. *Eur J Appl Physiol Occup Physiol* 60:86–90.

Arazi, H., F. Hassan, and S. Mohammadi. 2011. Anthropometric and physiological profiles of elite iranian junior rowers. *Middle East J Sci Res* 9:162–6.

Arngrimsson, S., E. M. Evans, M. J. Saunders et al. 2000. Validation of body composition estimates in male and female distance runners using estimates from a four-component model. *Am J Hum Biol* 12:301–14.

Arrese, A. L. and E. S. Ostariz. 2006. Skinfold thicknesses associated with distance running performance in highly trained runners. *J Sports Sci* 24:69–76.

Åstrand, P. O., K. Rodahl, H. A. Dahl, and S. B. Strømme. 2003. *Textbook of Work Physiology: Physiological Bases of Exercise*. Champaign, Illinois: Human Kinetics.

Bale, P., D. Bradbury, and E. Colley. 1986. Anthropometric and training variables related to 10 km running performance. *Br J Sports Med* 20:170–3.

Bale, P., S. Rowell, and E. Colley. 1985. Anthropometric and training characteristics of female marathon runners as determinants of distance running performance. *J Sports Sci* 3:115–26.

Ball, S., P. D. Swan, and R. DeSimone. 2004b. Comparison of anthropometry to dual energy X-ray absorptiometry: A new prediction equation for women. *Res Q Exerc Sport* 75:248–58.

Ball, S. D., T. S. Altena, and P. D. Swan. 2004a. Comparison of anthropometry to DXA: A new prediction equation for men. *Eur J Clin Nutr* 58:1525–31.

Bennell, K. L., S. A. Malcolm, K. M. Khan et al. 1997. Bone mass and bone turnover in power athletes, endurance athletes, and controls: A 12-month longitudinal study. *Bone* 20:477–84.

Bergh, U. and A. Forsberg. 1992. Influence of body mass on cross-country ski racing performance. *Med Sci Sports Exerc* 24:1033–9.

Berneis, K. and U. Keller. 2000. Bioelectrical impedance analysis during acute changes of extracellular osmolality in man. *Clin Nutr* 19:361–6.

Billat, V. L., A. Demarle, J. Slawinski, M. Paiva, and J. P. Koralsztein. 2001. Physical and training characteristics of top-class marathon runners. *Med Sci Sports Exerc* 33:2089–97.

Bosch, T. A., T. P. Burruss, N. L. Weir et al. 2014. Abdominal body composition differences in NFL football players. *J Strength Cond Res* 28:3313–9.

Bourgois, J., A. L. Claessens, J. Vrijens et al. 2000. Anthropometric characteristics of elite male junior rowers. *Br J Sports Med* 34:213–6; discussion 216–7.

Brozek, J., F. Grande, J. T. Anderson, and A. Keys. 1963. Densitometric analysis of body composition: Revision of some quantitative assumptions. *Ann NY Acad Sci* 110:113–40.

Burtscher, M. and H. Gatterer. 2013. Predictive importance of anthropometric and training data in recreational male Ironman triathletes and marathon runners: Comment on the study by Gianoli, et al. (2012). *Percept Mot Skills* 116:655–7.

Campion, F., A. M. Nevill, M. K. Karlsson et al. 2010. Bone status in professional cyclists. *Int J Sports Med* 31:511–5.

Carbuhn, A. F., T. E. Fernandez, A. F. Bragg, J. S. Green, and S. F. Crouse. 2010. Sport and training influence bone and body composition in women collegiate athletes. *J Strength Cond Res* 24:1710–7.

Carlsson, M., T. Carlsson, D. HammarstrOm, C. Malm, and M. Tonkonogi. 2014. Prediction of race performance of elite cross-country skiers by lean mass. *Int J Sports Physiol Perform* 9:1040–5.

Cheuvront, S. N., R. Carter, K. C. Deruisseau, and R. J. Moffatt. 2005. Running performance differences between men and women: An update. *Sports Med* 35:1017–24.

Cohen, B., P. J. Millett, B. Mist, M. A. Laskey, and N. Rushton. 1995. Effect of exercise training programme on bone mineral density in novice college rowers. *Br J Sports Med* 29:85–8.

Cosgrove, M. J., J. Wilson, D. Watt, and S. F. Grant. 1999. The relationship between selected physiological variables of rowers and rowing performance as determined by a 2000 m ergometer test. *J Sports Sci* 17:845–52.

Costill, D. L. 1967. The relationship between selected physiological variables and distance running performance. *J Sports Med Phys Fitness* 7:61–6.

Costill, D. L. 1972. Physiology of marathon running. *JAMA* 221:1024–9.

Costill, D. L., R. Bowers, and W. F. Kammer. 1970. Skinfold estimates of body fat among marathon runners. *Med Sci Sports* 2:93–5.

Coyle, E. F. 1995. Integration of the physiological factors determining endurance performance ability. *Exerc Sport Sci Rev* 23:25–63.

Coyle, E. F., M. E. Feltner, S. A. Kautz et al. 1991. Physiological and biomechanical factors associated with elite endurance cycling performance. *Med Sci Sports Exerc* 23:93–107.

Coyle, E. F., M. K. Hemmert, and A. R. Coggan. 1986. Effects of detraining on cardiovascular-responses to exercise—Role of blood-volume. *J Appl Physiol* 60:95–9.

Cureton, K. J., P. B. Sparling, B. W. Evans et al. 1978. Effect of experimental alterations in excess weight on aerobic capacity and distance running performance. *Med Sci Sports* 10:194–9.

Davy, K. P. and D. R. Seals. 1994. Total blood-volume in healthy-young and older men. *J Appl Physiol* 76:2059–62.

Dengel, D. R., T. A. Bosch, T. P. Burruss et al. 2014. Body composition and bone mineral density of national football league players. *J Strength Cond Res* 28(1):1–6.

Dengel, D. R., M. G. Flynn, D. L. Costill, and J. P. Kirwan. 1989. Determinants of success during triathlon competition. *Res Q Exerc Sport* 60(3):234–8.

DeRose, E. H., S. M. Crawford, D. A. Kerr, R. Ward, and W. D. Ross. 1989. Physique characteristics of Pan American Games lightweight rowers. *Int J Sports Med* 10:292–7.

Diversi, T., V. Franks-Kardum, and M. Climstein. 2016. The effect of cold water endurance swimming on core temperature in aspiring English Channel swimmers. *Extrem Physiol Med* 5:3. doi: 10.1186/s13728-016-0044-2.

Ebert, T. R., D. T. Martin, W. McDonald et al. 2005. Power output during women's World Cup road cycle racing. *Eur J Appl Physiol* 95:529–36.

Eisenman, P. A., S. C. Johnson, C. N. Bainbridge, and M. F. Zupan. 1989. Applied physiology of cross-country skiing. *Sports Med* 8:67–79.

Evans, E. M., D. A. Rowe, M. M. Misic, B. M. Prior, and S. A. Arngrimsson. 2005. Skinfold prediction equation for athletes developed using a four-component model. *Med Sci Sports Exerc* 37:2006–11.

Faria, E. W., D. L. Parker, and I. E. Faria. 2005. The science of cycling: Physiology and training—Part 1. *Sports Med* 35:285–312.

Faria, I. E., E. W. Faria, S. Roberts, and D. Yoshimura. 1989. Comparison of physical and physiological characteristics in elite young and mature cyclists. *Res Q Exerc Sport* 60:388–95.

Fehling, P. C., L. Alekel, J. Clasey, A. Rector, and R. J. Stillman. 1995. A comparison of bone mineral densities among female athletes in impact loading and active loading sports. *Bone* 17:205–10.

Fernandez-Garcia, B., J. Perez-Landaluce, M. Rodriguez-Alonso, and N. Terrados. 2000. Intensity of exercise during road race pro-cycling competition. *Med Sci Sports Exerc* 32:1002–6.

Fleck, S. J. 1983. Body composition of elite American athletes. *Am J Sports Med* 11:398–403.

Fleg, J. L. and E. G. Lakatta. 1988. Role of muscle loss in the age-associated reduction in VO_2max. *J Appl Physiol* 65:1147–51.

Fornetti, W. C., J. M. Pivarnik, J. M. Foley, and J. J. Fiechtner. 1999. Reliability and validity of body composition measures in female athletes. *J Appl Physiol* 87:1114–22.

Frisch, R. E. and J. W. McArthur. 1974. Menstrual cycles: Fatness as a determinant of minimum weight for height necessary for their maintenance or onset. *Science* 185:949–51.

Gardsell, P., O. Johnell, and B. E. Nilsson. 1990. The predictive value of forearm bone mineral content measurements in men. *Bone* 11:229–32.

Gianoli, D., B. Knechtle, P. Knechtle et al. 2012. Comparison between recreational male Ironman triathletes and marathon runners. *Percept Mot Skills* 115:283–99.

Gomez-Bruton, A., A. Gonzalez-Aguero, A. Gomez-Cabello, J. A. Casajus, and G. Vicente-Rodriguez. 2013. Is bone tissue really affected by swimming? A systematic review. *PLoS One* 8(8):e70119. doi: 10.1371/journal.pone.0070119.

Grassi, B., P. Cerretelli, M. V. Narici, and C. Marconi. 1991. Peak anaerobic power in master athletes. *Eur J Appl Physiol Occup Physiol* 62:394–9.

Gruber, J. J., M. L. Pollock, J. E. Graves, A. B. Colvin, and R. W. Braith. 1990. Comparison of Harpenden and Lange calipers in predicting body composition. *Res Q Exerc Sport* 61:184–90.

Gulbin, J. P. and P. T. Gaffney. 1999. Ultraendurance triathlon participation: Typical race preparation of lower level triathletes. *J Sports Med Phys Fitness* 39:12–5.

Haakonssen, E. C., L. M. Barras, L. M. Burke, D. G. Jenkins, and D. T. Martin. 2015. Body composition of female road and track endurance cyclists: Normative values and typical changes. *Eur J Sport Sci* 16:645–53.

Hagan, R. D., M. G. Smith, and L. R. Gettman. 1981. Marathon performance in relation to maximal aerobic power and training indices. *Med Sci Sports Exerc* 13:185–9.

Hagan, R. D., S. J. Upton, J. J. Duncan, and L. R. Gettman. 1987. Marathon performance in relation to maximal aerobic power and training indices in female distance runners. *Br J Sports Med* 21:3–7.

Hakkinen, K. and K. L. Keskinen. 1989. Muscle cross-sectional area and voluntary force production characteristics in elite strength- and endurance-trained athletes and sprinters. *Eur J Appl Physiol Occup Physiol* 59:215–20.

Hawley, J. A. and T. D. Noakes. 1992. Peak power output predicts maximal oxygen uptake and performance time in trained cyclists. *Eur J Appl Physiol Occup Physiol* 65:79–83.

Hebbelinck, M., W. D. Ross, J. E. Carter, and J. Borms. 1980. Anthropometric characteristics of female Olympic rowers. *Can J Appl Sport Sci* 5:255–62.

Heinonen, A., P. Oja, P. Kannus et al. 1993. Bone mineral density of female athletes in different sports. *Bone Miner* 23:1–4.

Heinonen, A., P. Oja, P. Kannus et al. 1995. Bone mineral density in female athletes representing sports with different loading characteristics of the skeleton. *Bone* 17:197–203.

Hetland, M. L., J. Haarbo, and C. Christiansen. 1998. Regional body composition determined by dual-energy X-ray absorptiometry. Relation to training, sex hormones, and serum lipids in male long-distance runners. *Scand J Med Sci Sports* 8:102–8.

Hew-Butler, T., B. T. Holexa, K. Fogard, K. J. Stuempfle, and M. D. Hoffman. 2015. Comparison of body composition techniques before and after a 161-km ultramarathon using DXA, BIS and BIA. *Int J Sports Med* 36:169–74.

Heyward, V. H. and D. R. Wagner. 2004. *Applied Body Composition Assessments.* Champaign, Illinois: Human Kinetics.

Hirsch, K. R., A. E. Smith-Ryan, E. T. Trexler, and E. J. Roelofs. 2016. Body composition and muscle characteristics of division I track and field athletes. *J Strength Cond Res* 30:1231–8.

Hoffman, M. D. 2008. Anthropometric characteristics of ultramarathoners. *Int J Sports Med* 29:808–11.

Holly, R. G., R. J. Barnard, M. Rosenthal, E. Applegate, and N. Pritikin. 1986. Triathlete characterization and response to prolonged strenuous competition. *Med Sci Sports Exerc* 18:123–7.

Holmberg, H. C., S. Lindinger, T. Stoggl, E. Eitzlmair, and E. Muller. 2005. Biomechanical analysis of double poling in elite cross-country skiers. *Med Sci Sports Exerc* 37:807–18.

Hunt, B. E., K. P. Davy, P. P. Jones et al. 1998. Role of central circulatory factors in the fat-free mass-maximal aerobic capacity relation across age. *Am J Physiol Heart Circ Physiol* 275:H1178–82.

Ingham, S. A., G. P. Whyte, K. Jones, and A. M. Nevill. 2002. Determinants of 2,000 m rowing ergometer performance in elite rowers. *Eur J Appl Physiol* 88:243–6.

Jackson, A. S. and M. L. Pollock. 1978. Generalized equations for predicting body density of men. *Br J Nutr* 40:497–504.

Jackson, A. S. and M. L. Pollock. 1985. Practical assessment of body composition. *Phys Sport Med* 13:76–90.

Jackson, A. S., M. L. Pollock, and A. Ward. 1980. Generalized equations for predicting body density of women. *Med Sci Sports Exerc* 12:175–81.

Johnson, G. O., L. J. Nebelsick-Gullett, W. G. Thorland, and T. J. Housh. 1989. The effect of a competitive season on the body composition of university female athletes. *J Sports Med Phys Fitness* 29:314–20.

Jurimae, J., J. Maestu, T. Jurimae, and E. Pihl. 1999. Relationship between rowing performance and different metabolic parameters in male rowers. *Medicina Dello Sport* 52:119–26.

Jurimae, J., J. Maestu, T. Jurimae, and E. Pihl. 2000. Prediction of rowing performance on single sculls from metabolic and anthropometric variables. *J Hum Movement Stud* 38:123–36.

Jurimae, J., P. Purge, T. Jurimae, and S. P. von Duvillard. 2006. Bone metabolism in elite male rowers: Adaptation to volume-extended training. *Eur J Appl Physiol* 97:127–32.

Kendall, K. L., D. H. Fukuda, P. N. Hyde, A. E. Smith-Ryan, J. R. Moon, and J. R. Stout 2017. Estimating fat-free mass in elite-level male rowers: A four-compartment model validation of laboratory and field methods. *J Sports Sci*: 35:1–10.

Knechtle, B., B. Baumann, P. Knechtle, and T. Rosemann. 2010a. Speed during training and anthropometric measures in relation to race performance by male and female open-water ultra-endurance swimmers. *Percept Mot Skills* 111:463–74.

Knechtle, B., B. Baumann, P. knechtle, and T. Rosemann. 2010b. What influences race performance in male open-water ultra-endurance swimmers: Anthropometry or training? *Hum Movement* 1:5–10.

Knechtle, B., B. Duff, G. Amtmann, and G. Kohler. 2007a. Cycling and running performance, not anthropometric factors, are associated with race performance in a Triple Iron Triathlon. *Res Sports Med* 15:257–69.

Knechtle, B., B. Duff, U. Welzel, and G. Kohler. 2009a. Body mass and circumference of upper arm are associated with race performance in ultraendurance runners in a multistage race—The Isarrun 2006. *Res Q Exerc Sport* 80:262–8.

Knechtle, B., P. Knechtle, J. L. Andonie, and G. Kohler. 2007b. Influence of anthropometry on race performance in extreme endurance triathletes: World Challenge Deca Iron Triathlon 2006. *Br J Sports Med* 41:644–8; discussion 648.

Knechtle, B., P. Knechtle, and T. Rosemann. 2009b. Skin-fold thickness and training volume in ultra-triathletes. *Int J Sports Med* 30:343–7.

Knechtle, B., P. Knechtle, and T. Rosemann. 2010c. Similarity of anthropometric measures for male ultra-triathletes and ultra-runners. *Percept Mot Skills* 111:805–18.

Knechtle, B., P. Knechtle, and T. Rosemann. 2011a. Upper body skinfold thickness is related to race performance in male Ironman triathletes. *Int J Sports Med* 32:20–7.

Knechtle, B., P. Knechtle, C. A. Rust, and T. Rosemann. 2011b. A comparison of anthropometric and training characteristics of Ironman triathletes and Triple Iron ultra-triathletes. *J Sports Sci* 29:1373–80.

Knechtle, B., P. Knechtle, I. Schulze, and G. Kohler. 2008. Upper arm circumference is associated with race performance in ultra-endurance runners. *Br J Sports Med* 42:295–9; discussion 299.

Knechtle, B. and G. Kohler. 2009. Running performance, not anthropometric factors, is associated with race success in a Triple Iron Triathlon. *Br J Sports Med* 43:437–41.

Knechtle, B. and T. Rosemann. 2009. No correlation of skin-fold thickness with race performance in male recreational mountain bike ultra-marathoners. *Med Sport* 13:152–6.

Knechtle, B., T. Rosemann, R. Lepers, and C. A. Rust. 2014. Women outperform men in ultradistance swimming: The Manhattan Island Marathon Swim from 1983 to 2013. *Int J Sports Physiol Perform* 9:913–24.

Knechtle, B., A. Wirth, B. Baumann, P. Knechtle, and T. Rosemann. 2010d. Personal best time, percent body fat, and training are differently associated with race time for male and female ironman triathletes. *Res Q Exerc Sport* 81:62–8.

Knechtle, B., A. Wirth, B. Baumann et al. 2010e. Differential correlations between anthropometry, training volume, and performance in male and female Ironman triathletes. *J Strength Cond Res* 24:2785–93.

Knechtle, B., A. Wirth, P. Knechtle, and T. Rosemann. 2009c. Increase of total body water with decrease of body mass while running 100 km nonstop—Formation of edema? *Res Q Exerc Sport* 80:593–603.

Knechtle, B., A. Wirth, P. Knechtle, and T. Rosemann. 2010f. Training volume and personal best time in marathon, not anthropometric parameters, are associated with performance in male 100-km ultrarunners. *J Strength Cond Res* 24:604–9.

Knechtle, B., A. Wirth, P. Knechtle, K. Zimmermann, and G. Kohler. 2009d. Personal best marathon performance is associated with performance in a 24-h run and not anthropometry or training volume. *Br J Sports Med* 43:836–9.

Knechtle, B., A. Wirth, and T. Rosemann. 2010g. Predictors of race time in male Ironman triathletes: Physical characteristics, training, or prerace experience? *Percept Mot Skills* 111:437–46.

Knechtle, B., A. Wirth, C. A. Rust, and T. Rosemann. 2011c. The relationship between anthropometry and split performance in recreational male Ironman triathletes. *Asian J Sports Med* 2:23–30.

Komi, P. V. 1987. Force measurements during cross-country skiing. *Int J Sport Biomech* 3:370–81.

Krawczyk, B., M. Sklad, and B. Majle. 1995. Body composition of male and female athletes representing various sports. *Biol Sport* 12:243–50.

Landers, G. J., B. A. Blanksby, T. R. Ackland, and D. Smith. 2000. Morphology and performance of world championship triathletes. *Ann Hum Biol* 27:387–400.

Lariviere, J. A., T. L. Robinson, and C. M. Snow. 2003. Spine bone mineral density increases in experienced but not novice collegiate female rowers. *Med Sci Sports Exerc* 35:1740–4.

Larsson, P. and K. Henriksson-Larsen. 2008. Body composition and performance in cross-country skiing. *Int J Sports Med* 29:971–5.

Laurenson, N. M., K. Y. Fulcher, and P. Korkia. 1993. Physiological characteristics of elite and club level female triathletes during running. *Int J Sports Med* 14:455–9.

Laursen, P. B., C. M. Shing, S. C. Tennant, C. M. Prentice, and D. G. Jenkins. 2003. A comparison of the cycling performance of cyclists and triathletes. *J Sports Sci* 21:411–8.

Leake, C. N. and J. E. Carter. 1991. Comparison of body composition and somatotype of trained female triathletes. *J Sports Sci* 9:125–35.

Lee, H., D. T. Martin, J. M. Anson, D. Grundy, and A. G. Hahn. 2002. Physiological characteristics of successful mountain bikers and professional road cyclists. *J Sports Sci* 20:1001–8.

Lee, R. C., Z. Wang, M. Heo et al. 2000. Total-body skeletal muscle mass: Development and cross-validation of anthropometric prediction models. *Am J Clin Nutr* 72:796–803.

Legaz Arrese, A., J. J. Gonzalez Badillo, and E. Serrano Ostariz. 2005. Differences in skinfold thicknesses and fat distribution among top-class runners. *J Sports Med Phys Fitness* 45:512–7.

Lohman, T. G., M. L. Pollock, M. H. Slaughter, L. J. Brandon, and R. A. Boileau. 1984. Methodological factors and the prediction of body fat in female athletes. *Med Sci Sports Exerc* 16:92–6.

Lucia, A., J. Pardo, A. Durantez, J. Hoyos, and J. L. Chicharro. 1998. Physiological differences between professional and elite road cyclists. *Int J Sports Med* 19:342–8.

Maciejczyk, M., M. Wiecek, J. Szymura et al. 2014a. Effect of body composition on respiratory compensation point during an incremental test. *J Strength Cond Res* 28:2071–7.

Maciejczyk, M., M. Wiecek, J. Szymura et al. 2014b. The influence of increased body fat or lean body mass on aerobic performance. *PLoS One* 9(4):e95797. doi: 10.1371/journal.pone.0095797.

Maimoun, L. and C. Sultan. 2011. Effects of physical activity on bone remodeling. *Metabolism* 60:373–88.

Malina, R. M. 2007. Body composition in athletes: Assessment and estimated fatness. *Clin Sports Med* 26:37–68.

Martin, D. T., B. McLean, C. Trewin et al. 2001. Physiological characteristics of nationally competitive female road cyclists and demands of competition. *Sports Med* 31:469–77.

Mayhew, J. L., F. C. Piper, and J. S. Ware. 1993. Anthropometric correlates with strength performance among resistance trained athletes. *J Sports Med Phys Fitness* 33:159–65.

McLean, S. P. and R. N. Hinrichs. 1998. Sex differences in the centre of buoyancy location of competitive swimmers. *J Sports Sci* 16:373–83.

Medelli, J., M. Shabani, J. Lounana, P. Fardellone, and F. Campion. 2009. Low bone mineral density and calcium intake in elite cyclists. *J Sports Med Phys Fitness* 49:44–53.

Melton, L. J., 3rd, E. J. Atkinson, M. K. O'Connor, W. M. O'Fallon, and B. L. Riggs. 1998. Bone density and fracture risk in men. *J Bone Miner Res* 13:1915–23.

Melvin, M. N., A. E. Smith-Ryan, H. L. Wingfield et al. 2014. Muscle characteristics and body composition of NCAA division I football players. *J Strength Cond Res* 28:3320–9.

Mikulic, P. 2008. Anthropometric and physiological profiles of rowers of varying ages and ranks. *Kinesiology* 40:80–8.

Mikulic, P. 2009. Anthropometric and metabolic determinants of 6,000-m rowing ergometer performance in internationally competitive rowers. *J Strength Cond Res* 23:1851–7.

Mikulic, P. and L. Ruzic. 2008. Predicting the 1000 m rowing ergometer performance in 12–13-year-old rowers: The basis for selection process? *J Sci Med Sport* 11:218–26.

Millet, G. P., P. Dreano, and D. J. Bentley. 2003. Physiological characteristics of elite short- and long-distance triathletes. *Eur J Appl Physiol* 88:427–30.

Minderico, C. S., A. M. Silva, K. Keller et al. 2008. Usefulness of different techniques for measuring body composition changes during weight loss in overweight and obese women. *Br J Nutr* 99:432–41.

Minderico, C. S., A. M. Silva, P. J. Teixeira et al. 2006. Validity of air-displacement plethysmography in the assessment of body composition changes in a 16-month weight loss program. *Nutr Metab (Lond)* 3:32.

Moon, J. R. 2013. Body composition in athletes and sports nutrition: An examination of the bioimpedance analysis technique. *Eur J Clin Nutr* 67(Suppl 1):S54–9.

Moon, J. R., J. M. Eckerson, S. E. Tobkin et al. 2009a. Estimating body fat in NCAA Division I female athletes: A five-compartment model validation of laboratory methods. *Eur J Appl Physiol* 105:119–30.

Moon, J. R., J. R. Stout, A. E. Smith-Ryan et al. 2013. Tracking fat-free mass changes in elderly men and women using single-frequency bioimpedance and dual-energy X-ray absorptiometry: A four-compartment model comparison. *Eur J Clin Nutr* 67(Suppl 1):S40–6.

Moon, J. R., S. E. Tobkin, P. B. Costa et al. 2008. Validity of the BOD POD for assessing body composition in athletic high school boys. *J Strength Cond Res* 22:263–8.

Moon, J. R., S. E. Tobkin, A. E. Smith et al. 2009b. Anthropometric estimations of percent body fat in NCAA division I female athletes: A 4-compartment model validation. *J Strength Cond Res* 23:1068–76.

Morris, F. L., W. R. Payne, and J. D. Wark. 1999. The impact of intense training on endogenous estrogen and progesterone concentrations and bone mineral acquisition in adolescent rowers. *Osteoporos Int* 10:361–8.

Morris, F. L., R. M. Smith, W. R. Payne, M. A. Galloway, and J. D. Wark. 2000. Compressive and shear force generated in the lumbar spine of female rowers. *Int J Sports Med* 21:518–23.

Mueller, S. M., E. Anliker, P. Knechtle, B. Knechtle, and M. Toigo. 2013. Changes in body composition in triathletes during an Ironman race. *Eur J Appl Physiol* 113:2343–52.

Mujika, I. and S. Padilla. 2001. Physiological and performance characteristics of male professional road cyclists. *Sports Med* 31:479–87.

Nevill, A. M., C. Beech, R. L. Holder, and M. Wyon. 2010. Scaling concept II rowing ergometer performance for differences in body mass to better reflect rowing in water. *Scand J Med Sci Sports* 20:122–7.

Ng, A. V., R. B. Demment, D. R. Bassett et al. 1988. Characteristics and performance of male citizen cross-country ski racers. *Int J Sports Med* 9:205–9.

Nichols, J. F., J. E. Palmer, and S. S. Levy. 2003. Low bone mineral density in highly trained male master cyclists. *Osteoporos Int* 14:644–9.

Niinimaa, V., M. Dyon, and R. J. Shephard. 1978. Performance and efficiency of intercollegiate cross-country skiers. *Med Sci Sports* 10:91–3.

Novak, L. P., R. E. Hyatt, and J. F. Alexander. 1968. Body composition and physiologic function of athletes. *JAMA* 205:764–70.

O'Connor, H. et al. 2007. Physique and performance for track and field events. *J Sports Sci* 25(Suppl 1):S49–60.

Olds, T. S., K. I. Norton, E. L. Lowe et al. 1995. Modeling road-cycling performance. *J Appl Physiol* 78:1596–611.

Ostojic, S. M. 2006. Estimation of body fat in athletes: Skinfolds vs bioelectrical impedance. *J Sports Med Phys Fitness* 46:442–6.

O'Toole, M. L., D. B. Hiller, L. O. Crosby, and P. S. Douglas. 1987. The ultraendurance triathlete: A physiological profile. *Med Sci Sports Exerc* 19:45–50.

Pace, N. and E. N. Rathbun. 1945. Studies on body composition. III. The body water and chemically combined nitrogen content in relation to fat content. *J Biol Chem* 158:685–91.

Padilla, S., I. Mujika, F. Angulo, and J. J. Goiriena. 2000a. Scientific approach to the 1-h cycling world record: A case study. *J Appl Physiol* 89:1522–7.

Padilla, S., I. Mujika, G. Cuesta, and J. J. Goiriena. 1999. Level ground and uphill cycling ability in professional road cycling. *Med Sci Sports Exerc* 31:878–85.

Padilla, S., I. Mujika, J. Orbananos, and F. Angulo. 2000b. Exercise intensity during competition time trials in professional road cycling. *Med Sci Sports Exerc* 32:850–6.

Palmer, G. S., J. A. Hawley, S. C. Dennis, and T. D. Noakes. 1994. Heart rate responses during a 4-d cycle stage race. *Med Sci Sports Exerc* 26:1278–83.

Palmeri, S. T., J. B. Kostis, L. Casazza et al. 2007. Heart rate and blood pressure response in adult men and women during exercise and sexual activity. *Am J Cardiol* 100:1795–801.

Pendergast, D. R., P. E. Di Prampero, A. B. Craig, Jr., D. R. Wilson, and D. W. Rennie. 1977. Quantitative analysis of the front crawl in men and women. *J Appl Physiol Respir Environ Exerc Physiol* 43:475–9.

Pettersson, U., H. Alfredson, P. Nordstrom, K. Henriksson-Larsen, and R. Lorentzon. 2000. Bone mass in female cross-country skiers: Relationship between muscle strength and different BMD sites. *Calcif Tissue Int* 67:199–206.

Pfeiffer, R. P., B. P. Harder, D. Landis, D. Barber, and K. Harper. 1993. Correlating indices of aerobic capacity with performance in elite women road cyclists. *J Strength Cond Res* 7:201–5.

Pichard, C., U. G. Kyle, G. Gremion, M. Gerbase, and D. O. Slosman. 1997. Body composition by x-ray absorptiometry and bioelectrical impedance in female runners. *Med Sci Sports Exerc* 29:1527–34.

Pipes, T. V. 1977. Body composition characteristics of male and female track and field athletes. *Res Q* 48:244–7.

Powers, S. K. and E. T. Howley. 2015. *Exercise Physiology: Theory and Application to Fitness and Performance* (9th Ed.), New York: McGraw-Hill.

Prior, B. M., C. M. Modlesky, E. M. Evans et al. 2001. Muscularity and the density of the fat-free mass in athletes. *J Appl Physiol* 90:1523–31.

Purge, P., J. Jurimae, and T. Jurimae. 2004. Body composition, physical performance and psychological factors contributing to 2000 m sculling in elite rowers. *J Hum Movement Stud* 47:367–78.

Rector, R. S., R. Rogers, M. Ruebel, and P. S. Hinton. 2008. Participation in road cycling vs running is associated with lower bone mineral density in men. *Metabolism* 57:226–32.

Risser, W. L., E. J. Lee, A. LeBlanc et al. 1990. Bone density in eumenorrheic female college athletes. *Med Sci Sports Exerc* 22:570–4.

Roelofs, E. J., A. E. Smith-Ryan, M. N. Melvin et al. 2015. Muscle size, quality, and body composition: Characteristics of division I cross-country runners. *J Strength Cond Res* 29:290–6.

Ross, R. and I. Janssen. 2005. Computed tomography and magnetic resonance imaging. In *Human Body Composition*, eds. S. B. Heymesfield, T. G. Lohman, Z. Wang, and S. B. Going, 89–108. Champaign, Illinois: Human Kinetics.

Rowbottom, D. G., D. Keast, P. Garcia-Webb, and A. R. Morton. 1997. Training adaptation and biological changes among well-trained male triathletes. *Med Sci Sports Exerc* 29:1233–9.

Rundell, K. W. and D. W. Bacharach. 1995. Physiological characteristics and performance of top U.S. biathletes. *Med Sci Sports Exerc* 27:302–10.

Rusko, H. 2003. Physiology of cross country skiing. In *Handbook of Sports Medicine and Science: Cross Country Skiing*, ed. H. Rusko, 1–31. Oxford, UK: Blackwell Science Ltd.

Russell, A. P., P. F. Le Rossignol, and W. A. Sparrow. 1998. Prediction of elite schoolboy 2000 m rowing ergometer performance from metabolic, anthropometric and strength variables. *J Sports Sci* 16:749–54.

Rust, C. A., B. Knechtle, P. Knechtle, and T. Rosemann. 2013. A comparison of anthropometric and training characteristics between recreational female marathoners and recreational female Ironman triathletes. *Chin J Physiol* 56:1–10.

Sabo, D., L. Bernd, J. Pfeil, and A. Reiter. 1996. Bone quality in the lumbar spine in high-performance athletes. *Eur Spine J* 5:258–63.

Schabort, E. J., S. C. Killian, A. St Clair Gibson, J. A. Hawley, and T. D. Noakes. 2000. Prediction of triathlon race time from laboratory testing in national triathletes. *Med Sci Sports Exerc* 32:844–9.

Schranz, N., G. Tomkinson, T. Olds, and N. Daniell. 2010. Three-dimensional anthropometric analysis: Differences between elite Australian rowers and the general population. *J Sports Sci* 28:459–69.

Schranz, N., G. Tomkinson, T. Olds, J. Petkov, and A. G. Hahn. 2012. Is three-dimensional anthropometric analysis as good as traditional anthropometric analysis in predicting junior rowing performance? *J Sports Sci* 30:1241–8.

Scofield, K. L. and S. Hecht. 2012. Bone health in endurance athletes: Runners, cyclists, and swimmers. *Curr Sports Med Rep* 11:328–34.

Secher, N. H. 1983. The physiology of rowing. *J Sports Sci* 1:23–53.

Secher, N. H. and O. Vaage. 1983. Rowing performance, a mathematical model based on analysis of body dimensions as exemplified by body weight. *Eur J Appl Physiol Occup Physiol* 52:88–93.

Shephard, R. J. 1998. Science and medicine of rowing: A review. *J Sports Sci* 16:603–20.

Silva, A. M., C. S. Minderico, P. J. Teixeira, A. Pietrobelli, and L. B. Sardinha. 2006. Body fat measurement in adolescent athletes: Multicompartment molecular model comparison. *Eur J Clin Nutr* 60:955–64.

Silva, D. A., T. R. Benedetti, E. P. Ferrari et al. 2012. Anthropometric profiles of elite older triathletes in the Ironman Brazil compared with those of young Portuguese triathletes and older Brazilians. *J Sports Sci* 30:479–84.

Siri, W. E. 1961. Body composition from fluid spaces and density: Analysis of methods. In *Techniques for Measuring Body Composition*, eds. J. Brozek and A. Henschel, 223–44. Washington, DC: National Academy of Sciences.

Slater, G. J., A. J. Rice, I. Mujika et al. 2005. Physique traits of lightweight rowers and their relationship to competitive success. *Br J Sports Med* 39:736–41.

Slemenda, C. W. and C. C. Johnston. 1993. High intensity activities in young women: Site specific bone mass effects among female figure skaters. *Bone Miner* 20:125–32.

Smathers, A. M., M. G. Bemben, and D. A. Bemben. 2009. Bone density comparisons in male competitive road cyclists and untrained controls. *Med Sci Sports Exerc* 41:290–6.

Staib, J. L., I. M. Joohee, Z. Caldwell, and K. W. Rundell. 2000. Cross-country ski racing performance predicted by aerobic and anaerobic double poling power. *J Strength Cond Res* 14:282–8.

Stanforth, P. R., B. N. Crim, D. Stanforth, and M. A. Stults-Kolehmainen. 2014. Body composition changes among female NCAA division 1 athletes across the competitive season and over a multiyear time frame. *J Strength Cond Res* 28:300–7.

Steinacker, J. M. 1993. Physiological aspects of training in rowing. *Int J Sports Med* 14:S3–10.

Stewart, A. and M. Marfell-Jones. 2006. In *International Standards for Anthropometric Assessment*. eds. A. D. Stewart and M. Marfell-Jones. The Secretary-General School of Physical Education, Exercise and Sport Studies The University of South Australia Holbrooks Rd, Underdale, SA, Australia, pp. 1–131 (Pages 137), ISBN: 0-620-36207-3.

Stewart, A. D. and J. Hannan. 2000. Total and regional bone density in male runners, cyclists, and controls. *Med Sci Sports Exerc* 32:1373–7.

Stoggl, T., J. Enqvist, E. Muller, and H. C. Holmberg. 2010. Relationships between body composition, body dimensions, and peak speed in cross-country sprint skiing. *J Sports Sci* 28:161–9.

Swain, D. P., J. R. Coast, P. S. Clifford, M. C. Milliken, and J. Stray-Gundersen. 1987. Influence of body size on oxygen consumption during bicycling. *J Appl Physiol* 62:668–72.

Szulc, P., F. Munoz, F. Marchand, R. Chapurlat, and P. D. Delmas. 2010. Rapid loss of appendicular skeletal muscle mass is associated with higher all-cause mortality in older men: The prospective MINOS study. *Am J Clin Nutr* 91:1227–36.

Taaffe, D. R., C. Snow-Harter, D. A. Connolly et al. 1995. Differential effects of swimming versus weight-bearing activity on bone mineral status of eumenorrheic athletes. *J Bone Miner Res* 10:586–93.

Tcheng, T. K. and C. M. Tipton. 1973. Iowa wrestling study: Anthropometric measurements and the prediction of a "minimal" body weight for high school wrestlers. *Med Sci Sports* 5:1–10.

Thorland, W. G., G. O. Johnson, G. D. Tharp, T. G. Fagot, and R. W. Hammer. 1984. Validity of anthropometric equations for the estimation of body density in adolescent athletes. *Med Sci Sports Exerc* 16:77–81.

Toth, M. J., A. W. Gardner, P. A. Ades, and E. T. Poehlman. 1994. Contribution of body-composition and physical-activity to age-related decline in peak VO_2 in men and women. *J Appl Physiol* 77:647–52.

Tsunawake, N., Y. Tahara, K. Yukawa et al. 1994. Classification of body shape of male athletes by factor analysis. *Ann Physiol Anthropol* 13:383–92.

Tsunawake, N., Y. Tahara, K. Yukawa et al. 1995. Characteristics of body shape of female athletes based on factor analysis. *Appl Human Sci* 14:55–61.

van Lieshout, J. J., F. Pott, P. L. Madsen, J. van Goudoever, and N. H. Secher. 2001. Muscle tensing during standing—Effects on cerebral tissue oxygenation and cerebral artery blood velocity. *Stroke* 32:1546–51.

Wang, Z. M., P. Deurenberg, S. S. Guo et al. 1998. Six-compartment body composition model: Inter-method comparisons of total body fat measurement. *Int J Obes Relat Metab Disord* 22:329–37.

Warner, S. E., J. M. Shaw, and G. P. Dalsky. 2002. Bone mineral density of competitive male mountain and road cyclists. *Bone* 30:281–6.

Williams, C. A. and P. Bale. 1998. Bias and limits of agreement between hydrodensitometry, bioelectrical impedance and skinfold calipers measures of percentage body fat. *Eur J Appl Physiol Occup Physiol* 77:271–7.

Withers, R. T., M. Borkent, and C. T. Ball. 1990. A comparison of the effects of measured, predicted, estimated and constant residual volumes on the body density of male athletes. *Int J Sports Med* 11:357–61.

Withers, R. T., N. P. Craig, P. C. Bourdon, and K. I. Norton. 1987a. Relative body fat and anthropometric prediction of body density of male athletes. *Eur J Appl Physiol Occup Physiol* 56:191–200.

Withers, R. T., N. O. Whittingham, K. I. Norton et al. 1987b. Relative body fat and anthropometric prediction of body density of female athletes. *Eur J Appl Physiol Occup Physiol* 56:169–80.

Wolman, R. L. 1990. Bone mineral density levels in elite female athletes. *Ann Rheum Dis* 49:1013–6.

Yoshiga, C. C. and M. Higuchi. 2003a. Bilateral leg extension power and fat-free mass in young oarsmen. *J Sports Sci* 21:905–9.

Yoshiga, C. C. and M. Higuchi. 2003b. Rowing performance of female and male rowers. *Scand J Med Sci Sports* 13:317–21.

11 Strength and Speed/Power Athletes

David H. Fukuda, Jay R. Hoffman, and Jeffrey R. Stout

CONTENTS

11.1 INTRODUCTION

A wide variety of sporting activities rely on the qualities of strength, speed, and power in order to maximize performance. Determining specific body composition characteristics may help identify athletic potential for success in sports. Strength and speed/power athletes tend to possess specific anthropometric features, a large fat-free mass to fat mass ratio, and have a predominance of type II muscle fibers. The primary outcomes for these competitors are based upon rapid production of force, maximal strength, and peak power output. While the importance of neuromuscular aspects of these activities cannot be understated, the primary focus of this chapter will be maintained on body composition in strength, speed, and power athletes.

Experience in training specifically for strength and speed/power activities influences the relationship between performance and body composition. For those training less than a year, lower extremity lean body mass is the primary determinant of explosive activities (throwing, jumping, and sprinting), whereas for those training between one and three years, anthropometric factors, muscle architecture of the vastus lateralis, and the cross-sectional area of type IIa/x muscle fibers are highly influential (Methenitis et al. 2016). For athletes training more than three years, explosive performance is related to fascicle length of the vastus lateralis, while additional factors for sprinting include type IIa/x muscle fiber area, while lower extremity lean body mass and type IIa muscle fiber area appear to be associated with throwing activities (Methenitis et al. 2016). These findings highlight the initial influence of lean body mass during training for strength and speed/power activities, which is overtaken by the influence of muscle morphology with additional years of experience (Methenitis et al. 2016).

In order to gain a clear understanding of body composition in strength and speed/power athletes, the first three sections of this chapter will be devoted to single-event (strength, speed, and jumping/throwing) athletes, while the fourth section will provide examples from team sport athletes. Throughout the text, the terms "endomorphy," "mesomorphy," and "ectomorphy" are used to describe body type and can generally be interpreted as the relative predominance of roundness/fatness, musculoskeletal development, and linearity, respectively (Housh et al. 2016).

11.2 STRENGTH ATHLETES

11.2.1 BRIEF DESCRIPTION

The strength athletes described in this section consist of Olympic weightlifting and powerlifting competitors. Both sets of athletes compete in multiple lifting events and are separated by weight categories. Olympic weightlifting competition is focused on the maximal performance of two dynamic multijoint lifts, the snatch and clean and jerk, whereas powerlifting competition consists of maximal performance of the squat, bench press, and deadlift. While each of these lifts is unique, they all result in large compressive and shear forces during their execution (Escamilla et al. 2000). Owing to stratification by body mass, the specific body composition of these athletes varies considerably. Furthermore, body composition values during training phases may not be reflective of those exhibited during competition with reported differences in body mass of 5%–10% between these periods (Storey and Smith 2012).

11.2.2 ANTHROPOMETRY/SOMATOTYPE

Lighter (≤85 kg) male Olympic weightlifting athletes demonstrate mesomorphic or ectomorphic features with lower body fat percentages (5%–10%) than heavier male athletes (>17%) who demonstrate endomorphic mesomorph features (Storey and Smith 2012). Conversely, powerlifters potentially possess greater body fat percentages (light/middleweights: 8%–17%; heavyweights: 20%–30%) while demonstrating primarily mesomorphic features, with higher endomorphic ratings in heavyweights, and similar skeletal proportions across weight classes (Keogh et al. 2007). Female Olympic weightlifters have substantially greater body fat percentages compared to male Olympic weightlifters, with body mass consisting of approximately 30% less contractile tissue (Ford et al. 2000), but are leaner than untrained controls (Stoessel et al. 1991; Storey and Smith 2012). In contrast, male and female powerlifting athletes possess relatively similar body fat percentages (Keogh et al. 2008). In addition to large amounts of muscle mass, both Olympic weightlifters and powerlifters tend to have shorter stature and limb lengths, resulting in an enhanced mechanical advantage compared to other strength/power athletes (Keogh et al. 2007; Storey and Smith 2012).

11.2.3 BODY COMPOSITION AND PERFORMANCE

World record holder strength athletes can lift two to four times their bodyweight, with lightweight athletes achieving greater relative values and heavyweight athletes achieving the greatest absolute values (Table 11.1). In order to achieve these remarkable performances, these athletes have a

TABLE 11.1

World Records (Absolute Values; Multiples of Body Weight) for Male and Female Strength Athletes[a]

	Powerlifting (Unequipped)			
	Men		Women	
Lift	Lightweight (−59 kg)	Heavyweight (120+ kg)	Lightweight (−47 kg)	Heavyweight (84+ kg)
Squat	226 kg; 3.9×	426 kg; 2.5×	152.5 kg; 3.3×	272.5 kg; 2.0×
Bench press	170 kg; 2.9×	270.5 kg; 1.9×	91.5 kg; 2.0×	147.5 kg; 1.1×
Deadlift	270.5 kg; 4.6×	375 kg; 2.6×	175 kg; 3.8×	237.5 kg; 2.0×
Total	661 kg; 11.4×	1008.5 kg; 6.0×	407.5; 8.8×	632.5 kg; 4.6×
	Olympic Lifting			
	Men		Women	
Lift	Lightweight (−56 kg)	Heavyweight (105+ kg)	Lightweight (−48 kg)	Heavyweight (75+ kg)
Snatch	137 kg; 2.4×	214 kg; 1.3×	98 kg; 2.1×	155 kg; 1.5×
Clean and jerk	171 kg; 3.1×	264 kg; 1.9×	121 kg; 2.5×	193 kg; 1.8×
Total	305 kg; 5.4×	475 kg; 3.4×	217 kg; 4.5×	348 kg; 3.3×

[a] Data gathered from http://www.powerlifting-ipf.com/ & http://www.iwf.net/

requisite need for large amounts of muscle mass and unique anthropometric features. In support, competition-winning Argentinian male powerlifters possess greater muscle to bone mass ratios compared to nonwinning powerlifters (5.3 vs. 4.7) (Lovera and Keogh 2015), while stronger power-lifters have shown to have greater levels of muscle mass per unit of height compared to weaker pow-erlifters (Keogh et al. 2009). For both men and women, elite-level Olympic weightlifting athletes have lower body fat percentages and greater lean body mass than their less competitive counterparts (Stone et al. 2005; Fry et al. 2006; Storey and Smith 2012).

Somatotype may be reflective of the level of competition in Olympic weightlifting, with a shift toward greater mesomorphy and lesser endomorphy in international competitors (Orvanova 1990). Furthermore, body mass index (BMI) and body fat percentage, coupled with measures of vertical jump and grip strength, have been reported as primary factors that can be used to discriminate between elite and nonelite Olympic lifting athletes (Fry et al. 2006). In addition, elite Olympic weightlifters have been reported to demonstrate greater force production relative to muscle cross-sectional area when compared to collegiate lifters, despite similarities with regard to muscle size (Funato et al. 2000). These findings reinforce the importance of lifting technique in the more experienced athletes.

Fat-free mass, derived from ultrasound measures, as well as site-specific muscle thicknesses, have been shown to be significantly correlated ($r = 0.61$ to $r = 0.91$) to powerlifting performance in Japanese athletes (Brechue and Abe 2002; Ikebukuro et al. 2011). Further, fascicle lengths of the triceps long-head and vastus lateralis (relative to respective limb lengths) are positively related to each of the powerlifting events, while pennation angle of the triceps long-head and medial gastroc-nemius are negatively associated with bench press and deadlift performance (relative to fat-free mass), respectively (Brechue and Abe 2002). More recently, both absolute and relative (to height) skeletal muscle mass estimations, derived from ultrasound measures, have been shown to be posi-tively related to bench press, squat, deadlift, and overall performance (Ye et al. 2013).

Powerlifters with higher total event (squat + bench press + deadlift) scores demonstrate greater muscle girths with no differences in segment lengths compared to weaker athletes (Lovera and Keogh 2015). Anthropometric ratios likely play a role in the expression of strength during powerlifting. For example, the contribution of specific body proportions may be related to success in individual events. Stronger powerlifters have been demonstrated to exhibit greater chest girth relative to height (Brugsch index) compared to weaker powerlifters (Keogh et al. 2009), which might be beneficial for bench press performance. Competition winners were reported to display greater lower leg length to thigh length (Crural index) compared to nonwinners (Lovera and Keogh 2015), which might indicate potential for success during squats. Furthermore, upper arm length relative to height has been suggested to be a factor to consider during deadlifts (Ye et al. 2013).

11.2.4 OTHER CONSIDERATIONS

In addition to the accumulation of skeletal muscle mass (Kanehisa et al. 1998b; Keogh et al. 2007), strength athletes also demonstrate a variety of unique adaptations with regard to body composition. While muscle fiber type percentages may be similar to nonstrength athletes, Olympic weightlifting and powerlifting athletes appear to have larger cross-sectional areas of type II fibers (Fry et al. 2003a,b; Storey and Smith 2012). The large bony breadths and bone mass reported in powerlifters (Johnson et al. 1990; Keogh et al. 2007) are likely needed to endure the heavy and consistent loading of the skeletal structure utilized during training and competition by these athletes. Site-specific bone mineral density is greater in competitive weightlifters compared to controls (Conroy et al. 1993; Karlsson et al. 1995b; Kanehisa et al. 1998a; Storey and Smith 2012), and this adaptation appears to have long-lasting effects with enhanced bone mass in retired weightlifters reported through the sixth decade of life (Karlsson et al. 1995a).

In a direct comparison with handball players, Olympic weightlifters were shown to have greater upper and lower body maximal strength, as well as greater lower body power output, but comparable upper body power output values (Izquierdo et al. 2002). The similarities between upper body power outputs between these different types of athletes demonstrate the greater contribution of the lower extremities during Olympic weightlifting movements as compared to the upper extremities (Izquierdo et al. 2002). In support, Japanese male collegiate Olympic weightlifting athletes were observed to have greater muscle cross-sectional areas of the thigh and lower leg, but similar upper arm and forearm values, compared to collegiate wrestlers (Kanehisa and Fukunaga 1999). Interestingly, the male collegiate weightlifters had greater thigh length to lower leg length ratios, but lower forearm length to lower leg length and upper arm length to thigh length ratios, than the collegiate wrestlers (Kanehisa and Fukunaga 1999). Taken together, these distinctions are likely attributed to specific adaptations to the activities required by each sport, but highlight the importance of lower body performance and anthropometric ratios within Olympic weightlifting.

With respect to maturation, younger Olympic weightlifting athletes (under the age of 17 years old) demonstrate more ectomorphic features, while older Olympic lifters exhibit an increase in mesomorphic features (Orvanova 1990). When examined within weight classes, the youngest athletes tended to possess more endomorphic and less mesomorphic features, and in the heaviest athletes, ectomorphic features become less prevalent (Orvanova 1990).

Despite the popularity of Olympic weightlifting and powerlifting, additional research is needed to provide greater clarity regarding the relationships between body composition, anthropometry, and performance in strength athletes. For example, little effort has been directed toward the direct comparison of powerlifters and Olympic lifters and few studies exist utilizing female athletes. While quality body composition research has been conducted within subsets of these populations (Keogh et al. 2007; Storey and Smith 2012), typically centered on national or continental champions, there is limited data comparing athletes worldwide with diverse ethnic backgrounds and competition levels.

11.2.5 SCALING FOR BODY MASS (AND AGE)

As is apparent from Table 11.1, discrepancies exist in regard to absolute strength and strength relative to body mass, a form of ratio scaling, with advantages conferred in heavier and lighter athletes, respectively. In order to address this potential dilemma, various mathematical models, such as allometric scaling and polynomial regression, have been proposed to compare strength athletes while accounting for body size (Batterham and George 1997; Dooman and Vanderburgh 2000; Cleather 2006; Markovic and Sekulic 2006). Detailed explanation of these investigations is beyond the scope of this chapter; however, a brief description of the currently used methods in the sports of Olympic weightlifting and powerlifting will be presented.

Individual lift and total lift values in powerlifting can also be calculated as Wilks points (Vanderburgh and Batterham 1999; Arandjelovic 2013). The Wilks formulas are reported to have been developed using a fifth-order polynomial estimating the relationship between expected performance (derived from male and female scores between 1987 and 1994) across weight categories and has been validated for bench press and total scores with respect to official elite performances (world records in 1998 and the top performances between 1996 and 1997 excluding heavyweights) (Vanderburgh and Batterham 1999). Coefficients generated from the Wilks performances are multiplied by individual event and overall scores to establish Wilks points that are used to identify the "Best Lifter" awards for men and women.

In Olympic weightlifting, Sinclair-adjusted scores serve a similar purpose as Wilks points (Sinclair 1985; Alberta Weightlifting Federation 2013). A new set of Sinclair coefficients are devised using a logarithmic model (with a specific adjustment for heavyweights) based upon the relationship between weight categories and world record totals from the previous Olympic quadrennial. The Sinclair coefficients are multiplied by individual event and overall scores to establish Sinclair-adjusted scores that are compared across weight categories and then used to establish rankings. Master athletes can use an additional adjustment, the Meltzer–Faber coefficient, to account for the age-related decline in muscular strength and power (Meltzer 1994; Baker and Tang 2010).

For the purpose of comparison, the Wilks points and Sinclair-adjusted world record values for male and female athletes are presented in Table 11.2. These values demonstrate relatively similar world record values for bench press and both Olympic movements between the lightweight and heavyweight categories, but divergent advantages for the squat and deadlift events with lightweights being superior in the squat and heavyweights being superior in the deadlift. As previously mentioned, discrepancies exist among these lifts, despite attempts to adjust for body size, which are likely related to specific anthropometric factors. Finally, the Wilks points appear to favor the lighter powerlifters, while the Sinclair adjustments appear to favor the heavier Olympic lifters.

TABLE 11.2
Wilks Points and Sinclair-Adjusted World Record Values for Male and Female Athletes

	Powerlifting (Unequipped); Wilks Points			
	Men		Women	
Lift	Lightweight (−59 kg)	Heavyweight (120+ kg)	Lightweight (−47 kg)	Heavyweight (84+ kg)
Bench press	149.38	150.59	123.25	115.29
Total (SQ + BP + DL)	579.90	548.12	551.43	494.36

	Olympic Lifting; Sinclair Adjustment			
	Men		Women	
Lift	Lightweight (−56 kg)	Heavyweight (105+ kg)	Lightweight (48 kg)	Heavyweight (75+ kg)
Snatch	214.03	214.10	161.24	161.80
Clean and jerk	267.72	274.01	198.78	201.47
Total	476.03	482.74	355.71	363.27

Note: SQ: squat; BP: bench press; DL: deadlift.

11.3 SPRINT ATHLETES

11.3.1 BRIEF DESCRIPTION

The athletes described in this section consist of sprint athletes competing in events of 400 m or less. Thus, the development of maximal speed/velocity becomes of paramount importance. Table 11.3 lists the winning and 6th place earning times, as well as stature and body weight, for male and female sprinters at the Olympic Games (2004–2012). Speed is a product of stride length and stride frequency. Both of these sprinting parameters are related to the athlete's height and/or limb length. Height is related with stride length in sprinters (Brechue 2011), while the influence of stride frequency is a function of the trade-off between the ability of the leg to maximize ground reaction forces and minimize moments of inertia (Watts et al. 2012). Increased height is often paired with greater body mass, particularly in team sport athletes, where the relationship with sprint performance tends to be diminished. Movement patterns in sports that require both speed and agility skills present added complexities to these relationships and will be briefly discussed later in this chapter. Despite the relative simplicity of sprinting events, and the aforementioned importance of height/limb length, body composition plays a crucial role in the start, acceleration/attainment of maximal velocity, and maintenance of velocity (Brechue 2011; Aerenhouts et al. 2012).

11.3.2 ANTHROPOMETRY/SOMATOTYPE

Height varies in sprint athletes depending on the event, and has reportedly increased in elite sprinters over the last decade (Watts et al. 2012). Body fat percentages in sprinters range between 6% and 12% in men and 10% and 20% in women (McArdle et al. 2006; Brechue 2011), with body mass values that tend to be less than the normal population (Uth 2005). The extremity (sum of triceps, thigh, and medial calf skinfolds) to trunk (sum of subscapular, suprailiac, and abdominal skinfolds) subcutaneous fat ratio differs between male and female sprinters, with women displaying higher values for 100 m (men: 0.866 ± 0.21; women: 1.459 ± 0.28) and 400 m (men: 0.808 ± 0.16; women: 1.334 ± 0.26) specialists (Legaz Arrese et al. 2005). Elite male sprinters are generally ectomorphic mesomorphs while female sprinters tend to have a more balanced somatotype (Aerenhouts et al. 2012). Furthermore, 100 m sprinters display greater mesomorphic features compared to 400 m sprinters who exhibit greater ectomorphic features (Figueirêdo et al. 2013).

With respect to ultrasound-derived muscle morphology, elite 100 m male sprinters possess long fascicle lengths of the vastus lateralis, but smaller pennation angles than distance runners that are comparable to controls (Abe et al. 2000). Female sprinters have comparable vastus lateralis and gastrocnemius fascicle lengths compared to male sprinters, but a smaller pennation angle for the vastus lateralis compared to controls (Abe et al. 2000, 2001; Kumagai et al. 2000). The enhanced shortening velocity of longer fascicle lengths coupled with the smaller physiological cross-sectional area of the thigh musculature, as indicated by the decreased pennation angle, demonstrate the potential for lower-body specific adaptations of sprint athletes (Abe et al. 2000). Male sprinters also have greater muscle thicknesses of both the upper and lower body compared to distance runners and controls (Abe et al. 2000). Interestingly, marked differences in muscle thickness between these groups were found in the most proximal, but not the most distal portion, of the anterior thigh (Abe et al. 2000). The performance implications of these findings will be presented in the next section.

11.3.3 BODY COMPOSITION AND PERFORMANCE

Body fat percentage in female Japanese sprinters ($16.7 \pm 1.8\%$) has been shown to be significantly related ($r = 0.62$) to personal best 100 m sprint times (12.21 ± 0.70 s) (Abe et al. 2001). While fat-free mass has shown to be correlated with running in team sport athletes and recreationally active individuals (Abe et al. 1999; Chelly and Denis 2001; Perez-Gomez et al. 2008; Brechue et al. 2010; Brechue 2011), this relationship does not appear to be present in elite sprinters (Kumagai et al. 2000;

TABLE 11.3
Winning and 6th Place Performances for Male and Female Sprinters at the Olympic Games (2004–2012)[a]

Event	Year	Men						Women					
		Gold			6th Place			Gold			6th Place		
		Height (m)	Weight (kg)	Time (s)	Height (m)	Weight (kg)	Time (s)	Height (m)	Weight (kg)	Time (s)	Height (m)	Weight (kg)	Time (s)
100 m	2012	1.96	86	9.63	1.88	80	9.98	1.6	52	10.75	1.67	54	10.94
	2008	1.96	86	9.69	1.7	67	9.97	1.6	52	10.78	1.63	60	11.14
	2004	1.85	83	9.85	1.8	77	10.00	1.76	62	10.93	1.63	59	11.07
200 m	2012	1.96	86	19.32	1.9	74	20.19	1.68	55	21.88	1.70	57	22.57
	2008	1.96	86	19.30	1.8	77	20.59	1.63	61	21.74	1.63	59	22.36
	2004	1.81	86	19.79	1.72	70	20.24	1.63	61	22.05	1.70	60	22.84
400 m	2012	1.8	66	43.94	1.8	67	44.83	1.73	62	49.55	1.68	59	50.17
	2008	1.88	84	43.75	1.98	79	45.12	1.75	70	49.62	1.74	59	50.11
	2004	1.88	71	44.00	1.78	78	44.83	1.68	59	49.42	1.73	62	50.19

[a] Data gathered from http://www.sports-reference.com/olympics/summer.

Abe et al. 2001). This discrepancy may be related to the overall influence of body mass on running speed and relative homogeneity of anthropometric specifications in sprint athletes compared to athletes with diverse specialties and playing positions (Brechue et al. 2010; Brechue 2011).

Differences with respect to body composition and performance likely exist among sprinters competing in different distances. For example, performance times in 100 m sprint athletes have been demonstrated to be significantly related to calf circumferences ($r = -0.55$), whereas 400 m sprint performance was significantly related to height ($r = -0.53$) in athletes that compete regularly in this event (Figueirêdo et al. 2013). Anthropometric ratios may be used as potential predictors of performance in sprint athletes; however, these measures also illustrate the complexity of these relationships. BMI ($kg \cdot m^{-2}$), a potential predictor of both adiposity and muscle mass, has been shown to be lower in elite sprinters as compared to the general population (Uth 2005). More recently, the reciprocal ponderal index ($m \cdot kg^{-0.333}$), a measure of linearity, has shown to exert a greater influence than BMI on sprint times in elite male and female 100 m sprint athletes (Watts et al. 2012). These relationships support the notion that height/limb length, potentially through altered stride length, is an important factor in sprint performance.

As indicated earlier, sprint events can be separated into several phases. In female sprinters, body fat percentage ($r = 0.51$) is significantly associated with the length of the first step during a 20 m sprint, while endomorphic rating is significantly associated with the first ($r = 0.44$) and fourth ($r = 0.74$) steps (Aerenhouts et al. 2012). The relationship between body fat percentage and sprint performance in female sprinters ($r = 0.62$), in the absence of similar associations with fat-free mass or BMI, has been previously corroborated by others (Abe et al. 2001). Sexual dimorphism appears to exist with respect to these comparisons, as calf girths of male sprint athletes corrected for skinfold thickness are significantly related to the first, third, fourth, and fifth steps during sprinting ($r = 0.38–0.76$) (Aerenhouts et al. 2012). The lack of any association between body fat percentage and sprint performance in male sprinters, despite having a greater body mass, suggests that the differences in sprint times between the genders may be related to the addition of fat-free mass in men compared to women.

The influence of muscle architecture on sprint times and personal best 100-m sprint performances has been shown to be related to muscle thickness ($r = -0.54$ to -0.62) of the knee extensors (Ikebukuro et al. 2011; Kubo et al. 2011). This is consistent with investigations comparing sprint and endurance athletes with controls. In these studies, sprint times in elite female sprinters were correlated with fascicle lengths of the vastus lateralis and lateral gastrocnemius (-0.51 and -0.44), but not pennation angle of these muscles (Abe et al. 2001). Male sprinters with 100 m sprint times below 10 s were demonstrated to have greater fascicle lengths and lesser pennation angles when compared to sprinters whose performance times exceeded 10 s (Kumagai et al. 2000). While the two groups had similar limb lengths, the faster sprinters demonstrated greater proximal muscle thickness in the vastus lateralis than the slower sprinters but comparable distal muscle thicknesses (Kumagai et al. 2000). These findings support the notion that sprinters may benefit more from enhanced shortening velocities generated by an increased fascicle length, as opposed to the greater physiological cross-sectional area associated with an increased pennation angle (Kumagai et al. 2000). Furthermore, the nonhomogenous adaptation of thigh musculature might confer benefits through alterations in the generation of force and moment of inertia during sprinting activities (Brechue 2011).

11.3.4 OTHER CONSIDERATIONS

Differences in skeletal muscle mass have been reported between junior and senior elite male sprinters, but not between junior and senior elite female sprinters (Aerenhouts et al. 2012). With respect to anthropometric changes, a shift toward more pronounced mesomorphic features occurs in male and female sprinters between the junior and senior ranks, while male sprinters only feature a significant decline in ectomorphic features (Aerenhouts et al. 2012). These developmental changes in sprinters ultimately result in the ectomorphic mesomorph and balanced ectomorph somatotypes previously described in male and female senior athletes, respectively (Aerenhouts et al. 2012).

In addition to unique anthropometric features and muscle architecture (increased fascicle length, decreased pennation angle) of the lower body, sprint athletes are known to possess high percentage of type II muscle fibers (Korhonen et al. 2006). The functional performance of type II muscle fibers in sprinters, and amount reflecting the MHC IIx isoform, likely differs from other athletes (Trappe et al. 2015). Maximal running velocity declines with aging in sprint athletes with concomitant decreases in leg length and stride length (Korhonen et al. 2009). Decreases in type II muscle fiber area (-4.5% per decade) and lower limb muscle thicknesses (-2% to -6% per decade) have been reported, with the latter being significantly associated with maximal running velocity ($r = 0.28$) and 60 m sprint times ($r = -0.26$) (Korhonen et al. 2009). Muscle thickness was also reported to be a strong predictor, accounting for 26% of the variance in the braking forces generated during sprinting (Korhonen et al. 2009). Interestingly, pennation angle of the vastus lateralis decreased with age ($r = -0.43$), while no change in the medial/lateral gastrocnemius or fascicle length of any of the evaluated muscles were observed (Korhonen et al. 2009). Thus, performance in aging sprinters appears to be compromised due to muscular atrophy and altered running biomechanics.

The repeated loading cycles associated with faster velocities of running result in greater increases in the magnitude of ground reaction forces and skeletal strain (Bennell et al. 1997). A mixed sample of male and female power athletes, including sprinters, hurdlers, jumpers, and multievent athletes, demonstrated greater bone mineral density in the upper and lower limbs compared to age-matched controls, as well as greater bone mineral density in the lumbar spine compared to endurance athletes and controls (Bennell et al. 1997). Competitive master sprint athletes (between the ages of 35 and 94 years) appear to possess greater bone mineral content/density of the tibial diaphysis and epiphysis than control subjects (Wilks et al. 2009). Interestingly, master athletes who competed in races of progressively longer distances displayed gradual decreases in tibial density (Wilks et al. 2009). These differences were evident in both male and female master sprint athletes, with greater bone strength values in men, but comparable tibial circumferences that were greater than controls (Wilks et al. 2009).

11.3.5 SCALING FOR BODY MASS

As discussed earlier, there does not appear to be a relationship between body mass and sprint performance in sprinters when compared to other athletes and untrained individuals. However, sprinters appear to be the largest of the track athletes in regard to both stature and body mass (Weyand and Davis 2005). Furthermore, increased muscle mass has been shown to be beneficial during the production of ground reaction forces, which are vital to achieving maximal velocities (Weyand and Davis 2005). However, to provide any benefit toward improving sprint performances, increases in muscle mass must be specific to areas of the body that improvements in power can be translated to greater speed without negatively impacting the power–velocity relationship (Slawinski et al. 2015). For example, excessive upper body mass would likely be detrimental (Arsac and Locatelli 2002), whereas the earlier-mentioned differences in proximal thigh muscle thickness may be beneficial, to sprinting performance.

Performance improvements in Olympic sprinting events appear to be related to changes in the power to body mass ratio exhibited by elite athletes (Stefani 2008, 2014; Slawinski et al. 2015). Table 11.4 lists the estimated power outputs and power to body mass ratios for the winning and 6th place male and female sprinters at the Olympic Games (2004–2012). Power output requirements and power to body mass ratios appear to decrease in athletes competing in the longer sprint events, though a large amount variability exists in these estimates. Several examples within this data, particularly in female Olympic sprint athletes, illustrate instances where the winning/fastest athlete generated lower power output, but a greater power to body mass ratio, than their slower competitor. This comparison reinforces the reported somatotypes of sprint athletes, specifically regarding

TABLE 11.4

Estimated Power Outputs[a] and Power to Body Mass Ratios for the Winning and 6th Place Male and Female Sprinters at the Olympic Games (2004–2012)

| | | Men | | | | Women | | | |
| | | Gold | | 6th Place | | Gold | | 6th Place | |
Event	Year	Power (W)	P:M_b (W/kg)	Power (W)	P:M_b (W/kg)	Power (W)	P:M_b (W/kg)	Power (W)	P:M_b (W/kg)
100 m	2012	613	7.1	550	6.9	332	6.4	339	6.3
	2008	609	7.1	461	6.9	331	6.4	369	6.2
	2004	578	7.0	528	6.9	389	6.3	366	6.2
200 m	2012	611	7.1	503	6.8	345	6.3	346	6.1
	2008	611	7.1	513	6.7	385	6.3	362	6.1
	2004	596	6.9	475	6.8	380	6.2	360	6.0
400 m	2012	412	6.2	410	6.1	343	5.5	323	5.5
	2008	527	6.3	480	6.1	387	5.5	323	5.5
	2004	443	6.2	477	6.1	328	5.6	339	5.5

[a] Estimated using the equations and assumptions outlined by Stefani (2008). P:M_b: power to body mass ratio.

leanness and muscularity, while giving guidance with respect to the selection of appropriate training and dietary interventions.

11.4 JUMPING AND THROWING ATHLETES

11.4.1 BRIEF DESCRIPTION

The athletes described in this section compete in the field events involving jumping (long jump, triple jump, high jump, pole vault) and throwing (discus, shot put, javelin, and hammer throw). These activities require competitors to project their bodies or objects with the intention of achieving either maximal distance or height. During jumping events, athletes generally utilize linear acceleration to achieve maximal approach speeds and horizontal/vertical takeoff forces (see Table 11.5), while throwing events utilize angular acceleration to achieve maximal angular speed and torque. These unique approaches result in drastically different body composition between competitors in field events with the first group tending to resemble sprint athletes and the second group resembling the heaviest strength athletes. Exceptions should be noted for pole vaulters, due to increased upper body strength/power requirements, and javelin throwers, due to an extended linear approach, who exhibit altered anthropometric and body composition requirements with respect to the jumping and throwing athletes, respectively.

11.4.2 ANTHROPOMETRY/SOMATOTYPE

Body fat percentages in male and female jumpers are reported to range between 7%–14% and 10%–20%, respectively (McArdle et al. 2006). A large group of male and female Czech, Slovak, and Danish high jumpers were assessed as being primarily ectomorphic mesomorphs from data collected over a 20-year period (Langer 2007). Female Greek youth jumping athletes displayed lower body mass, limb circumferences, skinfold thicknesses, and mesomorphic ratings compared to volleyball players (Rousanoglou et al. 2006). In addition to jump height, the sum of skinfold thicknesses, mid-thigh circumference, and knee breadth were found to be the best discriminators between jumpers, volleyball players, and a control group (Rousanoglou et al. 2006). Potentially reflective of the requirements of

TABLE 11.5
Winning and 6th Place Performances for Male and Female Jumping Athletes at the Olympic Games (2004–2012)[a]

Event	Year	Men						Women					
		Gold			6th Place			Gold			6th Place		
		Height (m)	Mass (kg)	Result (m)	Height (m)	Mass (kg)	Result (m)	Height (m)	Mass (kg)	Result (m)	Height (m)	Mass (kg)	Result (m)
Long jump	2012	1.88	84	8.31	1.97	81	8.07	1.73	62	7.12	1.75	64	6.76
	2008	1.83	70	8.34	1.90	82	8.16	1.73	61	7.04	1.72	58	6.70
	2004	1.85	73	8.59	1.85	73	8.24	1.7	61	7.07	1.85	70	6.80
High jump	2012	1.92	67	2.38	1.95	83	2.29	1.80	57	2.05	1.75	60	1.97
	2008	1.98	83	2.36	1.96	82	2.29	1.82	62	2.05	1.75	60	1.99
	2004	1.81	71	2.36	1.98	83	2.32	1.78	60	2.06	1.80	57	1.96

[a] Data gathered from http://www.sports-reference.com/olympics/summer.

their event, U.S. pole vaulters, ranging in age from 13–18 years, exhibited ectomorphic mesomorph features, which were similar across age groups (Sullivan et al. 1994).

While the heights and weights of jumping athletes tend to be similar to population averages and have remained relatively stable, throwing athletes benefit from greater body size and have been reported to be growing at an increasing rate, particularly with regard to body mass, compared to other athletes since 1970 (Norton and Olds 2001). Recently, dual-energy x-ray absorptiometry (DXA)-derived body composition data showed collegiate male and female jumpers, pole vaulters, and javelin throwers to have lower body mass, fat mass, body fat percentage, and trunk fat than collegiate throwing athletes (Hirsch et al. 2016). Throwers also demonstrated greater absolute lean mass and lean mass relative to body mass than other track and field athletes (Hirsch et al. 2016). Male and female throwing athletes have body fat percentages ranging between 12%–21% and 20%–30%, respectively, with endomorphic mesomorph features and low ectomorphic ratings (Kruger et al. 2006; McArdle et al. 2006; Terzis et al. 2010; Singh et al. 2012).

11.4.3 BODY COMPOSITION AND PERFORMANCE

Body composition plays a major role in performance for jumping athletes. Successful high jumpers appear to be taller, heavier, and have longer limbs with larger circumferences, as well as greater lean body mass, than their less successful counterparts (Singh et al. 2010). With respect to somatotype, better high jumpers can be characterized as having a greater mesomorphic and lesser endomorphic rating (Singh et al. 2010). Smaller skeletal structure, assessed by elbow and knee breadths, and skinfold thickness, combined with larger jumping ability and body mass, in youth jumpers compared to volleyball players highlight the different jumping requirements, projection-based versus stationary, respectively, between these groups of athletes (Rousanoglou et al. 2006).

Pole vaulting performance is highly correlated ($r = 0.88$) with the height of the top hand on the pole at the apex of the vault, but is also positively influenced by ectomorphic rating, limb circumferences, and skinfold thicknesses (Sullivan et al. 1994). In addition to running speed and strength/power, the placement of the hand during the vault is significantly related to body mass ($r = 0.71$), biceps circumference ($r = 0.66$), and calf circumference (0.61) (Sullivan et al. 1994). Thus, height, leanness, and muscle mass of the limbs likely contribute to the specific speed and strength/power capabilities needed to successfully compete in pole vaulting.

Despite evaluating a wide variety of anthropometric measures and body composition estimates, only mid-thigh girth and chest breadth were found to be different in world class (top 10) and competitive international (top 88) javelin throwers (Kruger et al. 2006). However, age, body mass, muscle mass percentage, mesomorphic rating, chest depth, chest breadth, and arm span were found to be significant discriminant variables between the groups of athletes (Kruger et al. 2006). Hammer throw performance is related to lean body mass ($r = 0.81$), leg lean mass ($r = 0.84$), trunk lean mass ($r = 0.85$), and the cross-sectional area of various muscle fiber types ($r \leq 0.90$) but not body fat, bone mineral density, body mass, or fiber type distribution (Terzis et al. 2010). The differences in the relationship between body mass and performance in javelin and hammer throwers may be a reflection of the running and rotational components, respectively, associated with the approach phase of these events.

More successful collegiate shot putters in India were taller with greater lean body mass, limb and chest circumferences, larger arm, shoulder, and hip circumferences, and lower endomorphic ratings than less successful shot putters (Singh et al. 2012). Technical variation may play a role in the influence of body composition during the shot put. Shot put performance from the power position has shown to be related to fat-free mass during both the preseason ($r = 0.76$) and competitive ($r = 0.66$) periods (Kyriazis et al. 2010). However, the positive correlation between shot put performance using the rotational style (spin technique), which may require a greater level of technical ability, and fat-free mass noted during the preseason ($r = 0.70$) appears to be diminished during the competitive period (Kyriazis et al. 2010). In support of the notion that technical improvements may limit this relationship, a 9-year case study on a Greek national champion reported no relationship between DXA-derived body composition values and shot put distances using the rotational style (Terzis et al. 2012).

With regard to muscle morphology in a mixed sample of throwing athletes, shot put performance from the power position (and rate of force development) was associated with fascicle length and muscle thickness, as well as appendicular, trunk, and total lean body mass values (Zaras et al. 2016). Furthermore, changes in the rate of force development following a 10-week periodized training program were related to changes in lean body mass, while changes in shot put performance were related to changes in vastus lateralis muscle thickness (Zaras et al. 2016). Interestingly, 53% of the variance reported in improvements in shot put performance could be attributed to changes in vastus lateralis muscle thickness and rate of force development (Zaras et al. 2016).

11.4.4 OTHER CONSIDERATIONS

With regard to muscle fiber type, experienced hammer throwers showed a greater percentage of type IIa fibers ($51.1 \pm 9.0\%$ vs. $34.4 \pm 6.0\%$), with comparable percentage of IIx fibers ($9.0 \pm 7.0\%$ vs. $14.3 \pm 7.0\%$), and a lesser percentage of type I fibers ($39.9 \pm 5.0\%$ vs. $51.4 \pm 7.0\%$) compared to untrained controls (Terzis et al. 2010). However, only the cross-sectional area of type IIa fibers (7703 ± 1171 μm^2 vs. 5676 ± 1270 μm^2) were found to be larger in the throwing athletes (Terzis et al. 2010). The hammer throwers also had significantly greater bone mineral density (1.484 ± 0.046 g/cm^2 vs. 1.264 ± 0.080 g/cm^2) than the control group (Terzis et al. 2010). Similar findings were reported in male collegiate shot putters with regard to total body and regional bone mineral densities (Whittington et al. 2009). Furthermore, male throwing athletes had greater bone mineral density than female throwing athletes, and regional bone mineral density values were significantly correlated with peak force ($r > 0.79$) and rate of force development ($r = 0.89$) generated during an isometric mid-thigh pull test as well as ball throw performance ($r > 0.81$) (Whittington et al. 2009). Interestingly, the combined group of shot put athletes showed bilateral differences in arm bone mineral density suggesting specific physiological adaptations to the athlete's dominant or throwing side (Whittington et al. 2009).

Former elite throwing and jumping athletes were reported to have greater lumbar bone mineral density than marathon athletes (Schmitt et al. 2005). Differences were found to persist despite consideration given to a variety of potential confounders, including age, BMI, training history, current physical activity levels, and degenerative spinal issues (Schmitt et al. 2005). These findings were attributed to self-selection, sport-specific loading, and the training methodologies employed by the athletes. Conversely, former elite throwers and high jumpers may display greater vertebral osteophytes than former runners and athletes competing in long/triple jump or pole vault. This may be related to the rotational requirements, and hyperextension in the case of the high jump, required in these events (Schmitt et al. 2004).

Muscle activation, strength/power characteristics, and muscle morphology have been reported to decrease with aging in a cross-sectional evaluation of master throwing athletes (Ojanen et al. 2007). Despite the general maintenance of body fat percentages (between 23% and 27%), 40-year-old throwing athletes have significantly greater muscle thickness of the leg extensors and triceps brachii compared to their 60- and 75-year-old counterparts (Ojanen et al. 2007). Middle-aged (52 years old) and older (~72 years old) Finnish master throwing athletes were reported to have greater lean body mass compared to age-matched controls, while older athletes had greater lean body mass than a middle-aged control group (~65 kg vs. ~55 kg, respectively) (Sallinen et al. 2008). Leg extensor strength relative to body mass was reported to be higher in older master athletes compared to both age-matched and young controls (~26 years old) (Sallinen et al. 2008). While no differences were seen in vastus lateralis muscle thickness between master throwing athletes or any of the control groups, leg extensor strength relative to vastus lateralis muscle thickness was greater in the middle-aged and older athletes compared to younger controls (Sallinen et al. 2008). Thus, master throwing athletes appear to maintain muscle mass and strength/power performance compared to nonathletes, but the age-related decline in these measures continues to occur.

TABLE 11.6

Estimated Power Outputs[a] and Power to Body Mass Ratios for the Winning and 6th Place Male and Female Jumping Athletes at the Olympic Games (2004–2012)

| | | Men | | | | Women | | | |
| | | Gold | | 6th Place | | Gold | | 6th Place | |
Event	Year	Power (W)	P:M$_b$ (W/kg)	Power (W)	P:M$_b$ (W/kg)	Power (W)	P:M$_b$ (W/kg)	Power (W)	P:M$_b$ (W/kg)
Long jump	2012	1372	16.3	1297	16.0	928	15.0	925	14.4
	2008	1146	16.4	1323	16.1	906	14.9	833	14.4
	2004	1219	16.7	1185	16.2	909	14.9	1016	14.5
High jump	2012	1663	24.8	1974	23.8	1264	22.2	1297	21.6
	2008	2017	24.3	1945	23.7	1368	22.1	1310	21.8
	2004	1790	25.2	1985	23.9	1344	22.4	1208	21.2

[a] Estimated using the equations and assumptions outlined by Stefani (2008). P:M$_b$: power to body mass ratio.

11.4.5 SCALING FOR BODY MASS

Similar to the discussion presented in sprinters, and in conjunction with the importance of muscle size and function with field event athletes, power to body mass ratios may also be useful when evaluating performance, particularly during jumping events. All of the jumping events contain a sprinting component during the initial approach, which provides the basis for increasing kinetic energy that can be transformed to potential energy (Stefani 2008). Owing to the limited time needed to complete the jumps, greater power outputs are produced during jumping events compared to running events and technical improvements likely play a greater role in performance (Stefani 2008). Nonetheless, the positive influence of lean body mass and potentially negative influence of total body mass can be illustrated by the estimated power to body mass ratios for Olympic jumpers presented in Table 11.6. It appears that male long jump and female high jump gold medalists have a tendency to exhibit greater power to body mass ratios than their less successful competitors despite lower overall power production during the event.

11.5 EXAMPLES FROM TEAM SPORTS

11.5.1 POSITION COMPARISONS: AMERICAN FOOTBALL

The activity/event-specific body composition illustrated in the sections devoted to strength, sprinting, and jumping/throwing athletes provide the basis for the comparison of team sport athletes stratified by playing position. Either through the selection process or through specific adaptations from sport- or position-specific stimuli, body composition varies greatly in team sports where athletes are assigned designated roles within the framework of the rules or strategies of the competition. However, it should be noted that the majority of the available body composition data has been collected in small groups and/or single teams (Snow et al. 1998; Kraemer et al. 2005; Pryor et al. 2014).

Changes in body composition of National Football League (NFL) players between 1980 and 2000 (Snow et al. 1998) appear to have somewhat stabilized with regard to whole body fat and fat-free mass (Anzell et al. 2013; Pryor et al. 2014). When classified by BMI values, the majority of these athletes can be classified as being overweight to severely obese (Dengel et al. 2014); however, body fat percentages from DXA vary greatly by position with offensive and defensive linemen (27 ± 6%; range: 12%–39%) being greater than linebackers, tight ends, and running backs (17 ± 4%; 8%–25%), which are greater than wide receivers and defensive backs (12% ± 3%; range 7%–23%)

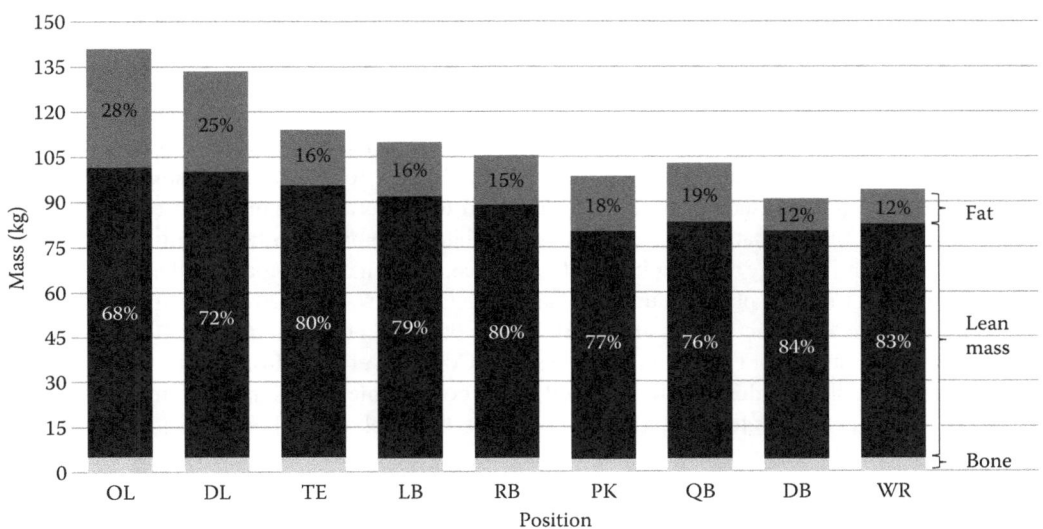

FIGURE 11.1   Dual x-ray absorptiometry (DXA)-derived body composition by position in National Football League players. OL: offensive line; DL: defensive line; TE: tight end; LB: linebacker; RB: running back; PK: place kicker; QB: quarterback; DB: defensive back; WR: wide receiver. (Adapted from Dengel, D. R., T. A. Bosch, T. P. Burruss et al. 2014. *J Strength Cond Res* 28:1–6.)

(Bosch et al. 2014). Select body composition values by position in NFL players are presented in Figure 11.1. Lean body mass and abdominal lean/fat mass appear to follow similar patterns between positions (Bosch et al. 2014; Dengel et al. 2014). These differences can be attributed to the roles of these athletes with linemen being tasked with blocking and/or impeding the opponent generally through inertia, whereas the other (skill) positions rely on varying degrees of strength and speed/power to outmaneuver or tackle the opponent using changes in momentum.

Additional comparisons reveal greater body fat percentages in offensive compared to defensive linemen, despite similar lean body mass and upper to lower body lean mass ratios. This has been suggested to be related to a greater emphasis on speed movements (e.g., pass rushing and chasing/tackling running backs) required on the part of defensive linemen (Dengel et al. 2014). Tight ends, who often have both receiving and blocking responsibilities on offense, display unique characteristics with fat mass values similar to running backs and linebackers, but greater upper body lean mass that is comparable to linemen (Dengel et al. 2014). Positional differences have also been reported in ultrasound-derived muscle cross-sectional area of the vastus lateralis in American collegiate football players with defensive linemen displaying greater values than wide receivers, placekickers, linebackers, and defensive backs, which mirrored significant differences in leg lean mass from DXA (Melvin et al. 2014).

11.5.2   REGIONAL MUSCLE MORPHOLOGY: SOCCER

The sport of soccer has a highly aerobic base but the ability to perform sprints of varying intensities and utilize strength/power characteristics during acceleration, change of direction, jumping, tackling, and kicking are likely determinants of success during competition (Stolen et al. 2005). Thus, the musculature of the lower body plays a major role in soccer and the morphological characteristics previously described in the sections covering strength, sprint, and jumping/throwing athletes should also be considered. Japanese youth soccer players (~16.5 years) have been demonstrated to exhibit greater lower leg length, lower leg circumference, and ultrasound-derived muscle thickness of the medial gastrocnemius in the dominant limb compared to university-aged controls (~18 years) (Kearns et al. 2001). Cross-sectional areas of various muscles (measured from magnetic resonance imaging [MRI]) within the thigh are reported to be larger in Japanese professional (~24 years) compared to elite-level youth (~17 years) soccer players (Hoshikawa et al. 2009). Despite no differences between above average and average Japanese university soccer players, upper leg muscle cross-sectional area has shown to be positively related ($r = 0.40–0.60$) to knee and hip isokinetic flexion/extension peak torque (Masuda et al. 2003). In regard to performance, maximal oxygen uptake, muscle thickness, and pennation angle of the vastus lateralis appear to be significant predictors ($R^2 = 0.978$) of high-intensity running in female American National Collegiate Athletic Association (NCAA) Division I soccer players during a game (McCormack et al. 2014). Furthermore, these muscle morphological characteristics are significantly related ($r = 0.893$ and $r = 0.740$, respectively) to fatigue rate measured from a 30-s Wingate test (McCormack et al. 2014).

In a comparison of individual and team-based speed/power athletes, Japanese Olympic swimmers and soccer players demonstrated unique lower body muscle morphological characteristics (Kanehisa et al. 2003). Within the vastus lateralis, the aquatic athletes had greater muscle thickness values than the soccer players; however, owing to between sex differences, only the male swimmers exhibited greater fascicle length and smaller pennation angle values than the male soccer players (Kanehisa et al. 2003). Comparisons of the medial gastrocnemius revealed similar muscle thicknesses between the different athletes, but swimmers had longer fascicle lengths and reduced pennation angle (Kanehisa et al. 2003). These relationships are depicted in Figure 11.2a and potentially demonstrate the relative importance of contraction velocity (increased stroke frequency) in swimming. A greater contraction velocity would be supported by longer fascicles in swimmers, while a greater emphasis on force production in soccer (specifically in the medial gastrocnemius) would be conferred by higher pennation angle yielding greater physiological cross-sectional area (Kanehisa et al. 2003). Interestingly, in female American collegiate soccer players, starters display similar muscle thickness values of the vastus lateralis, but greater pennation angle than nonstarters (Jajtner et al. 2013). In consideration for the relationships shown in Figure 11.2a, it might be assumed that the starters possessed longer fascicle lengths possibly related to differences in speed; however, these values were not reported. Furthermore, starters experienced greater decreases in muscle morphology compared to nonstarting athletes over the course of the competitive season (Jajtner et al. 2013). During a 15-week offseason resistance training program, female soccer athletes demonstrated increased vastus lateralis muscle thickness and fascicle length while maintaining pennation angle (Wells et al. 2014). This change is illustrated in Figure 11.2b. Furthermore, changes in 1RM squat strength were associated with changes in both muscle thickness ($r = 0.561$) and fascicle length ($r = 0.503$) (Wells et al. 2014).

Despite similar values for pennation angle in the medial gastrocnemius, the percentage difference between dominant and nondominant legs have shown to be significantly greater in Japanese youth soccer players compared to controls (Kearns et al. 2001). A comparison of the upper leg musculature in junior and senior Japanese soccer players reported no lateral dominance in MRI-derived muscle cross-sectional area, but showed that the younger players had a predominance of the quadriceps femoris cross-sectional area while the older players had a predominance of the hamstrings and adductors (Hoshikawa et al. 2009). This shift in predominance between junior and senior athletes was paired with an increase in the knee flexion to knee extension torque ratio and may be indicative of the importance of the hamstrings contribution to maximal speed and stabilization during kicking (Fried and Lloyd 1992; Delecluse 1997; Hoshikawa et al. 2009). Thus, these adaptations may be indicative of improved performance and potentially protective against injury.

11.6 CONCLUSION

The relationship between body composition and performance in strength and speed/power athletes is multifaceted. Lean body mass and muscle morphology may be associated with power output via enhanced force production and movement velocities, while anthropometrics likely contribute

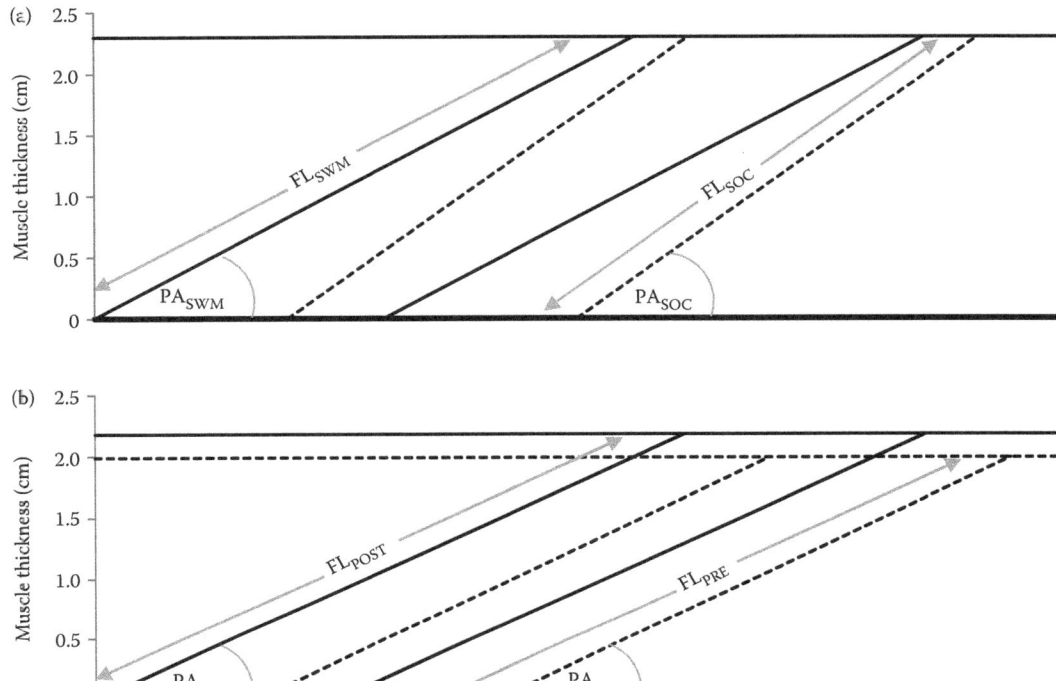

FIGURE 11.2 Schematic diagram comparing the muscle architectural characteristics of (A) the gastrocnemius medialis of elite soccer players (dashed line; SOC) and swimmers (solid line; SWM) and (B) the vastus lateralis of collegiate female soccer players before (dashed line; PRE) and after (solid line; POST) an offseason resistance training program. FL: fascicle length; PA: pennation angle. (Adapted from Kanehisa, H. et al 2003. *Int J Sports Med* 24:90–5; Jajtner, A. R. et al. 2013. *J Strength Cond Res* 27:2355–65; Wells, A. J. et al. 2014. *Muscle Nerve* 50:785–93.)

through biomechanical influences. Owing to the highly variable nature of sport and individual characteristics of athletes, as well as the limited data available, the ability to clearly define ranges of body composition values that are related to performance is limited. However, specific considerations, adjusted to the level of competition, should be given to fat-free to fat mass ratios and power to body mass ratios in these athletes. Furthermore, depending on the sport, certain anthropometric ratios may be of particular importance as appears to be the case in competitive weightlifting. Finally, further research is needed in order to fully utilize body composition parameters in the talent identification process and during the training and evaluation of strength and speed/power athletes.

REFERENCES

Abe, T., J. B. Brown, and W. F. Brechue. 1999. Architectural characteristics of muscle in black and white college football players. *Med Sci Sports Exerc* 31:1448–52.

Abe, T., S. Fukashiro, Y. Harada, and K. Kawamoto. 2001. Relationship between sprint performance and muscle fascicle length in female sprinters. *J Physiol Anthropol Appl Human Sci* 20:141–7.

Abe, T., K. Kumagai, and W. F. Brechue. 2000. Fascicle length of leg muscles is greater in sprinters than distance runners. *Med Sci Sports Exerc* 32:1125–9.

Aerenhouts, D., C. Delecluse, F. Hagman et al. 2012. Comparison of anthropometric characteristics and sprint start performance between elite adolescent and adult sprint athletes. *Eur J Sport Sci* 12:9–15.

Alberta Weightlifting Federation. 2013. Sinclair Coefficients 2013. http://www.iwf.net/wp-content/uploads/downloads/2013/02/Sinclair_Coefficients_2013.pdf. (accessed February 1, 2016).

Anzell, A. R., J. A. Potteiger, W. J. Kraemer, and S. Otieno. 2013. Changes in height, body weight, and body composition in American football players from 1942 to 2011. *J Strength Cond Res* 27:277–84.

Arandjelovic, O. 2013. On self-propagating methodological flaws in performance normalization for strength and power sports. *Sports Med* 43:451–61.

Arsac, L. M. and E. Locatelli. 2002. Modeling the energetics of 100-m running by using speed curves of world champions. *J Appl Physiol* 92:1781–8.

Baker, A. B. and Y. Q. Tang. 2010. Aging performance for masters records in athletics, swimming, rowing, cycling, triathlon, and weightlifting. *Exp Aging Res* 36:453–77.

Batterham, A. M. and K. P. George. 1997. Allometric modeling does not determine a dimensionless power function ratio for maximal muscular function. *J Appl Physiol* 83:2158–66.

Bennell, K. L., S. A. Malcolm, K. M. Khan et al. 1997. Bone mass and bone turnover in power athletes, endurance athletes, and controls: A 12-month longitudinal study. *Bone* 20:477–84.

Bosch, T. A., T. P. Burruss, N. L. Weir et al. 2014. Abdominal body composition differences in NFL football players. *J Strength Cond Res* 28:3313–9.

Brechue, W. F. 2011. Structure-function relationships that determine sprint performance and running speed in sport. *Int J Appl Sports Sci* 23:313–50.

Brechue, W. F. and T. Abe. 2002. The role of FFM accumulation and skeletal muscle architecture in powerlifting performance. *Eur J Appl Physiol* 86:327–36.

Brechue, W. F., J. L. Mayhew, and F. C. Piper. 2010. Characteristics of sprint performance in college football players. *J Strength Cond Res* 24:1169–78.

Chelly, S. M. and C. Denis. 2001. Leg power and hopping stiffness: Relationship with sprint running performance. *Med Sci Sports Exerc* 33:326–33.

Cleather, D. J. 2006. Adjusting powerlifting performances for differences in body mass. *J Strength Cond Res* 20:412–21.

Conroy, B. P., W. J. Kraemer, C. M. Maresh et al. 1993. Bone mineral density in elite junior Olympic weightlifters. *Med Sci Sports Exerc* 25:1103–9.

Delecluse, C. 1997. Influence of strength training on sprint running performance. Current findings and implications for training. *Sports Med* 24:147–56.

Dengel, D. R., T. A. Bosch, T. P. Burruss et al. 2014. Body composition and bone mineral density of National Football League players. *J Strength Cond Res* 28:1–6.

Dooman, C. S. and P. M. Vanderburgh. 2000. Allometric modeling of the bench press and squat: Who is the strongest regardless of body mass? *J Strength Cond Res* 14:32–6.

Escamilla, R. F., J. E. Lander, and J. Garhammer. 2000. Biomechanics of powerlifting and weightlifting exercises. In *Exercise and Sport Science*, eds. W. E. Garhammer and D. T. Kirkendall, 585–615. Philadelphia, PA: Lippincott Williams & Wilkins.

Figueirêdo, J. S., P. M. S. Dantas, M. I. Knackfuss, and E. S. T. Egito. 2013. How can somatotype become a tool to predict an anthropometric profile for high performance 100- and 400-meter runners? *Gazz Med Ital* 172:941–51.

Ford, L. E., A. J. Detterline, K. K. Ho, and W. Cao. 2000. Gender- and height-related limits of muscle strength in world weightlifting champions. *J Appl Physiol* 89:1061–4.

Fried, T. and G. J. Lloyd. 1992. An overview of common soccer injuries. Management and prevention. *Sports Med* 14:269–75.

Fry, A. C., D. Ciroslan, M. D. Fry et al. 2006. Anthropometric and performance variables discriminating elite American junior men weightlifters. *J Strength Cond Res* 20:861–6.

Fry, A. C., B. K. Schilling, R. S. Staron et al. 2003a. Muscle fiber characteristics and performance correlates of male Olympic-style weightlifters. *J Strength Cond Res* 17:746–54.

Fry, A. C., J. M. Webber, L. W. Weiss et al. 2003b. Muscle fiber characteristics of competitive power lifters. *J Strength Cond Res* 17:402–10.

Funato, K., H. Kanehisa, and T. Fukunaga. 2000. Differences in muscle cross-sectional area and strength between elite senior and college Olympic weight lifters. *J Sports Med Phys Fitness* 40:312–8.

Hirsch, K. R., A. E. Smith-Ryan, E. T. Trexler, and E. J. Roelofs. 2016. Body composition and muscle characteristics of division I track and field athletes. *J Strength Cond Res* 30:1231–8.

Hoshikawa, Y., T. Iida, M. Muramatsu et al. 2009. Differences in thigh muscularity and dynamic torque between junior and senior soccer players. *J Sports Sci* 27:129–38.

Housh, T. J., D. J. Housh, and H. A. DeVries. 2016. Anthropometric somatotyping determinations of body build characteristics. *Applied Exercise & Sport Physiology with Labs*, 264–78. Scottsdale, AZ: Holcomb Hathaway, Publishers.

Ikebukuro, T., K. Kubo, J. Okada, H. Yata, and N. Tsunoda. 2011. The relationship between muscle thickness in the lower limbs and competition performance in weightlifters and sprinters. *Jap J Phys Fit Sports Med* 60:401–11.

Izquierdo, M., K. Hakkinen, J. J. Gonzalez-Badillo, J. Ibanez, and E. M. Gorostiaga. 2002. Effects of long-term training specificity on maximal strength and power of the upper and lower extremities in athletes from different sports. *Eur J Appl Physiol* 87:264–71.

Jajtner, A. R., J. R. Hoffman, T. C. Scanlon et al. 2013. Performance and muscle architecture comparisons between starters and nonstarters in National Collegiate Athletic Association Division I women's soccer. *J Strength Cond Res* 27:2355–65.

Johnson, G. O., T. J. Housh, D. R. Powell, and C. J. Ansorge. 1990. A physiological comparison of female body builders and power lifters. *J Sports Med Phys Fitness* 30:361–4.

Kanehisa, H. and T. Fukunaga. 1999. Profiles of musculoskeletal development in limbs of college Olympic weightlifters and wrestlers. *Eur J Appl Physiol Occup Physiol* 79:414–20.

Kanehisa, H., S. Ikegawa, and T. Fukunaga. 1998a. Body composition and cross-sectional areas of limb lean tissues in Olympic weight lifters. *Scand J Med Sci Sports* 8:271–8.

Kanehisa, H., S. Ikegawa, and T. Fukunaga. 1998b. Comparison of muscle cross-sectional areas between weight lifters and wrestlers. *Int J Sports Med* 19:265–71.

Kanehisa, H., Y. Muraoka, Y. Kawakami, and T. Fukunaga. 2003. Fascicle arrangements of vastus lateralis and gastrocnemius muscles in highly trained soccer players and swimmers of both genders. *Int J Sports Med* 24:90–5.

Karlsson, M. K., O. Johnell, and K. J. Obrant. 1995a. Is bone mineral density advantage maintained long-term in previous weight lifters? *Calcif Tissue Int* 57:325–8.

Karlsson, M. K., P. Vergnaud, P. D. Delmas, and K. J. Obrant. 1995b. Indicators of bone formation in weight lifters. *Calcif Tissue Int* 56:177–80.

Kearns, C. F., M. Isokawa, and T. Abe. 2001. Architectural characteristics of dominant leg muscles in junior soccer players. *Eur J Appl Physiol* 85:240–3.

Keogh, J. W., P. A. Hume, S. N. Pearson, and P. Mellow. 2007. Anthropometric dimensions of male powerlifters of varying body mass. *J Sports Sci* 25:1365–76.

Keogh, J. W., P. A. Hume, S. N. Pearson, and P. Mellow. 2008. To what extent does sexual dimorphism exist in competitive powerlifters? *J Sports Sci* 26:531–41.

Keogh, J. W., P. A. Hume, S. N. Pearson, and P. J. Mellow. 2009. Can absolute and proportional anthropometric characteristics distinguish stronger and weaker powerlifters? *J Strength Cond Res* 23:2256–65.

Korhonen, M. T., A. Cristea, M. Alen et al. 2006. Aging, muscle fiber type, and contractile function in sprint-trained athletes. *J Appl Physiol* 101:906–17.

Korhonen, M. T., A. A. Mero, M. Alen et al. 2009. Biomechanical and skeletal muscle determinants of maximum running speed with aging. *Med Sci Sports Exerc* 41:844–56.

Kraemer, W. J., J. C. Torine, R. Silvestre et al. 2005. Body size and composition of National Football League players. *J Strength Cond Res* 19:485–9.

Kruger, A., J. H. de Ridder, H. W. Grobbelaar, and C. Underhay. 2006. A kinanthropometric profile and morphological prediction functions of elite international male javelin throwers. Paper presented at the Kinanthropometry IX: *Proceedings of the 9th International Conference of the International Society for the Advancement of Kinanthropometry*, eds. M. Marfell-Jones, A. Stewart and T. Olds, 36–48. London: Routledge.

Kubo, K., T. Ikebukuro, H. Yata, M. Tomita, and M. Okada. 2011. Morphological and mechanical properties of muscle and tendon in highly trained sprinters. *J Appl Biomech* 27:336–44.

Kumagai, K., T. Abe, W. F. Brechue et al. 2000. Sprint performance is related to muscle fascicle length in male 100-m sprinters. *J Appl Physiol* 88:811–6.

Kyriazis, T., G. Terzis, G. Karampatsos, S. Kavouras, and G. Georgiadis. 2010. Body composition and performance in shot put athletes at preseason and at competition. *Int J Sports Physiol Perform* 5:417–21.

Langer, F. 2007. Somatometric characteristics of high jumpers. *Acta Univ Patacki Olomuc Gymn* 37:37–47.

Legaz Arrese, A., E. Serrano Ostariz, J. A. Jcasajus Mallen, and D. Munguia Izquierdo. 2005. The changes in running performance and maximal oxygen uptake after long-term training in elite athletes. *J Sports Med Phys Fitness* 45:435–40.

Lovera, M. and J. Keogh. 2015. Anthropometric profile of powerlifters: Differences as a function of body-weight class and competitive success. *J Sports Med Phys Fitness* 55:478–87.

Markovic, G. and D. Sekulic. 2006. Modeling the influence of body size on weightlifting and powerlifting performance. *Coll Antropol* 30:607–13.

Masuda, K., N. Kikuhara, H. Takahashi, and K. Yamanaka. 2003. The relationship between muscle cross-sectional area and strength in various isokinetic movements among soccer players. *J Sports Sci* 21:851–8.

McArdle, W. D., F. I. Katch, and V. L. Katch. 2006. Body composition, obesity, and weight control. *Essentials of Exercise Physiology*, 559–65. Baltimore, MD: Lippincott Williams & Wilkins.

McCormack, W. P., J. R. Stout, A. J. Wells et al. 2014. Predictors of high-intensity running capacity in collegiate women during a soccer game. *J Strength Cond Res* 28:964–70.

Meltzer, D. E. 1994. Age dependence of Olympic weightlifting ability. *Med Sci Sports Exerc* 26:1053–67.

Melvin, M. N., A. E. Smith-Ryan, H. L. Wingfield et al. 2014. Muscle characteristics and body composition of NCAA division I football players. *J Strength Cond Res* 28:3320–9.

Methenitis, S. K., N. D. Zaras, K. M. Spengos et al. 2016. Role of muscle morphology in jumping, sprinting, and throwing performance in participants with different power training duration experience. *J Strength Cond Res* 30:807–17.

Norton, K. and T. Olds. 2001. Morphological evolution of athletes over the twentieth century: Causes and consequences. *Sports Med* 31:763–83.

Ojanen, T., T. Rauhala, and K. Hakkinen. 2007. Strength and power profiles of the lower and upper extremities in master throwers at different ages. *J Strength Cond Res* 21:216–22.

Orvanova, E. 1990. Somatotypes of weight lifters. *J Sports Sci* 8:119–37.

Perez-Gomez, J., G. V. Rodriguez, I. Ara et al. 2008. Role of muscle mass on sprint performance: Gender differences? *Eur J Appl Physiol* 102:685–94.

Pryor, J. L., R. A. Huggins, D. J. Casa et al. 2014. A profile of a National Football League team. *J Strength Cond Res* 28:7–13.

Rousanoglou, E., M. E. Nikolaidou, and K. Boudolos. 2006. Discrimination of young women athletes and nonathletes based on anthropometric jumping and muscular strength measures. *Percept Mot Skills* 102:881–95.

Sallinen, J., T. Ojanen, L. Karavirta, J. P. Ahtiainen, and K. Hakkinen. 2008. Muscle mass and strength, body composition and dietary intake in master strength athletes vs untrained men of different ages. *J Sports Med Phys Fitness* 48:190–6.

Schmitt, H., E. Dubljanin, S. Schneider, and M. Schiltenwolf. 2004. Radiographic changes in the lumbar spine in former elite athletes. *Spine (Phila Pa 1976)* 29:2554–9.

Schmitt, H., C. Friebe, S. Schneider, and D. Sabo. 2005. Bone mineral density and degenerative changes of the lumbar spine in former elite athletes. *Int J Sports Med* 26:457–63.

Sinclair, R. G. 1985. Normalizing the performances of athletes in Olympic weightlifting. *Can J Appl Sport Sci* 10:94–8.

Singh, K., P. Singh, and C. Singh. 2012. Anthropometric characteristics, body composition and somatotyping of high and low performer shot putters. *Int J Sports Sci Eng* 6:153–8.

Singh, S., K. Singh, and M. Singh. 2010. Anthropometric measurements, body composition and somatotyping of high jumpers. *Brazilian J Biomotricity* 4:266–71.

Slawinski, J., N. Termoz, G. Rabita et al. 2015. How 100-m event analyses improve our understanding of world-class men's and women's sprint performance. *Scand J Med Sci Sports*, doi: 10.1111/sms.12627.

Snow, T. K., M. Millard-Stafford, and L. B. Rosskopf. 1998. Body composition profile of NFL football players. *J Strength Cond Res* 12:146–9.

Stefani, R. 2008. The physics and evolution of Olympic winning performances. In *Statistical Thinking in Sports*, eds. J. Albert and R. H. Koning, 33–61. Boca Raton, FL: Taylor & Francis Group, LLC.

Stefani, R. 2014. The power-to-weight relationships and efficiency improvements of Olympic champions in athletics, swimming and rowing. *Int J Sports Sci Coaching* 9:271–85.

Stoessel, L., M. H. Stone, R. Keith, D. Marple, and R. Johnson. 1991. Selected physiological, psychological and performance characteristics of national-caliber United States women weightlifters. *J Strength Cond Res* 5:87–95.

Stolen, T., K. Chamari, C. Castagna, and U. Wisloff. 2005. Physiology of soccer: An update. *Sports Med* 35:501–36.

Stone, M. H., W. A. Sands, K. C. Pierce et al. 2005. Relationship of maximum strength to weightlifting performance. *Med Sci Sports Exerc* 37:1037–43.

Storey, A. and H. K. Smith. 2012. Unique aspects of competitive weightlifting: Performance, training and physiology. *Sports Med* 42:769–90.

Sullivan, J. J., R. G. Knowlton, R. K. Hetzler, and P. L. Woelke. 1994. Anthropometric characteristics and performance related predictors of success in adolescent pole vaulters. *J Sports Med Phys Fitness* 34:179–84.

Terzis, G., T. Kyriazis, G. Karampatsos, and G. Georgiadis. 2012. Muscle strength, body composition, and performance of an elite shot-putter. *Int J Sports Physiol Perform* 7:394–6.

Terzis, G., K. Spengos, S. Kavouras, P. Manta, and G. Georgiadis. 2010. Muscle fibre type composition and body composition in hammer throwers. *J Sports Sci Med* 9:104–9.

Trappe, S., N. Luden, K. Minchev et al. 2015. Skeletal muscle signature of a champion sprint runner. *J Appl Physiol* 118:1460–6.

Uth, N. 2005. Anthropometric comparison of world-class sprinters and normal populations. *J Sports Sci Med* 4:608–16.

Vanderburgh, P. M. and A. M. Batterham. 1999. Validation of the Wilks powerlifting formula. *Med Sci Sports Exerc* 31:1869–75.

Watts, A. S., I. Coleman, and A. Nevill. 2012. The changing shape characteristics associated with success in world-class sprinters. *J Sports Sci* 30:1085–95.

Wells, A. J., D. H. Fukuda, J. R. Hoffman et al. 2014. Vastus lateralis exhibits non-homogenous adaptation to resistance training. *Muscle Nerve* 50:785–93.

Weyand, P. G. and J. A. Davis. 2005. Running performance has a structural basis. *J Exp Biol* 208:2625–31.

Whittington, J., E. Schoen, L. L. Labounty et al. 2009. Bone mineral density and content of collegiate throwers: Influence of maximum strength. *J Sports Med Phys Fitness* 49:464–73.

Wilks, D. C., K. Winwood, S. F. Gilliver et al. 2009. Bone mass and geometry of the tibia and the radius of master sprinters, middle and long distance runners, race-walkers and sedentary control participants: A pQCT study. *Bone* 45:91–7.

Ye, X., J. P. Loenneke, C. A. Fahs et al. 2013. Relationship between lifting performance and skeletal muscle mass in elite powerlifters. *J Sports Med Phys Fitness* 53:409–14.

Zaras, N. D., A. N. Stasinaki, S. K. Methenitis et al. 2016. Rate of force development, muscle architecture, and performance in young competitive track and field throwers. *J Strength Cond Res* 30:81–92.

12 Weight-Sensitive Sports

Analiza M. Silva, Diana A. Santos, and Catarina N. Matias

CONTENTS

12.1 INTRODUCTION

12.1.1 OVERVIEW

Body composition plays a determinant role in sports with athletes, coaches, dietitians, and other sports professionals often looking into body weight and adiposity as an enemy to optimal performance. Several discussions on body composition in athletes focus on these aspects due to its potentially negative impact on performance (Ackland et al. 2012; Sundgot-Borgen et al. 2013). Some sports dictate to athletes to make changes in body weight and composition that may not be the best option for an individual athlete (Rodriguez et al. 2009). This issue has been particularly evident in weight-sensitive sports.

Weight-sensitive sports are defined as those in which extreme dieting, low adiposity, frequent weight fluctuation, and eating disorders have been reported in both the literature and practice

(Meyer et al. 2013). Weight-sensitive sports can be classified into three main groups (Ackland et al. 2012; Franchini et al. 2012; Meyer et al. 2013; Khodaee et al. 2015):

1. *Gravitational sports*, in which high body weight restricts performance due to mechanical (gravitational) reasons given that moving the body against gravity is an essential part of these sports. Among these sports are long-distance running, cross-country skiing, high and pole jumping, road and mountain bike cycling, climbing, or ski-jumping.
2. *Weight class sports*, in which athletic competitions are organized according to categories of body weight, anticipating an advantage when they are classified in a lower body weight category. This group includes combat sports such as wrestling, judo, boxing, taekwondo, jujitsu, martial arts, as well as weight lifting, lightweight rowing, or jockeying.
3. *Aesthetically judged sports*, in which athletes or their coaches expect higher scores when their body weight and shape conform to a perceived ideal body. This group includes rhythmic and artistic gymnastics, figure skating, diving and synchronized swimming, as well as freestyle aerials, or cheerleading.

Some athletes are genetically suited to the specific anthropometric demands of the sport in which they compete, but many elite athletes have to struggle with extreme dieting to meet the expectations of the sport itself and the demands of their coaches (Sundgot-Borgen and Garthe 2011; Sundgot-Borgen et al. 2013). As a consequence, male and female athletes with low-energy availability, very low body weight, and/or fat mass (FM), frequent weight fluctuations, disordered eating behaviors, and insufficient bone mineral density (BMD) are often found in weight-sensitive sports (Matzkin et al. 2015; Tenforde et al. 2015). Additionally, weight fluctuations and extreme dieting negatively impact performance (Sundgot-Borgen and Garthe 2011).

Medical staff, sports physicians, nutritionists, and exercise scientists, experience challenges in handling the issues of optimum body composition and dieting in elite athletes (Meyer et al. 2013; Sundgot-Borgen et al. 2013). In this chapter we will review the main issues and concerns about weight-loss strategies aimed to achieve a target weight and adiposity and its respective minimum values, highlight objective methodologies for energy expenditure assessment, and present and discuss the relevance of body composition in performance, and the major health consequences of athletes engaged in weight-sensitive sports. We expect to provide tools for sports professionals to counteract the currently used negative practices leading to enhanced health and performance of the athletes.

12.1.2 Minimum Weight and Fatness

Athletes competing in weight-sensitive sports commonly present a low weight and adiposity (Meyer et al. 2013; Khodaee et al. 2015). Despite the low weight and fatness, almost all athletes engaging at high competition level want or need to reduce their weight to obtain gravitational advantage (gravitational sports), to compete in a lower weight category (weight class sports) or, in the case of aesthetic sports, because extra adiposity may have a negative impact on judges' evaluation which will influence the final score. As a consequence, energy and fluid restriction along with weight-loss practices are often used for weight management with possible impairment of performance and/or health. On the other hand, these concerns may be related to the magnitude and duration of the weight-loss period and the recovery strategies that are used to regain weight between competitions (Sundgot-Borgen et al. 2013). Dieting and eating disorders are common practices in weight-sensitive sports (Ziegler et al. 1998a,b; Johnson et al. 1999; Smolak et al. 2000; Byrne and McLean 2002; Golden et al. 2003; Burke et al. 2004; Torstveit and Sundgot-Borgen 2005; Beals and Hill 2006; de Bruin et al. 2007; Rouveix et al. 2007; Sundgot-Borgen and Torstveit 2010; Dolan et al. 2011; Sundgot-Borgen and Garthe 2011; Dwyer et al. 2012; Sundgot-Borgen et al. 2013; Matzkin et al. 2015; Joy et al. 2016). Thus, a focus on minimizing the negative effect of chronic dieting and the recurring weight-loss processes, in both health and performance, establishing a minimum body weight, FM, or other body component, is mandatory. The use of a minimum body composition cutoff (e.g., %FM) could help ensuring the athletic health and well-being when competing in weight-sensitive sports. Conversely, due to methodological issues the implementation of a single body composition cutoff is not feasible (Clark et al. 2004; Sundgot-Borgen and Garthe 2011; Ackland et al. 2012). Different body composition techniques with varying accuracy and precision can be used to quantify body components, leading to different FM estimations that would be dependent on the method that is used. Additionally, many of the *in vivo* body composition methods rely on assumptions, such as the chemical composition of fat-free mass (FFM) that may not be valid in athletes, either to determine FM at a specific time point of the season or a given change over time, in- or off-season within and between athletes (Santos et al. 2010, b).

Meyer et al. (2013) reported the most common practices for assessing minimum weight or FM in athletes along with cutoff values used by sports trainers and coaches. This survey included athletes from weight-sensitive sports and non-weight-sensitive sports. The minimum values for %FM ranged from 4% to 10% for males and 9%–15% for female athletes and %FM was frequently determined by the use of skinfolds (SKF), or sex-specific and sport-specific sum of 6, 7, or 8 SKF. Minimum values of SKF using six sites were 30 mm for males and 40 mm for females. A minimum value of 18–21 kg/m^2 for body mass index (BMI) was also cited as an option to be used when evaluating body composition. Santos et al. (2014a) have recently developed normative values for athletes' body composition in a Portuguese top-level athletic population from several sports. For triathlon, a gravitational sport, the authors verified that the 5th percentile for BMI was 17.6 and 18.9 kg/m^2 for females and males, respectively. In the same triathletes, when using the sum of 7 SKF (triceps, subscapular, biceps, suprailiac, abdominal, thigh, and medial calf) the 5th percentile corresponded to 35.1 mm in females and 28.8 mm in males, values that are lower than the expected minimum when using the sum of 6SKF. When using dual x-ray energy absorptiometry (DXA), the 5th percentile for %FM in triathletes was 11.5% and 8.2% for females and males, respectively. Although lower levels of adiposity may bring competitive advantages in gravitational sports, Tanda and Knechtle (2015) verified that in marathoners and ultra-marathoners, a value less than 15%FM (estimated with SKF) was not associated with the time of the race.

In the gravitational sport of ski jumping, use of a mass index (MI: m is the jumper mass and s is the sitting height) less than = 0.28 m/s^2 was proposed to designate underweight. The MI has an advantage over BMI by considering the individual's leg length that plays a role in jump performance. Although the MI formula is similar to the BMI formula, height is replaced by the sitting height (s) with a factor of 0.28 representing an MI that is equal to BMI for persons with average leg length (Muller 2009a).

Regarding weight class sports, lower limits of adiposity corresponding to 5%FM for male athletes and 12%FM for female athletes have been suggested since the 1990s (Fogelholm 1994). The National Collegiate Athletic Association (NCAA) implemented a minimum weight based on 5%FM and the United States National Federation of State High School Associations (FSHSA) established a minimum of 7%FM for boys and 12%FM for girls (Alderman et al. 2004). A recent review addressed the current minimum %FM allowed in weight class sports (Khodaee et al. 2015), reporting 7%FM and 12%FM as the minimum allowed in male and female high school wrestlers, respectively, and a 5%FM and 12%FM minimum in male and female collegiate wrestlers, respectively. Minimum values of 6%FM and 12%FM were established in male and female jockeys, respectively. Santos et al. (2014a) reported that the 5th percentile for %FM in Portuguese elite wrestling and judo athletes, as assessed by DXA, corresponded to 7.2%, with the sum of 7SKF corresponding to 22 mm in these athletes.

Despite the apparent advantages in performance by competing with a lower body weight, a decreased weight or %FM to unrealistic values may compromise health and well-being, thus requiring the establishment of realistic boundaries (de Bruin et al. 2007). A review conducted by Sundgot-Borgen and Torstveit (2010) pointed out that athletes engaging in high intensity sports, including aesthetics sports (e.g., figure skating, gymnastics, and freestyle aerials), should maintain a weight of at least 90% of the expected mass corresponding to a %FM >6% for male athletes and >12% for female athletes, or an higher value, if prescribed by the multidisciplinary treatment team. It is important to mention that these estimations were based on body composition determinations derived from 2-component models and therefore are open to challenges, particularly within the athletic field.

Considering all the available literature, the ad hoc International Olympic Committee (IOC) group is presently gathering information regarding body composition measurements, proposed limit values for FM and guidelines for the appropriate %FM values for male and female athletes (Sundgot-Borgen and Garthe 2011; Sundgot-Borgen et al. 2013). Meanwhile, this group reports a range of 5%–7% in males and 12%–14% in female athletes as the most used minimum %FM levels. Once these values have not been determined by a reference methodology, its use should be performed cautiously and considering other aspects of health and athletic performance, instead of its blind implementation. The individual health profile and athletic performance should dictate its minimum weight/FM for competing in a specific sports event. For instance, a 7%FM may be the minimum value that does not compromise health or sports performance, for a given athlete, while for others 5% or 6%FM could be the most adequate value (Ackland et al. 2012). Accordingly, establishing an optimal competitive body weight and composition should be determined when an athlete is healthy and performing at his or her best (Ackland et al. 2012). Since, usually, the amount of FM or body weight, ideal for competition is less than the ideal for the health and well being of the athlete, the large variability in FM should be considered to avoid compromise health and sports performance (Garthe et al. 2011b). Therefore, some considerations have been proposed: (i) changes in body composition should be supervised (especially after the weight or the FM goal have been achieved, or whenever unintentional losses occurred, or when weight fluctuations are frequent); (ii) athletes involved in many competitions where a target weight is desired should attempt to maintain a weight/FM within 3% of the competition goal, during the season; (iii) athletes engaged in sports with less frequent competitions should try to keep weights and allow higher FM during the season, establishing a target weight only for the most relevant events of the season (Sundgot-Borgen and Garthe 2011; Sundgot-Borgen et al. 2013).

Considering health aspects related to the minimum weight, the ad hoc IOC research group completed an appraisal of rules and regulations applied to weight-sensitive sports (Sundgot-Borgen et al. 2013; Khodaee et al. 2015), and suggested, in 2013, some recommendations. These adjustments are related to weigh-in times, number of weight classes, use of BMI or other metrics or cutoff values for participating in a specific competition, and subjective judging. This group also reinforced the need for a "competition certificate" where the minimum body weight, FM, or sum of SKF is reported, and an appropriate hydration level is ensured.

The suggested changes were made after consideration of the results obtained by the application of procedures carried out by the United States men's collegiate wrestling in the 1990s. Apparently, these actions have been effective in reducing the prevalence of inappropriate behaviors with regard to weight loss and competitive equity (Davis et al. 2002; Oppliger et al. 2006).

A minimal competitive weight based on the preseason assessment of body composition was adopted. When weigh-in was moved to 2 h before the initial match, weight loss on the day before the tournament decreased from 3.7 ± 1.3 kg to 2.7 ± 1.4 kg (Scott et al. 1994, 2000). Similar results were observed by Ransone and Hughes, where the weight loss of 1.4 kg in the previous 24 hours to the weigh-in decreased to 1.1 kg (Ransone and Hughes 2004).

These results provided evidence to support the effectiveness of the new NCAA weight management rule that established a minimal competitive weight at the beginning of the season (Oppliger et al. 2006). Likewise, a survey completed in 1999 (Oppliger et al. 2003) found less extreme weight-loss practices among a sample of wrestlers from all three NCAA divisions of competition (i.e., Divisions I, II, and III).

In ski-jumping, the use of a minimum BMI for competition has been established and other regulatory changes have been suggested to avoid extreme leanness in athletes (Muller 2009a,b; Sundgot-Borgen et al. 2013). According to the specifications for competition of the International Ski Federation, the maximum ski length allowed for a skier is 145% of the height of the jumper. In order to be eligible for this maximum length, the competitor must have a minimum BMI of 21.0 kg/ m^2 (wearing ski suit and boots). For jumpers with less than this minimum value, a reduction in the ski length, in a proportion of 0.125 BMI per 0.5% ski length is applied. In respect to weight class sports, some recommendations were proposed by the IOC ad hoc group (Sundgot-Borgen et al. 2013), namely a weigh-in schedule of no more than 2–3 hours before competition has been suggested; tolerating some discretion in the weight allowance (e.g., 1–2 kg over the weight limit) in smaller tournaments; and disapproving changes between weight categories over the sports season. Additionally, it has been suggested that sports federations should have similar weight categories at national and international tournaments and should implement more weight categories in low- and middle-weight classes, particularly for female competitions.

In relation to aesthetic sports, the IOC ad hoc research group reported no published articles on the "risks" of judging in aesthetic sports. Nevertheless, athletes reported dieting due to judges' comments after competitive events (Sundgot-Borgen et al. 2013). As an example of good practice, the figure skating committee implemented a more objective judging system with the intent to de-emphasize the focus on leanness of aesthetic sports.

12.1.3 Most Commonly Used Weight-Loss Strategies

A "perfect" body type, shape, or weight is needed to compete in weight-sensitive sports, which frequently leads to dieting and other weight-loss procedures. Although a number of studies assessed nutrient intake among athletes, the real prevalence of abnormal eating behaviors among athletes representing weight-sensitive sports is unknown (Steen and Brownell 1990; Oppliger et al. 2003; Alderman et al. 2004; Slater et al. 2005; Artioli et al. 2010; Sundgot-Borgen and Garthe 2011; Franchini et al. 2012; Khodaee et al. 2015).

Overall, it is suggested that athletes, who intend to lose weight to achieve better gravitational performance, higher scores in aesthetic sports, or that may have physical advantage by competing in a lower weight class, should target FM loss without compromising FFM (Trexler et al. 2014). Weight loss is typically within 5%–10% of the athlete's weight and occurs normally in the week prior competition (Franchini et al. 2012).

Most athletes engaged in sports with enforced weight limits (e.g., wrestling, combat sports, etc.) want to achieve the lightest weight, as they expect to reach competitive advantage over the opponent by competing in a category below their normal body weight (Khodaee et al. 2015). Therefore, these athletes generally lose 2%–13% of the body weight before competition (Steen and Brownell 1990; Oppliger et al. 2003; Alderman et al. 2004; Slater et al. 2005; Artioli et al. 2010). Apparently, athletes competing in lower categories are more frequently engaged in extreme weight-loss approaches than athletes competing in middle or heavy weight categories (Oppliger et al. 2003). Most weight class athletes start to limit food and fluid intake a week before weigh-in (Artioli et al. 2010). Excessive and intense exercise (as running, jogging, cycling, and swimming) with or without wearing vapor impermeable suits, is another reported weight-loss strategy (Alderman et al. 2004). The use of diet pills to block appetite and/or use FM as a body store has been reported. Dehydration through wet or dry saunas, training in heated rooms, and training with plastic or rubberized suits is another weight-loss strategy reported by weight class sports that is generally used a couple of days before weigh-in (Khodaee et al. 2015). The dehydration process is known in the athletic community as the "drying out" and its popularity is due to the idea that body water can be easily and rapidly recovered by fluid intake after weigh-in (Oppliger et al. 1996, 2003). The use of laxatives or intentional vomiting is also reported to be used in the last days before weigh-in to help in reducing body weight (Filaire et al. 2001). Commonly, athletes use one or several methods at the same time, with food and fluid intake restrictions used as the main strategy.

Athletes engaged in aesthetic sports have a greater pressure to reduce weight on a daily basis from their coaches and judges (Nattiv et al. 2007; Sundgot-Borgen and Garthe 2011), especially when compared to other athletes competing in sports in which leanness or a target weight is considered less important for performance (Byrne and McLean 2002).

A meta-analysis, including 34 studies, scrutinized the overall relationship between athletic participation and eating disorders (Smolak et al. 2000). The authors hypothesized that a higher prevalence of eating disorders would be observed in athletes participating in aesthetic sports compared to a matched control group of non-athletes. Overall, the authors verified that, with the exception of gymnasts, athletes presented a higher risk than non-athletes for eating problems. Recently Dwyer et al. (2012), found that most competitive ice skaters had low-energy intakes and approximately 25% of the sample reported disordered attitudes and behaviors concerning eating patterns and weight control.

12.2   ENERGY EXPENDITURE AND WEIGHT-SENSITIVE SPORTS

12.2.1   Physical Activity and Energy Expenditure Components

To better understand energy expenditure in weight-sensitive sports it is determinant to clarify some concepts and definitions. Physical activity is defined as any bodily movement produced by skeletal muscles that result in energy expenditure. The term exercise has been used interchangeably with physical activity. In fact, both have a number of common elements, yet, exercise and physical activity are not synonyms; exercise is a subcategory of physical activity. Exercise is physical activity that is planned, structured, repetitive, and purposive in the sense that improvement or maintenance of one or more components of physical fitness is the goal. Both physical activity and exercise have in common a resulting increase in energy expenditure (Caspersen et al. 1985).

Total energy expenditure corresponds to the sum of resting energy expenditure, activity energy expenditure, and diet-induced thermogenesis (Donahoo et al. 2004). Resting energy expenditure represents the minimum amount of energy required to sustain vital bodily functioning in the post-absorptive awakened state (Gallagher and Elia 2005). Diet-induced thermogenesis is the increase in energy expenditure associated with the digestion, absorption, and storage of food and accounts for approximately 10% of total energy expenditure (D'Alessio et al. 1988). Physical activity energy expenditure can be further separated into exercise activity thermogenesis and non-exercise activity thermogenesis; the non-exercise activity thermogenesis is the energy expended in all activities that are not sleeping, eating or sports-like, which includes all occupation, leisure, sitting, standing, and ambulation (Levine 2004).

12.2.2   Energy Balance versus Energy Availability

Energy expenditure must equal energy intake (the sum of energy from foods, fluids, and supplements) to achieve energy balance (Rodriguez et al. 2009). Energy balance is usually calculated over longer periods of time and represents the difference between energy intake and total energy expenditure. When the energy balance is positive the athlete will gain weight, whereas if the athlete is under a negative energy balance weight loss will occur. Athletes are often under a negative energy balance for achieving a desirable body composition profile. However, a simple look at energy balance does not give a complete picture of the body composition profile as there may be differences in how the energy is stored in the body leading to different consequences in athletes' body composition and/or health. Any energy imbalance is partitioned between energy stored in FM or FFM. Using established energy densities for FM and FFM it is possible to quantify the average rate of changes in body energy stored or lost (energy balance) in kcal/day.

$$\text{Energy Balance (kcal/day)} = 1.0 \times \left(\frac{\Delta \text{FFM}}{\Delta t} \right) + 9.5 \times \left(\frac{\Delta \text{FM}}{\Delta t} \right) \qquad (12.1)$$

where ΔFFM and ΔFM correspond to changes in grams of FFM and FM from one time point to another, while Δt is the time length in days.

This equation has been validated to determine energy balance from the change in body energy stores (de Jonge et al. 2007; Pieper et al. 2011). There are considerable differences in the energy densities of FM and FFM, relying on rules about the chemical composition of FM and FFM changes. Energy density for FFM is expected to be about 1.0 kcal/g (Dulloo and Jacquet 1999) whereas for FM it is about 9.5 kcal/g (Merril and Watt 1973). Given the energy densities for FM and FFM, it is expected that for an athlete to lose a certain amount of weight as FM, a considerable greater deficit in net energy will be required. Also, the initial body composition plays a determinant role in weight loss (Forbes 2000) as the FFM contribution to weight loss is higher or smaller when a lower or higher initial FM is observed, respectively. Therefore any weight loss will be partitioned from FM but also from lean tissue (Hall 2007), although the presence of high-intensity physical activity may somehow preserve FFM during weight-loss periods.

Santos et al. (2010) have verified that, in a sample of Portuguese elite male judo athletes from a period of weight stability to prior competition (Δt = 37 days) a mean change of −0.42 kg of FM and −0.45 of FFM, estimated with DXA, occurred. Using Equation 12.1 it is possible to conclude that for about the same weight loss as FM and FFM, the imbalance to lose FM corresponded to about −108 kcal/day whereas for FFM the imbalance was −12 kcal, with a total required imbalance of −120 kcal/day (−1.4 kcal/kg/day) to lose 0.87 kg in 37 days. In this sample of athletes only 48% of the weight loss resulted from the FM component whereas in terms of energy balance 90% of the imbalance occurred from the contribution of FM, as expected given the higher energy density associated with this body store component.

When using Equation 12.1 to estimate energy balance there may be some methodological limitations in assessing baseline and changes in body composition (FM and FFM) which preclude an accurate quantification of the actual energy imbalance required. Thus, selection of a valid body composition method to estimate changes in FM and FFM is determinant to accurately determine the rate of change in body energy stores. However, the accuracy of the main available body composition methods to detect small differences is very limited, requiring the development and validation of further methods. Although the portions of FM and FFM in energy balance can differentially impact health and performance in athletes, to date, there are no studies that focus on energy partition models in sports that emphasize leanness.

Another important concept for athletic health is the term energy availability; the use of the term energy availability considers that the body uses energy in many physiological processes that include thermoregulation, growth, cellular maintenance, reproduction, immunity, or locomotion; when energy is expended in one of this metabolic processes it will not be available for another (Loucks 2004; Loucks et al. 2011). Energy availability is defined as the amount of dietary energy for all physiologic functions after accounting for energy expenditure from exercise training. Operationally, it can be calculated as energy intake minus exercise energy expenditure normalized to FFM. More than energy balance, energy availability is the factor that impairs the reproductive and skeletal health (Nattiv et al. 2007), as an athlete can be in energy balance (stable body weight) while energy availability is low. The health consequences of low-energy availability will be further detailed ahead in this chapter.

Figure 12.1 illustrates the concept of energy balance versus energy availability. In the example, the athlete from the left is in a neutral state of energy balance. However, due to the increased energy expenditure from exercise training, her energy availability is below 30 kcal/day/kg of FFM. Athletes who aim to reduce body weight, and therefore are in negative energy balance, should follow diet and exercise programs that are associated with energy availabilities between 30 and 45 kcal/day/kg FFM (Loucks et al. 2011). The athlete from the right panel is under a negative energy balance and loses weight; nevertheless, given the fact that the energy expenditure associated with exercise training is considerably lower than the athlete from the left, the energy availability will be higher with a value between 30 and 45 kcal/day/kg FFM. Notwithstanding, a severe weight loss may result from long-term negative energy imbalance which will also impact health and energy availability.

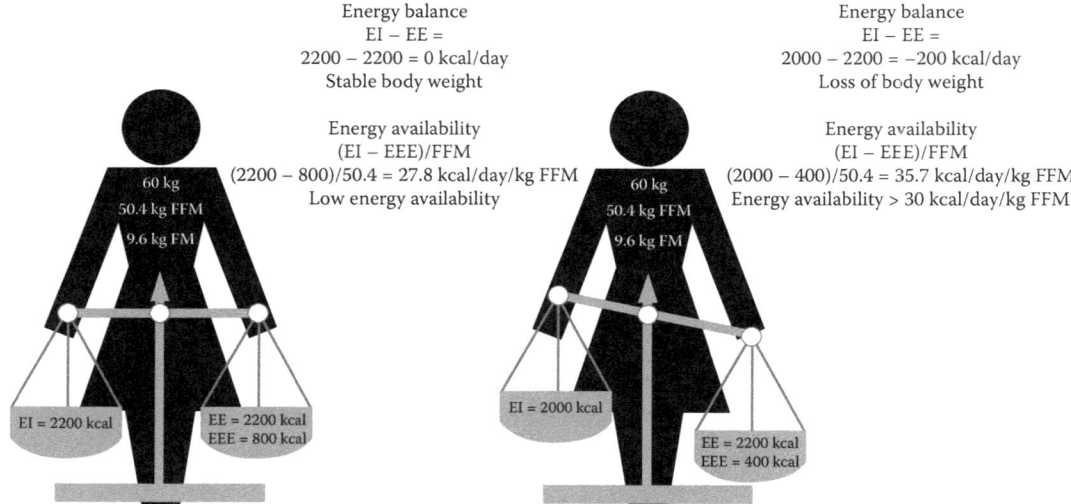

FIGURE 12.1 Difference between energy balance and energy availability. FFM, fat-free mass; FM, fat mass; EI, energy intake; EE, energy expenditure; EEE, exercise energy expenditure.

Some athletes reduce energy availability by increasing exercise energy expenditure more than energy intake while others focus on decreasing energy intake (with or without eating disorders) (Ebine et al. 2000). To estimate energy balance and energy availability, apart from knowing energy intake (through reported measures or by a prescribed diet) one must accurately estimate total energy expenditure and exercise energy expenditure.

12.2.3 ESTIMATING ENERGY REQUIREMENTS IN WEIGHT-SENSITIVE SPORTS

Many athletes are chronically energy deficient and it is therefore determinant to characterize athletes' energy expenditure in order to identify individual energy requirements in accordance to their individual goals (Loucks 2004). These concerns have been more directed to weight-sensitive sports and also to female athletes (Nattiv et al. 2007; Nazem and Ackerman 2012). Regardless, it is important to estimate energy requirements for both males and females, which will depend on individual factors related to the duration, frequency, and intensity of exercise, and prior nutritional status (Rodriguez et al. 2009).

The methods to estimate human energy expenditure are diverse; the doubly-labeled water (DLW) technique is relatively noninvasive and allows quantification of total energy expenditure over a prolonged period of time (usually 1 week in highly active individuals), and, as a result, it is considered the gold standard for total energy expenditure assessment under free-living conditions. The technique is based on the administration of an oral dose of two stable isotopes of water (^2H_2O and $H_2^{18}O$). These two isotopes are used as tracers and the slightly heavier atoms ^2H (deuterium) and ^{18}O can be measured in urine. The ^2H is lost from the body in water alone, whereas the ^{18}O is lost in water and breath ($C^{18}O_2$). The differences between the two tracer excretion rates represent the CO_2 production rate. The more rapid the drop in ^{18}O relative to the drop in ^2H, the higher the energy expenditure is. Along with the information of the fuel oxidized, total energy expenditure can be calculated (Speakman 1997). Additionally, if we are able to assess resting energy expenditure, for example by using indirect calorimetry, and assuming that diet-induced thermogenesis is 10% of total energy expenditure, we are able to estimate physical activity energy expenditure.

$$PAEE = TEE - REE - 0.1\,TEE$$

(12.2)

where PAEE is physical activity energy expenditure, TEE is total energy expenditure, and REE is resting energy expenditure.

The main advantage of this technique is that it does not interfere with daily activities which allow athletes to engage in their normal training regimens and, consequently, unbiased measures of free-living conditions can be obtained. Furthermore, measures can be conducted over prolonged periods allowing the estimation of daily energy expenditure under free-living conditions and, consequently, estimation of individual energy requirements if the person is under a neutral energy balance (Speakman 1997). Regardless, the analytical procedures that are required are time-consuming, expensive, and involve complex methods and specialized technicians, limiting its routine use for energy expenditure assessment (Schoeller and van Santen 1982).

The use of energy intake from self-reported measures could be considered an alternative to estimate energy requirements since energy intake generally corresponds to energy expenditure when the body weight is stable. However, underreporting of nutritional intakes by athletes engaged in weight-sensitive sports (Edwards et al. 1993; Hill and Davies 2002) will result in difficulties to accurately recommend energy requirements and, consequently, health and performance may be affected. Energy intake is consistently underreported by athletes (Table 12.1). It has been previously speculated that low-energy intake in physically active women with increased energy expenditure could be a result of adaptation to chronically high levels of activity or due to genetic circumstances that turn athletes into a "more efficient machine" (Mulligan and Butterfield 1990). Expansion of the DLW technique to the sports field provided an opportunity to deconstruct this theory and to underline that the cause of low-energy intake was attributed to underreporting (Edwards et al. 1993). This underreporting of energy intake has been the main focus of investigations regarding the energy balance in athletes (Edwards et al. 1993; Ebine et al. 2000, 2002; Hill and Davies 2001b; Silva et al. 2013). In fact, exercise training itself has been shown to affect the accuracy of dietary recording in healthy nonobese adults and adolescents. Westerterp et al. (1992) studied individuals at the beginning and end of a 40-week training intervention program. All subjects were previously non-exercisers and the initial difference between the subjects' self-reported intake and expenditure from DLW was 25%. However, by the end of the training program, the discrepancy between the measurements increased to 219%. Also, van Etten et al. (1997) found an increased underreporting over the 18-weeks of a weight-training program (from 21% to 34%). Silva et al. (2013) observed that in elite junior basketball during a weight maintenance period the energy intake reported only explained 34% of the total energy expenditure from the DLW method.

To solve the limitations of underreporting energy intake, particularly during weight-loss periods, one can calculate energy intake by rearranging the energy balance equation (energy balance = energy intake − energy expenditure). This approach is commonly known as the DLW/DXA method (Equation 12.3) (Schoeller 2009).

$$\text{Energy Intake (kcal/day)} = \text{Energy Expenditure (kcal/day)} + \text{Energy Balance (kcal/day)}$$

$$(12.3)$$

In Equation 12.3, energy expenditure can be obtained with the DLW technique and energy balance is calculated from the changes in energy stores, as demonstrated in Equation 12.1. The use of this technique provides a valid objective measure of energy intake during both negative and positive energy balance (de Jonge et al. 2007; Redman et al. 2009). Nonetheless, to calculate energy intake it is necessary to know body composition changes, accordingly it will be required to estimate a target FM and FFM before using Equation 12.3. At this point it is important to remember that although losses in FFM may be attenuated in the presence of exercise, a weight restriction period is expected to result in weight-loss partitioned from both FM and FFM (Hall 2007).

TABLE 12.1
Total and Resting Energy Expenditure, Physical Activity Level, and Energy Intakes in Different Weight-Sensitive Sports Determined by the DLW Method, Including Energy Intake (If Available)

Sample	Sex	TEE, kJ/day (kcal/day)	REE, kJ/day (kcal/day)	PAL	EI, kJ/day (kcal/day)	Reference
Elite *lightweight rowers* during high intensity and volume training (n = 7)	F	16,567 ± 5103 (3957 ± 1219)	5815 ± 142 (1389 ± 34)	2.9 ± 0.9	9270 ± 1310 (2214 ± 313)	Hill and Davies (2002)
Elite *synchronized swimmers*, after competition when athletes engaged normal training regimens (n = 9)	F	11,500 ± 2800 (2747 ± 669)	5200 ± 300 (1242 ± 72)	2.2 ± 0.4	8900 ± 1700 (2126 ± 406)	Ebine et al. (2000)
Elite *endurance runners* in peak physical condition (n = 9)	M	14,611 ± 1043 (3490 ± 249)	6408 ± 224 (1531 ± 54)	2.3 ± 0.1	13,241 ± 1330 (3163 ± 318)	Fudge et al. (2006)
Adolescent *speed skaters* living at a boarding school for young athletes at a preseason period (n = 8)	M	16,900 ± 2900 (4037 ± 693)	8400 ± 500 (2006 ± 119)	2.0 ± 0.2	NR	Ekelund et al. (2002)
Cyclists during the Tour de France, week 1 (n = 4)	M	29,375 ± 991 (7016 ± 237)	6845 ± 412 (1635 ± 98)	4.3 ± 0.2	24,525 ± 1596 (5858 ± 381)	Westerterp et al. (1986)
Cyclists during the Tour de France, week 2 (n = 4)	M	36,025 ± 1802 (8604 ± 430)	6798 ± 404 (1624 ± 96)	5.3 ± 0.6	26,275 ± 854 (6276 ± 204)	
Cyclists during the Tour de France, week 3 (n = 4)	M	35,650 ± 2199 (8515 ± 525)	6763 ± 393 (1615 ± 94)	5.3 ± 0.3	23,225 ± 1305 (5547 ± 312)	
Highly trained *endurance runners*, 7 eumenorrheic and 2 oligomenorrheic (n = 9)	F	12,516 ± 1737 (2989 ± 415)	NR	NR	8527 ± 1246 (2037 ± 298)	Edwards et al. (1993)
Elite *distance runners* (n = 9)	F	11,832 ± 1306 (2826 ± 312)	6025 ± 950 (1439 ± 227)	1.99 ± 0.30	9182 ± 1951 (2193 ± 466)	Schulz et al. (1992)
Elite *cross-country skiers* during a preseason period with high-volume training (n = 4)	F	18,300 ± 2200 (4371 ± 525)	5500 ± 300[a] (1314 ± 72)	3.4 ± 0.3	18,200 ± 1900 (4347 ± 454)	Sjodin et al. (1994)
Elite *cross-country skiers* during a preseason period with high-volume training (n = 4)	M	30,200 ± 4200 (7213 ± 1003)	7600 ± 300[a] (1815 ± 72)	4.0 ± 0.5	30,200 ± 4600 (7213 ± 1099)	
Ultra-marathon running (7 month run around Australia) (n = 1)	M	26,088 (6231)	6686[a] (1597)	3.9	NR	Hill and Davies (2001a)

Note: TEE, total energy expenditure; REE, resting energy expenditure (by indirect calorimetry); PAL, physical activity level (PAL = TEE/REE); EI, energy intake (self-reported, weighed record, or food diary kept over); M, males; F, females; NR, not reported.

[a] REE estimated from equation.

The use of a physical activity level (PAL), which represents the ratio of total to resting energy expenditure, is also a commonly used form to represent energy expenditure, as it allows comparing athletes with different body sizes by adjusting for resting energy expenditure. The average PAL lies between 1.4 and 1.7 in the general population with a sedentary or light activity lifestyle (FAO/WHO/UNU Expert Consultation 2011). All athletes have in common the fact that they are more physically active than the general population and consequently they have higher daily energy expenditure. Table 12.1 summarizes energy expenditure (total and resting and PAL) values that have been reported in the literature for weight-sensitive sports and also, if available, the energy intake reported by the athletes.

Other objective measurements of energy expenditure in free-living conditions have been developed including motion sensors, or devices that assess physiological responses to exercise such as heart rate, body heat loss, and galvanic skin response. Devices combining two or more of these measures have been developed to estimate energy expenditure in free-living conditions. However, investigations have been conducted revealing that the currently available objective measures of energy expenditure may not provide reliable measurements in free-living conditions. Motion sensors are not capable of detecting upper body movements, changes in grade during walking and running, and free-weight exercises (Bassett 2000), and evidence exists that the relation between accelerometry and physical activity intensity is affected at higher intensities (Brage et al. 2004; Matthew 2005). Heart rate is often used as a physiological objective variable, directly associated with oxygen consumption (Ceesay et al. 1989; Schoeller and Racette 1990). The main limitation of the use of heart rate to estimate energy expenditure is the almost flat slope of the relationship at low expenditure levels. At rest, slight movements can increase heart rate while energy expenditure remains almost the same (Achten and Jeukendrup 2003). On the other hand, heart rate does not present a good accuracy in estimating energy expenditure of individuals with high PALs (Schoeller and Racette 1990; Boulay et al. 1994) and the estimation of energy expenditure from heart rate is sport-specific; it has been well documented that the type of activity and posture can influence the relationship between energy expenditure and heart rate (Achten and Jeukendrup 2003). Even electronic devices that combine different objective measures have been shown to provide inaccurate estimates of energy expenditure, particularly for individual assessment in those with high PALs (Assah et al. 2011; Koehler et al. 2011). Also, in weight-sensitive sports limitations have been reported; Koehler et al. (2011) verified that a portable electronic device that synchronically assesses biaxial accelerometry, body heat loss, and galvanic skin response did not provide valid results of total and activity energy expenditure in endurance athletes due to an underestimation of energy expenditure at higher exercise intensities. Nichols et al. (2010) tested the accuracy of a combined heart rate and uniaxial motion sensor and observed that the equipment may have limited use estimating total energy expenditure in a sample of young female competitive runners. Santos et al. (2013) verified that the use of a combined heart rate and motion sensor was not valid to estimate individual energy expenditure in elite junior male and female basketball players. In this framework, it is still necessary to validate new methods or to develop new algorithms for available physical activity electronic devices. It remains a continuing goal to develop and evaluate methods to estimate energy expenditure that are also affordable and minimally invasive. Regardless, contrarily to the DLW method, the use of motion sensors or devices that assess physiological parameters allow energy expenditure estimation in a particular time period, such as during exercise training, which is necessary to calculate energy availability.

Other subjective instruments are available to estimate exercise energy expenditure. The use of the physical activity compendium (Ainsworth et al. 2011) allows the quantification of the energy expenditure in a range of activities, but the use of estimated energy costs during training in athletes should be avoided. Also, Melin et al. (2014) have recently developed a screening tool, *the Low Energy Availability in Females Questionnaire (LEAF-Q)* with the objective of identifying females at risk for the female athlete triad, however, this tool has not been further validated.

12.3   BODY COMPOSITION AND PERFORMANCE

Body composition assessment is relevant for monitoring athletic performance and training regimens (Ackland et al. 2012). With extreme energy restrictions, often associated with weight-sensitive sports, losses of FFM and its components, and an extremely low FM may adversely influence performance. Individualized assessment of an athlete's body composition and body weight or body image may be advantageous for the improvement of athletic performance. Although quantifying FM has been the prime focus of attention, many coaches and scientists working with elite athletes are starting to recognize that knowledge of the amount and distribution of other body components can be as important to sports performance (Ackland et al. 2012).

Athletes exposed to long periods of low-energy availability, with or without eating disorders, may experience health and physical performance impairment (Nattiv et al. 2007; Rodriguez et al. 2009; Sundgot-Borgen et al. 2013). Data on the relationship between sports participation, use of extreme weight-loss methods, and their effect on health and performance are inconsistent, varying by sport, level of athletic performance, and the methodology used in different studies (Sundgot-Borgen and Torstveit 2010; Sundgot-Borgen et al. 2013). The effect of weight loss on sports performance depends on the initial %FM, the magnitude and time exposed to the weight-loss process, and the strategy used for weight-loss and recovery (Table 12.2). Reduced stimulus for muscle growth combined with negative energy balance is likely to cause a reduction in muscle mass and may impair strength and performance (Koutedakis et al. 1994; Koral and Dosseville 2009). Since most studies on the effect of extreme weight loss have methodological weaknesses, namely small samples, undefined performance level, unclear and uncontrolled diet and recovery methods, as well as questionable performance test parameters, it is difficult to systematize the effects of body composition on performance (Sundgot-Borgen and Torstveit 2010; Sundgot-Borgen and Garthe 2011; Franchini et al. 2012; Sundgot-Borgen et al. 2013). Nevertheless, a compilation of the main results from longitudinal and cross-sectional studies that analyze the relationship between body composition and performance are displayed in Tables 12.2 and 12.3, respectively.

12.3.1   GRAVITATIONAL SPORTS

In gravitational sports body weight may restrict performance due to mechanical reasons, since moving the body against gravity is an essential part of these sports (Meyer et al. 2013). Among gravitational sports are long-distance running, cross-country skiing, high and pole jumping, road and mountain bike cycling, climbing, or ski jumping. In jumping sports, at which the athletes need to lift the body, a lower weight may result in higher speed (Muller 2009b). In climbing, a low body weight may be advantageous for competition given that performance may be largely determined by the relation of force applicable through the fingers and toes to the body weight (Muller 2009b). Conversely, Mermier et al. (2000) verified that a climber does not necessarily possess specific anthropometric characteristics to be successful in climbing. On the contrary, Barbieri et al. (2012) verified that in elite mountain climbers, anthropometric characteristics may play a determinant role. Even at younger ages there seems to be differences in body characteristics between climbers and athletes from other sports (Watts et al. 2003); young climbers appear to be more linear in body type with narrow shoulders relative to hips, and even though there are no differences in BMI there are considerable differences in adiposity as estimated by the sum of the chest, midaxillar, triceps, subscapular, suprailiac, abdominal, and thigh SKF (climbers: $\Sigma7SKF = 50.4 \pm 14.5$ mm; non-climbers: $\Sigma7SKF = 76.7 \pm 33.4$ mm). When considering individual SKF sites the authors verified that, with the exception of the subscapular and midaxillar sites, where no differences were reported, SKF thicknesses were lower in climbers compared to non-climbers or controls. Although summing SKFs are often used, assessing the individual value of each site seems to have a major importance in gravitational sports. Legaz and Eston (2005) verified that 3 years of intense athletic conditioning in high-level runners resulted in an enhanced performance concomitant with decreases in $\Sigma6SKF$;

TABLE 12.2
Body Composition and Performance in Weight-Sensitive Sports, Longitudinal Studies

Study	Sports/Sex/Level of Competition	% of Reduction	Body Composition Variables	Performance Variables	Influence of BC Changes in Performance	Body Composition Characteristics (Method)
Fogelholm et al. (1993)	Wrestlers and judo/male/international; national	WL 5% (2.4 d)	BW	Sprint (30 m), Wingate test, and vertical jump height with extra load	→ Sprint , Wingate test, and vertical jump height with extra load	n.a.
	Wrestlers and judo/male/international; national	WL 6% (3 wk)		Sprint (30 m), Wingate test, and vertical jump height with extra load	→ Sprint (30 m) and Wingate test ↑ Vertical jump height	
Artioli et al. (2010)	Judo/male/≥regional level	WL 5% (7 d)	BW, FM	Specific judo exercise, 5-minute judo combat, and three bouts of the Wingate test	→ Specific judo exercise, 5-minute judo combat ↑ Wingate test	*Baseline* FM, kg = 8.8 ± 2.6 BW, kg = 77.9 ± 12.2 *After WL* FM, kg = 8.0 ± 2.3 BW, kg = 74.1 ± 11.4 (UWW)
Smith et al. (2001)	Boxers/male/amateur	WL 3% (5 d)	BW	Boxing ergometer with 3 × 3 minute rounds with 1 minute rest	→ Boxing ergometer	n.a.
Reljic et al. (2015)	Boxers/male/elite	WL 5.5% (7 d)	BW, FM	Peak treadmill-running and VO$_2$peak	→ Peak treadmill-running and VO$_2$peak	*Baseline* %FM = 12.4 ± 4.8 *1–2 d before competition* %FM = 11.6 ± 4.6 *Post-competition* %FM = 11.8 ± 4.6 (SKF)
Marttinen et al. (2011)	Wrestlers/male/collegiate	WL 8.1% (10 d)	BW	Grip strength and lower-body power (Wingate test)	→ Grip strength and Wingate test	n.a.

(Continued)

TABLE 12.2 (Continued)
Body Composition and Performance in Weight-Sensitive Sports, Longitudinal Studies

Study	Sports/Sex/Level of Competition	% of Reduction	Body Composition Variables	Performance Variables	Influence of BC Changes in Performance	Body Composition Characteristics (Method)
Koral and Dosseville (2009)	Judo/male and female/elite	WL 4% (4 wk)	BW, FM	Countermovement jump, squat jump, 5 s and 30 s repetitions of judo movements, and rowing with extra load	→ Countermovement jump, squat jump, 5 s repetitions of judo movements, and rowing with extra load ↓30 s repetitions of judo movements	Diet Group *Baseline* Males %FM = 11.8 ± 2.8 Females %FM = 22.5 ± 7.5 *After WL* Males %FM = 10.4 ± 2.1 Females %FM = 20.5 ± 2.6 (SKF)
Horswill et al. (1990a)	Wrestlers/male/collegiate	2× WL 6% (4 d)	BW, SKF	Arm cranking ergometer and 8 bouts of 15 s maximal effort intervals with 30 s of easy pace between	→ Arm cranking ergometer and 8 bouts of 15 s maximal effort intervals with 30 s of easy pace between (high carb diet) ↓Arm cranking ergometer and 8 bouts of 15 s maximal effort intervals with 30 s of easy pace between (low carb diet)	High carbohydrate diet *Baseline* ∑7SKF,mm = 57.6 ± 3.6 *After WL* ∑7SKF,mm = 53.1 ± 3.5 low carbohydrate diet *Baseline* ∑7SKF,mm = 58.1 ± 3.3 *After WL* ∑7SKF,mm = 53.4 ± 3.5
Filaire et al. (2001)	Judo/male/national	WL 4.9% (7 d)	BW, FM	Left arm strength and 30 s jumping test, 7 s jumping test	→ Left arm strength 7 s jumping test ↓30 s jumping test	*Baseline* %FM = 17.3 ± 2.1 *After 7 d food restriction* %FM = 16.8 ± 1.4 (SKF)
Webster et al. (1990)	Wrestlers/male/intercollegiate	WL 3.8% (36 h)	BW, Bd, FM	Strength, anaerobic power, anaerobic capacity, the lactate threshold, and peak aerobic power	↓Strength, anaerobic power, anaerobic capacity, the lactate threshold, and peak aerobic power	*Baseline* Bd = 1.073 (%FM = 11.2) *After WL* Bd = 1.074 (%FM = 11.2) (UWW)

(Continued)

TABLE 12.2 (*Continued*)
Body Composition and Performance in Weight-Sensitive Sports, Longitudinal Studies

Study	Sports/Sex/Level of Competition	% of Reduction	Body Composition Variables	Performance Variables	Influence of BC Changes in Performance	Body Composition Characteristics (Method)
Hall and Lane (2001)	Boxers/male/amateur	WL 5.2% (1 wk)	BW	Difference between the number of repetitions set as goal by each individual and the number of repetitions performed, in a 4 × 2 minute circuit training	→ Number of repetitions	n.a.
Degoutte et al. (2006)	Judo/male/national	WL 5% (7 d)	BW, FM	Handgrip and maximal strength, a 30 s rowing task, and simulated competition (5 × 5 minute bouts)	↓ Handgrip and maximal strength, 30 s rowing task, and simulated competition	Diet group *Baseline* %FM = 15.8 ± 1.1 *After 7 d food restriction* %FM = 15.0 ± 1.0 (SKF)
Silva et al. (2010)	Judo/male/elite	WL 1.1 kg (1 mo)	TBW, ICW, ECW, FM, LST, BW	Upper-body power	↓ Upper-body power	*Baseline* %FM = 12.1 ± 3.1 *Pre-competition* %FM = 11.7 ± 2.8 (DXA)
Silva et al. (2011)	Judo/male/elite	WL 1.1 kg (1 mo)	TBW, ICW, ECW, FM, BW	Grip strength	↓ Grip strength	*Baseline* %FM = 12.1 ± 3.1 *Pre-competition* %FM = 11.7 ± 2.8 (DXA)
Slater et al. (2006)	Rowers/male and female/national	WL 3.9% (24 h)	BW	3 × 1800 m time trials under cool conditions, 48 h apart each trial.	→ Time trials under cool conditions	n.a.
Slater et al. (2005)	Rowers/male and female/national	WL 4.3% (24 h)	BW	Ergometer trials	↓ Ergometer trials	n.a.

(Continued)

TABLE 12.2 (*Continued*)
Body Composition and Performance in Weight-Sensitive Sports, Longitudinal Studies

Study	Sports/Sex/Level of Competition	% of Reduction	Body Composition Variables	Performance Variables	Influence of BC Changes in Performance	Body Composition Characteristics (Method)
Koutedakis et al. (1994)	Lightweight rowers/ male and female/ international	WL 6% (8 wk)	BW, FFM, FM	Maximal oxygen intake consumption (VO_2max), respiratory anaerobic threshold (T_{vent}), upper body anaerobic peak power (PP) and mean power (MP) outputs, and knee flexor (KF) and extensor (KE) isokinetic peak torques	$\rightarrow VO_2max$, PP, MP, and KE $\downarrow T_{vent}$ and KF	*Baseline* %FFM = 86.6 ± 4.9 (%FM = 13.4%) *8 wk* %FFM = 88.0 ± 5.7 (%FM = 12.0%) (TBK)
Koutedakis et al. (1994)	Lightweight rowers/ female/international	WL 7.4% (16 wk)	BW, FFM, FM	Maximal oxygen consumption (VO_2max), respiratory anaerobic threshold (T_{vent}), upper body anaerobic peak power (PP) and mean power (MP) outputs, and knee flexor (KF) and extensor (KE) isokinetic peak torques	$\uparrow VO_2max$, T_{vent}, PP, and KF $\rightarrow$ MP and KE	*Baseline* %FFM = 86.0 ± 5.4 (%FM = 14.0%) *16 wk* %FFM = 88.3 ± 5.2 (%FM = 11.7%) (TBK)
Wilson et al. (2014)	Jockeys/male/ professional	WL 2% (45 minute)	BW	Chest strength, leg strength, simulated riding performance, and simple reaction time	$\downarrow$ Chest strength, leg strength, simulated riding performance $\rightarrow$ simple reaction time	n.a.
Dolan et al. (2013)	Jockeys/male/ professional	WL 3.6% (48 h)	BW, FM	VO_2peak and peak work capacity	$\downarrow$ Peak work $\rightarrow VO_2$peak	*Baseline* %FM = 9.1 ± 1.4 *Retrial* %FM = 8.9 ± 1.4 (SKF)

(*Continued*)

TABLE 12.2 (Continued)
Body Composition and Performance in Weight-Sensitive Sports, Longitudinal Studies

Study	Sports/Sex/Level of Competition	% of Reduction	Body Composition Variables	Performance Variables	Influence of BC Changes in Performance	Body Composition Characteristics (Method)
Garthe et al. (2011a)	Athletes[a]/male and female/elite	WL 5.3% (5 weeks)	FM, LST, BW	Countermovement jump, 1 RM squat, bench press, bench pull, and 40-m sprint	→ Countermovement jump, bench press, bench pull, and 40-m sprint ↑ 1 RM squat	Baseline *Slow-rate WL* Male %FM = 17.0 ± 5.0 Female %FM = 27.0 ± 5.0 *Fast-rate WL* Male %FM = 16.0 ± 3.0 Female %FM = 30.0 ± 5.0 (DXA)
Garthe et al. (2011a)	Athletes[a]/male and female/elite	WL 5.6% (9 weeks)	FM, LST, BW	Countermovement jump, 1 RM squat, bench press, bench pull, and 40-m sprint	↑ Countermovement jump, 1 RM squat, bench press, bench pull → 40-m sprint	Baseline *Slow-rate WL* Male %FM = 17.0 ± 5.0 Female %FM = 27.0 ± 5.0 *Fast-rate WL* Male %FM = 16.0 ± 3.0 Female %FM = 30.0 ± 5.0 (DXA)
Garthe et al. (2011b)	Athletes[a]/male and female/elite	6 mo after WL	FM, LST, BW	1 RM squat, bench press, and bench pull	→ 1 RM squat, bench press, and bench pull	Baseline *Ad libitum* %FM = 13.0 ± 6.0
Garthe et al. (2011b)	Athletes[a]/male and female/elite	12 mo after WL		1 RM squat, bench press, and bench pull	→ 1 RM squat, bench press, and bench pull	*Nutritional counselling* %FM = 11.0 ± 4.0 (DXA)

(Continued)

TABLE 12.2 (*Continued*)
Body Composition and Performance in Weight-Sensitive Sports, Longitudinal Studies

Study	Sports/Sex/Level of Competition	% of Reduction	Body Composition Variables	Performance Variables	Influence of BC Changes in Performance	Body Composition Characteristics (Method)
Ingjer and Sundgot-Borgen (1991)	Long-distance runners and long-distance runners/female/elite	2 mo WL (2 mo) 9.4%	BW, FM	VO_2max Running speed	↓VO_2max (only in the cases) ↓Running speed (only in the cases)	*Baseline:* cases %FM = 17.4 ± 2.2; controls %FM = 14.8 ± 0.5 *After 2 mo dieting:* cases %FM = 11.5 ± 3.2; controls %FM = 14.6 ± 0.4 *After 1 year:* Cases %FM = 12.1 ± 3.2; controls %FM = 14.6 ± 0.4 (SKF)

Note: BW, body weight; WL, weight loss; WR, weight gain; BW, body weight; SKF, skinfold; FM, fat mass; FFM, fat-free mass; LST, lean-soft tissue; TBW, total body water; ECW, extracellular water; ICW, intracellular water; UWW, underwater weighting; DXA, dual x-ray absorptiometry; TBK, total body potassium; d, days; wk, weeks; mo, months; n.a., data not available (authors only reported body weight);→, performance remained unchanged after weight change; ↑ performance increased after weight change; ↓ performance decreased after weight change.

[a] Includes cross-country skiing, judo, jujitsu, taekwondo, water-skiing, motocross, cycling, track and field, kickboxing, gymnastics, alpine skiing, ski-jumping, freestyle sports dancing, skating, biathlon, and ice hockey.

TABLE 12.3

Body Composition and Performance in Gravitational and Aesthetic Sports (Cross-Sectional Studies)

Study	Sports/Sex/1evel of Competition	Variables of Body Composition Assessed	Performance Variables	Association of BC with Performance	Body Composition (Method)
Claessens et al. (1991)	Rhythmic gymnastics/male/ international	BW, height, sitting height, leg and forearm length, humerus and femur width, girths, and SKF	Scores	SKF (−) Other (0)	n.a
Claessens et al. (1999)	Rhythmic gymnastics/male/ international	SKF and somatotype	Scores	SKF (−) Endomorphic (−)	n.a
Di Cagno et al. (2008)	Rhythmic gymnastics/ female/elite + sub-elite	Anthropometric variables, FFM	Height of hopping	FFM (+) anthropometric variables (0)	*Elite* FM, kg = 4.8 ± 0.7 BW, kg = 47.9 ± 3.4
			Countermovement jump	FFM (0) anthropometric variables (0)	*Sub-Elite* FM, kg = 4.2 ± 1.3 BW, kg = 39.8 ± 6.7 (SKF)
Silva and Paiva (2015)	Rhythmic gymnasts/female/ elite	WC/HC, WC, BMI, FM, FFM, TBW	Scores	WC/HC (−) WC (+)	*Highest scores* %FM = 9.2 ± 2.2 *Lowest scores* %FM = 8.9 ± 2.0 (BIA)
Knechtle et al. (2012)	Half-marathon, marathon, and ultra-marathon/males/ master athletes	SMM, FM	Race time	FM (+) SMM (0)	*Half-marathoners* %FM = 18.2 ± 4.4 *Marathoners* %FM = 16.9 ± 3.4 *100-km ultra-Marathoners* %FM = 18.2 ± 4.4 (SKF)

(Continued)

TABLE 12.3 (*Continued*)
Body Composition and Performance in Gravitational and Aesthetic Sports (Cross-Sectional Studies)

Study	Sports/Sex/Level of Competition	Variables of Body Composition Assessed	Performance Variables	Association of BC with Performance	Body Composition (Method)
Tanaka and Matsuura (1982)	Middle and long-distance runners/male/well-trained	Several anthropometric variables	Race time 5000	Chest girth (−) Leg length (−) Upper leg length (−) Thigh girth (−) Waist girth (−)	%FM = 10.6 ± 1.1 Σ2SKF,mm = 13.5 ± 2.3~ (SKF)
			Race time 10,000 m	Upper arm girth (+) Forearm girth (+) Rohrer index (+) BMI (+)	
Knechtle et al. (2010)	Ultra-marathoners/male/	BW, BMI, %FM, Circumference: Upper arm, thigh, calf, leg length	Race time	BW (+) BMI (+) %FM (+) Circumference: Upper arm (+), thigh (0), calf (0) Leg length (0)	%FM = 16.1 ± 4.3 (SKF)
Barandun et al. (2012)	Marathoners/male/ recreational	BW, %FM, Σ8SKF, SMM	Race time	BW (0) %FM (+) Σ8SKF (+) SMM (0)	%FM = 16.3 ± 5.6 Σ8SKF,mm = 88.4 ± 26.2 (SKF)

(Continued)

TABLE 12.3 (Continued)
Body Composition and Performance in Gravitational and Aesthetic Sports (Cross-Sectional Studies)

Study	Sports/Sex/Level of Competition	Variables of Body Composition Assessed	Performance Variables	Association of BC with Performance	Body Composition (Method)
Tanda and Knechtle (2015), Barandun et al. (2012), Knechtle et al. (2010)	Marathoners and ultra-marathoners/male	%FM	Race pace	%FM (+)	*Marathoners:* %FM = 16.3 ± 3.6 *Ultra-marathoners* %FM = 16.1 ± 4.3 (SKF)
Stoggl et al. (2010)	Male sprint skiers/male/elite	BW, total and regional body composition	Double poling	BW (+) LST, kg (+) Trunk mass (+) Trunk LST (+) Trunk FM (−)	%FM = 12.5 ± 2.4 %LST = 83.4 ± 2.3 (DXA)
			Diagonal stride	LST (+) FM (−) Trunk LST (+) Trunk FM (−) Arms and legs LST (+)	

Note: BW, body weight; SKF, skinfold; FM, fat mass; FFM, fat-free mass; LST, lean-soft tissue; SMM; skeletal muscle mass; TBW, total body water; WC, waist circumference; HC, hip circumference; BMI, body mass index; DXA, dual x-ray absorptiometry; n.a., data not available (authors only reported body weight); (+), positive association; (−), negative association; (0); no association.

interestingly the authors also verified that the loss of adiposity seems to be specific of the muscular groups used during training, and that improvements in performance were consistently related to decreases in lower limbs SKF. In this regard, Knechtle (2014) has reviewed the relationship between anthropometric characteristics with race performance in endurance and ultra-endurance athletes. In this work the author verified that, depending on the race distance and duration, specific single SKF thickness are related to the running pace. In another review, Knechtle et al. (2015) reported that in the Ironman triathlon there are sex differences in the association between individual SKF thickness and performance.

In ski-jumping, body weight is associated with the jump length and the velocity of motion; lighter athletes may benefit by flying further, and the touch down is facilitated by a lower landing velocity (Muller 2009a). To achieve a competitive advantage, a considerable number of underweight athletes with eating disorders were observed among ski-jumpers in the past, fortunately new competition regulations have now helped to reduce this prevalence. Muller (2009b) has reviewed body composition issues in ski-jumping and stated that the mean BMI in ski-jumpers has considerably changed from 23.6 kg/m² in the 1970s to 19.4 kg/m² in 2002. The author mentions that this 4.2 kg/m² reduction in mean BMI can theoretically lead to an increase up to 20 m in jumping length on a large hill in a 180 cm tall athlete. Regardless, a low body weight may also cause a negative influence in performance because of a reduction in muscle strength, general weakness, reduced ability to cope with pressure, and increased susceptibility to disease.

In endurance sports, a lower body weight may be advantageous as mechanical work required for accelerating the body is expected to be lower when related to heavier athletes (Muller 2009b). Regardless the impact of a low body weight or a low BMI in endurance performance is not consensual (Knechtle 2014). On the other hand, the composition of body weight seems to play an important role; in master long-distance athletes, including half-marathoners, marathoners, and ultra-marathoners, FM, and not skeletal muscle mass was associated with race time (Knechtle et al. 2012). Combining data from different studies, Tanda and Knechtle (2015) verified that in marathoners and ultra-marathoners adiposity was associated with a worst performance, with the race pace (seconds per km) increasing linearly with %FM (r = 0.60 for marathoners and r = 0.51 for ultra-marathoners). Interestingly, when considering only athletes with lower levels of adiposity (%FM < 15%) there was no association between adiposity and race pace in these endurance athletes, with race time being predicted uniquely by training characteristics. Knechtle (2014) has recently reviewed the importance of body composition and anthropometric characteristics in road and mountain bike cyclists, and in runners and triathletes over different distances and verified that a low FM was among the most important predictor variables for ultra-endurance race performance.

In cross-country skiing there is a tendency for heavier skiers to be more successful than light ones (Bergh and Forsberg 1992) although body weight does not seem to be associated with either maximal or submaximal oxygen uptake in this group of athletes. Regardless, a reduced %FM (Niinimaa et al. 1978) and greater amounts of lean tissue, particularly in the arms, are of great importance for cross-country skiing performance (Larsson and Henriksson-Larsen 2008). On the other hand, it has also been observed that in cross-country skiing the association between performance and body composition depends on the technique and on the type of track; skiers who are light will have advantage on steep uphill slopes, whereas heavier skiers will be favored in the other parts of the track (Bergh 1987). Stoggl et al. (2010) verified that cross-country skiers should look for a body composition profile with lower adiposity and a higher percentage of lean whereas different body composition profiles are associated with different techniques required during the competition.

Considering the possible positive impact of low levels of adiposity in endurance sports there are several athletes aiming to reduce their body weight for competition periods. A case-control study (Ingjer and Sundgot-Borgen 1991) with seven elite female endurance athletes, including three middle- and long-distance runners and four cross-country skiers undergoing a weight-loss period (18–26 years) investigated the relationship of weight reduction on maximal oxygen consumption and running speed. Pathogenic weight-control methods were reported by all athletes with a weight-loss period of 2 months (stable body weight the rest of the year), when compared with controls, which maintained a stable weight. Differences in %FM were observed between groups and these athletes presented a significant decrease in performance when compared to controls. The authors concluded that a period of about 1-year would be required to regain performance. Of importance is the fact that the sample in this study included two athletes diagnosed with anorexia athletica and two with bulimia nervosa.

12.3.2 WEIGHT CLASS SPORTS

To qualify for a given weight category, many athletes from weight class sports undertake remarkable weight changes preceding the competition (Oppliger et al. 1996, 2003, 2006). Studies indicate that muscle endurance and prolonged aerobic and anaerobic work capacity are likely to be diminished by rapid weight loss. Gradual weight loss seems to be the method with the smallest impairment in performance in these athletes (Garthe et al. 2011a). Yet, the extent of the impairment seems to depend on the time from weigh-in to competition and the recovery strategy used (Sundgot-Borgen and Garthe 2011).

The most common studies regarding weight class sports have been conducted to understand the impact of short-term weight reductions on body composition and on athletes' performance. Fogelholm et al. (1993) studied the effect of a gradual and a rapid weight loss, both from energy restriction (gradual 3: weeks and rapid: 2.4 day) in the performance of wrestlers and judo athletes, evaluated by a sprint (30 m), Wingate test, and vertical jump height with extra load. The authors concluded that weight-loss, regardless of the method, impaired experienced athletes' performance (with the exception of vertical jump height which improved 6%–8% in the gradual weight-loss process).

Artioli et al. (2010) examined the effects of rapid (7 days) weight loss (5% body weight reduction by self-determined regimen) followed by a 4-hour recovery on judo-related performance. Weight loss resulted in a discrete, however significant, decrease in FM and in a marked decrease in FFM in the weight-loss group. Performance was tested through a specific judo exercise, a 5-minute judo combat, and by three Wingate tests. Performance in both judo athletes engaged in a weight reduction intervention and in judo athletes from the control group (no weight reduction), remained unchanged in sport-specific exercises and had a slight improvement in Wingate test.

The impact of repeated weight reductions, induced by fluid and energy restriction, on performance in male amateur boxers was studied by Smith et al. (2001). Performance was assessed in a boxing ergometer with bouts of 3, 3 minute rounds with 1 minute rest. Authors concluded that energy and fluid restrictions in amateur boxers do not lead to a significant decrease in performance, but because of the small sample size and large variations in individual performances, these findings should be interpreted cautiously.

In a study of 28 well-trained combat athletes, Reljic et al. (2015) reported no significant change in aerobic performance capacity assessed by peak treadmill-running and oxygen consumption (VO$_2$peak) in a group that performed rapid weight loss, compared to the control group, despite a significant decrease in hemoglobin caused by impaired erythropoiesis and increased hemolysis. Total body water declined significantly during weight loss, which was due to both a loss in extracellular and intracellular water. FFM and %FM also decreased in the group that lost weight.

Marttinen et al. (2011) found that the self-selected rapid weight-loss strategy (weight loss during 10 days before competition) did not impair performance regarding grip strength and lower-body power (Wingate test), among 16 male collegiate wrestlers.

In a sample of judo athletes, Koral and Dosseville (2009) examined the impact of a combination of a gradual and a rapid body weight loss on performance, in a 4-week period. Athletes were split into a diet group (self-restricted diet) and a non-diet group. The diet group significantly reduced FM. The chosen indicators of performance were countermovement jump, squat jump, 5 and 30 s repetitions of judo movements, and rowing with extra load. No differences between groups were observed for all performance parameters, with the exception of the 30 s repetitions of judo movements which decreased in the diet group.

Male wrestlers were randomized into two weight-loss processes over 4 days, one with a low carbohydrate diet and one with a high carbohydrate diet. Performance was assessed after the two weight-loss processes by arm cranking ergometer and eight bouts of 15 s maximal effort intervals with 30 s of easy pace between. The sum of SKF showed a reduction by ~4.5 mm in both groups after intervention, nevertheless, results suggested that performance was maintained with the high carbohydrate diet and impaired with the low carbohydrate diet. Additionally, performance decreased more in the second weight-loss process (Horswill et al. 1990a).

Filaire et al. (2001) studied the dietary intake, plasma lipids, lipoprotein and apolipoprotein levels, anthropometric measurements, and anaerobic performance of judo athletes during a period of weight stability and after a 7-day food restriction, resulting in weight loss. FFM showed a tendency to decrease. Regarding performance tests, left arm strength and 30 s jumping test decreased while the 7 s jumping test was not affected by the diet restriction.

An investigation conducted by Webster et al. (1990) studied the effects of weight loss (36 hours) through dehydration techniques on performance parameters (strength, anaerobic power, anaerobic capacity, the lactate threshold, and peak aerobic power), in intercollegiate wrestlers. Weight loss only occurred during the 12 hour prior to weigh-in and resulted in a reduction in upper body but not lower body strength parameters (peak torque and average work per repetition). Additionally, anaerobic power, anaerobic capacity, VO$_2$peak, and treadmill time to exhaustion were also reduced at the end of the weight loss. With these results in hand, authors concluded that wrestling weight-loss techniques result in impairment of strength, anaerobic power, anaerobic capacity, lactate threshold, and aerobic power.

Hall and Lane (2001) studied the impact of a rapid and self-selected strategy for weight loss in the performance of amateur boxers. The authors assessed the performance as the difference between the number of repetitions set as a goal by each individual and the number of repetitions performed, in a 4×2 minute circuit training (1-minute recovery between rounds). Results indicated that athletes failed to reach their subjective expected level of performance after losing weight.

The effects of weight loss induced by energy and fluid intake restriction on physiology, psychology, and physical performance of judo athletes were studied by Degoutte et al. (2006), in two groups: a 5% weight loss intervention and a control group. Weight loss was completed through self and individual determined approaches during the week before the competition. The weight-loss group showed a significant decline in %FM and FFM, while no changes occurred in the control group. Performance testing included handgrip and maximal strength, a 30 s rowing task (to assess anaerobic capacity of the upper limbs) and a simulated competition (5×5 minute bouts). This study showed that food restriction was associated with poor performance and that the combination of energy restriction and intense exercise training adversely affected performance before the competition.

In judo athletes a significant mean reduction of 1.1 kg was observed in body weight from a period of weight maintenance to before a competition but no mean changes were found in FM, FFM, lean soft tissue (LST), total, extracellular, and intracellular water (Silva et al. 2010, 2011). The authors verified that total body water and intracellular water changes were positively related to upper-body power variation and that reduction in intracellular water increased the risk of losing grip strength in these judo athletes. It is important to mention that total and extracellular water were assessed by dilution methods, which are state-of-the-art techniques for body water assessment.

To assess the impact of moderate (4%) but acute (24 hours) weight loss compared to no weight restriction on rowing performance, Slater et al. (2006) performed a 3×1800 m time trials under cool conditions, 48 hours apart each trial. Weight loss showed no significant (however a tendency was observed) effect on the on-water time trial performance compared with unrestricted body weight. Therefore, authors settled that acute weight loss of ~4% over 24 hours, combined with aggressive weight loss strategies, can be undertaken with minimal impact on on-water rowing performance, in cool conditions.

The impact of acute weight loss on rowing performance was also assessed by Slater et al. (2005) in another research study. Competitive rowers completed four ergometer trials, each separated by 48 hours: two trials after a 4% body weight loss in the previous 24 hours and two after no weight restrictions. Each weight condition was performed in a thermoneutral environment and in the heat. Results indicated that performance was impaired by weight loss, which was further exacerbated when exercise was performed in the heat.

Weight loss, resulting from energy restriction, in female elite lightweight rowers was associated with performance indicators (Koutedakis et al. 1994). Weight loss was associated with performance over an 8- and a 16-week period. Performance parameters included maximal oxygen consumption (VO_2max), respiratory anaerobic threshold (T_{vent}), upper body anaerobic peak power and mean power outputs, and knee flexor and extensor isokinetic peak torques. In the two weight-reduction periods, FFM contributed by approximately 50% to the weight loss. The authors concluded that (i) at the end of an 8-week weight-reduction period, T_{vent} and knee flexor decreased; (ii) at the end of a 16-week period weight loss, VO_2max and peak power increased.

Regarding jockeys, Wilson et al. (2014) tested the effect of weight loss on performance, namely in chest strength, leg strength, simulated riding performance, and simple reaction time after performing 45 minutes of exercise. Authors reported a significant impairment in maximum pushing frequency (due to a reduction in chest and leg strength) and in the simulated riding performance.

Male jockeys and controls were evaluated in order to understand the effect of weight loss on aerobic work capacity (cycle ergometer test) and cognitive processes. Jockeys reduced weight two times, 4% each, within 48 hours. The $VO_{2\,peak}$ remained unaltered between trials but the peak power output (watts and watts/kg) at which this peak was achieved was significantly reduced. The authors concluded that reductions in body weight below 4% of the initial weight caused a decrease in aerobic work capacity (Dolan et al. 2013).

12.3.3 AESTHETIC SPORTS

Leanness is generally viewed in aesthetic sports as an enhancer of the performance and final scores, with heavier athletes expected to be slower and less flexible (Smolak et al. 2000). The type of pressure that aesthetic athletes are submitted might lead to a drive for thinness, preoccupation with weight and shape, adoption of extreme methods to lose weight, and, eventually, serious eating problems (Smolak et al. 2000). In these sports a reduced body weight is regularly observed, especially in female athletes.

A relation between body type characteristics and performance in gymnasts was assessed (Claessens et al. 1991, 1999). Male athletes were separated according to performance scores obtained in the 24th World Championship, with athletes that obtained higher scores presenting lower mean values of SKF (Claessens et al. 1991). In female athletes, performance scores were positively associated with SKF or an endomorph somatotype; Gymnasts with higher mean values of SKF or a more endomorphic somatotype tend to have lower performance scores (Claessens et al. 1999).

Body composition and performance (assessed by jumping ability) were correlated in elite and non-elite gymnastics. Elite gymnasts had significantly higher FFM values and jumping height, but no significant differences in countermovement jump between two groups were found (Di Cagno et al. 2008). Elite and non elite rhythmic gymnastics were evaluated to understand the physiological and anthropometric predictors of performance (assessed by the obtained scores in a national competition). The authors reported that aerobic power, flexibility, and explosive strength were the most important determinants of performance in this sport (Douda et al. 2008).

Silva and Paiva (2015) evaluated the relationship between body composition, sleep, precompetitive anxiety, and dietary intake on elite female gymnasts' performance prior to an international competition. Gymnasts' performance (assessed by competition scores) was positively correlated with waist circumference; however, it was negatively related with the waist-to-hip ratio, energy availability, and exercise energy expenditure.

12.3.4 MIXED WEIGHT-SENSITIVE SPORTS

A study combining athletes of several weight-sensitive sports including, cross-country skiing, judo, jujitsu, taekwondo, water-skiing, motocross, cycling, track and field, kickboxing, gymnastics, alpine skiing, ski jumping, freestyle sports, dancing, skating, biathlon, and ice hockey investigated weight loss obtained through controlled diet intervention, at two different rates demonstrating an improvement of performance in the majority of physical tests (Garthe et al. 2011a). Weight was reduced by 5.6% in the slow rate group and by 5.3% in the fast rate group. There was a significant decrease in FM in both groups by 31.2% and 23.4%, respectively, for the slow rate group and fast rate group. Total LST increased significantly by 2.0% in the slow rate group and a nonsignificant increase of 1.1% was observed in the fast rate group. Results of the slow rate intervention showed performance improvements in countermovement jump, one-repetition maximum (1RM) squat, bench press and pull, and unchanged results for 40-m sprint. Regarding the fast rate intervention, performance remained unchanged in all the above parameters with the exception of a significant improvement in 1RM squat.

A follow-up after 6 and 12 months of the aforementioned investigation (Garthe et al. 2011b) was also conducted. Six months after the initial intervention, the slow rate group regained 77% of the weight lost, whereas the fast rate group regained 14%. Twelve months after the initial intervention, both groups had returned to their initial body weights. The FM component showed a tendency to decrease more in the slow rate than in the fast rate group during the intervention. Twelve months after the intervention, both groups regained their original FM. Total LST returned to baseline after 6 and 12 months and there was no significant difference in total LST between groups over time. Due to the small sample size, countermovement jump and 40-m sprint data analysis were excluded. Over time no significant changes in performance were observed in the fast rate group. The 1RM squat in the slow rate group returned to baseline values at 6 and 12 months after intervention. Bench press performance in the slow rate group was still higher at 12 months' post-intervention compared to baseline.

12.4 BODY COMPOSITION AND HEALTH

Athletes involved in weight-sensitive sports, where leanness or a specific target weight is relevant for performance are at a higher pressure compared to other non-weight-sensitive sports (de Bruin et al. 2007). As such, to meet their sports requirements and enhance performance the pressure to achieve an ideal body weight or shape is likely to occur, on a daily basis, from judges and coaches (Sundgot-Borgen 1994; Nattiv et al. 2007), or if a target weight is required prior competition.

As a consequence, risky weight management methods, disordered eating behaviors, and a compromised health and performance is expected to achieve their dieting goals (Oppliger et al. 2003; Nattiv et al. 2007; Slater et al. 2014).

The impact of extreme weight-control techniques on performance and health differs by sport, level of physical performance, and the methodology employed by several studies, limiting a general and accurate conclusion for diverse weight-sensitive sports (Sundgot-Borgen and Garthe 2011). The female athlete triad (Sundgot-Borgen 1994; Sundgot-Borgen and Torstveit 2004; Torstveit and Sundgot-Borgen 2005; Nattiv et al. 2007), dehydration, cognitive function, stress and inflammatory markers, compromised growth and maturation are common health-related consequences of the extreme dieting methods that these athletes are exposed to (Sundgot-Borgen and Garthe 2011).

Currently, dieting patterns and rapid weight loss in athletes competing in sports where leanness or a lower body weight is desired for the sport-specific demands, meet the criteria for clinical eating disorders (Rosendahl et al. 2009).

12.4.1 The Female Athlete Triad

The benefits of participating in sports are recognized among adolescents and adult female athletes but it is important to assure adequate nutrition to avoid compromising reproductive and skeletal health.

In fact, amenorrhea is expected to occur when female athletes are exposed to low-energy availability, insufficient to meet the sport-specific energy requirements and remaining physiological needs (Loucks et al. 1989, 1992). The most evident sign of such energy deficit is the disruption of the reproductive cycle that leads to absent or irregular menses. Accordingly, the need for achieving a certain level of FM leads to extreme dieting processes and disordered eating, that ultimately ends up in clinical eating disorders, such as anorexia or bulimia nervosa. The resulting energy deficit along with a reduction in estrogen levels may cause remodeling imbalance in the bone, which will lead to low bone mass or osteoporosis (Drinkwater et al. 1984; Ihle and Loucks 2004). The insufficient energy intake for the demands of a specific sport will decrease the energy availability, which in turn leads to menstrual dysfunction and, as a consequence, to a low BMD, a sequence of events that is known as the "Female Athlete Triad."

The female triad was formally recognized due to the rise in the rates of stress fractures, menstrual dysfunction, and low BMD in apparently healthy female athletes, being first characterized by the presence of an eating disorder, amenorrhea, and osteoporosis (Otis et al. 1997). Another position stand in 2007, on the female athlete triad acknowledged this syndrome as the result of complex and interrelated conditions, specifically energy availability, menstrual status, and BMD, with varied clinical manifestations, comprising eating disorders, functional hypothalamic amenorrhea, and osteoporosis (Nattiv et al. 2007), as displayed in Figure 12.2.

12.4.1.1 Components of the Triad

12.4.1.1.1 Energy Availability

Female athletes involved in sports that emphasize leanness and aesthetics, such as gymnastics, figure skating, or ballet dancing, are at higher risk of developing the female athlete triad. Food restriction, diuretic abuse, binging or purging, laxatives, enemas or/and excessive exercise are likely to occur in these athletes resulting in low-energy availability (Nattiv et al. 2007). Even though the presence of eating behavior disorders is not required to activate the cascade of harmful events that characterize the female athlete triad, abnormal eating behaviors, false beliefs about eating, and unreasonable fear of gaining body weight contribute to a low-energy availability (Sundgot-Borgen 1993; Johnson et al. 1999; Beals and Hill 2006). Eating disorders are potentially chronic conditions associated with a range of medical, psychosocial, and psychological consequences. Anorexia nervosa, bulimia, and other eating disorders not otherwise specified are the most common eating disorders (American Psychiatric Association 2013). This chapter, however, is not intended to cover this topic but a detailed review is provided in a recent update on eating disorders in athletes (Joy et al. 2016).

12.4.1.1.2 Menstrual Status

The most frequent menstrual dysfunction in female athletes is amenorrhea, or the lack of menstrual cycle, and that can be categorized as primary and secondary amenorrhea (Medicine 2008). In young athletic females, primary amenorrhea, or late menarche, may occur in those that started their training prior puberty, if by the age of 15 years the menstrual cycle is still absent though normal secondary sexual characteristics are presented (Roupas and Georgopoulos 2011). Postmenarchal female athletes missing three or more cycles after menarche, consecutively (if not pregnant), are

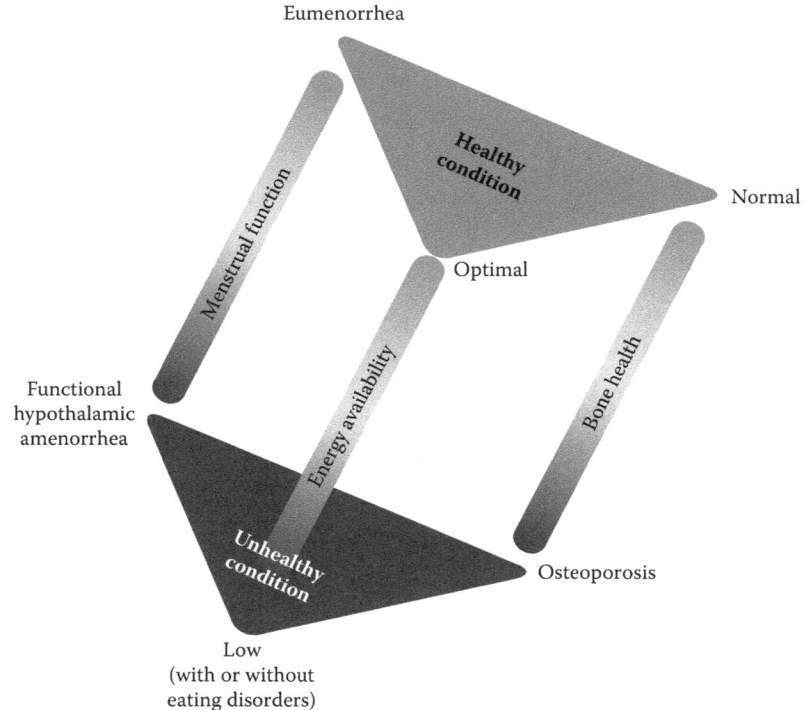

FIGURE 12.2 Female athlete triad: middle, left, and right spectral lines represent energy availability, menstrual function, and bone health, respectively, along which female athletes are distributed. According to diet and exercise habits, an athlete's condition moves along each spectral line at a different rate or direction. (Adapted from Nattiv, A. et al. 2007. *Med Sci Sports Exerc* 39:1867–82.)

classified as presenting a secondary amenorrhea (Roupas and Georgopoulos 2011). Oligomenorrhea, describes menstrual cycles longer than 35 days or menstrual intervals of 45–90 days (Roupas and Georgopoulos 2011) and is also common in athletic girls and women involved in intensive exercise (Warren and Perlroth 2001). Anovulation and a luteal phase defect is also likely to occur in female athletes due to concomitant lower production of progesterone during the luteal phase and estrogen production in the early follicular phase (De Souza et al. 1998).

Menstrual cycle problems result from abnormal hypothalamic gonadotrophin-releasing hormone (GnRH) pulsatility that in turn influences the gonadotropin pulsatility leading to a decrease secretion of luteinizing hormone (LH) and follicle stimulating hormone (FSH). As a consequence, the ovarian function is not stimulated, leading to a drop in progesterone and estrogens levels.

Several factors have been related to menstrual dysfunction, such as weight, body composition, physical and psychological stress, energy balance, dietary intake, type of sport, and the maturity of reproductive system (Roupas and Georgopoulos 2011).

12.4.1.1.3 Weight and Body Composition

Frisch and MacArthur (1974) theorized in 1939 that a "critical threshold" of FM, specifically 17% of body weight, is required to achieve the onset of menarche and that a fall in FM below 22% of body weight leads to menstruation disturbances. In their theory, Frisch and MacArthur (1974) pointed out that decreases in metabolic rate and alterations in the sensitivity of the hypothalamus to gonadal steroids occurs at a critical percentage of FM. Accordingly, a low body weight and body composition alterations have been accepted as the most rational explanation for menstrual dysfunction in athletes. However, this theory dysfunction has been challenged (Trussell 1980; Bronson and Manning

1991; Loucks 2003), and a focus on adipose tissue as an active endocrine organ has increased. Relevant investigations pointed out the role of specific adipokines, secreted by the adipocyte, as signals of energy balance, reproductive function, insulin action, and inflammatory processes. Actually, reproductive function has been strongly related with leptin levels whereas growing interest has been directed to adiponectin as a mediator in metabolism and reproduction.

The body composition hypothesis has gained relevance after leptin was discovered. In fact, leptin has an important role as a mediator between the relation of FM and the reproductive system (Moschos et al. 2002). Levels of leptin reflect energy balance status; an accentuated reduction in leptin has been addressed following restrictions in dieting and fasting state, whereas rises after overfeeding and refeeding following energy restriction occur. Nevertheless, even in extreme underfed females, leptin seems to mediate the preservation of neuroendocrine control of the reproductive system (Miller et al. 2004). These observations reveal that a critical serum leptin level is required for menstrual function (Kopp et al. 1997). Highly trained athletes reported declines in levels of leptin and the secretion of the diurnal patterns of leptin was absent in amenorrheic but not in eumenorrheic female athletes (Laughlin and Yen 1997).

Adiponectin is inversely related with FM levels, presenting a noticeable decline in obesity, but with increases in substantial weight lost and prolonged fasting. In addition to the role in cardiovascular protection, inflammatory process, and metabolism, it has been suggested that adiponectin has a possible role in neuroendocrine reproductive regulation (Michalakis and Segars 2010). Therefore, along with leptin, the role of adiponectin as a link between adipocyte and the reproductive system is expected. As a result, if levels of adiponectin are high (as observed in energy restricted athletic women) LH suppression levels and chronic anovulation may occur.

Moreover, a reduction in LH pulsatility is also caused by high ghrelin levels (Kluge et al. 2007). Greater levels of ghrelin have been observed in amenorrheic compared to eumenorrheic exercising individuals, suggesting that higher levels of ghrelin may be related with hypogonadotropic hypogonadism (De Souza et al. 2004).

12.4.1.1.4 *Physical Stress*

The hypothesis that stress due to exercise may lead to menstrual dysfunction has been sustained by investigations conducted in athletes with amenorrhea. Untrained women who present a regular menstrual cycle developed menstrual disturbances when exposed to vigorous exercise (Bullen et al. 1985). Indeed, these women when exposed to higher amounts of aerobic exercise raised the prevalence of anovulation and defects on luteal phase. Likewise, levels of cortisol slightly increase in amenorrheic athletes (Ding et al. 1988).

Athletes with significant menstrual dysfunction display a larger activation of hypothalamic–pituitary–adrenal (HPA) axis (Loucks et al. 1989; Laughlin and Yen 1996; Chrousos et al. 1998), which denotes an endocrine mechanism of reproductive disturbances in athletes. Cortisol is able to suppress the secretion of gonadotropins (LH and FSH) produced by the pituitary (Ding et al. 1988), whereas corticotrophin-releasing hormone (CRH) is able to suppress the secretion of GnRH through the inhibition of hypothalamic opiate (Gindoff and Ferin 1987). Catecholamines are also implicated in reproductive function as it may interfere with pulsatile LH release which in turn may lead to menstrual dysfunction (Chin et al. 1987). Other hormones, including thyroxine, growth hormone, and insulin-like growth factor, may also affect menstrual function (Loucks et al. 1992; Jenkins et al. 1993; Waters et al. 2001).

12.4.1.1.5 *Psychological Stress*

There is still a lack of data that supports psychological stress as a determinant factor in the etiology and pathogenesis of menstrual dysfunction in athletes, even though a correlation between behavioral and psychological parameters in female non-athletes with functional hypothalamic amenorrhea is documented (Marcus et al. 2001). In fact, a comparable psychological profile is observed between amenorrheic and menstruating athletes (Schwartz et al. 1981).

12.4.1.1.6 Energy Availability

In female athletes, energy availability, as previously described, has been documented as a determinant factor in the pathogenesis of reproductive disturbances rather than weight or exercise stress (Loucks 2003). If brain energy availability is reduced its function is altered, disrupting GnRH pulsatility. Researchers studying monkeys concluded that exercise-induced amenorrhea was reversed by diet and caloric supplementation, without any modification in their exercise regimen (Williams et al. 2001). Apparently, when energy is depleted LH pulsatility is suppressed as observed in exercising women exposed to a restrictive energy availability (Loucks et al. 1998). Therefore, the detrimental effects in reproductive function of females may not result from exercise per se but rather from a compromised energy balance.

12.4.1.1.7 Diet

There is paucity of available data in athletes about the role of diet composition in menstrual dysfunction. In fact, controversial results aimed to analyze the association of menstrual dysfunction incidence and the types of diet (specifically vegetarian diets) have been observed (Pirke et al. 1986; Barr et al. 1994). Hence, attention should be given in studies about the synergic effect of energy balance, exercise training, and stress when testing the influence of diet composition on the reproductive system.

12.4.1.1.8 Training Methods/Sports Characteristics

The specific requirements of sports, age of the training onset, somatotype, and the exercise training dose (intensity, frequency, duration, and volume) induce restriction on diet and an expected metabolic and energy profile that will have an expected impact on menstrual function in athletes.

Detrimental effects on menstrual function occur if a vigorous exercise training load starts abruptly in comparison with a gradual exercise training load (De Souza and Metzger 1991).

Additionally, menstrual function is more affected by long-term exercise training at an intensity level above the lactate threshold compared to long-term exercise training at or below the lactate threshold (Rogol et al. 1992). It is notwithstanding that that the prevalence of menstrual disorders is higher in weight-sensitive sports (Redman and Loucks 2005).

12.4.1.1.9 Reproductive Maturity

An intense exercise training has higher effect on menstrual function in premenarcheal adolescents than in formerly sedentary and menstruating females (Bonen 1992). A possible explanation is the higher sensitivity to the harmful effects of vigorous exercise in females who are reproductively immature. Nonetheless, it is challenging to isolate reproductive maturity as a determinant factor in the pathogenesis of menstrual disturbances independently of body weight, FM, and energy availability (Loucks 2003).

12.4.1.1.10 Bone Health

Bone health is the third component of the female triad in a spectrum covering optimum bone health, low BMD, and osteoporosis (Figure 12.2). In female athletes, osteoporosis can be described as premature bone loss and inadequate bone formation, causing low BMD, increased skeletal fragility, microarchitectural deterioration, and a higher incidence of stress fractures (Beals and Manore 2002; Ackerman and Misra 2011). Healthy athletes show higher BMD than non-athletes, due to the positive effect of exercise on bone architecture and accrual (Lambrinoudaki and Papadimitriou 2010). Nevertheless, it is recognized that amenorrheic athletes present lower values of BMD compared to their eumenorrheic colleagues (Drinkwater et al. 1984; Myburgh et al. 1993). Hence, menstrual dysfunction can compromise bone health, contributing to abnormal low values of BMD (osteopenia) and osteoporosis (Lindberg et al. 1984; McGee 1997; Warren et al. 2002).

Official positions from the International Society for Clinical Densitometry (ISCD) were published recommending that for premenopausal women and children, the WHO criteria for diagnosing osteopenia and osteoporosis should not be applied (Lewiecki et al. 2008). Alternatively, in these populations ISCD recommended the use of Z-scores to express BMD for comparing individuals to age- and sex-matched controls. ISCD indicated that Z-scores below −2.0 should be designated as "low bone density below the expected range for age" in premenopausal women and as "low bone density for chronological age" in children. In addition, ISCD recommended that osteopenia should not be used and osteoporosis diagnostic involved the presence of low BMD values with secondary clinical risk factors that reveal a high risk of bone loss and fracture, at a short term. Chronic malnutrition, hypogonadism, eating disorders, glucocorticoid exposure, and previous fractures are considered secondary risk factors. The American Society for Bone and Mineral Research, the American Association of Clinical Endocrinologists, and the International Osteoporosis Foundation endorsed the recommendations from ISCD.

A 5%–15% higher BMD is observed in athletes involved in weight-bearing sports compared to non-athletes (Risser et al. 1990; Fehling et al. 1995; Robinson et al. 1995). Hence, if a BMD Z-score below −1.0 is found in an athlete, additional study is required, even though no previous fracture has occurred. A "low BMD" is defined by the ACSM as a BMD Z-score value between −1.0 and −2.0 along with past nutritional deficiencies, stress fractures, hypoestrogenism, and/or additional secondary clinical risk factors for fracture (Nattiv et al. 2007). To reveal a higher risk of fragility fracture, "osteoporosis" is defined by ACSM as BMD Z-scores of ≤ −2.0 together with secondary clinical risk factors for fracture (Nattiv et al. 2007). Detailed description about the criteria for who and what site should be considered for having a DXA scan and how often this scan should be performed is provided by the female athlete triad coalition consensus statement on treatment and return to play of the female athlete triad (De Souza et al. 2014a). This consensus statement includes a set of recommendations developed following the International Symposia on the female athlete triad (De Souza et al. 2014a).

The risk for stress fractures is observed among female athletes exposed to menstrual cycle dysfunction, with a documented incidence higher among amenorrheic and oligomenorrheic female athletes as compared to their eumenorrheic counterparts (Warren et al. 1986; Wilson and Wolman 1994; Bennell et al. 1999).

Estrogen deficiency along with a decrease in energy availability suppresses markers of bone formation and increases markers of bone resorption (De Souza et al. 2008). Even if estrogenic status is normal, it is not possible to fully compensate the energy restricted environment as changes in bone formation remain apparent (De Souza et al. 2008). Although, the concurrent increase in body weight that occurs with alteration of diet and exercise and resumption of menses improves BMD in previously amenorrheic athletes (Drinkwater et al. 1986; Lindberg et al. 1987; Fredericson and Kent 2005) this change is not immediate and does not always fully undo the negative effects of amenorrhea on bone health, and the loss of BMD may never be completely restored (Warren et al. 2002). In fact, increases in BMD are small and short-lived if not achieved at a young enough age and sustained (Keen and Drinkwater 1997).

In fact, low-energy availability may lead to an insufficient intake of macronutrients, in particular essential amino acids and fatty acids and micronutrients, such as calcium and vitamin D, which are necessary for bone health (Manore et al. 2007; Constantini et al. 2010; McClung et al. 2014). Additionally, the low-energy availability may also disturb bone formation by influencing cortisol and leptin (Loucks et al. 1989; Laughlin and Yen 1996, 1997; Miller et al. 1998; Zanker and Swaine 1998). Depending on site, peak bone mass occurs by the end of the second decade or very early in the third decade (Baxter-Jones et al. 2011), which underscores the risk of the presence of the female athlete triad components in adolescent athletes to avoid compromising bone health.

12.4.1.2 Evidence for a Parallel with the Female Triad in Male Athletes

Health concerns comparable to those associated with the female athlete may be experienced by male athletes, particularly in those involved in weight-sensitive sports. Studies have addressed that low-energy availability with or without eating disorders, hypogonadotropic hypogonadism, and low BMD are also present in males (Burge et al. 1997; Thienpont et al. 2000) and may increase the risk of bone stress.

There is evidence suggesting hypogonadotropic hypogonadism substitutes the triad component, that is functional hypothalamic amenorrhea (Hackney 2001). In fact, the combination of a low-energy availability, hypogonadotropic hypogonadism, and low BMD may occur in a subset of male athletes in parallel with the female athlete triad (Tenforde et al. 2016).

12.4.1.2.1 Low-Energy Availability

Nutritional deficiencies, though understudied, have been observed in specific athletes, compromising an adequate energy availability (Tenforde et al. 2016).

A large study about the diet and nutritional intake in 419 male and female elite athletes involved in endurance, team sports, and strength was performed using 4- to 7-day food logs (van Erp-Baart et al. 1989). Overall, the findings revealed that insufficient levels of carbohydrate were consumed across sports, with dieting and under-eating occurring in male and female athletes competing in weight-sensitive sports (van Erp-Baart et al. 1989).

Studies conducted in male adolescent athletes participating in team sports, such as soccer, football, and ice hockey, pointed out adequate energy intake, ranging from nearly 40 to 60 kcal/kg (Hickson et al. 1987; Rankinen et al. 1995; Rico-Sanz et al. 1998; Petrie et al. 2004). Contrarily, periods of low-energy intake or nutritional deficits were observed in athletes involved in weight-sensitive sports, where leanness or weight-control behaviors are required (wrestling, judo, and horse-racing) (Horswill et al. 1990b; Fogelholm et al. 1993; Dolan et al. 2011) and in endurance sports such as cycling (Julian-Almarcegui et al. 2013) and running (Eden and Abernethy 1994; Glace et al. 2002; Pfeiffer et al. 2012). These findings advocate that weight-sensitive sports, especially endurance and weight class sports are at risk of nutritional deficiencies, eating disorders, and disordered eating (Tenforde et al. 2016).

An epidemiological study to assess the prevalence of eating disorders, including anorexia nervosa, bulimia nervosa, eating disorder not otherwise specified, and anorexia athletica, was conducted in 687 athletes and 629 non-athletes (Sundgot-Borgen and Torstveit 2004). The main results indicated a higher prevalence of eating disorders in male athletes (8%) compared to non-athletes (0.5%), specifically in weight-sensitive sports (12.9%), than in athletes participating in non-weight-sensitive sports (4.6%), including ball games, power, and motor sports (Sundgot-Borgen and Torstveit 2004). These findings are similar to those observed in female athletes (Sundgot-Borgen and Torstveit 2004). A recent meta-analysis, observed that wrestlers displayed a significant higher incidence of disordered eating (even more than aesthetic and mass-dependent sports) compared with non-athlete control individuals (Chapman and Woodman 2016). Weight-control techniques, as described earlier, have been observed in male wrestlers (Oppliger et al. 1998, 2003), judoists (Rouveix et al. 2007), professional jockeys (Moore et al. 2002; Dolan et al. 2012), and in endurance sports (cycling and running) (Wheeler et al. 1986; DiGioacchino DeBate et al. 2002; Ferrand and Brunet 2004; Tenforde et al. 2011), whereas restraint eating (Pietrowsky and Straub 2008) and subclinical eating disorders (Thiel et al. 1993) were observed in lightweight rowers.

12.4.1.2.2 Hypogonadotropic Hypogonadism

As a result of low-energy availability female athletes may develop functional hypothalamic amenorrhea (Nattiv et al. 2007). Based on the magnitude of energy deficit, women may develop luteal-phase defects and anovulation, which are difficult to identify whereas menstrual disorders (oligomenorrhea or amenorrhea) can be detected more easily (Williams et al. 2015). Likewise, assessing reproductive function changes in male athletes involves sophisticated procedures that may make the detection of a parallel syndrome in males difficult. Sperm and fertility exams may be required to assess any reproductive impairment in males as clinical symptoms are limited (De Souza and Miller 1997). A number of studies in male athletes reported changes in measurable hormones that impact reproduction and metabolism, namely at the hypothalamic-pituitary-gonadal axis (HPG) axis (Hackney et al. 1988; McColl et al. 1989; Roberts et al. 1993). Male athletes can be exposed to low-energy availability, either by an increase in endurance training or an insufficient energy intake for the exercise demands. Still, little previous research assessed energy intake and endocrine function in male athletes (Gomez-Merino et al. 2002). Male athletes involved in endurance sports, such as running and cycling, display a small amount of reproductive hormones (Hackney et al. 1988; McColl et al. 1989; Wheeler et al. 1991; Arce et al. 1993; Roberts et al. 1993; Bennell et al. 1996; Gomez-Merino et al. 2002). Significant lower testosterone levels were reported in endurance athletes compared to sedentary males (Hackney et al. 1998). Using a limited number of endurance runners (N = 5 to 11 athletes per study) involved in high-volume training (more than 100 km/week), four studies out of five presented 10%–30% lower levels of testosterone compared with sedentary controls (MacConnie et al. 1986; Hackney et al. 1988, 1990; Arce et al. 1993; De Souza et al. 1994). In contrast only two out of six studies assessing runners performing training volumes of less than 100 km/week (N = 6 to 20 athletes per study) observed serum levels of testosterone significantly lower than controls (Ayers et al. 1985; Gutin et al. 1985; Mathur et al. 1986; McColl et al. 1989; Bagatell and Bremner 1990; De Souza et al. 1994). In this regard, a "volume threshold hypothesis" was proposed to understand the results of changes in the reproductive function of runners who exceed 100 km/week (De Souza and Miller 1997).

In addition to the aforementioned cross-sectional studies, decreases in the level of testosterone were also observed in prospective research (Griffith et al. 1990; Wheeler et al. 1991; Roberts et al. 1993).

Elite endurance runners that participated in overtraining protocol reduced testosterone and sperm counts by 40% and 43%, respectively (Roberts et al. 1993), though 3 months after continuing with their normal training volume the levels of testosterone achieved the initial values. Sedentary males after 6 months of running 56 km/week decreased body weight and testosterone (Wheeler et al. 1991). In another study, an inverse dose-response between running distance and levels of testosterone was observed (Wheeler et al. 1986). Griffith et al. (1990) observed that levels of testosterone decreased by 12% in endurance athletes with a volume of 1–2 h each day during 6–7 days a week. It is important to note that in the aforementioned studies, though the levels of testosterone decreased, the values were within a normal physiological levels range. Similar findings of lower levels of testosterone were also found in male triathletes (Smith and Rutherford 1993), lightweight rowers (Vinther et al. 2008), and cyclists (Maimoun et al. 2003), compared to age-matched controls. It has been documented that besides lower or reduced levels of testosterone, male athletes participating in high-volume endurance training display other changes in the endocrine system that may reflect the contribution of the HPG axis (Bennell et al. 1996; De Souza and Miller 1997).

Though a proposed alteration in the hypothalamic–pituitary–testicular axis of male endurance athletes has been advanced (Hackney 2001, 2008; Hackney et al. 1988, 1998) the exact mechanisms of disturbances in the neuroendocrine axis require further investigation, due to the cross-sectional design or limited prospective researches. A lower amplitude and frequency LH pulse was found in six elite male marathon runners training 125–200 km/week compared to healthy controls (MacConnie et al. 1986). Also, in six male runners performing a minimum of 80 km/week, a decrease in LH with no disturbances in the frequency and amplitude of LH pulse was observed when compared to baseline values (McColl et al. 1989). Likewise, in male recreational athletes a reduction in the concentrations of LH and FSH after 2 weeks of vigorous exercise sessions, 4 times a week, on a cycle ergometer was displayed compared to baseline values and to matched controls (Vaamonde et al. 2006). Overall, these findings indicate possible changes in HPG axis that in turn could potentially elucidate the lower levels of testosterone observed in male endurance athletes.

In female athletes, a dose–response association between HPG function markers and energy availability, comprising decreases in LH pulse frequency and concentration of estradiol were observed with rising energy deficit (Loucks and Thuma 2003; Ihle and Loucks 2004). In men there is a paucity of related studies though endurance athletes exposed to high volume of exercise or to sudden increases in training demands contribute to an insufficient energy availability that could potentially suppress the HPG function (De Souza et al. 1994; De Souza and Miller 1997; Gomez-Merino et al. 2002).

Soldiers exposed to intense combat training inducing a negative energy balance of 1800 kcal/day decreased serum levels of testosterone, leptin, and insulin with increases in norepinephrine and dopamine compared to initial values (Gomez-Merino et al. 2002), linking energy deficit with decreases in testosterone.

The decrease in leptin is comparable to that observed in female athletes exposed to an energy availability of 10 kcal/kg FFM/day (Hilton and Loucks 2000). The contribution of leptin in energy deficit status may be revealed by the preservation in the function of the HPG axis, together with normal concentrations of LH pulsatility and testosterone during fast in males, after the administration of recombinant leptin (Chan et al. 2003). Leptin may work as a sign of insufficient energy for the brain and hypothalamus, inducing adaptations in hypothalamic–pituitary growth, gonadal, adrenal hormone, and thyroid axes in the presence of low-energy availability (Chan and Mantzoros 2005).

12.4.1.2.3 Low BMD

In male athletes, alike females, to optimize bone strength and resistance and decrease the risk of fracture it is required that a peak bone mass is accrued and maintained. Genetics, behavioral and environmental influences, such as diet and exercise, play a determinant role in bone metabolism (Nattiv et al. 2007). A relevant factor to develop bone mass and strength is the type of loading applied to bone (Tenforde and Fredericson 2011), as described by the Wolff law (Wolf 1995). Several physiological stressors such as the ground reaction forces exerted to bone during exercise promote bone adaption (Wolf 1995). High-impact activities with multidirectional loading to bone, such as soccer, volleyball, basketball, and martial arts, promote an increased bone mineralization that explains the higher BMD found in athletes compared to non-athletes (Dias Quiterio et al. 2011; Tenforde and Fredericson 2011). In addition athletes involved in ball sports or high-impact activities exhibit higher BMD than athletes competing in endurance sports with repetitive lower impact loads, namely long-distance running, or nonimpact activities such as cycling or swimming (Andreoli et al. 2001; Morel et al. 2001; Fredericson et al. 2007; Tenforde and Fredericson 2011). In men, the rate of peak accrual occurs between 13 and 15 years and achieves the highest value by the age of 20 years (Heaney et al. 2000). Hence, high-impact activities and ball sports are recommended in the beginning of the adolescent period and for at least 2 years, around the peak accrual rate to maximize bone mass and protect against stress fractures (Milgrom et al. 2000; Chen et al. 2013; Tenforde et al. 2013).

Indeed, both male and female endurance athletes (cycling and running) may present "low BMD" as defined by ACSM using Z-scores, and previously mentioned in athletic and physically active premenopausal women and children (Nattiv et al. 2007). In men below the age of 50 years, Z-scores are used, as well, and osteoporosis diagnosis needs to include the presence of risk factors and low BMD Z-scores (Lewiecki et al. 2008).

A low bone mass or osteoporosis have been documented in male athletes involved in weight-sensitive sports or in activities promoting low-impact loads exerted to bone. A lower BMD is found in male jockeys (Dolan et al. 2012), adolescent runners with BMD values below a Z-score of −1 (Tenforde et al. 2015), and in male cyclists (Smathers et al. 2009; Nichols and Rauh 2011). A compromised lumbar spine has been observed in male runners (Fredericson et al. 2007), of both sexes (Stewart and Hannan 2000; Smathers et al. 2009; Nichols and Rauh 2011). In a 5-year prospective study, track and field athletes exhibit a higher percentage of bone stress injuries in trabecular regions (pubic bone, femoral neck, and sacrum) in comparison with cortical sites (Nattiv et al. 2013).

The prevalence of low BMD in males is still unknown but the prevalence of impaired bone health is higher among male athletes involved in weight-sensitive sports, specifically in gravitational sports (running and cycling) and weight class sports (wrestlers and judo) (Tenforde et al. 2015). In elite male runners, when a cutoff for low BMD is considered using a Z-score or T-score below −1.0, respectively, the prevalence among these athletes range between 19% and 40% (Hind et al. 2006; Fredericson et al. 2007; Tenforde et al. 2015) and between 25% and 89% for male cyclists (Smathers et al. 2009; Nichols and Rauh 2011). Since the prevalence of a low BMD or osteoporosis comprised small sample sizes, wide range of ages, and a reduced number of studies that provided the number of athletes presenting a threshold cutoff for low BMD, the exact prevalence of low BMD is still unidentified, which limits the generalizability to the whole male athletic population. It is also important to mention that many studies used values of T-score thresholds from −1 to −2.5, and as previously mentioned the use of Z-scores to assess bone health in athletes are currently recommended (Nattiv et al. 2007; Lewiecki et al. 2008). In addition, it is still unknown if a Z-score of −1 should be used to define BMD in males given the reduced research studies conducted in this population. Nevertheless, weight-sensitive sports, particularly in gravitational sports (runners and cyclers) present an increased risk of a compromised bone health as observed by the low BMD Z-scores and T-scores in comparison with healthy controls.

In female athletes with the triad, level of reproductive hormones explains their compromised bone health (Ihle and Loucks 2004; Nattiv et al. 2007). Likewise, in male athletes a decrease in testosterone and other sex hormones may justify the lower BMD values found (Bilanin et al. 1989; Bennell et al. 1996; Ackerman et al. 2012). However, a cross-sectional study with male wrestlers and runners observed that levels of estradiol are more predictive of BMD than levels of testosterone (Ackerman et al. 2012). Another research study revealed the role of energy balance in bone mass preservation in male runners (Zanker and Swaine 2000). As well the lower values of BMD in male jockeys may be related with the adoption of restrictive diets observed in these athletes to remain with a low weight for performance related advantages (Dolan et al. 2011, 2012).

Therefore, either a low-energy availability or a lower production of sex hormones may impact bone health in a male athletic population. However, the lack of experimental studies testing these effects on bone health in male athletes as opposed with females do not allow to a fully characterization of these factors though males involved in weight-sensitive sports may be exposed to a higher risk of low BMD.

Tenforde et al. (2016) reviewed adverse health issues in the male athletic population that parallel the female athlete triad, namely the low-energy availability with or without eating disorders, hypogonadotropic hypogonadism, and bone health disturbances. However, in male athletes there is still limited research on the clinical sequelae severity associated with energy deficiency. Regardless, the impact of an insufficient dietary intake on compromised health in male and female athletes has been underscored by the IOC with a proposed definition "Relative Energy Deficiency in Sport (RED-S)" (Mountjoy et al. 2014). Still, more research is required to apply this term collectively to both sexes (De Souza et al. 2014b). Therefore, authors that have been involved in studying the female athlete triad in the past decades recommended to preserve the term, the "Female Athlete Triad," whereas ongoing efforts should be made to develop knowledge about the mechanisms, relationships, and outcomes in male athletes that seem to be comparable to the triad (De Souza et al. 2014b). Evidence-based recommendations to propose best practices in male athletes at risk of developing a parallel to the female triad are only possible if additional knowledge of these mechanisms is further examined.

12.4.2 Health Consequences

12.4.2.1 Triad Health-Related Concerns

Athletes exposed to chronic energy deficit are at higher risk of adverse effects on health and performance, in particular with the presence of a clinical eating disorders (De Souza and Williams 2004). The role of low-energy availability is recognized to impact gonadal function in both females and males (Bullen et al. 1985; Williams et al. 2001). Hypoestrogenemia along with a suppressed reproductive function can adversely influence musculoskeletal and cardiovascular health (Rickenlund et al. 2005; O'Donnell et al. 2007; De Souza et al. 2008).

A chronic energy deficit can have an additional negative musculoskeletal effect regardless of hypoestrogenism (De Souza and Williams 2005; De Souza et al. 2008). Bone stress injuries, comprising the range of stress reactions and fractures, are more prevalent in athletic females with menstrual disturbances and/or low BMD (Kelsey et al. 2007; Field et al. 2011; Duckham et al. 2012; Nattiv et al. 2013; Tenforde et al. 2013; Barrack et al. 2014) as well as in female military recruits (Lauder et al. 2000; Rauh et al. 2006) but recently a risk of a reduced low BMD has been observed in male athletes involved in endurance sports (Andreoli et al. 2001; Morel et al. 2001; Fredericson et al. 2007; Tenforde and Fredericson 2011). According to Rauh et al. (2014) a higher risk of musculoskeletal injury at lower extremities is related with the triad in cross-country and track adolescent females using a prospective design. The main findings revealed that the athletes who present amenorrhea or oligomenorrhea with reduced BMD are more prone to musculoskeletal injuries. In another study, a higher skeletal muscle was related with greater values of bone mineral content and BMD in Division I cross-country runners (Roelofs et al. 2015). In addition, performance may be reduced in the presence of bone stress injuries and has been recognized in swimming performance with ovarian suppression and low-energy status markers (Vanheest et al. 2014).

Anorexia-related hypogonadal conditions are associated with body composition changes, liver enzymes, hematological and hemodynamic parameters (Misra et al. 2004). Likewise, athletic activity is related with greater levels of aspartate aminotransferase, while lower values of total and regional FM and higher alanine aminotransferase levels are linked to menstrual dysfunction (Singhal et al. 2014).

Maestu et al. (2010) observed that insulin changes were associated with FM and lean body weight changes in bodybuilders before competition. Likewise, concentrations of anabolic pathways are decreased with extreme reductions in body energy stores due to severe restrictions in energy intake. Changes in the concentrations of insulin growth factor (IGF-1) and insulin should be tracked to avoid reductions in skeletal muscle as a result of exposure to high-energy restriction.

Furthermore, findings using a combined energy imbalance with high-volume exercise training in rowers showed acute postexercise changes in neuropeptide Y, leptin, and ghrelin levels and decreases in leptin in the fasted state (Ramson et al. 2012).

Additional discussion of adverse health effects from the triad is provided elsewhere (Nattiv et al. 2007; Barrack et al. 2013).

12.4.2.2 Hydration Changes, Adipose, and Skeletal Muscle Tissues Lost

Plasma volume is decreased and peripheral blood flow and sweating rate are reduced in athletes presenting a dehydrated state. Thermoregulatory function is impaired and may increase health risks (Shirreffs et al. 2004). Therefore, dehydration along with exercise performed in a sweat suit or sauna, common weight-loss techniques, or hot and humid environments, compromise heat dissipation and ultimately causes death (Grundstein et al. 2012).

A reduction of weight is commonly detected among ultra-endurance athletes, such as those involved in ultra-running (Skenderi et al. 2006), ultra-triathlon (Lehmann et al. 1995; Gastmann et al. 1998), and ultra-cycling (Neumayr et al. 2003, 2005). The body weight reduction is essentially due to FM decreases (Raschka et al. 1991; Raschka and Plath 1992; Helge et al. 2003), though skeletal muscle loss has also been reported (Bircher et al. 2006; Knechtle and Kohler 2007; Knechtle et al. 2008) in ultra-endurance performances. A body weight reduction along with FM and skeletal muscle loss and a total body water increase was observed in runners who performed a continuous 100 km race (Knechtle et al. 2009). Water increases may reveal edema formation, further complicating a valid determination of the actual weight, FM, and skeletal muscle mass change right after an ultra-endurance performance.

Another study (Weitkunat et al. 2012) observed that fluid intake patterns, plasma volume changes, plasma sodium, and urine specific gravity, particularly in females, may be linked to the occurrence of a combined fluid shift from blood vessels to interstitial tissue, enabled by a damage in skeletal muscle along with exercise-related hyponatremia. A sexual dimorphism was also observed in changes in body composition and hydration status in open-water ultra-endurance swimmers (Weitkunat et al. 2012).

In 2013, Schutz et al. (2013) using a mobile magnetic resonance imaging (MRI) field, observed that ultra-marathon athletes lost adipose tissue by more than a half. Likewise, the volume of skeletal muscle tissue reduced as a result of inevitable chronic energy deficits over the race (Schutz et al. 2013). The fastest and deepest reduction was observed in visceral adipose tissue (VAT) in comparison with somatic adipose soft tissue (total adipose tissue minus adipose bone marrow and VAT) and compartments of lean tissue.

12.4.2.3   Inadequate Intake of Macro- and Micronutrients

The risk of insufficient intake of essential fatty acids, carbohydrates, and protein is present in athletes involved in severe energy restriction and fasting. Carbohydrates reductions will lead to depletion of glycogen, insufficient recovery, and fatigue, among sessions of exercise training (Burke et al. 2004). Moreover, a protein intake decrease is expected to lead to higher lean tissue losses through weight loss (Mettler et al. 2010). Intake of calcium and iron and other micronutrients below the adequate levels occur in athletes exposed to weight loss (Sandoval et al. 1989; Fogelholm et al. 1993; Filaire et al. 2001). In turn, specifically when recurrent weight-loss episodes exist, athletes are likely to compromise minerals and vitamins intake over the season.

12.4.2.4   Cognitive Function and Psychological Factors

Athletes exposed to a very restrictive energy and dehydration will be prone to fatigue and to a perceived increase of effort (Horswill et al. 1990a). Increased feelings of tension, anger, anxiety, and compromised memory at the short term are common in athletes experiencing rapid weight loss (Steen and Brownell 1990; Choma et al. 1998; Filaire et al. 2001; Hall and Lane 2001; Degoutte et al. 2006).

It is important to underscore that athletes are exposed to constant levels of stress by contradicting hunger, struggling over body weight, and food obsession. Apprehensiveness of increasing body weight is emotionally arduous. Likewise, this obsession affects the athlete's daily activities, training, and competition. As previously mentioned, athletes exposed to extensive low-energy availability periods, regardless the presence or absence of disordered eating, can harm health and performance (Nattiv et al. 2007).

12.4.2.5   Increased Stress and Impaired Immune Function

Athletes involved in high training loads along with low-energy or carbohydrate intake are at greater risk of injuries, oxidative stress, and chronic fatigue, and may compromise immune function (Gleeson et al. 2004; Yanagawa et al. 2010). If athletes are exposed to such conditions for a long term, more recurrent injuries and illness events are expected. In endurance male rowers Jurimae et al. (2015) observed that skeletal muscle mass and FFM were inversely associated with serum levels of interferon-gamma, while cardiorespiratory fitness was inversely correlated to serum levels of interleukin-8 (Jurimae et al. 2015). Evidence exists for an increased risk of upper respiratory tract infections because of negative changes in immune function in long-distance runners due to marathon training and racing (Sparling et al. 1993).

12.4.2.6   Metabolic Changes

Athletes under low-energy availability, from increased exercise or restrictions in energy intake, exhibit energy expenditure conservation as a result of metabolic, hormonal, and functional disorders (Loucks 2004). In weight-cycling athletes it has been hypothesized that a lower resting metabolic rate would be seen compared to their counterparts not involved in weight-cycling (Brownell et al. 1987; Steen et al. 1988). Nevertheless, prospective research studies indicate that resting metabolic rate decreases over the season but at post-season an increase to initial values is observed. Hence, it seems that these metabolic rate changes will not be long-lasting (Melby et al. 1990) and may be reversible, though long-term adverse health effects may occur if athletes are exposed to repeated dieting processes. In fact, weight class athletes who commonly use risky techniques for "making weight" may experience growing complications in the upcoming years favoring the use of more extreme methods to achieve their competitive target weight. It is still unknown if this is the result of changes in resting metabolic rate or other, biological, psychological, or physiological factors. Using elite gymnasts and runners, Deutz et al. (2000) evaluated body composition and energy balance. The authors suggest that within-day energy deficits are related with higher adiposity in both aerobic and anaerobic highly trained athletes, advancing a potential adaptive reduction in resting metabolic rate. Energy deficiency with resting energy expenditure reductions has been documented in endurance athletes, in particular long-distance runners (Myerson et al. 1991; Lebenstedt et al. 1999). Endurance athletes exposed to long-term exercise may downregulate thyroid hormone levels reducing resting energy expenditure (Simsch et al. 2002; Steinacker et al. 2005; Perseghin et al. 2009). These studies may suggest that athletes following restrained diets to achieve a target body composition should be discouraged.

In another study, Campos et al. (2012) found that heart rate recovery was inversely related with absolute and relative values of FM but not with VO_{2max}, whereas excess post oxygen consumption (EPOC) was positively associated with adiposity and FFM and negatively related with heart rate recovery. Thus, greater body composition values, regardless of FM or FFM, may raise EPOC. Still, after the effort FM obstructs heart rate recovery and delays oxygen consumption recovery in highly trained athletes.

12.4.2.7 Growth and Maturation

It is recognized that aesthetic sports exercise training begins early, and high intensity starts quickly, regular, and long-term, keeping in mind the maintenance of minimal values of adiposity. Throughout the growth period insufficient nutrient and energy intakes can cause a delayed growth and pubertal development (Soric et al. 2008). Late menarche, retardation of bone growth, reduced weight, fatness, and height have been documented in gymnasts (Weimann et al. 2000). Athletes exposed to short-term weight loss may display disturbances on hormonal parameters and blood biochemistry (Karila et al. 2008). If prolonged over a season, weight loss may cause adverse health consequences in adolescent athletes. Despite the fact that several months may be required, it has been reported that a catch-up of bone and FFM growth subsequently to a weight-loss period in young athletes may occur (Roemmich and Sinning 1997; Caine et al. 2001). Studies also reveal that eating disorders are related with the demands of training in specific sports at early ages (Sundgot-Borgen 1994), with children beginning their practice at 3 or 4 years of age. It is documented that girls aged 5–7 years, involved in aesthetic sports present superior concerns with weight in comparison with girls practicing non-aesthetic sports or not participating in sports (Davison et al. 2002). Elite female artistic gymnasts, exposed to a greater and more sustained energy output than rhythmic gymnasts, present a more pronounced delay in both pubertal development and skeletal maturation with a deterioration of growth potential (Georgopoulos et al. 2002; Theodoropoulou et al. 2005).

Nonetheless, well designed research is lacking in exploring the long-term consequences of engaging in recurrent weight instability and energy restriction on growth and development.

12.5 CONCLUSION AND PERSPECTIVES

Athletes involved in weight-sensitive sports often experience weight fluctuations that may impact their performance and increase the risk of adverse health effects, specifically when considering the energy imbalance that they are exposed to, which is commonly in parallel to a low-energy availability.

Medical staff, sports physicians, nutritionists, exercise scientists, and other stakeholders should focus on accurate estimations of athletes' energy requirements in order to avoid the severe health consequences that are associated with low-energy availability. At this regard, when an athlete needs to lose weight it must be kept in mind that an energy availability between 30 and 45 kcal/kg FFM/day is mandatory. An accurate assessment of body composition is also required to enhance performance and to help prevent and treat the health consequences of chronic energy deficiency. The use of DXA to monitor body composition and objective methods to assess energy expenditure may provide useful and valid information to understand energy balance, regulation, and availability. However, to detect body composition changes, specifically in athletes with lower FM levels and expected small changes in this component, more precise and accurate methods should be developed and validated for athletes competing in weight-sensitive sports.

Although efforts have been made to establish a minimum body weight and body composition there is still no consensus, with values depending on the sport and also on the body composition method. It is noteworthy to mention that sports federations are becoming aware of the leanness problem in weight-sensitive sports, and many have started establishing regulations on a minimum weight for competition. More research is required to establish a body composition profile in weight-sensitive sports in order to inform decision makers in sports federations.

Long-term reduced energy availability, as observed in endurance athletes such as long-distance runners, may compromise the cardiovascular, endocrine, reproductive, skeletal, gastrointestinal, renal, and central nervous systems (Becker et al. 1999; American Psychiatric Association Work Group on Eating Disorders 2000; Golden et al. 2003; Rome et al. 2003). A recognized and prevalent syndrome in females competing in weight-sensitive sports is the female athlete triad that results from complex and interrelated conditions, specifically energy availability, menstrual status, and bone mineral, with varied clinical manifestations. Adverse health issues that parallel the female athlete triad, including low-energy availability with or without eating disorders, hypogonadotropic hypogonadism, and bone health disturbances have also been observed in the male athletic population. However, to propose evidence-based recommendations in male athletes at risk of developing a parallel of the female triad, additional research is required.

Although a lower body weight may bring competition advantages, medical staff, nutritionists, coaches, and athletes need to consider the two sides of the scale. If by one side a lower weight may be associated with competition benefits, on the other side of the scale, particularly in the long term, there are severe health consequences that need to be recognized. Additionally, although at a first glance athletes who are lighter may succeed in competition, extreme leanness and decreases in FFM occur that are associated with decreases in sports performance.

Preventing, recognizing, and treating clinical conditions associated with chronic energy deficit should be a major concern for professionals who work with athletes in a multidisciplinary team, specifically those competing in weight-sensitive sports, to ensure they maximize performance and avoid risk of injury and illness.

REFERENCES

Achten, J., and A. E. Jeukendrup. 2003. Heart rate monitoring: Applications and limitations. *Sports Med* 33:517–38.

Ackerman, K. E., and M. Misra. 2011. Bone health and the female athlete triad in adolescent athletes. *Phys Sportsmed* 39:131–41.

Ackerman, K. E., G. S. Skrinar, E. Medvedova, M. Misra, and K. K. Miller. 2012. Estradiol levels predict bone mineral density in male collegiate athletes: A pilot study. *Clin Endocrinol (Oxf)* 76:339–45.

Ackland, T. R., T. G. Lohman, J. Sundgot-Borgen et al. 2012. Current status of body composition assessment in sport: Review and position statement on behalf of the ad hoc research working group on body composition health and performance, under the auspices of the I.O.C. Medical Commission. *Sports Med* 42:227–49.

Ainsworth, B. E., W. L. Haskell, S. D. Herrmann et al. 2011. Compendium of physical activities: A second update of codes and MET values. *Med Sci Sports Exerc* 43:1575–81.

Alderman, B., D. M. Landers, J. Carlson, and J. R. Scott. 2004. Factors related to rapid weight loss practices among international-style wrestlers. *Med Sci Sports Exerc* 36:249–52.

American Psychiatric Association Work Group on Eating Disorders. 2000. Practice guideline for the treatment of patients with eating disorders (revision). *Am J Psychiatry* 157:1–39.

Andreoli, A., M. Monteleone, M. Van Loan, L. Promenzio, U. Tarantino, and A. De Lorenzo. 2001. Effects of different sports on bone density and muscle mass in highly trained athletes. *Med Sci Sports Exerc* 33:507–11.

Arce, J. C., M. J. De Souza, L. S. Pescatello, and A. A. Luciano. 1993. Subclinical alterations in hormone and semen profile in athletes. *Fertil Steril* 59:398–404.

Artioli, G. G., R. T. Iglesias, E. Franchini et al. 2010. Rapid weight loss followed by recovery time does not affect judo-related performance. *J Sports Sci* 28:21–32.

Assah, F. K., U. Ekelund, S. Brage, A. Wright, J. C. Mbanya, and N. J. Wareham. 2011. Accuracy and validity of a combined heart rate and motion sensor for the measurement of free-living physical activity energy expenditure in adults in Cameroon. *Int J Epidemiol* 40:112–20.

American Psychiatric Association. 2013. *Diagnostic and Statistical Manual of Mental Disorders* (5th Ed.), Arlington, VA: American Psychiatric Publishing.

Ayers, J. W., Y. Komesu, T. Romani, and R. Ansbacher. 1985. Anthropomorphic, hormonal, and psychologic correlates of semen quality in endurance-trained male athletes. *Fertil Steril* 43:917–21.

Bagatell, C. J., and W. J. Bremner. 1990. Sperm counts and reproductive hormones in male marathoners and lean controls. *Fertil Steril* 53:688–92.

Barandun, U., B. Knechtle, P. Knechtle et al. 2012. Running speed during training and percent body fat predict race time in recreational male marathoners. *Open Access J Sports Med* 3:51–8.

Barbieri, D., L. Zaccagni, A. Cogo, and E. Gualdi-Russo. 2012. Body composition and somatotype of experienced mountain climbers. *High Alt Med Biol* 13:46–50.

Barr, S. I., K. C. Janelle, and J. C. Prior. 1994. Vegetarian vs nonvegetarian diets, dietary restraint, and subclinical ovulatory disturbances: Prospective 6-mo study. *Am J Clin Nutr* 60:887–94.

Barrack, M. T., K. E. Ackerman, and J. C. Gibbs. 2013. Update on the female athlete triad. *Curr Rev Musculoskelet Med* 6:195–204.

Barrack, M. T., J. C. Gibbs, M. J. De Souza et al. 2014. Higher incidence of bone stress injuries with increasing female athlete triad-related risk factors: A prospective multisite study of exercising girls and women. *Am J Sports Med* 42:949–58.

Bassett, D. R., Jr. 2000. Validity and reliability issues in objective monitoring of physical activity. *Res Q Exerc Sport* 71:S30–6.

Baxter-Jones, A. D., R. A. Faulkner, M. R. Forwood, R. L. Mirwald, and D. A. Bailey. 2011. Bone mineral accrual from 8 to 30 years of age: An estimation of peak bone mass. *J Bone Miner Res* 26:1729–39.

Beals, K. A., and A. K. Hill. 2006. The prevalence of disordered eating, menstrual dysfunction, and low bone mineral density among US collegiate athletes. *Int J Sport Nutr Exerc Metab* 16:1–23.

Beals, K. A., and M. M. Manore. 2002. Disorders of the female athlete triad among collegiate athletes. *Int J Sport Nutr Exerc Metab* 12:281–93.

Becker, A. E., S. K. Grinspoon, A. Klibanski, and D. B. Herzog. 1999. Eating disorders. *N Engl J Med* 340:1092–8.

Bennell, K. L., P. D. Brukner, and S. A. Malcolm. 1996. Effect of altered reproductive function and lowered testosterone levels on bone density in male endurance athletes. *Br J Sports Med* 30:205–8.

Bennell, K., G. Matheson, W. Meeuwisse, and P. Brukner. 1999. Risk factors for stress fractures. *Sports Med* 28:91–122.

Bergh, U. 1987. The influence of body mass in cross-country skiing. *Med Sci Sports Exerc* 19:324–31.

Bergh, U., and A. Forsberg. 1992. Influence of body mass on cross-country ski racing performance. *Med Sci Sports Exerc* 24:1033–9.

Bilanin, J. E., M. S. Blanchard, and E. Russek-Cohen. 1989. Lower vertebral bone density in male long distance runners. *Med Sci Sports Exerc* 21:66–70.

Bircher, S., A. Enggist, T. Jehle, and B. Knechtle. 2006. Effects of an extreme endurance race on energy balance and body composition—A case study. *J Sports Sci Med* 5:154–62.

Bonen, A. 1992. Recreational exercise does not impair menstrual cycles: A prospective study. *Int J Sports Med* 13:110–20.

Boulay, M. R., O. Serresse, N. Almeras, and A. Tremblay. 1994. Energy expenditure measurement in male cross-country skiers: Comparison of two field methods. *Med Sci Sports Exerc* 26:248–253.

Brage, S., N. Brage, P. W. Franks et al. 2004. Branched equation modeling of simultaneous accelerometry and heart rate monitoring improves estimate of directly measured physical activity energy expenditure. *J Appl Physiol* 96:343–51.

Bronson, F. H., and J. M. Manning. 1991. The energetic regulation of ovulation: A realistic role for body fat. *Biol Reprod* 44:945–50.

Brownell, K. D., S. N. Steen, and J. H. Wilmore. 1987. Weight regulation practices in athletes: Analysis of metabolic and health effects. *Med Sci Sports Exerc* 19:546–56.

Bullen, B. A., G. S. Skrinar, I. Z. Beitins, G. von Mering, B. A. Turnbull, and J. W. McArthur. 1985. Induction of menstrual disorders by strenuous exercise in untrained women. *N Engl J Med* 312:1349–53.

Burge, M. R., R. A. Lanzi, S. T. Skarda, and R. P. Eaton. 1997. Idiopathic hypogonadotropic hypogonadism in a male runner is reversed by clomiphene citrate. *Fertil Steril* 67:783–5.

Burke, L. M., B. Kiens, and J. L. Ivy. 2004. Carbohydrates and fat for training and recovery. *J Sports Sci* 22:15–30.

Byrne, S., and N. McLean. 2002. Elite athletes: Effects of the pressure to be thin. *J Sci Med Sport* 5:80–94.

Caine, D., R. Lewis, P. O'Connor, W. Howe, and S. Bass. 2001. Does gymnastics training inhibit growth of females? *Clin J Sport Med* 11:260–70.

Campos, E. Z., F. N. Bastos, M. Papoti, I. F. Freitas Junior, C. A. Gobatto, and P. Balikian Jr. 2012. The effects of physical fitness and body composition on oxygen consumption and heart rate recovery after high-intensity exercise. *Int J Sports Med* 33:621–6.

Caspersen, C. J., K. E. Powell, and G. M. Christenson. 1985. Physical activity, exercise, and physical fitness: Definitions and distinctions for health-related research. *Public Health Rep* 100:126–31.

Ceesay, S. M., A. M. Prentice, K. C. Day et al. 1989. The use of heart rate monitoring in the estimation of energy expenditure: A validation study using indirect whole-body calorimetry. *Br J Nutr* 61:175–86.

Chan, J. L., K. Heist, A. M. DePaoli, J. D. Veldhuis, and C. S. Mantzoros. 2003. The role of falling leptin levels in the neuroendocrine and metabolic adaptation to short-term starvation in healthy men. *J Clin Invest* 111:1409–21.

Chan, J. L., and C. S. Mantzoros. 2005. Role of leptin in energy-deprivation states: Normal human physiology and clinical implications for hypothalamic amenorrhoea and anorexia nervosa. *Lancet* 366:74–85.

Chapman, J., and T. Woodman. 2016. Disordered eating in male athletes: A meta-analysis. *J Sports Sci* 34:101–9.

Chen, Y. T., A. S. Tenforde, and M. Fredericson. 2013. Update on stress fractures in female athletes: Epidemiology, treatment, and prevention. *Curr Rev Musculoskelet Med* 6:173–81.

Chin, N. W., F. E. Chang, W. G. Dodds, M. H. Kim, and W. B. Malarkey. 1987. Acute effects of exercise on plasma catecholamines in sedentary and athletic women with normal and abnormal menses. *Am J Obstet Gynecol* 157:938–44.

Choma, C. W., G. A. Sforzo, and B. A. Keller. 1998. Impact of rapid weight loss on cognitive function in collegiate wrestlers. *Med Sci Sports Exerc* 30:746–9.

Chrousos, G. P., D. J. Torpy, and P. W. Gold. 1998. Interactions between the hypothalamic-pituitary-adrenal axis and the female reproductive system: Clinical implications. *Ann Intern Med* 129:229–40.

Claessens, A. L., J. Lefevre, G. Beunen, and R. M. Malina. 1999. The contribution of anthropometric characteristics to performance scores in elite female gymnasts. *J Sports Med Phys Fitness* 39:355–60.

Claessens, A. L., J. Lefevre, G. Beunen, V. Stijnen, H. Maes, and F. M. Veer. 1991. Gymnastic performance as related to anthropometric and somatotype characteristics in male gymnasts. *Anthrop Kozl* 33:243–7.

Clark, R. R., C. Bartok, J. C. Sullivan, and D. A. Schoeller. 2004. Minimum weight prediction methods cross-validated by the four-component model. *Med Sci Sports Exerc* 36:639–47.

Constantini, N. W., R. Arieli, G. Chodick, and G. Dubnov-Raz. 2010. High prevalence of vitamin D insufficiency in athletes and dancers. *Clin J Sport Med* 20:368–71.

D'Alessio, D. A., E. C. Kavle, M. A. Mozzoli et al. 1988. Thermic effect of food in lean and obese men. *J Clin Invest* 81:1781–9.

Davis, S. E., G. B. Dwyer, K. Reed, C. Bopp, J. Stosic, and M. Shepanski. 2002. Preliminary investigation: The impact of the NCAA Wrestling Weight Certification Program on weight cutting. *J Strength Cond Res* 16:305–7.

Davison, K. K., M. B. Earnest, and L. L. Birch. 2002. Participation in aesthetic sports and girls' weight concerns at ages 5 and 7 years. *Int J Eat Disord* 31:312–7.

de Bruin, A. P., R. R. D. Oudejans, and F. C. Bakker. 2007. Dieting and body image in aesthetic sports: A comparison of Dutch female gymnasts and non-aesthetic sport participants. *Psychol Sport Exerc* 8:507–20.

Degoutte, F., P. Jouanel, R. J. Begue et al. 2006. Food restriction, performance, biochemical, psychological, and endocrine changes in judo athletes. *Int J Sports Med* 27:9–18.

de Jonge, L., J. P. DeLany, T. Nguyen et al. 2007. Validation study of energy expenditure and intake during calorie restriction using doubly labeled water and changes in body composition. *Am J Clin Nutr* 85:73–9.

De Souza, M. J., J. C. Arce, L. S. Pescatello, H. S. Scherzer, and A. A. Luciano. 1994. Gonadal hormones and semen quality in male runners. A volume threshold effect of endurance training. *Int J Sports Med* 15:383–91.

De Souza, M. J., H. J. Leidy, E. O'Donnell, B. Lasley, and N. I. Williams. 2004. Fasting ghrelin levels in physically active women: Relationship with menstrual disturbances and metabolic hormones. *J Clin Endocrinol Metab* 89:3536–42.

De Souza, M. J., and D. A. Metzger. 1991. Reproductive dysfunction in amenorrheic athletes and anorexic patients: A review. *Med Sci Sports Exerc* 23:995–1007.

De Souza, M. J., and B. E. Miller. 1997. The effect of endurance training on reproductive function in male runners. A 'volume threshold' hypothesis. *Sports Med* 23:357–74.

De Souza, M. J., B. E. Miller, A. B. Loucks et al. 1998. High frequency of luteal phase deficiency and anovulation in recreational women runners: Blunted elevation in follicle-stimulating hormone observed during luteal-follicular transition. *J Clin Endocrinol Metab* 83:4220–32.

De Souza, M. J., A. Nattiv, E. Joy et al. 2014a. 2014 Female Athlete Triad Coalition consensus statement on treatment and return to play of the female athlete triad. 1st International Conference, San Francisco, CA, May 2012, and 2nd International Conference, Indianapolis, IN, May 2013. *Clin J Sport Med* 24:96–119.

De Souza, M. J., S. L. West, S. A. Jamal, G. A. Hawker, C. M. Gundberg, and N. I. Williams. 2008. The presence of both an energy deficiency and estrogen deficiency exacerbate alterations of bone metabolism in exercising women. *Bone* 43:140–8.

De Souza, M. J., and N. I. Williams. 2004. Physiological aspects and clinical sequelae of energy deficiency and hypoestrogenism in exercising women. *Hum Reprod Update* 10:433–8.

De Souza, M. J., and N. I. Williams. 2005. Beyond hypoestrogenism in amenorrheic athletes: Energy deficiency as a contributing factor for bone loss. *Curr Sports Med Rep* 4:38–44.

De Souza, M. J., N. I. Williams, A. Nattiv et al. 2014b. Misunderstanding the female athlete triad: Refuting the IOC consensus statement on Relative Energy Deficiency in Sport (RED-S). *Br J Sports Med* 48:1461–5.

Deutz, R. C., D. Benardot, D. E. Martin, and M. M. Cody. 2000. Relationship between energy deficits and body composition in elite female gymnasts and runners. *Med Sci Sports Exerc* 32:659–68.

Dias Quiterio, A. L., E. A. Carnero, F. M. Baptista, and L. B. Sardinha. 2011. Skeletal mass in adolescent male athletes and nonathletes: Relationships with high-impact sports. *J Strength Cond Res* 25:3439–47.

Di Cagno, A., C. Baldari, C. Battaglia et al. 2008. Leaping ability and body composition in rhythmic gymnasts for talent identification. *J Sports Med Phys Fitness* 48:341–6.

DiGioacchino DeBate, R., H. Wethington, and R. Sargent. 2002. Sub-clinical eating disorder characteristics among male and female triathletes. *Eat Weight Disord* 7:210–20.

Ding, J. H., C. B. Sheckter, B. L. Drinkwater, M. R. Soules, and W. J. Bremner. 1988. High serum cortisol levels in exercise-associated amenorrhea. *Ann Intern Med* 108:530–4.

Dolan, E., N. Crabtree, A. McGoldrick, D. T. Ashley, N. McCaffrey, and G. D. Warrington. 2012. Weight regulation and bone mass: A comparison between professional jockeys, elite amateur boxers, and age, gender and BMI matched controls. *J Bone Miner Metab* 30:164–70.

Dolan, E., S. Cullen, A. McGoldrick, and G. D. Warrington. 2013. The impact of making weight on physiological and cognitive processes in elite jockeys. *Int J Sport Nutr Exerc Metab* 23:399–408.

Dolan, E., H. O'Connor, A. McGoldrick, G. O'Loughlin, D. Lyons, and G. Warrington. 2011. Nutritional, lifestyle, and weight control practices of professional jockeys. *J Sports Sci* 29:791–9.

Donahoo, W. T., J. A. Levine, and E. L. Melanson. 2004. Variability in energy expenditure and its components. *Curr Opin Clin Nutr Metab Care* 7:599–605.

Douda, H. T., A. G. Toubekis, A. A. Avloniti, and S. P. Tokmakidis. 2008. Physiological and anthropometric determinants of rhythmic gymnastics performance. *Int J Sports Physiol Perform* 3:41–54.

Drinkwater, B. L., K. Nilson, C. H. Chesnut, 3rd, W. J. Bremner, S. Shainholtz, and M. B. Southworth. 1984. Bone mineral content of amenorrheic and eumenorrheic athletes. *N Engl J Med* 311:277–81.

Drinkwater, B. L., K. Nilson, S. Ott, and C. H. Chesnut, 3rd. 1986. Bone mineral density after resumption of menses in amenorrheic athletes. *JAMA* 256:380–2.

Duckham, R. L., N. Peirce, C. Meyer, G. D. Summers, N. Cameron, and K. Brooke-Wavell. 2012. Risk factors for stress fracture in female endurance athletes: A cross-sectional study. *BMJ Open* 2: e001920.

Dulloo, A. G., and J. Jacquet. 1999. The control of partitioning between protein and fat during human starvation: Its internal determinants and biological significance. *Br J Nutr* 82:339–56.

Dwyer, J., A. Eisenberg, K. Prelack, W. O. Song, K. Sonneville, and P. Ziegler. 2012. Eating attitudes and food intakes of elite adolescent female figure skaters: A cross sectional study. *J Int Soc Sports Nutr* 9:53.

Ebine, N., J. Y. Feng, M. Homma, S. Saitoh, and P. J. Jones. 2000. Total energy expenditure of elite synchronized swimmers measured by the doubly labeled water method. *Eur J Appl Physiol* 83:1–6.

Ebine, N., H. H. Rafamantanantsoa, Y. Nayuki et al. 2002. Measurement of total energy expenditure by the doubly labelled water method in professional soccer players. *J Sports Sci* 20:391–7.

Eden, B. D., and P. J. Abernethy. 1994. Nutritional intake during an ultraendurance running race. *Int J Sport Nutr* 4:166–74.

Edwards, J. E., A. K. Lindeman, A. E. Mikesky, and J. M. Stager. 1993. Energy balance in highly trained female endurance runners. *Med Sci Sports Exerc* 25:1398–404.

Ekelund, U., A. Yngve, K. Westerterp, and M. Sjostrom. 2002. Energy expenditure assessed by heart rate and doubly labeled water in young athletes. *Med Sci Sports Exerc* 34:1360–6.

FAO/WHO/UNU Expert Consultation. 2011. *Human Energy Requirements: Report of a Joint FAO/WHO/UNU Expert Consultation*. Rome: Food and Agriculture Organization (FAO).

Fehling, P. C., L. Alekel, J. Clasey, A. Rector, and R. J. Stillman. 1995. A comparison of bone mineral densities among female athletes in impact loading and active loading sports. *Bone* 17:205–10.

Ferrand, C., and E. Brunet. 2004. Perfectionism and risk for disordered eating among young French male cyclists of high performance. *Percept Mot Skills* 99:959–67.

Field, A. E., C. M. Gordon, L. M. Pierce, A. Ramappa, and M. S. Kocher. 2011. Prospective study of physical activity and risk of developing a stress fracture among preadolescent and adolescent girls. *Arch Pediatr Adolesc Med* 165:723–8.

Filaire, E., F. Maso, P. Degoutte, P. Jouanel, and G. Lac. 2001. Food restriction, performance, psychological state and lipid values in judo athletes. *Int J Sports Med* 22:454–9.

Fogelholm, G. M., R. Koskinen, J. Laakso, T. Rankinen, and I. Ruokonen. 1993. Gradual and rapid weight loss: Effects on nutrition and performance in male athletes. *Med Sci Sports Exerc* 25:371–7.

Fogelholm, M. 1994. Effects of bodyweight reduction on sports performance. *Sports Med* 18:249–67.

Forbes, G. B. 2000. Body fat content influences the body composition response to nutrition and exercise. *Ann N Y Acad Sci* 904:359–65.

Franchini, E., C. J. Brito, and G. G. Artioli. 2012. Weight loss in combat sports: Physiological, psychological and performance effects. *J Int Soc Sports Nutr* 9:52.

Fredericson, M., K. Chew, J. Ngo, T. Cleek, J. Kiratli, and K. Cobb. 2007. Regional bone mineral density in male athletes: A comparison of soccer players, runners and controls. *Br J Sports Med* 41:664–8; discussion 668.

Fredericson, M., and K. Kent. 2005. Normalization of bone density in a previously amenorrheic runner with osteoporosis. *Med Sci Sports Exerc* 37:1481–6.

Frisch, R. E., and J. W. McArthur. 1974. Menstrual cycles: Fatness as a determinant of minimum weight for height necessary for their maintenance or onset. *Science* 185:949–51.

Fudge, B. W., K. R. Westerterp, F. K. Kiplamai, V. O. Onywera, M. K. Boit, B. Kayser, and Y. P. Pitsiladis. 2006. Evidence of negative energy balance using doubly labelled water in elite Kenyan endurance runners prior to competition. *Br J Nutr* 95:59–66.

Gallagher, D., and M. Elia. 2005. Body composition, organ mass, and resting energy expenditure. In *Human Body Composition*, edited by S. B. Heymsfield, T. G. Lohman, Z. Wang and S. B. Going, 219–39. Champaign, IL: Human Kinetics.

Garthe, I., T. Raastad, P. E. Refsnes, A. Koivisto, and J. Sundgot-Borgen. 2011a. Effect of two different weight-loss rates on body composition and strength and power-related performance in elite athletes. *Int J Sport Nutr Exerc Metab* 21:97–104.

Garthe, I., T. Raastad, and J. Sundgot-Borgen. 2011b. Long-term effect of weight loss on body composition and performance in elite athletes. *Int J Sport Nutr Exerc Metab* 21:426–35.

Gastmann, U., F. Dimeo, M. Huonker et al. 1998. Ultra-triathlon-related blood-chemical and endocrinological responses in nine athletes. *J Sports Med Phys Fitness* 38:18–23.

Georgopoulos, N. A., K. B. Markou, A. Theodoropoulou, D. Benardot, M. Leglise, and A. G. Vagenakis. 2002. Growth retardation in artistic compared with rhythmic elite female gymnasts. *J Clin Endocrinol Metab* 87:3169–73.

Gindoff, P. R., and M. Ferin. 1987. Endogenous opioid peptides modulate the effect of corticotropin-releasing factor on gonadotropin release in the primate. *Endocrinology* 121:837–42.

Glace, B. W., C. A. Murphy, and M. P. McHugh. 2002. Food intake and electrolyte status of ultramarathoners competing in extreme heat. *J Am Coll Nutr* 21:553–9.

Gleeson, M., D. C. Nieman, and B. K. Pedersen. 2004. Exercise, nutrition and immune function. *J Sports Sci* 22:115–25.

Golden, N. H., D. K. Katzman, R. E. Kreipe et al. 2003. Eating disorders in adolescents: Position paper of the Society for Adolescent Medicine. *J Adolesc Health* 33:496–503.

Gomez-Merino, D., M. Chennaoui, C. Drogou, D. Bonneau, and C. Y. Guezennec. 2002. Decrease in serum leptin after prolonged physical activity in men. *Med Sci Sports Exerc* 34:1594–9.

Griffith, R. O., R. H. Dressendorfer, C. D. Fullbright, and C. E. Wade. 1990. Testicular function during exhaustive endurance training. *Phys Sportsmed* 18:54–64.

Grundstein, A. J., C. Ramseyer, F. Zhao et al. 2012. A retrospective analysis of American football hyperthermia deaths in the United States. *Int J Biometeorol* 56:11–20.

Gutin, B., D. Alejandro, T. Duni, K. Segal, and G. B. Phillips. 1985. Levels of serum sex hormones and risk factors for coronary heart disease in exercise-trained men. *Am J Med* 79:79–84.

Hackney, A. C. 2001. Endurance exercise training and reproductive endocrine dysfunction in men: Alterations in the hypothalamic-pituitary-testicular axis. *Curr Pharm Des* 7:261–73.

Hackney, A. C. 2008. Effects of endurance exercise on the reproductive system of men: The "exercise-hypogonadal male condition". *J Endocrinol Invest* 31:932–8.

Hackney, A. C., C. L. Fahrner, and T. P. Gulledge. 1998. Basal reproductive hormonal profiles are altered in endurance trained men. *J Sports Med Physical Fitness* 38:138–41.

Hackney, A. C., W. E. Sinning, and B. C. Bruot. 1988. Reproductive hormonal profiles of endurance-trained and untrained males. *Med Sci Sports Exerc* 20:60–5.

Hackney, A. C., W. E. Sinning, and B. C. Bruot. 1990. Hypothalamic-pituitary-testicular axis function in endurance-trained males. *Int J Sports Med* 11:298–303.

Hall, C. J., and A. M. Lane. 2001. Effects of rapid weight loss on mood and performance among amateur boxers. *Br J Sports Med* 35:390–5.

Hall, K. D. 2007. Body fat and fat-free mass inter-relationships: Forbes's theory revisited. *Br J Nutr* 97:1059–63.

Heaney, R. P., S. Abrams, B. Dawson-Hughes, A. Looker, R. Marcus, V. Matkovic, and C. Weaver. 2000. Peak bone mass. *Osteoporos Int* 11:985–1009.

Helge, J. W., C. Lundby, D. L. Christensen et al. 2003. Skiing across the Greenland icecap: Divergent effects on limb muscle adaptations and substrate oxidation. *J Exp Biol* 206:1075–83.

Hickson, J. F., Jr., M. A. Duke, W. L. Risser, C. W. Johnson, R. Palmer, and J. E. Stockton. 1987. Nutritional intake from food sources of high school football athletes. *J Am Diet Assoc* 87:1656–9.

Hill, R. J., and P. S. Davies. 2001a. Energy expenditure during 2 wk of an ultra-endurance run around Australia. *Med Sci Sports Exerc* 33:148–51.

Hill, R. J., and P. S. Davies. 2001b. The validity of self-reported energy intake as determined using the doubly labelled water technique. *Br J Nutr* 85:415–30.

Hill, R. J., and P. S. Davies. 2002. Energy intake and energy expenditure in elite lightweight female rowers. *Med Sci Sports Exerc* 34:1823–9.

Hilton, L. K., and A. B. Loucks. 2000. Low energy availability, not exercise stress, suppresses the diurnal rhythm of leptin in healthy young women. *Am J Physiol (Endocrinol Metab)* 278:E43–9.

Hind, K., J. G. Truscott, and J. A. Evans. 2006. Low lumbar spine bone mineral density in both male and female endurance runners. *Bone* 39:880–5.

Horswill, C. A., R. C. Hickner, J. R. Scott, D. L. Costill, and D. Gould. 1990a. Weight loss, dietary carbohydrate modifications, and high intensity, physical performance. *Med Sci Sports Exerc* 22:470–6.

Horswill, C. A., S. H. Park, and J. N. Roemmich. 1990b. Changes in the protein nutritional status of adolescent wrestlers. *Med Sci Sports Exerc* 22:599–604.

Ihle, R., and A. B. Loucks. 2004. Dose-response relationships between energy availability and bone turnover in young exercising women. *J Bone Miner Res* 19:1231–40.

Ingjer, F., and J. Sundgot-Borgen. 1991. Influence of body weight reduction on maximal oxygen uptake in female elite athlete. *Scand J Med Sci Sports* 1:141–6.

Jenkins, P. J., X. Ibanez-Santos, J. Holly et al. 1993. IGFBP-1: A metabolic signal associated with exercise-induced amenorrhoea. *Neuroendocrinology* 57:600–4.

Johnson, C., P. S. Powers, and R. Dick. 1999. Athletes and eating disorders: The National Collegiate Athletic Association study. *Int J Eat Disord* 26:179–88.

Joy, E., A. Kussman, and A. Nattiv. 2016. 2016 update on eating disorders in athletes: A comprehensive narrative review with a focus on clinical assessment and management. *Br J Sports Med* 50:154–62.

Julian-Almarcegui, C., A. Gomez-Cabello, A. Gonzalez-Aguero et al. 2013. The nutritional status in adolescent Spanish cyclists. *Nutr Hosp* 28:1184–9.

Jurimae, J., V. Tillmann, P. Purge, and T. Jurimae. 2015. Body composition, maximal aerobic performance and inflammatory biomarkers in endurance-trained athletes. *Clin Physiol Funct Imaging*. September 16, 2015. Doi: 10.1111/cpf.12299. [Epub ahead of print], https://www.ncbi.nlm.nih.gov/pubmed/26373614

Karila, T. A., P. Sarkkinen, M. Marttinen, T. Seppala, A. Mero, and K. Tallroth. 2008. Rapid weight loss decreases serum testosterone. *Int J Sports Med* 29:872–7.

Keen, A. D., and B. L. Drinkwater. 1997. Irreversible bone loss in former amenorrheic athletes. *Osteoporos Int* 7:311–5.

Kelsey, J. L., L. K. Bachrach, E. Procter-Gray et al. 2007. Risk factors for stress fracture among young female cross-country runners. *Med Sci Sports Exerc* 39:1457–63.

Khodaee, M., L. Olewinski, B. Shadgan, and R. R. Kiningham. 2015. Rapid weight loss in sports with weight classes. *Curr Sports Med Rep* 14:435–41.

Kluge, M., P. Schussler, M. Uhr, A. Yassouridis, and A. Steiger. 2007. Ghrelin suppresses secretion of luteinizing hormone in humans. *J Clin Endocrinol Metab* 92:3202–5.

Knechtle, B. 2014. Relationship of anthropometric and training characteristics with race performance in endurance and ultra-endurance athletes. *Asian J Sports Med* 5:73–90.

Knechtle, B., B. Duff, G. Amtmann, and G. Kohler. 2008. An ultratriathlon leads to a decrease of body fat and skeletal muscle mass—the Triple Iron Triathlon Austria 2006. *Res Sports Med* 16:97–110.

Knechtle, B., P. Knechtle, T. Rosemann, and R. Lepers. 2010. Predictor variables for a 100-km race time in male ultra-marathoners. *Percept Mot Skills* 111:681–93.

Knechtle, B., R. Knechtle, M. Stiefel, M. A. Zingg, T. Rosemann, and C. A. Rust. 2015. Variables that influence Ironman triathlon performance—What changed in the last 35 years? *Open Access J Sports Med* 6:277–90.

Knechtle, B., and G. Kohler. 2007. Running 338 kilometres within five days has no effect on body mass and body fat but reduces skeletal muscle mass—The Isarrun 2006. *J Sports Sci Med* 6:401–7.

Knechtle, B., C. A. Rust, P. Knechtle, and T. Rosemann. 2012. Does muscle mass affect running times in male long-distance master runners? *Asian J Sports Med* 3:247–56.

Knechtle, B., A. Wirth, P. Knechtle, and T. Rosemann. 2009. Increase of total body water with decrease of body mass while running 100 km nonstop—formation of edema? *Res Q Exerc Sport* 80:593–603.

Koehler, K., H. Braun, M. de Marees, G. Fusch, C. Fusch, and W. Schaenzer. 2011. Assessing energy expenditure in male endurance athletes: Validity of the SenseWear Armband. *Med Sci Sports Exerc* 43:1328–33.

Kopp, W., W. F. Blum, S. von Prittwitz et al. 1997. Low leptin levels predict amenorrhea in underweight and eating disordered females. *Mol Psychiatry* 2:335–40.

Koral, J., and F. Dosseville. 2009. Combination of gradual and rapid weight loss: Effects on physical performance and psychological state of elite judo athletes. *J Sports Sci* 27:115–20.

Koutedakis, Y., P. J. Pacy, R. M. Quevedo et al. 1994. The effects of two different periods of weight-reduction on selected performance parameters in elite lightweight oarswomen. *Int J Sports Med* 15:472–7.

Lambrinoudaki, I., and D. Papadimitriou. 2010. Pathophysiology of bone loss in the female athlete. *Ann N Y Acad Sci* 1205:45–50.

Larsson, P., and K. Henriksson-Larsen. 2008. Body composition and performance in cross-country skiing. *Int J Sports Med* 29:971–5.

Lauder, T. D., S. Dixit, L. E. Pezzin, M. V. Williams, C. S. Campbell, and G. D. Davis. 2000. The relation between stress fractures and bone mineral density: Evidence from active-duty Army women. *Arch Phys Med Rehabil* 81:73–9.

Laughlin, G. A., and S. S. Yen. 1996. Nutritional and endocrine-metabolic aberrations in amenorrheic athletes. *J Clin Endocrinol Metab* 81:4301–9.

Laughlin, G. A., and S. S. Yen. 1997. Hypoleptinemia in women athletes: Absence of a diurnal rhythm with amenorrhea. *J Clin Endocrinol Metab* 82:318–21.

Lebenstedt, M., P. Platte, and K. M. Pirke. 1999. Reduced resting metabolic rate in athletes with menstrual disorders. *Med Sci Sports Exerc* 31:1250–6.

Legaz, A., and R. Eston. 2005. Changes in performance, skinfold thicknesses, and fat patterning after three years of intense athletic conditioning in high level runners. *Br J Sports Med* 39:851–6.

Lehmann, M., M. Huonker, F. Dimeo et al. 1995. Serum amino acid concentrations in nine athletes before and after the 1993 Colmar ultra triathlon. *Int J Sports Med* 16:155–9.

Levine, J. A. 2004. Non-exercise activity thermogenesis (NEAT). *Nutr Rev* 62:S82–97.

Lewiecki, E. M., C. M. Gordon, S. Baim et al. 2008. International society for clinical densitometry 2007 adult and pediatric official positions. *Bone* 43:1115–21.

Lindberg, J. S., W. B. Fears, M. M. Hunt, M. R. Powell, D. Boll, and C. E. Wade. 1984. Exercise-induced amenorrhea and bone density. *Ann Intern Med* 101:647–8.

Lindberg, J. S., M. R. Powell, M. M. Hunt, D. E. Ducey, and C. E. Wade. 1987. Increased vertebral bone mineral in response to reduced exercise in amenorrheic runners. *West J Med* 146:39–42.

Loucks, A. B. 2003. Energy availability, not body fatness, regulates reproductive function in women. *Exerc Sport Sci Rev* 31:144–8.

Loucks, A. B. 2004. Energy balance and body composition in sports and exercise. *J Sports Sci* 22:1–14.

Loucks, A. B., B. Kiens, and H. H. Wright. 2011. Energy availability in athletes. *J Sports Sci* 29(Suppl 1):S7–15.

Loucks, A. B., G. A. Laughlin, J. F. Mortola, L. Girton, J. C. Nelson, and S. S. Yen. 1992. Hypothalamic-pituitary-thyroidal function in eumenorrheic and amenorrheic athletes. *J Clin Endocrinol Metab* 75:514–8.

Loucks, A. B., J. F. Mortola, L. Girton, and S. S. Yen. 1989. Alterations in the hypothalamic-pituitary-ovarian and the hypothalamic-pituitary-adrenal axes in athletic women. *J Clin Endocrinol Metab* 68:402–11.

Loucks, A. B., and J. R. Thuma. 2003. Luteinizing hormone pulsatility is disrupted at a threshold of energy availability in regularly menstruating women. *Journal of Clinical Endocrinology & Metabolism* 88:297–311.

Loucks, A. B., M. Verdun, and E. M. Heath. 1998. Low energy availability, not stress of exercise, alters LH pulsatility in exercising women. *J Appl Physiol* 84:37–46.

MacConnie, S. E., A. Barkan, R. M. Lampman, M. A. Schork, and I. Z. Beitins. 1986. Decreased hypothalamic gonadotropin-releasing hormone secretion in male marathon runners. *N Engl J Med* 315:411–7.

Maestu, J., A. Eliakim, J. Jurimae, I. Valter, and T. Jurimae. 2010. Anabolic and catabolic hormones and energy balance of the male bodybuilders during the preparation for the competition. *J Strength Cond Res* 24:1074–81.

Maimoun, L., S. Lumbroso, J. Manetta, F. Paris, J. L. Leroux, and C. Sultan. 2003. Testosterone is significantly reduced in endurance athletes without impact on bone mineral density. *Horm Res* 59:285–92.

Manore, M. M., L. C. Kam, and A. B. Loucks. 2007. The female athlete triad: Components, nutrition issues, and health consequences. *J Sports Sci* 25(Suppl 1):S61–71.

Marcus, M. D., T. L. Loucks, and S. L. Berga. 2001. Psychological correlates of functional hypothalamic amenorrhea. *Fertil Steril* 76:310–6.

Marttinen, R. H., D. A. Judelson, L. D. Wiersma, and J. W. Coburn. 2011. Effects of self-selected mass loss on performance and mood in collegiate wrestlers. *J Strength Cond Res* 25:1010–5.

Mathur, D. N., A. L. Toriola, and O. A. Dada. 1986. Serum cortisol and testosterone levels in conditioned male distance runners and nonathletes after maximal exercise. *J Sports Med Phys Fitness* 26:245–50.

Matthew, C. E. 2005. Calibration of accelerometer output for adults. *Med Sci Sports Exerc* 37:S512–22.

Matzkin, E., E. J. Curry, and K. Whitlock. 2015. Female athlete triad: Past, present, and future. *J Am Acad Orthop Surg* 23:424–32.

McClung, J. P., E. Gaffney-Stomberg, and J. J. Lee. 2014. Female athletes: A population at risk of vitamin and mineral deficiencies affecting health and performance. *J Trace Elem Med Biol* 28:388–92.

McColl, E. M., G. D. Wheeler, P. Gomes, Y. Bhambhani, and D. C. Cumming. 1989. The effects of acute exercise on pulsatile LH release in high-mileage male runners. *Clin Endocrinol (Oxf)* 31:617–21.

McGee, C. 1997. Secondary amenorrhea leading to osteoporosis: Incidence and prevention. *Nurse Pract* 22:38, 41–5, 48 passim.

Medicine, Practice Committee of American Society for Reproductive. 2008. Current evaluation of amenorrhea. *Fertil Steril* 90:S219–25.

Melby, C. L., W. D. Schmidt, and D. Corrigan. 1990. Resting metabolic rate in weight-cycling collegiate wrestlers compared with physically active, noncycling control subjects. *Am J Clin Nutr* 52:409–14.

Melin, A., A. B. Tornberg, S. Skouby et al. 2014. The LEAF questionnaire: A screening tool for the identification of female athletes at risk for the female athlete triad. *Br J Sports Med* 48:540–5.

Mermier, C. M., J. M. Janot, D. L. Parker, and J. G. Swan. 2000. Physiological and anthropometric determinants of sport climbing performance. *Br J Sports Med* 34:359–65; discussion 366.

Merril, A. L. and B. K. Watt. 1973. *Energy Value of Foods, Basis and Derivation (Agriculture Handbook no 74)*. Agriculture Handbook No. 74. Washington, DC: ARS United States Department of Agriculture.

Mettler, S., N. Mitchell, and K. D. Tipton. 2010. Increased protein intake reduces lean body mass loss during weight loss in athletes. *Med Sci Sports Exerc* 42:326–37.

Meyer, N. L., J. Sundgot-Borgen, T. G. Lohman et al. 2013. Body composition for health and performance: A survey of body composition assessment practice carried out by the Ad Hoc Research Working Group on Body Composition, Health and Performance under the auspices of the IOC Medical Commission. *Br J Sports Med* 47:1044–53.

Michalakis, K. G., and J. H. Segars. 2010. The role of adiponectin in reproduction: From polycystic ovary syndrome to assisted reproduction. *Fertil Steril* 94:1949–57.

Milgrom, C., A. Simkin, A. Eldad, M. Nyska, and A. Finestone. 2000. Using bone's adaptation ability to lower the incidence of stress fractures. *Am J Sports Med* 28:245–51.

Miller, K. K., S. Grinspoon, S. Gleysteen et al. 2004. Preservation of neuroendocrine control of reproductive function despite severe undernutrition. *J Clin Endocrinol Metab* 89:4434–8.

Miller, K. K., M. S. Parulekar, E. Schoenfeld et al. 1998. Decreased leptin levels in normal weight women with hypothalamic amenorrhea: The effects of body composition and nutritional intake. *J Clin Endocrinol Metab* 83:2309–12.

Misra, M., A. Aggarwal, K. K. Miller et al. 2004. Effects of anorexia nervosa on clinical, hematologic, biochemical, and bone density parameters in community-dwelling adolescent girls. *Pediatrics* 114:1574–83.

Moore, J. M., A. F. Timperio, D. A. Crawford, C. M. Burns, and D. Cameron-Smith. 2002. Weight management and weight loss strategies of professional jockeys. *Int J Sport Nutr Exerc Metab* 12:1–13.

Morel, J., B. Combe, J. Francisco, and J. Bernard. 2001. Bone mineral density of 704 amateur sportsmen involved in different physical activities. *Osteoporos Int* 12:152–7.

Moschos, S., J. L. Chan, and C. S. Mantzoros. 2002. Leptin and reproduction: A review. *Fertil Steril* 77:433–44.

Mountjoy, M., J. Sundgot-Borgen, L. Burke et al. 2014. The IOC consensus statement: Beyond the female athlete triad—Relative Energy Deficiency in Sport (RED-S). *Br J Sports Med* 48:491–7.

Muller, W. 2009a. Determinants of ski-jump performance and implications for health, safety and fairness. *Sports Med* 39:85–106.

Muller, W. 2009b. Towards research-based approaches for solving body composition problems in sports: Ski jumping as a heuristic example. *Br J Sports Med* 43:1013–9.

Mulligan, K., and G. E. Butterfield. 1990. Discrepancies between energy intake and expenditure in physically active women. *Br J Nutr* 64:23–36.

Myburgh, K. H., L. K. Bachrach, B. Lewis, K. Kent, and R. Marcus. 1993. Low bone mineral density at axial and appendicular sites in amenorrheic athletes. *Med Sci Sports Exerc* 25:1197–202.

Myerson, M., B. Gutin, M. P. Warren et al. 1991. Resting metabolic rate and energy balance in amenorrheic and eumenorrheic runners. *Med Sci Sports Exerc* 23:15–22.

Nattiv, A., G. Kennedy, M. T. Barrack et al. 2013. Correlation of MRI grading of bone stress injuries with clinical risk factors and return to play: A 5-year prospective study in collegiate track and field athletes. *Am J Sports Med* 41:1930–41.

Nattiv, A., A. B. Loucks, M. M. Manore et al. 2007. American college of sports medicine position stand. The female athlete triad. *Med Sci Sports Exerc* 39:1867–82.

Nazem, T. G., and K. E. Ackerman. 2012. The female athlete triad. *Sports Health* 4:302–11.

Neumayr, G., R. Pfister, H. Hoertnagl et al. 2003. The effect of marathon cycling on renal function. *Int J Sports Med* 24:131–7.

Neumayr, G., R. Pfister, H. Hoertnagl, G. Mitterbauer, W. Prokop, and M. Joannidis. 2005. Renal function and plasma volume following ultramarathon cycling. *Int J Sports Med* 26:2–8.

Nichols, J. F., H. Aralis, S. G. Merino, M. T. Barrack, L. Stalker-Fader, and M. J. Rauh. 2010. Utility of the actiheart accelerometer for estimating exercise energy expenditure in female adolescent runners. *Int J Sport Nutr Exerc Metab* 20:487–95.

Nichols, J. F., and M. J. Rauh. 2011. Longitudinal changes in bone mineral density in male master cyclists and nonathletes. *J Strength Cond Res* 25:727–34.

Niinimaa, V., M. Dyon, and R. J. Shephard. 1978. Performance and efficiency of intercollegiate cross-country skiers. *Med Sci Sports* 10:91–3.

O'Donnell, E., P. J. Harvey, J. M. Goodman, and M. J. De Souza. 2007. Long-term estrogen deficiency lowers regional blood flow, resting systolic blood pressure, and heart rate in exercising premenopausal women. *Am J Physiol (Endocrinol Metab)* 292:E1401–9.

Oppliger, R. A., H. S. Case, C. A. Horswill, G. L. Landry, and A. C. Shelter. 1996. American college of sports medicine position stand. Weight loss in wrestlers. *Med Sci Sports Exerc* 28:ix–xii.

Oppliger, R. A., G. L. Landry, S. W. Foster, and A. C. Lambrecht. 1998. Wisconsin minimum weight program reduces weight-cutting practices of high school wrestlers. *Clin J Sport Med* 8:26–31.

Oppliger, R. A., S. A. Steen, and J. R. Scott. 2003. Weight loss practices of college wrestlers. *Int J Sport Nutr Exerc Metab* 13:29–46.

Oppliger, R. A., A. C. Utter, J. R. Scott, R. W. Dick, and D. Klossner. 2006. NCAA rule change improves weight loss among national championship wrestlers. *Med Sci Sports Exerc* 38:963–70.

Otis, C. L., B. Drinkwater, M. Johnson, A. Loucks, and J. Wilmore. 1997. American College of Sports Medicine position stand. The female athlete triad. *Med Sci Sports Exerc* 29:i–ix.

Perseghin, G., G. Lattuada, F. Ragogna, G. Alberti, A. La Torre, and L. Luzi. 2009. Free leptin index and thyroid function in male highly trained athletes. *Eur J Endocrinol* 161:871–6.

Petrie, H. J., E. A. Stover, and C. A. Horswill. 2004. Nutritional concerns for the child and adolescent competitor. *Nutrition* 20:620–31.

Pfeiffer, B., T. Stellingwerff, A. B. Hodgson, R. Randell, K. Pottgen, P. Res, and A. E. Jeukendrup. 2012. Nutritional intake and gastrointestinal problems during competitive endurance events. *Med Sci Sports Exerc* 44:344–51.

Pieper, C., L. Redman, S. Racette et al. 2011. Development of adherence metrics for caloric restriction interventions. *Clin Trials* 8:155–64.

Pietrowsky, R., and K. Straub. 2008. Body dissatisfaction and restrained eating in male juvenile and adult athletes. *Eat Weight Disord* 13:14–21.

Pirke, K. M., U. Schweiger, R. Laessle, B. Dickhaut, M. Schweiger, and M. Waechtler. 1986. Dieting influences the menstrual cycle: Vegetarian versus nonvegetarian diet. *Fertil Steril* 46:1083–8.

Ramson, R., J. Jurimae, T. Jurimae, and J. Maestu. 2012. The effect of 4-week training period on plasma neuropeptide Y, leptin and ghrelin responses in male rowers. *Eur J Appl Physiol* 112:1873–80.

Rankinen, T., M. Fogelholm, U. Kujala, R. Rauramaa, and M. Uusitupa. 1995. Dietary intake and nutritional status of athletic and nonathletic children in early puberty. *Int J Sport Nutr* 5:136–50.

Ransone, J., and B. Hughes. 2004. Body-weight fluctuation in collegiate wrestlers: Implications of the National Collegiate Athletic Association Weight-Certification Program. *J Athl Train* 39:162–5.

Raschka, C., and M. Plath. 1992. Body fat compartment and its relationship to food intake and clinical chemical parameters during extreme endurance performance. *Schweiz Z Sportmed* 40:13–25.

Raschka, C., M. Plath, R. Cerull, W. Bernhard, K. Jung, and C. Leitzmann. 1991. The body muscle compartment and its relationship to food absorption and blood chemistry during an extreme endurance performance. *Z Ernahrungswiss* 30:276–88.

Rauh, M. J., M. Barrack, and J. F. Nichols. 2014. Associations between the female athlete triad and injury among high school runners. *Int J Sports Phys Ther* 9:948–58.

Rauh, M. J., C. A. Macera, D. W. Trone, R. A. Shaffer, and S. K. Brodine. 2006. Epidemiology of stress fracture and lower-extremity overuse injury in female recruits. *Med Sci Sports Exerc* 38:1571–7.

Redman, L. M., L. K. Heilbronn, C. K. Martin et al. 2009. Metabolic and behavioral compensations in response to caloric restriction: Implications for the maintenance of weight loss. *PLoS One* 4:e4377.

Redman, L. M., and A. B. Loucks. 2005. Menstrual disorders in athletes. *Sports Med* 35:747–55.

Reljic, D., J. Feist, J. Jost, M. Kieser, and B. Friedmann-Bette. 2016. Rapid body mass loss affects erythropoiesis and hemolysis but does not impair aerobic performance in combat athletes. *Scand J Med Sci Sports*. 26(5):507–17.

Rickenlund, A., M. J. Eriksson, K. Schenck-Gustafsson, and A. L. Hirschberg. 2005. Amenorrhea in female athletes is associated with endothelial dysfunction and unfavorable lipid profile. *J Clin Endocrinol Metab* 90:1354–9.

Rico-Sanz, J., W. R. Frontera, P. A. Mole, M. A. Rivera, A. Rivera-Brown, and C. N. Meredith. 1998. Dietary and performance assessment of elite soccer players during a period of intense training. *Int J Sport Nutr* 8:230–40.

Risser, W. L., E. J. Lee, A. LeBlanc, H. B. Poindexter, J. M. Risser, and V. Schneider. 1990. Bone density in eumenorrheic female college athletes. *Med Sci Sports Exerc* 22:570–4.

Roberts, A. C., R. D. McClure, R. I. Weiner, and G. A. Brooks. 1993. Overtraining affects male reproductive status. *Fertil Steril* 60:686–92.

Robinson, T. L., C. Snow-Harter, D. R. Taaffe, D. Gillis, J. Shaw, and R. Marcus. 1995. Gymnasts exhibit higher bone mass than runners despite similar prevalence of amenorrhea and oligomenorrhea. *J Bone Miner Res* 10:26–35.

Rodriguez, N. R., N. M. Di Marco, and S. Langley. 2009. American college of sports medicine position stand. Nutrition and athletic performance. *Med Sci Sports Exerc* 41:709–31.

Roelofs, E. J., A. E. Smith-Ryan, M. N. Melvin, H. L. Wingfield, E. T. Trexler, and N. Walker. 2015. Muscle size, quality, and body composition: Characteristics of division I cross-country runners. *J Strength Cond Res* 29:290–6.

Roemmich, J. N., and W. E. Sinning. 1997. Weight loss and wrestling training: Effects on nutrition, growth, maturation, body composition, and strength. *J Appl Physiol* 82:1751–9.

Rogol, A. D., A. Weltman, J. Y. Weltman et al. 1992. Durability of the reproductive axis in eumenorrheic women during 1 yr of endurance training. *J Appl Physiol (1985)* 72:1571–80.

Rome, E. S., S. Ammerman, D. S. Rosen et al. 2003. Children and adolescents with eating disorders: The state of the art. *Pediatrics* 111:e98–108.

Rosendahl, J., B. Bormann, K. Aschenbrenner, F. Aschenbrenner, and B. Strauss. 2009. Dieting and disordered eating in German high school athletes and non-athletes. *Scand J Med Sci Sports* 19:731–9.

Roupas, N. D., and N. A. Georgopoulos. 2011. Menstrual function in sports. *Hormones (Athens)* 10:104–16.

Rouveix, M., M. Bouget, C. Pannafieux, S. Champely, and E. Filaire. 2007. Eating attitudes, body esteem, perfectionism and anxiety of judo athletes and nonathletes. *Int J Sports Med* 28:340–5.

Sandoval, W. M., V. H. Heyward, and T. M. Lyons. 1989. Comparison of body composition, exercise and nutritional profiles of female and male body builders at competition. *J Sports Med Phys Fitness* 29:63–70.

Santos, D. A., J. A. Dawson, C. N. Matias et al. 2014a. Reference values for body composition and anthropometric measurements in athletes. *PLoS One* 9:e97846.

Santos, D. A., C. N. Matias, P. M. Rocha et al. 2014b. Association of basketball season with body composition in elite junior players. *J Sports Med Phys Fitness* 54:162–73.

Santos, D. A., A. M. Silva, C. N. Matias, D. A. Fields, S. B. Heymsfield, and L. B. Sardinha. 2010. Accuracy of DXA in estimating body composition changes in elite athletes using a four compartment model as the reference method. *Nutr Metab (Lond)* 7:22.

Santos, D. A., A. M. Silva, C. N. Matias et al. 2013. Validity of a combined heart rate and motion sensor for the measurement of free-living energy expenditure in very active individuals. *J Sci Med Sport* 17:387–93.

Schoeller, D. A. 2009. The energy balance equation: Looking back and looking forward are two very different views. *Nutr Rev* 67:249–54.

Schoeller, D. A., and S. B. Racette. 1990. A review of field techniques for the assessment of energy expenditure. *J Nutr* 120:1492–5.

Schoeller, D. A., and E. van Santen. 1982. Measurement of energy expenditure in humans by doubly labeled water method. *J Appl Physiol* 53:955–9.

Schulz, L. O., S. Alger, I. Harper, J. H. Wilmore, and E. Ravussin. 1992. Energy expenditure of elite female runners measured by respiratory chamber and doubly labeled water. *J Appl Physiol* 72:23–8.

Schutz, U. H., C. Billich, K. Konig et al. 2013. Characteristics, changes and influence of body composition during a 4486 km transcontinental ultramarathon: Results from the TransEurope FootRace mobile whole body MRI-project. *BMC Med* 11:122.

Schwartz, B., D. C. Cumming, E. Riordan, M. Selye, S. S. Yen, and R. W. Rebar. 1981. Exercise-associated amenorrhea: A distinct entity? *Am J Obstet Gynecol* 141:662–70.

Scott, J. R., C. A. Horswill, and R. W. Dick. 1994. Acute weight gain in collegiate wrestlers following a tournament weigh-in. *Med Sci Sports Exerc* 26:1181–5.

Scott, J. R., R. A. Oppliger, A. C. Utter, and C.G. Kerr. 2000. Body weight changes at the national tournaments-the impact of rules governing wrestling weight management. *Med Sci Sports Exerc* 32:S131, Supplement, #532.

Shirreffs, S. M., L. E. Armstrong, and S. N. Cheuvront. 2004. Fluid and electrolyte needs for preparation and recovery from training and competition. *J Sports Sci* 22:57–63.

Silva, A. M., D. A. Fields, S. B. Heymsfield, and L. B. Sardinha. 2010. Body composition and power changes in elite judo athletes. *Int J Sports Med* 31:737–41.

Silva, A. M., D. A. Fields, S. B. Heymsfield, and L. B. Sardinha. 2011. Relationship between changes in total-body water and fluid distribution with maximal forearm strength in elite judo athletes. *J Strength Cond Res* 25:2488–95.

Silva, M. G., and T. Paiva. 2015. Poor precompetitive sleep habits, nutrients' deficiencies, inappropriate body composition and athletic performance in elite gymnasts. *Eur J Sport Sci* 16:726–35.

Silva, A. M., D. A. Santos, C. N. Matias, C. S. Minderico, D. A. Schoeller, and L. B. Sardinha. 2013. Total energy expenditure assessment in elite junior basketball players: A validation study using doubly labeled water. *J Strength Cond Res* 27:1920–7.

Simsch, C., W. Lormes, K. G. Petersen et al. 2002. Training intensity influences leptin and thyroid hormones in highly trained rowers. *Int J Sports Med* 23:422–7.

Singhal, V., M. de Lourdes Eguiguren, L. Eisenbach et al. 2014. Body composition, hemodynamic, and biochemical parameters of young female normal-weight oligo-amenorrheic and eumenorrheic athletes and nonathletes. *Ann Nutr Metab* 65:264–71.

Sjodin, A. M., A. B. Andersson, J. M. Hogberg, and K. R. Westerterp. 1994. Energy balance in cross-country skiers: A study using doubly labeled water. *Med Sci Sports Exerc* 26:720–4.

Skenderi, K. P., S. A. Kavouras, C. A. Anastasiou, N. Yiannakouris, and A. L. Matalas. 2006. Exertional Rhabdomyolysis during a 246-km continuous running race. *Med Sci Sports Exerc* 38:1054–7.

Slater, G., A. Rice, D. Jenkins, and A. Hahn. 2014. Body mass management of lightweight rowers: Nutritional strategies and performance implications. *Br J Sports Med* 48:1529–33.

Slater, G. J., A. J. Rice, K. Sharpe et al. 2005. Impact of acute weight loss and/or thermal stress on rowing ergometer performance. *Med Sci Sports Exerc* 37:1387–94.

Slater, G., A. J. Rice, R. Tanner et al. 2006. Acute weight loss followed by an aggressive nutritional recovery strategy has little impact on on-water rowing performance. *Br J Sports Med* 40:55–9.

Smathers, A. M., M. G. Bemben, and D. A. Bemben. 2009. Bone density comparisons in male competitive road cyclists and untrained controls. *Med Sci Sports Exerc* 41:290–6.

Smith, M., R. Dyson, T. Hale, M. Hamilton, J. Kelly, and P. Wellington. 2001. The effects of restricted energy and fluid intake on simulated amateur boxing performance. *Int J Sport Nutr Exerc Metab* 11:238–47.

Smith, R., and O. M. Rutherford. 1993. Spine and total body bone mineral density and serum testosterone levels in male athletes. *Eur J Appl Physiol Occup Physiol* 67:330–4.

Smolak, L., S. K. Murnen, and A. E. Ruble. 2000. Female athletes and eating problems: A meta-analysis. *Int J Eat Disord* 27:371–80.

Soric, M., M. Misigoj-Durakovic, and Z. Pedisic. 2008. Dietary intake and body composition of prepubescent female aesthetic athletes. *Int J Sport Nutr Exerc Metab* 18:343–54.

Sparling, P. B., D. C. Nieman, and P. J. O'Connor. 1993. Selected scientific aspects of marathon racing. An update on fluid replacement, immune function, psychological factors and the gender difference. *Sports Med* 15:116–32.

Speakman, J. R. 1997. *Doubly Labelled Water: Theory and Practice*. London, UK: Chapman & Hall.

Steen, S. N., and K. D. Brownell. 1990. Patterns of weight loss and regain in wrestlers: Has the tradition changed? *Med Sci Sports Exerc* 22:762–8.

Steen, S. N., R. A. Oppliger, and K. D. Brownell. 1988. Metabolic effects of repeated weight loss and regain in adolescent wrestlers. *JAMA* 260:47–50.

Steinacker, J. M., M. Brkic, C. Simsch et al. 2005. Thyroid hormones, cytokines, physical training and metabolic control. *Horm Metab Res* 37:538–44.

Stewart, A. D., and J. Hannan. 2000. Total and regional bone density in male runners, cyclists, and controls. *Med Sci Sports Exerc* 32:1373–7.

Stoggl, T., J. Enqvist, E. Muller, and H. C. Holmberg. 2010. Relationships between body composition, body dimensions, and peak speed in cross-country sprint skiing. *J Sports Sci* 28:161–9.

Sundgot-Borgen, J. 1993. Prevalence of eating disorders in elite female athletes. *Int J Sport Nutr* 3:29–40.

Sundgot-Borgen, J. 1994. Risk and trigger factors for the development of eating disorders in female elite athletes. *Med Sci Sports Exerc* 26:414–9.

Sundgot-Borgen, J., and I. Garthe. 2011. Elite athletes in aesthetic and olympic weight-class sports and the challenge of body weight and body compositions. *J Sports Sci* 29(Suppl 1):S101–14.

Sundgot-Borgen, J., N. L. Meyer, T. G. Lohman et al. 2013. How to minimise the health risks to athletes who compete in weight-sensitive sports review and position statement on behalf of the Ad Hoc Research Working Group on Body Composition, Health and Performance, under the auspices of the IOC Medical Commission. *Br J Sports Med* 47:1012–22.

Sundgot-Borgen, J., and M. K. Torstveit. 2004. Prevalence of eating disorders in elite athletes is higher than in the general population. *Clin J Sport Med* 14:25–32.

Sundgot-Borgen, J., and M. K. Torstveit. 2010. Aspects of disordered eating continuum in elite high-intensity sports. *Scand J Med Sci Sports* 20(Suppl 2):112–21.

Tanaka, K., and Y. Matsuura. 1982. A multivariate analysis of the role of certain anthropometric and physiological attributes in distance running. *Ann Hum Biol* 9:473–82.

Tanda, G., and B. Knechtle. 2015. Effects of training and anthropometric factors on marathon and 100 km ultramarathon race performance. *Open Access J Sports Med* 6:129–36.

Tenforde, A. S., M. T. Barrack, A. Nattiv, and M. Fredericson. 2016. Parallels with the female athlete triad in male athletes. *Sports Med* 46:171–82.

Tenforde, A. S., and M. Fredericson. 2011. Influence of sports participation on bone health in the young athlete: A review of the literature. *PM R* 3:861–7.

Tenforde, A. S., M. Fredericson, L. C. Sayres, P. Cutti, and K. L. Sainani. 2015. Identifying sex-specific risk factors for low bone mineral density in adolescent runners. *Am J Sports Med* 43:1494–504.

Tenforde, A. S., L. C. Sayres, M. L. McCurdy, H. Collado, K. L. Sainani, and M. Fredericson. 2011. Overuse injuries in high school runners: Lifetime prevalence and prevention strategies. *PM R* 3:125–31; quiz 131.

Tenforde, A. S., L. C. Sayres, M. L. McCurdy, K. L. Sainani, and M. Fredericson. 2013. Identifying sex-specific risk factors for stress fractures in adolescent runners. *Med Sci Sports Exerc* 45:1843–51.

Theodoropoulou, A., K. B. Markou, G. A. Vagenakis et al. 2005. Delayed but normally progressed puberty is more pronounced in artistic compared with rhythmic elite gymnasts due to the intensity of training. *J Clin Endocrinol Metab* 90:6022–7.

Thiel, A., H. Gottfried, and F. W. Hesse. 1993. Subclinical eating disorders in male athletes. A study of the low weight category in rowers and wrestlers. *Acta Psychiatr Scand* 88:259–65.

Thienpont, E., J. Bellemans, I. Samson, and G. Fabry. 2000. Stress fracture of the inferior and superior pubic ramus in a man with anorexia nervosa and hypogonadism. *Acta Orthop Belg* 66:297–301.

Torstveit, M. K., and J. Sundgot-Borgen. 2005. The female athlete triad exists in both elite athletes and controls. *Med Sci Sports Exerc* 37:1449–59.

Trexler, E. T., A. E. Smith-Ryan, and L. E. Norton. 2014. Metabolic adaptation to weight loss: Implications for the athlete. *J Int Soc Sports Nutr* 11:7.

Trussell, J. 1980. Statistical flaws in evidence for the Frisch hypothesis that fatness triggers menarche. *Hum Biol* 52:711–20.

Vaamonde, D., M. E. Da Silva, M. S. Poblador, and J. L. Lancho. 2006. Reproductive profile of physically active men after exhaustive endurance exercise. *Int J Sports Med* 27:680–9.

van Erp-Baart, A. M., W. H. Saris, R. A. Binkhorst, J. A. Vos, and J. W. Elvers. 1989. Nationwide survey on nutritional habits in elite athletes. Part I. Energy, carbohydrate, protein, and fat intake. *Int J Sports Med* 10(Suppl 1):S3–10.

Van Etten, L. M., K. R. Westerterp, F. T. Verstappen, B. J. Boon, and W. H. Saris. 1997. Effect of an 18-wk weight-training program on energy expenditure and physical activity. *J Appl Physiol* 82:298–304.

Vanheest, J. L., C. D. Rodgers, C. E. Mahoney, and M. J. De Souza. 2014. Ovarian suppression impairs sport performance in junior elite female swimmers. *Med Sci Sports Exerc* 46:156–66.

Vinther, A., I. L. Kanstrup, E. Christiansen, C. Ekdahl, and P. Aagaard. 2008. Testosterone and BMD in elite male lightweight rowers. *Int J Sports Med* 29:803–7.

Warren, M. P., J. Brooks-Gunn, R. P. Fox, C. C. Holderness, E. P. Hyle, and W. G. Hamilton. 2002. Osteopenia in exercise-associated amenorrhea using ballet dancers as a model: A longitudinal study. *J Clin Endocrinol Metab* 87:3162–8.

Warren, M. P., J. Brooks-Gunn, L. H. Hamilton, L. F. Warren, and W. G. Hamilton. 1986. Scoliosis and fractures in young ballet dancers. Relation to delayed menarche and secondary amenorrhea. *N Engl J Med* 314:1348–53.

Warren, M. P., and N. E. Perlroth. 2001. The effects of intense exercise on the female reproductive system. *J Endocrinol* 170:3–11.

Waters, D. L., C. R. Qualls, R. Dorin, J. D. Veldhuis, and R. N. Baumgartner. 2001. Increased pulsatility, process irregularity, and nocturnal trough concentrations of growth hormone in amenorrheic compared to eumenorrheic athletes. *J Clin Endocrinol Metab* 86:1013–9.

Watts, P. B., L. M. Joubert, A. K. Lish, J. D. Mast, and B. Wilkins. 2003. Anthropometry of young competitive sport rock climbers. *Br J Sports Med* 37:420–4.

Webster, S., R. Rutt, and A. Weltman. 1990. Physiological effects of a weight loss regimen practiced by college wrestlers. *Med Sci Sports Exerc* 22:229–34.

Weimann, E., C. Witzel, S. Schwidergall, and H. J. Bohles. 2000. Peripubertal perturbations in elite gymnasts caused by sport specific training regimes and inadequate nutritional intake. *Int J Sports Med* 21:210–5.

Weitkunat, T., B. Knechtle, P. Knechtle, C. A. Rust, and T. Rosemann. 2012. Body composition and hydration status changes in male and female open-water swimmers during an ultra-endurance event. *J Sports Sci* 30:1003–13.

Westerterp, K. R., G. A. Meijer, E. M. Janssen, W. H. Saris, and F. Ten Hoor. 1992. Long-term effect of physical activity on energy balance and body composition. *Br J Nutr* 68:21–30.

Westerterp, K. R., W. H. Saris, M. van Es, and F. ten Hoor. 1986. Use of the doubly labeled water technique in humans during heavy sustained exercise. *J Appl Physiol* 61:2162–7.

Wheeler, G. D., M. Singh, W. D. Pierce, W. F. Epling, and D. C. Cumming. 1991. Endurance training decreases serum testosterone levels in men without change in luteinizing hormone pulsatile release. *J Clin Endocrinol Metab* 72:422–5.

Wheeler, G. D., S. R. Wall, A. N. Belcastro, P. Conger, and D. C. Cumming. 1986. Are anorexic tendencies prevalent in the habitual runner? *Br J Sports Med* 20:77–81.

Williams, N. I., D. L. Helmreich, D. B. Parfitt, A. Caston-Balderrama, and J. L. Cameron. 2001. Evidence for a causal role of low energy availability in the induction of menstrual cycle disturbances during strenuous exercise training. *J Clin Endocrinol Metab* 86:5184–93.

Williams, N. I., H. J. Leidy, B. R. Hill, J. L. Lieberman, R. S. Legro, and M. J. De Souza. 2015. Magnitude of daily energy deficit predicts frequency but not severity of menstrual disturbances associated with exercise and caloric restriction. *Am J Physiol Endocrinol Metab* 308:E29–39.

Wilson, G., M. B. Hawken, I. Poole et al. 2014. Rapid weight-loss impairs simulated riding performance and strength in jockeys: Implications for making-weight. *J Sports Sci* 32:383–91.

Wilson, J. H., and R. L. Wolman. 1994. Osteoporosis and fracture complications in an amenorrhoeic athlete. *Br J Rheumatol* 33:480–1.

Wolf, J. H. 1995. Julis Wolff and his "law of bone remodeling." *Orthopade* 24:378–86.

Yanagawa, Y., T. Morimura, K. Tsunekawa et al. 2010. Oxidative stress associated with rapid weight reduction decreases circulating adiponectin concentrations. *Endocr J* 57:339–45.

Zanker, C. L., and I. L. Swaine. 1998. Bone turnover in amenorrhoeic and eumenorrhoeic women distance runners. *Scand J Med Sci Sports* 8:20–6.

Zanker, C. L., and I. L. Swaine. 2000. Responses of bone turnover markers to repeated endurance running in humans under conditions of energy balance or energy restriction. *Eur J Appl Physiol* 83:434–40.

Ziegler, P., S. Hensley, J. B. Roepke, S. H. Whitaker, B. W. Craig, and A. Drewnowski. 1998a. Eating attitudes and energy intakes of female skaters. *Med Sci Sports Exerc* 30:583–6.

Ziegler, P. J., C. S. Khoo, B. Sherr, J. A. Nelson, W. M. Larson, and A. Drewnowski. 1998b. Body image and dieting behaviors among elite figure skaters. *Int J Eat Disord* 24:421–7.

13 Mathematical Modeling of Anthropometrically Based Body Fat for Military Health and Performance Applications

Col. Karl E. Friedl

CONTENTS

The average normal man represents the mean between the two extremes of the emaciated, half-starved individual, disinclined to physical or mental work, and the over-fed, obese epicure, both extremes being relatively low in vital activity and in productivity.

Francis Benedict (1915)

The specific gravity or weight of tissue per unit volume gives a true index of proper weight and not the standard tables which interpret weight in relation to height. These findings together with accurate measurements of thoracic and abdominal circumferences and diameters provide information as to the physical characteristics associated with rugged physique and unusual fitness.

Lt. W. C. Welham and Lt. Cdr. A. R. Behnke (1942)

13.1   INTRODUCTION

Body composition has been used as a marker of soldier fitness and physical capability for centuries. Originally, armies sought to exclude recruits who were chronically malnourished or diseased because they were more likely to struggle under the physical demands of load carriage and other common military tasks. It was also advantageous to have impressively large soldiers who looked like a force to be reckoned with. With improved medicine and nutrition of the past century, this focus on underweight soldiers shifted to identification of seriously overweight soldiers who were at increased risk for health issues, such as type 2 diabetes, and might also be unable to meet military physical demands. The most important reason today for military body composition standards is to ensure that soldiers are ready to perform their military duties on short notice, where they may have to deploy anywhere in the world within 24 hours. Body fat standards serve this purpose as motivators of regular physical activity and good nutrition habits, providing a practical marker of chronic behavior that affects soldier health and performance. For this purpose, methods must be consistent and reproducible but do not require a research level of accuracy for total body fat content analysis; although criterion methods of total body fat assessment have been used for calibration of the military circumference-based equations, they are not appropriate for military body composition standards enforcement (the point is highlighted in this chapter). The military body fat standards also differ from physical fitness standards; these are assessed separately with physical performance tests. Both the body fat and physical fitness standards relate to physical activity habits and promotion of health fitness habits. Regular physical activity habits are important even for the modern cyber-warrior because of the profound benefits to mental performance (neurocognition, mood, and brain health) that may be especially important to the technologically enabled soldier (Friedl et al. 2016). Nevertheless, there is currently a move to ease the body fat standards that have been in force for the U.S. military since the 1980s. This is because of the increasing difficulty in recruiting and retaining young men and women who meet these standards.

This chapter summarizes the scientific basis of military body composition standards and military contributions to the science of body composition assessment. There is an emphasis on the Army perspective, representing the largest service by number of personnel.

13.2   ORIGIN OF MILITARY BODY COMPOSITION STANDARDS

Military physical standards involved some version of weight-for-height tables for most of the twentieth century (Friedl 1992; Johnson 1997). In World War I, a man simply had to be at least 64 in. tall, be between 128 and 190 lb, and have a chest circumference (at expiration) to be at least half of the height measurement; the standards varied for special jobs, such as cavalrymen who could not exceed 165 lb (Orr 1917). Obesity standards were not necessarily rigidly enforced; 75,000 men were rejected for military service due to being underweight, while only 4211 were rejected for obesity because excessive weight tended to be a "variation correctable with proper food and physical training" (Love and Davenport 1920). This assumption that overweight recruits would lose weight during the rigors of basic training continued into World War II. The tables used in World War II were derived from the 1912 medico-actuarial tables and represented desirable weights (Newman 1952). This put the focus on mortality risk. Men were unacceptable if they were less than 105 lb or "overweight which is greatly out of proportion to the height," but could still be considered if, in the opinion of the examiner, the variation was correctable with proper food and physical training (Foster et al. 1967).

Nevertheless, in 1942, Cdr. Albert Behnke made the observation that military weight-for-height tables might select out lean recruits who were large but strong and potentially ideal military performers (Welham and Behnke 1942). In an article published in the *Journal of the American Medical Association*, Behnke, a leader in diving medicine research, noted that body density measured by underwater weighing could distinguish big and muscular from big and fat recruits (Behnke et al.

1942). They demonstrated this big-but-lean concept with data from 25 professional football players (average weight: 200 lb, body density: 1.080 g/cm^3) (Welham and Behnke 1942). At the other extreme, the issue of underweight recruits who might not hold up under the rigors of training and military service was addressed after World War II, when Congress passed the School Lunch Act. In the 1946 Act, national security concerns were specifically cited with mention of the large number of recruits who were turned away from military service during the war because of chronic malnutrition.

Weight-for-height tables continued to guide military recruitment through the 1970s. After World War II, the weight tables for women became progressively more stringent than the original tables established for World War II nurses, and the weight standards for men became more liberal (Karpinos 1958). These tables also formed the basis of "retention" standards, the standards for minimal fitness to remain on active duty in the military services. Regulations included guidance that overweight service members would be referred for medical examination to determine if they were obese and should be discharged from the military. These were subjective standards that were inconsistently applied. Physicians who may themselves have been overweight made the decision about whether or not a soldier's level of obesity was inconsistent with being able to perform one's military duties. The inadequacy of relative weight as an objective standard to distinguish big and fat from big and muscular soldiers was already well documented (Behnke et al. 1942; Selzer et al. 1970).

The post-Vietnam era Army of the late 1970s was demoralized and without an active wartime mission. Fitness of the services had fallen to a low point. One anecdote described a nationally televised ceremony in the capital where the television cameras panned down the ample pot bellies of an honor guard representing all of the military services, with news commentators speculating about the physical ability of these men to defend the country (David D. Schnakenberg, personal communication 1989). In 1980, President Carter directed the military services to conduct a review of fitness in the military and to establish new standards to ensure a higher level of fitness (Study of the Military Services' Physical Fitness 1981). This was not unprecedented, as President Theodore Roosevelt had called for a similar review of a peacetime Army, which led to establishment of the annual test ride for cavalrymen (General Orders No. 181 1907). In 1980, a combined group of physiologists and line officers met and drew up new recommendations that formed the basis of a Department of Defense (DoD) Directive on service fitness standards. They recommended the use of body fat assessments to distinguish lean and fat soldiers, with upper limits for young men and women of 20% and 30% body fat. The panel arrived at these values based on the average body fat of fit young men and women (15% and 25%, respectively) and a five-point statistical window above these means to encompass the majority of healthy, fit individuals. This fit, young male value of 20% body fat was further verified against satisfactory aerobic fitness level representing the mean for a large group of male soldiers, and 20% served as the anchor point for later age- and sex-specific body fat standards (Friedl 2012). These were remarkably prescient recommendations that have stood the test of time and verified with new data.

The DoD Directive that was issued as a result of the recommendations established DoD-wide goals but did not prescribe specific percent body fat thresholds for action. The directive simply stated that "the DoD goal is 20% body fat for males and 26% for females," and that "services are authorized to set more stringent standards." The panel consensus of 30% body fat as the most stringent standard for young women had been adjusted down by the authors of the DoD Directive to a lower 26% body fat goal. This was a reflection of the prevailing perception that service women were simply men with too much fat and, that by legislating lower fat levels, their physical performance might move closer to that of men. In fact, initial considerations by the Army had been for a single 25% body fat standard regardless of sex (Johnson 1997). A later update to the DoD Directive set upper limits of body fat standards at 26% and 36% body fat for men and women (U.S. Department of Defense 1995a,b). The DoD Instruction was amended to provide an acceptable range for the services to choose from that included 26%–36% body fat for women and 18%–26% body fat for men (U.S. Department of Defense 2002). These values reflected the Marine Corps standards at the lower

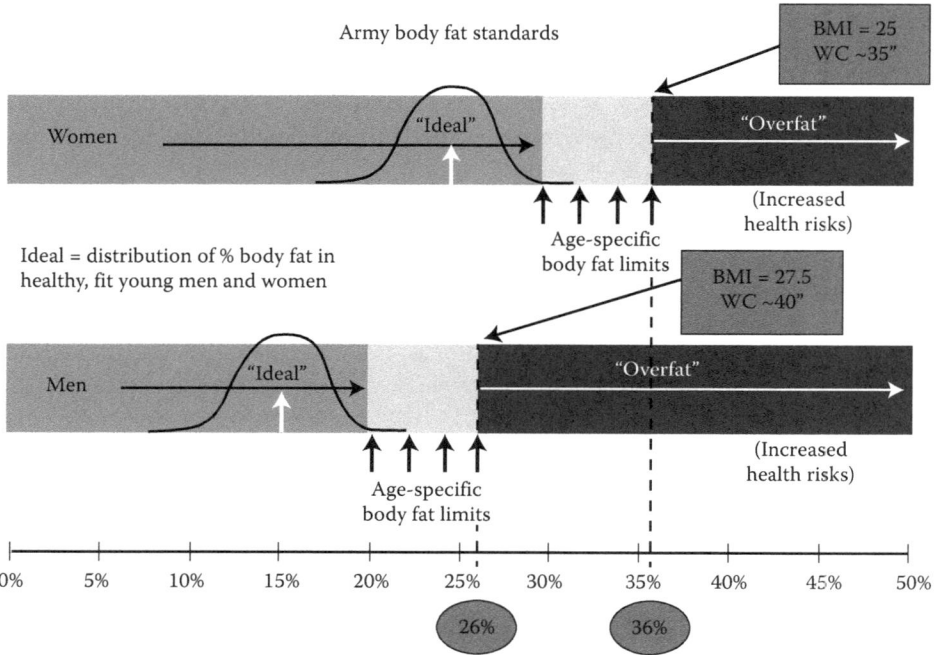

FIGURE 13.1 Basis for the DoD body fat limits was anchored in the limit set for young men, with a 15% body fat average for fit young men and an upper limit set at 20% body fat. A comparable alignment for women with 25% body fat average for fit young women provided a fixed sex difference of 10%. To accommodate age-related increases in relative body fat, the Army set an upper limit of 26% and 36% body fat for men and women over age 40, directly related to health risk thresholds. Incremental age allowances between the least and most stringent standards were random gradations.

end (18% and 26% body fat) and the over-age-40 health-based thresholds used by the Army at the upper end (26% and 36% body fat) (Figure 13.1).

13.3 DEVELOPMENT OF SERVICE-SPECIFIC ANTHROPOMETRIC EQUATIONS

13.3.1 THE 1980 REVIEW OF FITNESS IN THE SERVICES

All of the services were encouraged to follow the model of the Marine Corps with a practical circumference-based body fat measurement technique. The DoD Directive that resulted from the panel recommendations mandated that each of the services would set body fat standards according to their requirements and that "height to weight tables may be used by all Military Services as the first line screening technique until validated body composition measurement techniques are in place service wide" (U.S. Department of Defense 1981a,b). Later, this was changed to state that body fat standards would be based on a "circumference measurement technique" and that "this technique must have a reliability coefficient of 0.85 or greater compared to hydrostatic weighing" (U.S. Department of Defense 1987). In recommendations to the services, the DoD Directive stated that services should conduct validation analyses against measures of military performance and that "it is possible that standards should be different for males and females." These efforts led to the establishment of body fat standards that have been in force for the military services for nearly 30 years. The DoD Directive specified that weight-for-height tables could be useful first level screening tools but were not to be used as the standard. Individuals exceeding service weight tables would then be assessed for body fat to determine if they met standards. These military standards specifically target overweight individuals who are determined to be overfat by the circumference-based body fat equations (Figure 13.2).

Each of the four military services sought to establish their own methods for body fat estimation, using the argument that the individual makeup of each of the services differed and might require different equations (Table 13.1). In retrospect, this is nonsensical if the goal was to produce generalizable methods of body fat estimation that would be free of important bias on the basis of race/ethnicity or any other physical characteristic. It took nearly 20 years for the DoD to resolve the methodological differences that were originally permitted. In the 2002 revision of the DoD Instruction, the methods were finally consolidated into a single set of male and female equations representing the best circumference-based method. This was the one developed for the Navy by James Hodgdon at the Naval Health Research Center. The instruction acknowledged that "circumference methods are inextricably linked to the military body fat standards" and stated that "no alternative method of body fat assessment will be allowed" (U.S. Department of Defense 2002). This consolidation was precipitated by a U.S. Government Accountability Office (GAO) review of the

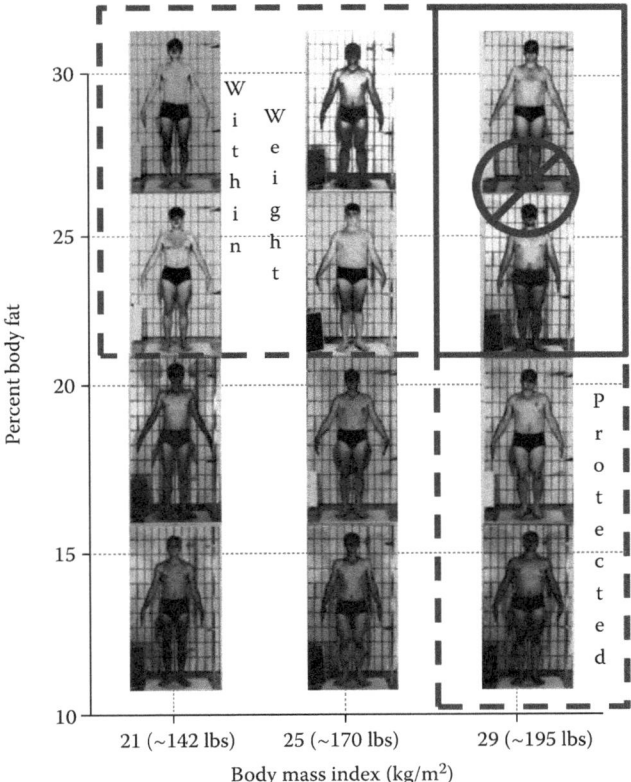

FIGURE 13.2 The "twelve zorros" represent a sample of young (~18–20-year-old) soldiers of similar height approximately 69" selected from the 1984-5 Army Body Composition Study database to illustrate a range of BMI (retention weight = 25 kg/m²; accession weight = 29 kg/m²) and % body fat, based on underwater weighing (derived from Friedl et al. 1989). The four soldiers in the column on the right would be measured for body fat because they exceed BMI 25 kg/m² and the two overfat soldiers at the top of the column would be targeted for weight loss, while the other two would be protected as large but not excessively fat. The other four young soldiers exceeding body fat standards (upper left) would not usually be identified, but this group represents a very small proportion of "within weight but overfat" soldiers. The underweight but 30% body fat soldier in the upper left is particularly rare. The same soldiers in Class A uniforms are more difficult to distinguish by visual inspection.

TABLE 13.1

Circumference-Based Equations Originally Developed for Each of the Military Services

Men

Army (Vogel et al. 1988; modified to equation actually used)

%body fat = 76.5 × Log10 (abdomen II − neck)−68.7 × Log10 (height) + 43.7

Navy (Hodgdon and Beckett 1984a)

Density = −0.191 × Log10 (abdomen II − neck) + 0.155 × Log10 (height) + 1.032

Marine Corps (Wright et al. 1980)

%body fat = 0.740 × abdomen II − 1.249 × neck + 40.985

U.S. Air Force (Fuchs et al. 1978)

FFM = 0.018 × flexed biceps + 0.514 × height − 49.67

Women

Army (Vogel et al. 1988)

%body fat = 105.3 × Log10 (weight) − 0.200 × wrist − 0.533 × neck − 1.574 × forearm + 0.173 × hip − 0.515 × height − 35.6

Navy (Hodgdon and Beckett 1984b)

Density = −0.350 × Log10 (abdomen I + hip + neck) + 0.221 × Log10 (height) + 1.296

Marine Corps (Wright et al. 1981)

%body fat = 1.051 × biceps − 1.522 × forearm − 0.879 × neck + 0.326 × abdomen II + 0.597 × thigh + 0.707

Air Force (Brennen 1979)

FFM = 1.619 × forearm + 0.311 × height − 47.76

Note: In a cross validation of the equations, the Navy equations for men and women were superior based on standard error of the estimate, mean difference, and correlation coefficients, compared to the criterion method of hydrostatic weighing (Hodgdon 1992). The DoD equation currently in use is based on the Navy equations and provides %body fat estimates from English units (Hodgdon and Friedl 1999). Circumference measurements and height are in cm; abdomen I is measured in women at the thinnest part of the waist, usually about midway between the edge of the sternum and the umbilicus; abdomen II is measured at the umbilicus; thigh circumference is taken in women at the upper end of the thigh, just below the gluteal fold; FFM = fat-free mass; density is converted with the Siri equation (Siri 1961).

body composition standards of the services, where a 42-year-old female GAO employee was used as a test subject and yielded body fat estimations that ranged from 27% to 40% body fat using the various female-specific equations developed by each of the services (GAO 1998). Individuals were not held to standards of their service based on the equations of another service, but this significant discrepancy in the estimations provided by the various female equations where each service used different measurement sites called into question the validity of any body fat testing.

13.3.2 U.S. Marine Corps: Fitness Standard Leaders

The Marines were the first to implement a set of circumference-based body fat standards. These grew out of a long line of research in the United States and Great Britain, primarily sponsored by the military to find practical anthropometric predictors of density, body fat and lean mass, developed against the criterion method of underwater weighing. Among these pioneers, Jack Wilmore and Albert Behnke concluded that neck and abdominal ("abd2" = abdomen at the level of the navel) circumferences were among the most promising predictive anthropometric variables for body density and for lean mass of healthy young men (Wilmore and Behnke 1969). A subsequent study by Maj. Howell Wright using a large sample of Marines as test subjects provided the first neck–waist circumferences for the Marine Corps (Wright and Wilmore 1974). The same procedures were used with 226 female Marines to derive an equation using neck, biceps, forearm, waist, and thigh circumferences to predict body fat in Marine Corps women (U.S. Department of the Navy 1980; Wright et al. 1980).

Additional attempts with nonlinear relationships failed to improve the equation for overestimate at the low end of body fat and underestimate at the upper end (Wright et al. 1981). This has proven to a common observation with anthropometric predictions, where smaller amounts of intra-abdominal fat are not readily distinguishable by an abdominal circumference measurement, and at the higher levels of body fat, inconsistent fat distribution to other body sites is not assessed by an abdominal circumference measurement. Thus, the circumference equations are well suited to classification of individuals that begin to exceed levels of intra-abdominal fat in the detectable range.

The Marines later adopted the Hodgdon equations developed for the Navy. The Navy equations improved on the original Marine Corps equations with the addition of stature as a variable, eliminating discrimination against tall Marines (Figure 13.3). The original Marine Corps female

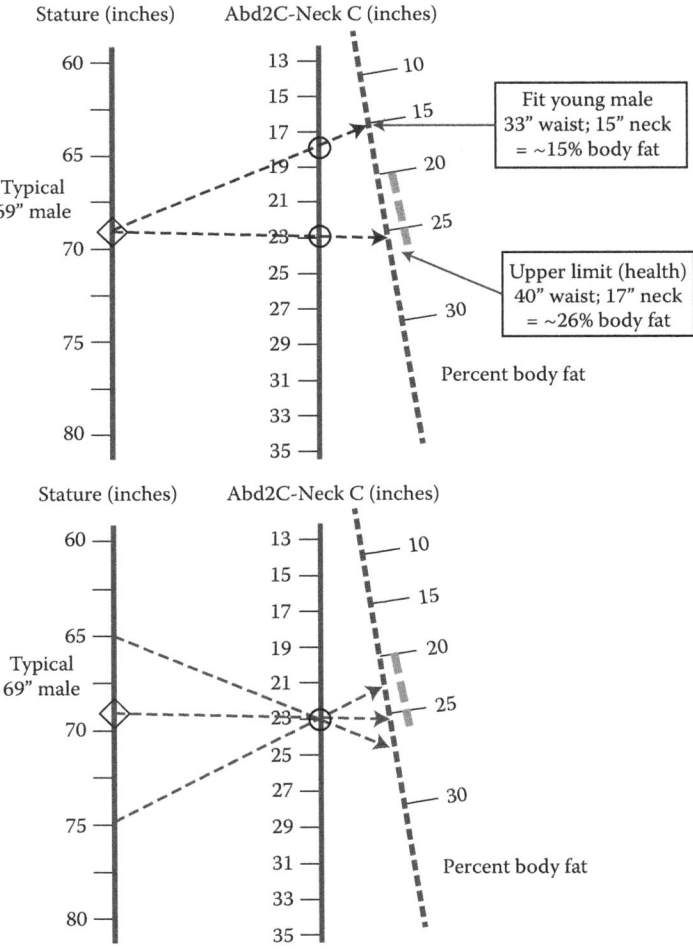

FIGURE 13.3 Military body fat standards rely on equations that focus on abdominal circumference, with adjustments for stature and body size (neck circumference). This nomogram for the DoD male equation illustrates (upper graph) how a typical young recruit might compute and how an older (>age 40) soldier reaching the upper limit for age (26%) might be assessed. The lower graph illustrates the effect of stature on body fat estimates for tall and short soldiers. A fixed waist circumference standard would be biased against taller but leaner soldiers.

equation was substantially simplified, including elimination of the high thigh measurement, which was considered invasive and measured a fat site that is less influenced by exercise and nutrition habits of the individual. The Marine Corps male and female body fat thresholds were set at 18% and 26%, respectively. Until a change in 1998, older Marines were not assessed for body fat.

13.3.3   U.S. AIR FORCE: OVERTHINKING THE PROBLEM

The Air Force was already concerned about obesity even before the 1980 review of fitness in the services after it was determined that many older airmen were within weight-for-height limits but exceeded 23% body fat; 15% body fat was the mean for healthy young airmen (Theis 1975). The Air Force used sophisticated criterion techniques to develop simplified anthropometric estimates of body fat and ultimately adopted a height-corrected flexed biceps circumference as the method for men (Allen 1963; Fuchs et al. 1978). This was based on a sample of 198 Air Force crewmen tested in a series of studies against state-of-the-art methods, including tritium dilution, potassium-40 counting, and the air displacement measurement of density invented by Allen (Fuchs et al. 1978). The goal of this study was to find a practical circumferential method that would include a less difficult measurement site than the abdomen. The flexed bicep was considered to be a more reproducible and reliable measure than the abdominal region, which is susceptible to variations associated with respiration (Fuchs et al. 1978). The equation was developed to predict fat-free mass instead of providing a direct estimate of relative body fat, because this was regarded as an extension of height-weight tables, and fat-free mass correlated with height, while body fat did not (Fuchs et al. 1978). A similar equation using a height-corrected flexed forearm circumference was used for Air Force women. This was based on a sample of 38 women compared to underwater weighing and reported in an unpublished master's thesis (Brennen 1974). The regulation used nomograms to establish a maximum allowable weight based on the upper limits of body fat permitted by the Air Force standards (Air Force Regulation 35-11 1985). The limits were set at 20% and 24% body fat for men and 26% and 30% for women, with body fat allowance increases at age 30.

The Air Force was also the only service that provided base commander discretion in the final determination of actions against an overfat service member, essentially taking the teeth out of the body composition regulation (Air Force Regulation 35-11 1985). Other services required automatic enrollment in a weight management program, and service members risked elimination from military service for failure to meet body fat standards.

More recently, the Air Force Instruction changed to include a waist circumference as part of a composite fitness score that includes physical fitness testing measures. A requested waiver from the prescribed DoD methodology was granted to the Air Force to be allowed to use only an abdominal circumference (measured at the iliac crest) as one component of a weighted fitness score (Department of the Air Force Memorandum 2003). Airmen fail this part of their fitness assessment when they exceed abdominal circumference measurements (at the iliac crest) of 39 in. and 35.5 in. for men and women across all ages (U.S. Department of the Air Force 2013). The basis for the scoring has not been published (GAO 1998).

13.3.4   U.S. NAVY: EQUATIONS THAT ARE JUST RIGHT FOR THE MILITARY

The Navy took a holistic approach to the establishment of fitness standards that carefully considered military performance and appearance outcomes and included fitness test measures. This history has been previously reviewed by James Hodgdon (1992). Part of Hodgdon's objective was to produce the simplest equations with the easiest measurements that would provide reasonably accurate estimations for the weight control standards enforcement. The Wright equations developed for the Marine Corps provided a starting point for reexamination and improvement.

The Navy equations were developed in studies comparing anthropometry to underwater weighing, using active duty Navy men ($n = 602$) and women ($n = 214$) (Hodgdon and Beckett 1984a,b).

The equations were validated with additional samples of men ($n = 100$) and women ($n = 146$) and also later validated on the Army sample collected for the development of the Army equations. The equations have been subsequently retested and validated even against a four-compartment model method (Hodgdon and Friedl 1999). The anthropometric equations developed by the Navy for men and women were later adopted for use by all military services as the single most practical and valid method (Figure 13.3) (U.S. Department of Defense 2004).

In 1999, the Navy relaxed their enforcement of their body fat standards due to recruitment and retention issues. The Navy was eliminating approximately 2000 active duty personnel per year, which represents a relatively large proportion of Navy personnel. For comparison, the Army has nearly twice as many personnel and eliminated a similar absolute number of soldiers (~2000 per year between 1988 and 1999) for failing to meet Army body fat standards; this Army rate decreased precipitously after 1999 during the large personnel deployments in support of Operation Enduring Freedom and Operation Iraqi Freedom (Betty D. Maxfield, personal communication 2009). Military physical standards have always been adjusted according to available manpower and the needs of the military (Wheeler 1965).

In 2015, the Navy unilaterally chose to relax their body fat standards and move to a new standard that had been recommended to them by the Air Force: a waist circumference measure of 39 in. for all men and 35 in. for all women, regardless of age (Friedl 2015; Peterson 2015). The basis for the Navy change was that recruitment was too difficult for the Navy due to the growing prevalence of overfat young men and women in the U.S. population. The DoD Directive will likely be revised to officially endorse this broadening range of service fitness standards.

13.3.5   U.S. Army: Experimental Challenges and Over Fitted Equations

The Army conducted experiments with soldiers to develop their own predictive equations. This was directed by the Deputy Chief of Staff of the Army, Lieutenant General Maxwell Thurman, and managed from the Office of the Surgeon General by Col. James Kirkpatrick. The U.S. Army Research Institute of Environmental Medicine, representing the largest intramural performance physiology laboratory in the federal government, planned a comprehensive test that would also satisfy DoD guidance to conduct validation analyses against measures of military performance (Vogel et al. 1988). This was one of the largest body composition and anthropometry studies ever reported. In addition to the body composition measures, a large number of other variables were collected, including aerobic and strength testing; physical fitness test scores; appearance documented in side, front, and back photographs in uniforms and swimsuits, and detailed questionnaires about health and fitness habits (Fitzgerald et al. 1986). The testing used substantially similar methods employed in the Navy testing, and there was an active collaboration that included swapping final data sets for cross validation of equations. The initial test sample comprised 1194 male and 319 female soldiers obtained primarily from a convenience sample at Fort Hood, Texas, and included a smaller sample of older soldiers from Carlisle Barracks, Pennsylvania.

While the equations were being developed, the Army adopted an interim method using skinfolds and the equations of Durnin and Womersley (Durnin and Womersley 1974; U.S. Department of the Army, 1983a). James Vogel, the Army's chief physiologist who was responsible for Army fitness and body composition standards research, had conducted research at the British Army research lab in Farnborough using skinfold measurements in studies of British Army recruits (Haisman 1970; Vogel and Crowdy 1979). Although the Durnin and Womersley skinfold equations were developed using a homogeneous white Scottish cohort, the relationships between skinfold thicknesses, and body fat derived from the Siri equation (with model assumptions that were appropriate to this population) proved to be highly generalizable in an ethnically more diverse population in the U.S. Army (Durnin and Womersley 1974; Friedl and Vogel 1991). Derivation of skinfold equations from a diverse Army sample would likely not have been as successful because of the assumptions of fat-free mass density, which are not accurate for a sample of black and Hispanic subjects (Friedl and

Vogel 1991). Unfortunately, measurement of skinfold thickness was not a method that could be used efficiently across the Army, and there were 6-month waiting lists for soldiers to be assessed for body fat by the personnel trained in caliper use from the Army Medical Specialist Corps (physical therapists and dietitians) (U.S. Department of the Army, 1983a). The reliable use of skinfold calipers by a large group of individuals with varied experience proved challenging and provided many lessons in the use of a technique that required practiced skill, as well as a standardization and monitoring process (Friedl et al. 1987; Vogel et al. 1988).

The final selection of the Army equations from a family of generated models was further complicated in two ways (U.S. Department of the Army 1986). The equations generated from the sample of women did not achieve the required correlation coefficient of 0.80, and the equation that was finally adopted was one derived only from the subsample of white women (Vogel et al. 1988). At least part of the rationale for using this subsample of women was the observation that a very high proportion of black soldiers were nonswimmers and had more difficulty performing the maneuvers required for underwater weighing. The most extreme cases of individuals who could not perform the underwater weighing test included 10% of the white female sample and 23% of the black female sample (Vogel et al. 1988). The female equation adopted by the Army was also unnecessarily complex, requiring four circumference measurements including neck, abd1, forearm, and wrist; height and weight were also both factors in the equation. The inclusion of the weight factor may make this a better predictor of body composition change, as noted in a sample of 150 women before and after basic training (compared to dual x-ray absorptiometry [DXA]), but ultimately the equation for women originally adopted by the Army was not as accurate as the simpler Navy equation (Hodgdon 1999; Friedl et al. 2001).

Another problem that was not generally appreciated at the time was the interpretation of body fat from body density with populations that violated the assumptions of the Siri equation, developed from white males. In the Army Body Composition Study, black men and women represented 28% and 38% of the sample, with an additional approximately 10% representation by Hispanic soldiers. This is notable because the assumptions of the Siri equation for a fat-free mass density of 1.1 do not hold up for black and Hispanic subjects and would tend to produce underestimates of the percent body fat in these subjects. Appropriate adjustments would have to be made with direct measurement of bone mineral content in each subject, but this technique was not readily available at the time of these studies.

Another problem with the equations was a reported error in the male equation that was implemented for use by the Army. The mistake resulted in an Army body fat calculation that produced an underestimate of 3.15% body fat relative to the intended equation (Vogel et al. 1988). However, this error was never resolved and the "incorrect" equation adopted by the Army was left in place without correction as it produced results that closely matched other measurement techniques, including the Navy equation (K. E. Friedl, unpublished 1989; Friedl and Vogel 1997). Both of the Army equations (male and female) were replaced by the Navy equations in 2004 (U.S. Department of the Army 2006; Bathalon et al. 2006).

The Army screening weights, based on body mass index (BMI) relationships, were adjusted to more appropriately target individuals likely to exceed the fat standards. The most important change was the acknowledgement that a BMI of 25 kg/m^2 was too stringent for males and would misclassify many soldiers, with at least half of all Army males exceeding this weight but not carrying excessive fat (Leu and Friedl 2002; Bathalon et al. 2006). The Army (and DoD) upper limit for weight screening was pushed up to 27.5 kg/m^2 for males to accommodate this difference in the soldier population compared to their civilian peers (Bathalon et al. 2006). This was driven in part by commanders' complaints that too many lean soldiers were being singled out for body fat assessment by the weight tables. The Army culture of physical fitness and self-selection factors that favor more physically oriented recruits explains the difference in adiposity–BMI relationships for soldiers compared to their civilian peers. For women, the tables were pushed out to 26 kg/m^2 simply to maintain a semblance of symmetry in the Army regulation. Men were appropriately screened for increasing body fat standards across four age groups by tables that ranged from 25 to 27.5 kg/m^2, while women were all properly screened for increasing body fat standards across the same four age groups by a single 25 kg/m² cutoff. The Army Surgeon General at the time could not contemplate a set of screening tables that was asymmetrical between men and women.

In 1982, General Thurman had proposed a standard of 24% and 32% for men and women, with no testing of personnel after age 40. Ultimately, the Army adopted age-related body fat standards that ranged between the standards appropriate for healthy, fit, young men and women (the most stringent standards) and the more liberal, health-based standards for over-age-40 men and women. This was spread across four separate age groups so that adjustments were graduated and did not make a sudden 6% body fat jump in a single birthday (Figure 13.1). In these categories, the Army made an unconventional break at age 27 instead of a more typical decade-based category of age 30. This age represented a functional change in soldier jobs to increased supervisory positions, typically the increase in rank from Sergeant to Staff Sergeant and Lieutenant to Captain.

Adjustments to the body fat standards provided a 2% increase in the threshold levels for women. This was actually a correction that returned to the original recommendation of the 1980 panel that the strictest body fat standard for men and women should be 20% and 30% body fat, respectively. The original DoD Directive reduced the desired goal from 30% to 26% for body fat in women. The Army had split the difference and adopted body fat standards of 20% and 28% as the most stringent (under age 21) standards (U.S. Department of the Army 1983b). This seemingly trivial remaining difference of 2% for women (28% instead of 30%) had a very significant impact on a large number of female soldiers because the distribution of women by percent body fat was much more kurtotic than the very broad distribution for men (~5% to over 30% body fat) (Friedl et al. 1989). A correction to these body fat standards (+2% body fat at each of the four age groups) was approved after a presentation to the Deputy Chief of Staff for Personnel (Lt. Gen. William Reno). This presentation included a photograph of a young, elite female distance runner at the U.S. Military Academy, who was obviously lean yet was on a fasting diet in order to meet body fat standards. The cadet standards at the time were set 2% lower than the Army standards in order to ensure that new officers did not exceed Army standards as new leaders, that is, 26%. The 2% increase provided relief to a large number of Army women previously held to a physiologically inappropriate standard (Friedl et al. 1989).

A greater difficulty came in the acceptance of a shift for the upper limit for older female soldiers, from 34% to 36% body fat. It was bad enough that 30% body fat, considered in male terms, was already noted to be "obese." This difficulty in appreciating human sexual dimorphism was also managed by personal demonstration, using a trim and fit female officer on Reno's staff, known as a model of daily fitness training habits. With her permission at the briefing, the General was shown her body fat estimated by six different methods, including underwater weighing, bioelectrical impedance analysis (BIA), skinfold thicknesses, female circumference equation, DXA, and total body water (TBW). In a stroke of luck, these six estimates had turned out to be unusually consistent, ranging between 30% and 31% body fat, with the anthropometric methods slightly lower. Reno approved the increase in female body fat limits across all age groups on the spot (this female staff officer later became the Army Surgeon General).

13.4 BASIS FOR MILITARY BODY FAT STANDARDS

13.4.1 MILITARY GOALS

The 1980 expert review emphasized three key purposes of DoD body fat standards: (1) to ensure suitable military appearance, with the pot belly as a focus; (2) to ensure physical readiness; and (3) to promote health of the force (U.S. Department of Defenses 1981b). The panel agreed that the most stringent thresholds would be associated with appearance and the most liberal with long-term health considerations. The emphasis on any of these goals and the actual body fat standards were to be set according to service requirements and, indeed, each service took a different approach.

What is clear is that the abdominal circumference method is an inextricable part of the standard because of the convergence on abdominal fat on the three intended goals and as the primary anthropometric predictor of body fat. There are many different anthropometric methods to estimate body fat, but a crucial point was that the abdominal circumference (and hip circumference, for the assessment of women) also targets the site(s) that are changeable with exercise and diet. Norwegian and U.S. Ranger trainees provide an extreme example of this, where 8 weeks of semi-starvation further reduced the abdominal circumference in fit, young men by an average 10 cm (Friedl et al. 1994). Fat biopsies from three sites in the Norwegian model of 7 days of food deprivation during training demonstrated substantial reduction of lipids stored in adipocytes from the abdomen and gluteal regions but not from the thigh (Rognum et al. 1982). Fat deposited in locations other than the abdomen and hips, such as upper back and arms, thighs, etc., is less influenced by exercise and diet and more influenced by genetics and hormones (Friedl 2012). Alternate methods that provide more accurate total body fat measurements are irrelevant to the purposes of the military standards. In fact, this measurement of fat in other locations simply makes the standard less appropriate to military readiness objectives and makes the method less generalizable and unfair for some subsets of service members. Any further refinement of the Hodgdon equations should be developed against the appropriate gold standard of fat assessment that is relevant to military objectives; this would be an abdominal computed tomography scan (Kvist et al. 1988; Després et al. 1991; Matsuzawa et al. 1992; Camhi et al. 2011).

13.4.2 Military Appearance

An important aspect of any military force is to appear to be a formidable and even intimidating opponent. The appearance of a strong military force is a deterrent to aggression. The Army preferentially selects larger imposing members. For example, military police were previously selected on the basis of height, with a minimum height requirement of 5 ft 9 in (men) and 5 ft 4 in (women) set on the basis of the average height of the population for psychological advantage (Gordon and Friedl 1994). This interpretation of dominant and assertive leaders based on physical features permeates society even at a subconscious level. For example, tall men have an advantage in job advancement, where the tallest members of the West Point class of 1950 reached the highest ranks (Mazur et al. 1984).

Body fat and military bearing was specifically investigated in the Army Body Composition Study. Soldiers in the study were photographed in three views (front, side, and rear) in anthropometric poses wearing swimsuits, and this was repeated in Class A (formal) uniforms (Figure 13.2 is derived from this photographic data set) (Fitzgerald et al. 1986). An experienced group of military raters estimated percent body fat in male and female soldiers in swimsuits with a correlation of 0.78 (men) and 0.72 (women) compared to percent body fat by hydrostatic weight (Hodgdon et al. 1990). Military appearance ratings had lower correlations with percent body fat for soldiers in swimsuits and substantially lower correlations for soldiers in properly fitted Class A uniforms. For both men and women, disproportionately large abdominal circumferences (and small wrist circumferences) were key distinguishing factors in the rating of poor military appearance, in and out of uniform (Friedl 2004). It was also remarkable that the break points where average ratings fell from "good" to "fair/poor" coincided with each of the age-specific body fat thresholds for men (i.e., at 20%, 22%, 24% body fat for men aged <21, 21–27, and 27–39, respectively) and for women (i.e., 30%, 32% body fat for women aged <21, 21–27, respectively). Inadequate sample sizes for higher fat soldiers in the older age categories prevented a more complete analysis (Friedl, unpublished observations 1989). This suggests that a visual calibration has occurred between military appearance expectations and current age-related limits of body fat. Excess fat is associated with poorer ratings of military appearance, and abdominal fat is the main offender of military appearance in overweight or over fat soldiers.

13.4.3 Performance

Percent body fat is not a good predictor of physical performance (Marriott and Grumstrup-Scott 1992). Associations between adiposity and some aspects of physical performance can be demonstrated with inclusion of lean and fat extremes, but specific relationships are difficult to demonstrate within the range of fatness for most soldiers.

In the Army Body Composition Study, strength performance was measured with an incremental dynamic lift device (a machine version of a clean) and aerobic performance was measured with a treadmill-based maximal aerobic test. There was no relationship between adiposity and either lift or aerobic capacity but there were strong correlations with fat-free mass for both these aspects of physical performance (Vogel and Friedl 1992; Friedl 2004). Aerobic performance (expressed per kg body weight) and strength performance from this same dataset demonstrated opposite relationships with BMI (Harman and Frykman 1992). Some of the strongest soldiers are the biggest (and sometimes fattest), and Olympic power lifters tend to be relatively fat compared to athletes in many other specialties; there may even be an intra-abdominal fat advantage during the Valsalva maneuver used to complete a clean (Harman et al. 1989). In aerobic performance, every additional amount of fat counts as extra weight that must be moved through space; this provides a disadvantage, especially in distance running, where the thinnest, lightest phenotype benefits in terms of energy cost and thermoregulation (Marriott and Grumstrup-Scott 1992).

As physical fitness performance and percent body fat are not directly related, there have been several proposals to link physical fitness scores to a sliding scale for a minority of soldiers who exceed their body fat standards (Leu and Friedl 2002).

Thermoregulatory advantages and disadvantages of increased body fat have been examined and modeled, with smaller and leaner men and women predicted to have lower core temperatures during work in the heat (Yokota et al. 2008, 2012).

13.4.4 Health

Morbid obesity, generally defined as BMI >30 kg/m^2, has strong associations with increased musculoskeletal disease, such as arthritis and degenerative joint disease, presumably through mechanical strains produced by the increased mass. A relationship to musculoskeletal injury at both the lowest and highest levels of BMI has been well described in soldiers by retired Col. Bruce Jones (Jones et al. 1992). He also reported increased rates of injury for the fattest men and the leanest women. There are also strong associations of excess weight and particular patterns of fat distribution with metabolic diseases, such as type 2 diabetes (Krotkiewski et al. 1983; Larsson et al. 1984; Ohlson et al. 1985). This was documented by Jean Vague (1956) and many others since then. These health risk associations of excess weight and abdominal fat distribution have been quantified in various national health goals over the past 30 years (Kuczmarski and Flegal 2000). At the time of the 1980 expert panel on fitness in the services, the Dietary Guidelines were just being issued with new BMI guidance to stay below approximately 25 kg/m^2. This was followed in 1985 by the National Institutes of Health (NIH) Consensus Development Panel recommendations for an upper desirable limit at the 85th percentile of the National Health and Nutritional Examination Survey (NHANES) data (i.e., BMI 27.8 and 27.3 for men and women, respectively). In 1998, the National Heart, Lung, and Blood Institute (NHLBI) Expert Panel published their recommendations for an upper limit of 25 kg/m^2, along with new abdominal circumference guidelines of 40 and 35 in for men and women. The original DoD panel discussion revolved around the original 25 kg/m^2 recommendation; by the time of the 1998 NHLBI guidelines, the Army standards were already converging on upper limits of body fat at 26% and 36% body fat for men and women that approximate the NHLBI abdominal circumference thresholds of 40 and 35 in (Figures 13.1 and 13.3). These are the most liberal body fat standards that are allowed, applied to soldiers age 40 and over. Thus, initial standards are more stringent, with the expectation that age-related body fat accretion will occur but with nobody permitted to exceed the health-related threshold.

More recent data suggest that the weight thresholds at 25 kg/m^2 were overly stringent health recommendations. In a careful analysis of nationally representative data from the NHANES surveys, Katherine Flegal demonstrated that relative risks for mortality are no different or even slightly less in the weight range of 25–30 kg/m^2 compared to the group in the original NHLBI-defined "healthy" weights below BMI 25 kg/m^2 (actually 18.5–25 kg/m^2). In this USARIEM-funded study, mortality risk only increased above BMI 30 kg/m^2 (Flegal et al. 2005). These data supported the elevation of the upper limit of the DoD weight screen for men from 25 to 27.5 kg/m^2. Half of the male soldier population exceeds 25 kg/m^2 and, with greater variability in the fat-free mass in men compared to women, many of these are not high fat or unhealthy (Friedl and Vogel 1997). National and international definitions now generally classify BMI >30 as obese and are less prescriptive about weights below this level (Kuczmarski and Flegal 2000).

The associations between health consequences and abdominal fat were already well known in 1980 at the time of the review of fitness in the services. This was even recognized in the 1930s, when the insurance industry concluded that a greater than 2-in. excess abdominal circumference compared to an expanded chest circumference was a significant marker of morbidity and mortality (Metropolitan Life Insurance Company 1937) and in a study of the "cardiac" type, based on annual physical records over 20-year periods in Army officers (Reed and Love 1932). Jean Vague popularized the importance of "male type" abdominal fat distribution in the 1950s (Vague 1956), and this began a wide range of abdominal measurements and indices, such as the waist-to-hip ratio, abdominal thickness, and measurements corrected for stature, such as a waist/height index.

In an analysis of NHANES data, NHLBI upper limit goals for Americans for waist circumference (40 and 35 in for men and women, respectively) were shown to be too liberal for health risk associations, with lower levels associated with diminishing levels of cardiovascular health risk markers (serum lipids and high blood pressure) in otherwise healthy individuals (Flegal 2007). Healthy individuals in this NHANES sample had median waist circumferences of approximately 35 in. (men) and approximately 31 in. (women). This is closer to the national standards of Japan implemented in 2008 in the "Metabo Law," which mandates annual waist circumference measurements for all men and women between the ages of 40 and 74 (44% of the population of Japan). Individuals exceeding upper limits established by the Japanese Diabetes Society (85 cm or 33.5 in. for men; 90 cm or 35.4 in. for women) must enroll in weight management programs and employers are penalized by poor compliance rates. This law is intended to prevent the rise of obesity and obesity-related illnesses, such as type 2 diabetes.

13.5 ARMY EXPERIENCE WITH 30 YEARS OF BODY FAT STANDARDS

13.5.1 Effect of the Standards

Although there is still no good longitudinal data on body composition in the military, several effects of the enforced body fat standards can be demonstrated. Senior noncommissioned officers attending the U.S. Army Sergeant Major Academy were tested for body fat (regardless of their weight status) as part of a health risk factors study; the upper limit for body fat for these older career soldiers was 26%. There was a neat linear correlation between the Army circumference-based method body fat and DXA body fat up to 26% body fat, and then there was a flat line relationship above 26%, where total body fat measured by DXA continued to increase beyond 30% (Friedl 2004). These data demonstrate retention of senior soldiers who have been successful in maintaining a trim waist girth, even if they carry more fat elsewhere on the body, such as typical subcutaneous distributions across the back and extremities. Older soldiers are also substantially leaner than their civilian peers. Cross-sectional surveys of soldier populations demonstrate that, especially at the upper age range typically involving career soldiers, their body fat does not exceed the median value for older Americans (i.e., older soldiers fall in the lower half of the distribution of the U.S. population for body fat) (Leu and Friedl 2002; Bathalon et al. 2006). A third line of evidence that the standards have an impact on weight gain restraint is the large weight gain of soldier veterans within the first few years of retirement, catching up to or even exceeding obesity in the civilian population (Littman et al. 2013). This is actually a special health risk problem for veterans that indicates the need to establish health and fitness habits in soldiers that will be sustainable after retirement, as part of the "soldier for life" concept. A fourth line of evidence for standards-motivated changes is the recurrent observation from commanders that increasingly fewer soldiers assessed as overweight are actually overfat; this represents an enrichment of large, lean individuals in the population, where overfat soldiers have lost weight or have been eliminated. Without a longitudinal fitness database, the relative contribution of successful weight management versus elimination of soldiers (from discharges for failure to meet standards, bars to reenlistment, or simply failure to retain soldiers because of the standards) cannot be determined. At the start of the program, in an analysis of records at Fort Lewis, at least half of all soldiers appeared to be successful in coming off the weight control program (Friedl et al. 1987). In three major attempts to establish comprehensive fitness databases, it was apparent that there are many challenges to body fat standards tracking and enforcement, including an Army post-wide effort with active duty soldiers, a geographically distributed Army reserve unit, and an entire state Army National Guard unit (Williamson et al. 2009; Newton et al. 2011; Stewart et al. 2011).

13.5.2 IMPLEMENTATION ISSUES

The method of body fat assessment has been challenged on a regular basis and in a periodic cycle of institutional amnesia. One typical complaint has been that soldiers with large necks can "beat the tape" and that soldiers are effectively increasing their neck size with neck exercises (e.g., Army Inspector General 1989). The hypertrophy of the male neck was tested in an Army-funded study at the Naval Health Research Center. In a 12 week supervised neck strength training program, 10 men increased neck circumference from 38.8 to 40.2 cm, but the change and comparison with the control group was not significant (Taylor et al. 2006). Although neck hypertrophy was difficult to demonstrate, isometric and dynamic strength increased significantly, even by 4 weeks; this was likely due to neural mechanisms in addition to hypertrophy of very specific pairs of muscles, as demonstrated in previous studies (Conley et al. 1997). Even assuming soldiers could produce a consistent training effect that increased neck circumference by 0.5 in., this would only provide a reduction in the body fat prediction of about 1 body fat unit. The individuals would also have benefitted from spending some extra time engaged in physical training, a key goal of the body fat standards.

Ultimately, the main complaints center on suspicion that a 50 cent tape measure could not possibly produce results as meaningful as an expensive, technologically sophisticated method such as DXA, BIA, or TBW, leading to one suggestion that the Army purchase $2000 tape measures to increase acceptability of the technique. This issue is raised with regularity, especially every time leaders at the Army War College are exposed to another body fat testing methodology as part of their health and wellness education (e.g., bioelectrical impedance, body volume/air displacement plethysmography).

Procedural issues, such as the use of a tension tape for circumference measurements, are periodically raised. The variability in tissue compressibility between individuals increases the variability in the measurements compared to a simple instruction to pull the tape snugly around the person, flat against the skin, and without creating an indentation. It is difficult to ensure standardized tension on these devices, and the springs stretch with continued use. Seemingly trivial methodological issues gain huge importance when the method is required to be applied fairly across a diverse group of hundreds of thousands of individuals and where careers are on the line.

With minimum training, the precision of the measurement technique is 1% body fat for repeated measures and measures between observers following the instructions in the regulation. The original worksheet for body fat calculation in the Army regulation carried body fat measurements out to two decimal places, implying an impossible level of precision in the method. Humans vary in body water content by 2% body weight without even triggering thirst mechanisms, and 1% body fat variability is an easily normal biological variation; thus, no values should be expressed with greater significance than rounding down to the nearest integer.

It is doubtful that there has ever been a waiver request submitted for a soldier assessed as overfat where there was disagreement that the soldier could indeed benefit from some diet and exercise modification. The estimates from anthropometric equations err on the side of soldiers who are in the zone above the body fat limits by underestimating total body fat (Figure 13.4). Questions periodically raised by fit lean soldiers at the other end of the spectrum question the validity of military equations that overestimate their body fat. This implies that it may misclassify everyone; however, these soldiers, who are below their fat limits, should not be at risk (Figure 13.4). When overfat soldiers are tested by alternate methods, such as density-based methods (e.g., volume displacement), body water-based methods (e.g., BIA, water dilution), and DXA, they generally obtain even higher values, if significant amounts of fat are also distributed to sites other than the abdominal/hip region that is targeted by the military standards. Density-based assessments produce incorrectly low body fat estimations if the assumptions of the Siri equation are not valid for the fat-free mass density (i.e., the fat-free body mass [FFM] density exceeds 1.100 g/cm^3) (Siri 1961). This is a typical problem for many black and Hispanic soldiers and it can even produce nonsensical negative body fat estimations for the leanest individuals (unpublished data on Army champion body builder 1985).

Some soldiers at or above their fat standard still have excellent performance on their physical fitness test, and it has been suggested that the standards could be linked with a sliding scale for some slightly overfat soldiers (Leu and Friedl 2002). This concept was briefed to the Army DCSPER, Lieutenant General Timothy Maude, who was considering it but was concerned about adding complexity to the Army standards. General Maude was killed in the Pentagon in September 2001 before a final decision was made, and the issue has not been revisited.

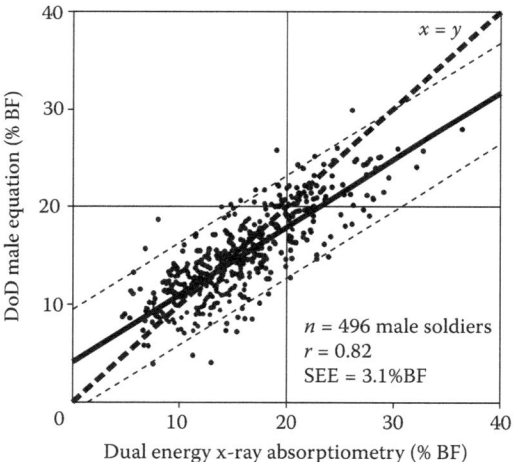

FIGURE 13.4 Scatterplot of a sample of male soldiers measured for body fat using the DoD equation and by dual energy x-ray absorptiometry (DXA). The circumference-based equations cannot distinguish modest differences in intra-abdominal fat at the lower end, overestimating body fat in the leanest individuals. These regionally based equations also cannot detect fat distributed to other body sites and underestimate body fat in the fattest individuals. The same trends are observed for the DoD equation for women. This gives service members the benefit of doubt in their assessment for compliance with fat standards. (Adapted from Friedl, K. E. and J. A. Vogel. 1997. *Mil Med* 162:194–200.)

13.6 EARLIER MILITARY CONTRIBUTIONS TO THE SCIENCE OF BODY COMPOSITION ASSESSMENT

The military has been a pace setter in body composition studies and development of methodologies that have been vital to modern nutrition research. With these breakthrough advances, it is ironic that the military is such a poor environment for sustaining institutional knowledge that could guide continuous improvement instead of experiencing cycles of reinvention. The U.S. Navy had specific problems in diving medicine that required new methods in body fat composition analysis to measure sequestered nitrogen and study its contribution to decompression sickness. Modern day body composition tools emerged from these programs. Capt. Alfred Behnke and his dive researchers evolved underwater weighing to estimate the fat compartment and Cdr. Nello Pace developed the body water dilutional techniques as another approach (Behnke et al. 1942; Pace and Rathbun 1945). A watershed meeting at Natick Army Labs in 1959 produced recommendations for standardization of body composition techniques, including two- and three-compartment models using underwater weighing and body water determination (Brozek and Henschel 1961). Early concepts of roentgenographic analyses that included imaging bone (Garn 1957; Brozek et al. 1958) preceded the DXA techniques that emerged from specific bone density measurement needs in endocrinology. Later efforts provided the foundation for air displacement plethysmography methods (Allen 1963); four-compartment model estimates, including estimated bone content (Allen et al. 1959); and methods specifically estimating total nitrogen and muscle mass components, such as potassium-40 in soldiers at Fort Carson, Colorado (Krzywicki and Chinn 1967). More recent studies have involved multicenter trials on bioelectrical impedance validation (Hodgdon and Fitzgerald 1987; Segal et al. 1988) and four-compartment model studies (Friedl et al. 1992; Sun et al. 2003). Other specific components of body composition have been charted by Army-sponsored research, notably the detailed bone composition and structure studies in military trainees (Jepsen et al. 2011). The research on semi-starvation, commissioned by the Office of the Army Surgeon General, to understand refeeding of returning prisoners of war at the end of World War II is an example of some of the seminal work related to body composition research in the DoD (Keys et al. 1950). These have been important contributions to the field that came out of research to meet national security needs.

13.7 CONCLUSION AND PERSPECTIVES

The U.S. military stands out from other armies in the world with a weight control policy that enforces an abdominal circumference-based body fat standard. The main parallel to this attempt to prevent the "inching" up of population waist girths is the 2008 "Metabo Law" in Japan that enforces an absolute waist circumference limit for the older population. The military standards were put in place in the 1980s to ensure readiness of service members to perform their mission anywhere anytime. The standards apply to all active duty military members and are intended to reinforce regular physical activity and good nutrition habits, which in turn serves three key goals: (1) promoting physical and mental optimization (performance); (2) reducing health consequences in older soldiers (health); and (3) ensuring that the force appears to be formidably fit and capable (appearance). The anthropometric method of fat estimation is inextricably linked to the goals of the military; thus, the method is the standard. The military equations are essentially corrected abdominal circumferences that have been calibrated to body fat. This abdominal measure provides the single most important predictor of adiposity in men and, when combined with hip circumference, is also the strongest predictor of adiposity in women, and there is a convergence on this abdominal site as the key marker of military weight control goals for military appearance, modifiable exercise and nutrition habits, and long-term health outcomes.

ACKNOWLEDGMENTS

This work was prepared by the author as a paid Fellow in the Knowledge Preservation Program, Oak Ridge Institute for Research and Education, funded by the Biophysics and Biomedical Modeling Division, U.S. Army Research Institute of Environmental Medicine. The editing assistance of Ms. Mallory E. Roussel is gratefully acknowledged. The opinions and assertions in this chapter are solely those of the author and do not necessarily represent any official view or position of the Department of the Army.

REFERENCES

Allen, T. H. 1963. Measurement of body fat: A quantitative method suited for use by aviation medical officers. *Aerosp Med* 34:907–9.

Allen, T. H., H. J. Krzywicki, and J. E. Roberts. 1959. Density, fat, water and solids in freshly isolated tissues. *J Appl Physiol* 14:1005–8.

Army Inspector General. Special Inspection of Management of Personnel Readiness. Memorandum from Army Inspector General to Office of the Deputy Chief of Staff for Personnel. Washington, DC, July 14, 1989.

Bathalon, G. P., S. M. McGraw, M. A. Sharp, D. A. Williamson, A. J. Young, and K. E. Friedl. 2006. The effect of proposed improvements to the Army Weight Control Program on female soldiers. *Mil Med* 171:800–5.

Behnke, A. R., B. G. Feen, and W. C. Welham. 1942. The specific gravity of healthy men: Body weight divided by volume as an index of obesity. *J Am Med Assoc* 118:495–8.

Benedict, F. G., H. W. Goodall, J. E. Ash, H. S. Langfeld, A. I. Kendall, and H. L. Higgins. 1915. *A Study of Prolonged Fasting (No. 203)*, 12. Washington, DC: Carnegie Institution for Science.

Brennen, E. H. 1974. Development of a binomial involving anthropometric measurements for predicting lean mass in young women. *Master of Science Thesis*, Incarnate Word College, San Antonio, Texas.

Brozek, J. and A. Henschel. 1961 (eds.). *Conference on Techniques for Measuring Body Composition (1959: Natick, Mass.)*. Washington, DC: National Academy of Sciences.

Brozek, J., H. Mori, and A. Keys. 1958. Estimation of total body fat from roentgenograms. *Science* 128:901–3.

Camhi, S. M., G. A. Bray, C. Bouchard et al. 2011. The relationship of waist circumference and BMI to visceral, subcutaneous, and total body fat: Sex and race differences. *Obesity* 19:402–8.

Committee on Nutritional Research, Institute of Medicine. 1992. In *Body Composition and Physical Performance: Applications for the Military Services*, eds. B. M. Marriott and J. Grumstrup-Scott. Washington, DC: National Academies Press, 356 pp.

Conley, M. S., M. H. Stone, M. Nimmons, and G. A. Dudley. 1997. Specificity of resistance training responses in neck muscle size and strength. *Eur J Appl Physiol Occup Physiol* 75:443–8.

U.S. Department of the Navy. 1980. *Weight Control and Military Appearance*. Marine Corps Order 6100.10. Washington, DC: Headquarters United States Marine Corps, October 23.

Després, J. P., D. Prud'homme, M. C. Pouliot, A. Tremblay, and C. Bouchard. 1991. Estimation of deep abdominal adipose-tissue accumulation from simple anthropometric measurements in men. *Am J Clin Nutr* 54:471–7.

Durnin, J. V. G. A. and J. Womersley. 1974. Body fat assessed from total body density and its estimation from skinfold thickness: Measurements on 481 men and women aged from 16 to 72 years. *Br J Nutr* 32:77–97.

Fitzgerald, P. I., J. A. Vogel, W. L. Daniels et al. 1986. *The body composition project: A summary report and descriptive data*. Technical Report T5-87, AD A177-679. Natick, Massachusetts: U.S. Army Research Institute of Environmental Medicine.

Flegal, K. M. 2007. Waist circumference of healthy men and women in the United States. *Int J Obes* 31:1134–9.

Flegal, K. M., B. I. Graubard, D. F. Williamson, and M. H. Gail. 2005. Excess deaths associated with underweight, overweight, and obesity. *J Am Med Assoc* 293:1861–7.

Foster, W. B., I. L. Hellman, D. Hesford, and D. G. McPherson. 1967. *Physical Standards in World War II*. Washington, DC: Office of the Surgeon General, Department of the Army.

Friedl, K. E. 1992. Body composition and military performance: Origins of the Army standards. In *Body Composition and Physical Performance: Applications for the Military Services*, eds. B. M. Marriott and J. Grumstrup-Scott, 31–55. Washington, DC: National Academies Press.

Friedl, K. E. 2004. Can you be large and not obese? The distinction between body weight, body fat, and abdominal fat in occupational standards. *Diab Technol Ther* 6:732–49.

Friedl, K. E. 2012. Body composition and military performance—Many things to many people. *J Strength Cond Res* 26:S87–S100.

Friedl, K. E. 2015. Letter to the editor: Navy contributions to body composition standards. *Mil Med* 180:vi.

Friedl, K. E., T. J. Breivik, R. Carter III et al. 2016. Soldier health and performance and the metabolically optimized brain. *Mil Med* 181:e1499.

Friedl, K. E., J. P. DeLuca, L. J. Marchitelli, and J. A. Vogel. 1992. Reliability of body-fat estimations from a four-compartment model by using density, body water, and bone mineral measurements. *Am J Clin Nutr* 55:764–70.

Friedl, K. E., C. M. DeWinne, and R. L. Taylor. 1987. The use of the Durnin–Womersley generalized equations for body fat estimation and their impact on the Army Weight Control Program. *Mil Med* 152:150–5.

Friedl, K. E., R. J. Moore, L. E. Martinez-Lopez, J. A. Vogel, E. W. Askew, L. J. Marchitelli, R. W. Hoyt, and C. C. Gordon. 1994. Lower limits of body fat in healthy active men. *J Appl Physiol* 77:933–40.

Friedl, K. E. and J. A. Vogel. 1991. Looking for a few good generalized body-fat equations. *Am J Clin Nutr* 53:795–7.

Friedl, K. E. and J. A. Vogel. 1997. Validity of percent body fat predicted from circumferences: Classification of men for weight control regulations. *Mil Med* 162:194–200.

Friedl, K. E., J. A. Vogel, M. W. Bovee, and B. H. Jones. 1989. *Assessment of body weight standards in male and female Army recruits.* Technical Report T15-90, AD-A224 586. Natick, Massachusetts: U.S. Army Research Institute of Environmental Medicine.

Friedl, K. E., K. A. Westphal, L. J. Marchitelli, J. F. Patton, W. C. Chumlea, and S. S. Guo. 2001. Evaluation of anthropometric equations to assess body-composition changes in young women. *Am J Clin Nutr* 73:268–75.

Fuchs, R. J., C. F. Theis, and M. C. Lancaster. 1978. A nomogram to predict lean body mass in men. *Am J Clin Nutr* 31:673–8.

Garn, S. M. 1957. Fat weight and fat placement in the female. *Science* 125:1091–2.

General Orders No. 181. 1907. *President Theodore Roosevelt's Message to the Secretary of War Expressing His Concern about Officer Physical Fitness, with Accompanying Orders to Implement Army Fitness Policy.* General Orders No. 181. Washington, DC, August 30.

Gordon, C. C. and K. E. Friedl. 1994. Anthropometry in the U.S. Armed Forces. In *Anthropometry in the Individual and the Population*, eds. S. J. Ulijaszek and C. G. N. Mascie-Taylor, 179–210. Cambridge: Cambridge University Press.

Government Accounting Office. 1998. *Gender Issues: Improved Guidance and Oversight are Needed to Ensure Validity and Equity of Fitness Standards.* NSIAD-99-9. Washington, DC: Government Accounting Office, November 17.

Haisman, M. F. 1970. The assessment of body fat content in young men from measurements of body density and skinfold thickness. *Hum Biol* 42:679–88.

Harman, E. A. and P. N. Frykman. 1992. The relationship of body size and composition to the performance of physically demanding military tasks. In *Body Composition and Physical Performance: Applications for the Military Services*, eds. B. M. Marriott and J. Grumstrup-Scott, 105–118. Washington, DC: National Academies Press.

Harman, E. A., R. M. Rosenstein, P. N. Frykman, and G. A. Nigro. 1989. Effects of a belt on intra-abdominal pressure during weight lifting. *Med Sci Sport Exerc* 21:186–90.

Hodgdon, J. A. 1992. Body composition in the military services: Standards and methods. In *Body Composition and Physical Performance: Applications for the Military Services*, eds. B. M. Marriott and J. Grumstrup-Scott, 57–70. Washington, DC: National Academies Press.

Hodgdon, J. A. 1999. *A History of the U.S. Navy Physical Readiness Program From 1976 to 1999.* Technical Report No. NHRC-TD-99-6F San Diego, California: Naval Health Research Center.

Hodgdon, J. A. and M. A. Beckett. 1984a. *Prediction of percent body fat for U.S. Navy men from body circumferences and height.* Technical Report No. 84-11. San Diego, California: U.S. Naval Health Research Center.

Hodgdon, J. A. and M. A. Beckett. 1984b. *Prediction of percent body fat for U.S. Navy women from body circumferences and height.* Technical Report No. 84-29. San Diego, California: U.S. Naval Health Research Center.

Hodgdon, J. A. and P. I. Fitzgerald. 1987. Validity of impedance predictions at various levels of fatness. *Hum Biol* 59:281–98.

Hodgdon, J. A., P. I. Fitzgerald, and J. A. Vogel. 1990. *Relationships between body fat and appearance ratings of U.S. soldiers.* Technical Report T12-90. Natick, Massachusetts: U.S. Army Research Institute of Medicine.

Hodgdon, J. A. and K. Friedl. 1999. *Development of the DoD Body composition estimation equations.* Technical Report No. NHRC-TD-99-2B. San Diego, California: Naval Health Research Center.

Jepsen, K. J., A. Centi, G. F. Duarte et al. 2011. Biological constraints that limit compensation of a common skeletal trait variant lead to inequivalence of tibial function among healthy young adults. *J Bone Miner Res* 26:2872–85.

Johnson, N. A. 1997. The history of the Army weight standards. *Mil Med* 162:564–70.

Jones, B. H., M. W. Bovee, and J. J. Knapik. 1992. Associations among body composition, physical fitness, and injury in men and women Army trainees. In *Body Composition and Physical Performance: Applications for the Military Services*, eds. B. M. Marriott and J. Grumstrup-Scott, 141–174. Washington, DC: National Academies Press.

Karpinos, B. D. 1958. Weight-height standards based on World War II experience. *Am Stat Assoc J* 53:408–19.

Keys, A., J. Brožek, A. Henschel, O. Mickelsen, and H. L. Taylor. 1950. *The Biology of Human Starvation* (2 vols). Minneapolis, Minnesota: University of Minnesota Press.

Krotkiewski, M., P. Björntorp, L. Sjöström, and U. Smith. 1983. Impact of obesity on metabolism in men and women: Importance of regional adipose tissue distribution. *J Clin Invest* 72:1150–62.

Krzywicki, H. J. and K. S. Chinn. 1967. Body composition of a military population, Fort Carson, 1963 I: Body density, fat, and potassium-40. *Am J Clin Nutr* 20:708–15.

Kuczmarski, R. J. and K. M. Flegal. 2000. Criteria for definition of overweight in transition: Background and recommendations for the United States. *Am J Clin Nutr* 72:1074–81.

Kvist, H., B. Chowdhury, U. Grangård, U. Tylen, and L. Sjöström. 1988. Total and visceral adipose-tissue volumes derived from measurements with computed tomography in adult men and women: Predictive equations. *Am J Clin Nutr* 48:1351–61.

Larsson, B., K. Svärdsudd, L. Welin, L. Wilhelmsen, P. Björntorp, and G. Tibblin. 1984. Abdominal adipose tissue distribution, obesity, and risk of cardiovascular disease and death: 13 year follow up of participants in the study of men born in 1913. *Br Med J* 288:1401–4.

Leu, J. R. and K. E. Friedl. 2002. Body fat standards and individual physical readiness in a randomized Army sample: Screening weights, methods of fat assessment, and linkage to physical fitness. *Mil Med* 167:994–1000.

Littman, A. J., I. G. Jacobson, E. J. Boyko, T. M. Powell, and T. C. Smith. 2013. Weight change following U.S. military service. *Int J Obes* 37:244–53.

Love, A. G. and C. B. Davenport. 1920. *Defects Found in Drafted Men: Statistical Information Compiled from the Draft Records Showing the Physical Condition of the Men Registered and Examined in Pursuance of the Requirements of the Selective Service Act*. Washington, DC: War Department, U.S. Government Printing Office.

Matsuzawa, Y., S. Fujioka, K. Tokunaga, and S. Tarui. 1992. Classification of obesity with respect to morbidity. *Exp Biol Med* 200:197–201.

Mazur, A., J. Mazur, and C. Keating, 1984. Military rank attainment of a West Point class: Effects of cadets' physical features. *Am J Sociol* 90:125–50.

Metropolitan Life Insurance Company. 1937. Girth and death. *Stat Bull Metrop Life Insur Co* 18:2–5.

Newman, R. W. 1952. *The assessment of military personnel by 1912 height-weight standards*. Report no. 194. Lawrence, Massachusetts: U.S. Army Quartermaster Climatic Research Laboratories.

Newton, R. L., H. Han, T. M. Stewart, D. H. Ryan, and D. A. Williamson. 2011. Efficacy of a pilot internet-based weight management program (HEALTH) and longitudinal physical fitness data in Army Reserve soldiers. *J Diab Sci Technol* 5:1255–62.

Ohlson, L. O., B. Larsson, K. Svärdsudd et al. 1985. The influence of body fat distribution on the incidence of diabetes mellitus: 13.5 years of follow-up of the participants in the study of men born in 1913. *Diabetes* 34:1055–8.

Orr, H. D. 1917. Examination of recruits for the Army and militia. *Am J Public Health* 7:485–8.

Pace, N. and E. N. Rathbun. 1945. Studies on body composition: III. The body water and chemically combined nitrogen content in relation to fat content. *J Biol Chem* 158:685–91.

Peterson, D. D. 2015. History of the U.S. Navy body composition program. *Mil Med* 180:91–6.

Reed, L. J. and A. G. Love. 1932. Biometric studies on U.S. Army officers: Somatological norms, correlations, and changes with age. *Hum Biol* 4:509–24.

Rognum, T. O., K. Rodahl, and P. K. Opstad. 1982. Regional differences in the lipolytic response of the subcutaneous fat depots to prolonged exercise and severe energy efficiency. *Eur J Appl Physiol Occup Physiol* 49:401–8.

Segal, K. R., M. Van Loan, P. I. Fitzgerald, J. A. Hodgdon, and T. B. Van Itallie. 1988. Lean body mass estimation by bioelectrical impedance analysis: A four-site cross-validation study. *Am J Clin Nutr* 47:7–14.

Seltzer, C. C., H. W. Stoudt, B. Bell, and J. Mayer. 1970. Reliability of relative body weight as a criterion of obesity. *Am J Epidemiol* 92:339–50.

Siri, W. E. 1961. Body composition from fluid spaces and density: Analysis of methods. In *Conference on Techniques for Measuring Body Composition (1959: Natick, Mass.)*, eds. J. Brozek and A. Henschel, 223–244. Washington, DC: National Academy of Sciences.

Stewart, S. T., H. Han, H. R. Allen, G. Bathalon, D. H. Ryan, R. L. Newton, and D. A. Williamson. 2011. HEALTH: Efficacy of an internet/population-based behavioral weight management program for the US Army. *J Diab Sci Technol* 5:178–87.

Sun, S. S., W. C. Chumlea, S. B. Heymsfield et al. 2003. Development of bioelectrical impedance analysis prediction equations for body composition with the use of a multicomponent model for use in epidemiologic surveys. *Am J Clin Nutr* 77:331–40.

Taylor, Lt. Gen. George Peach, Surgeon General. 2003. *Request for Waiver of Body Fat Measurement Methodology in DoDI 1308.3, DoD Physical Fitness and Body Fat Procedures*. Memorandum for Deputy Under Secretary of Defense (Personnel and Readiness) from Lieutenant General George Peach Taylor, Surgeon General. Washington, DC: Department of the Air Force, October 10.

Taylor, M. K., J. A. Hodgdon, L. Griswold, A. Miller, D. E. Roberts, and R. F. Escamilla. 2006. Cervical resistance training: Effects on isometric and dynamic strength. *Aviat Space Environ Med* 77:1131–5.

Theis, C. F. 1975. *Analysis of human body composition data as related to height and age*. Technical Report SAM-TR-75-38. Brooks Air Force Base, San Antonio, Texas: U.S. Air Force School of Aerospace Medicine.

U.S. Department of the Air Force. 2013. *Fitness Program*. Air Force Instruction 36-2905. Washington, DC: Department of the Air Force, October 21.

U.S. Department of Defense. 1981a. *DoD Physical Fitness and Weight Control Program*. Department of Defense Directive 1308.1. Washington, DC: U.S. Department of Defense, June 29.

U.S. Department of Defense. 1981b. *Study of the Military Services Physical Fitness*. Washington, DC: Office of the Assistant Secretary of Defense for Manpower, Reserve Affairs and Logistics, April 3.

U.S. Department of Defense. 1987. *Physical Fitness and Weight Control Programs*. Department of Defense Directive 1308.1, Change 1. Washington, DC: U.S. Department of Defense, January 15.

U.S. Department of Defense. 1995a. *DoD Physical Fitness and Body Fat Program*. Department of Defense Directive 1308.1. Washington, DC: U.S. Department of Defense, July 20.

U.S. Department of Defense. 1995b. *DoD Physical Fitness and Body Fat Programs Procedures*. Department of Defense Instruction 1308.3. Washington, DC: U.S. Department of Defense, August 30.

U.S. Department of Defense. 2002. *DoD Physical Fitness and Body Fat Programs Procedures*. Department of Defense Instruction 1308.3. Washington, DC: U.S. Department of Defense, November 5.

U.S. Department of Defense. 2004. *DoD Physical Fitness and Body Fat Program*. Department of Defense Directive 1308.1. Washington, DC: U.S. Department of Defense, June 30.

U.S. Department of the Air Force. 1985. *Military Personnel: The Air Force Weight and Fitness Programs*. Air Force Regulation 35-11. Washington, DC: Department of the Air Force, April 10.

U.S. Department of the Army. 1983a. *Army Medical Department Support of the Army Weight Control Program*. HQDA Letter 40-83-7. Washington, DC: U.S. Department of the Army, April 1.

U.S. Department of the Army. 1983b. *The Army Weight Control Program*. Army Regulation 600-9. Washington, DC: U.S. Department of the Army, February 15.

U.S. Department of the Army. 1986. *The Army Weight Control Program*. Army Regulation 600-9. Washington, DC: Department of the Army, September 1.

U.S. Department of the Army. 2006. *The Army Weight Control Program*. Army Regulation 600-9. Washington, DC: U.S. Department of the Army, November 17.

Vague, J. 1956. The degree of masculine differentiation of obesities: A factor determining predisposition to diabetes, atherosclerosis, gout, and uric calculous disease. *Am J Clin Nutr* 4:20–34.

Vogel, J. A. and J. P. Crowdy. 1979. Aerobic fitness and body fat of young British males entering the Army. *Eur J Appl Physiol Occup Physiol* 40:73–83.

Vogel, J. A. and K. E. Friedl. 1992. Body fat assessment in women: Special considerations. *Sports Med* 13:245–69.

Vogel, J. A., J. W. Kirkpatrick, P. I. Fitzgerald, J. A. Hodgdon, and E. A. Harman. 1988. *Derivation of anthropometry based body fat equations for the Army's weight control program*. Technical Report T17-88, AD-A197 706. Natick, Massachusetts: U.S. Army Research Institute of Medicine.

Welham, W. C. and A. R. Behnke. 1942. The specific gravity of healthy men: Body weight divided by volume and other physical characteristics of exceptional athletes and of Naval personnel. *J Am Med Assoc* 118:498–501.

Williamson, D. A., G. P. Bathalon, L. D. Sigrist et al. 2009. Military services fitness database: Development of a computerized physical fitness and weight management database for the U.S. Army. *Mil Med* 174:1–8.

Wilmore, J. H. and A. R. Behnke. 1969. An anthropometric estimation of body density and lean body weight in young men. *J Appl Physiol* 27:25–31.

Wheeler, D. C. 1965. Physical standards in allied and enemy armies during World War II. *Mil Med* 130:899–916.

Wright, H. F., C. O. Dotson, and P. O. Davis. 1980. An investigation of assessment techniques for body composition of women Marines. *US Navy Med* 71:15–26.

Wright, H. F., C. O. Dotson, and P. O. Davis. 1981. A simple technique for measurement of percent body fat in man. *US Navy Med* 72:23–7.

Wright, H. F. and J. H. Wilmore. 1974. Estimation of relative body fat and lean body weight in a United States Marine Corps population. *Aerosp Med* 45:301–6.

Yokota, M., G. P. Bathalon, and L. G. Berglund. 2008. Assessment of male anthropometric trends and the effects on simulated heat stress responses. *Eur J Appl Physiol* 104:297–302.

Yokota, M., L. G. Berglund, and G. P. Bathalon. 2012. Female anthropometric variability and their effects on predicted thermoregulatory responses to work in the heat. *Int J Biometeorol* 56:379–85.

14 Body Composition and Public Safety
The Industrial Athlete

Paul O. Davis and Mark G. Abel

CONTENTS

14.1 INTRODUCTION

Emergency Services, by definition, connotes a certain element of urgency. In the employment sector of workaday North America, law enforcement and fire suppression are among the few jobs that still require vigorous levels of physical exertion (Lemon and Hermiston 1977; Haskell et al. 1989). The construction trades, long a sector where manual labor meant exactly that, have moved to hydraulics and electrification to do much of the heavy lifting. Subduing fleeing and combative felons and gaining entry to burning buildings and suppression of structural fires are essential functions that make Emergency Service occupations unique. Unlike the sport athlete, there is no "finish line" for the industrial athlete, and the nature of the job drives the metabolic requirement.

As sport science would expand the knowledge of the underpinnings of human performance, the 1970s and beyond represented a significant rise in the number of studies examining professions outside of sport (Moulson-Litchfield and Freedson 1986). Public safety, including law enforcement, fire, rescue, and EMS, comprises occupations with clear requirements for physical abilities. Thus, this chapter explores a variety of body composition topics with regard to law enforcement officers (LEO) and firefighters, including the relationship between body composition versus health outcomes, occupational performance, and risk of injury. This chapter concludes with a description of factors that influence the body composition of industrial athletes and a discussion of strategies to manage body composition.

14.2 LAW ENFORCEMENT

14.2.1 BODY COMPOSITION AND HEALTH OUTCOMES

Cardiovascular disease (CVD) is a health concern in law enforcement. In fact, research indicates that there is a greater prevalence of CVD among LEO compared to other occupations (Calvert et al. 1999). Although there may be several factors responsible for this trend, unfavorable body composition is likely one of the culprits. Multiple investigations report that obesity rates among LEO exceeds 40% (Hartley et al. 2011; Can and Hendy 2014). A meta-analysis of body composition in LEO examined nutritional status across 23 studies (Da Silva et al. 2014). The majority of the officers identified in the study were overweight as evidenced by expanded girths with a higher risk of chronic disease. A longitudinal investigation of body composition changes among LEO indicated that the increase in relative body fat (percentage body fat) was approximately 5% over a 12.5-year period (Boyce et al. 2008). Over the same period of time, a comparison, by race, indicated that black LEO experienced a greater increase in relative body fat compared to white officers (6.6% vs. 4.5%, respectively, p = 0.01). There was no difference between black and white female officers (5.7% vs. 4.6%, respectively; Boyce et al. 2008). In addition, the study demonstrated that male LEO who have lower relative body fat were less likely to become obese. Finally, the study noted that male LEO experienced greater increases in lean body mass (LBM) compared to female officers (5.7 vs. 2.5 kg, p= 0.001; Boyce et al. 2008), despite no difference in the change in fat mass between genders. Although it is unclear what produced the enhanced LBM among male and female officers in this study, it is important for both sexes to participate in activities (e.g., resistance training, adequate dietary protein intake) that will increase LBM and limit fat mass to enhance occupational performance and health outcomes. Collectively, these findings underscore the importance of incorporating weight management programs throughout the career of a LEO, especially those who are already obese.

A recent investigation identified a relationship between obesity and markers associated with CVD in LEO. Specifically, the study reported a significant correlation between leptin levels and low frequency heart rate variability (HRV), especially among LEO with increased adiposity (Charles et al. 2015). Although not causal, these novel findings indicate that there is a relationship between leptin, a marker of CVD (Hasan-Ali et al. 2011), and HRV, an indicator of stress and increased CVD risk (Tsuji et al. 1996). Relationships between body composition surrogates and other negative health outcomes have been noted in LEO. Specifically, Violanti et al. (2011) noted a positive relationship between male officers' BMI and depression symptom scores. Collectively, these findings suggest that excess body fat increases an officer's risk of negative health outcomes.

14.2.2 BODY COMPOSITION VERSUS OCCUPATIONAL PERFORMANCE AND PHYSICAL FITNESS

Body composition and anthropometric measurements were associated with occupational performance in LEO (Dawes et al. 2014; Beck et al. 2015). Dawes et al. (2014) reported a positive relationship between the sum of three skinfolds and time to complete an obstacle course composed of occupational tasks. Beck et al. (2015) reported that body mass and waist and hip circumferences were positively correlated with occupational physical ability. Interestingly, after adjusting for the confounding effect of age, relative body fat was not correlated to occupational physical ability suggesting that the location of the fat depot (i.e., waist or hip) and the absolute amount of fat may have a greater impact on occupational physical ability than the relative amount of fat.

In a Canadian study, 98 officers volunteered to participate in the Police Officer's Physical Abilities Test (POPAT) with a passing criterion of 4 minutes and 15 seconds. While 16% of the women passed, 68% of the males passed (Rhodes and Farenholtz 1992). Body composition was not a statistically significant predictor of performance. Certainly, with a more robust sample, in all likelihood, body composition would have entered the regression equations. Given the discrepancy between the sexes in the pass rate, this study may suggest that, in addition to physical fitness, the stature or fat-free body mass of an officer may affect occupational performance. In another investigation, a small sample (n= 12) of British officers was tested on a battery of health and fitness constructs, including body composition (Spitier et al. 1987). The males' and females' relative body fat (determined via skinfold assessment) was 24.4 ± 7.1% and 30.9 ± 1.2%, respectively. Interestingly, despite these rather high relative body fat values, all of the officers were able to complete the job-related physical ability test. Discrepancies between the pass rates of various studies may be due to a variety of factors in addition to body composition including the test composition, tactical gear worn, environmental factors, etc.

The above findings suggest that fat and lean mass likely play a role in law enforcement occupational performance. However, a variety of physical fitness attributes are necessary to successfully complete essential occupational tasks and fat and lean mass may impact fitness attributes differently. For instance, Dawes et al. (2016) reported that percentage body fat was correlated with upper body muscular endurance, relative upper body strength (1 repetition maximum/body mass), and lower-body power (vertical jump height). Interestingly, the investigators further reported that the analysis of lean mass and fat mass further identified functional relationships between body composition and performance outcomes. Specifically, lean mass was positively correlated with push-up performance, vertical jump height and peak power, and maximum (absolute and relative) bench press performance. Whereas, absolute fat mass was inversely correlated with vertical jump height, 1.5 mile (3,740 m) run time, and relative maximum oxygen uptake (Dawes et al. 2016). These findings suggest that LEO should focus on utilizing training and dietary strategies to increase LBM to improve muscular endurance, power, and strength attributes. Likewise, LEO may consider decreasing fat mass and train to improve metabolic fitness to enhance aerobic and anaerobic performance attributes (Dawes et al. 2016).

In other tactical populations (e.g., military personnel) it has been demonstrated that relative body fat was the strongest predictor of aerobic performance while wearing 11 kg of body armor (Ricciardi et al. 2007). Furthermore, relative body fat was inversely correlated with pull-ups to fatigue in men (Ricciardi et al. 2007). These findings support the supposition that greater relative body fat decreases physical performance.

A 15-year longitudinal study of 103 Finnish police officers revealed expected trends in added body weight (0.5 kg/year) and nominal losses in muscular fitness (Sorensen et al. 2000). Aerobic fitness was strongly predicted by activity in early adulthood, suggesting a rationale for pre-selection of applicants with a penchant toward fitness. Waist circumference emerged as an easily obtained anthropometric measure with predictive value on job-related fitness tasks.

14.2.2.1 Relationship of Body Mass to Load Carriage Capabilities

Because LEO are required to carry tactical equipment weighing approximately 5.5 kg (comprised of body armor, Sam Browne belt with flashlight, cuffs, baton, magazines, radio, pistol, and holster), it seems reasonable that reduced fat mass and increased LBM is advantageous for occupational physical ability (i.e., performing explosive tasks). Lewinski et al. (2015) demonstrated that wearing a 9.07 kg (equivalent to 11.5 ± 1.6% of body mass) weighted belt decreased sprint stride velocity by 5% in male law enforcement students. Interestingly, Carlton et al. (2014) reported that there might be a dose–response relationship with regard to load carriage magnitude versus body mass on occupational performance. Specifically, specialist police officers' occupational physical ability was not affected when carrying loads less than 25% of body mass, but was significantly impaired when carrying loads greater than 25% of body mass. The tasks included a 10 m linear sprint, movement through two doorways, stair descent, movement through a third doorway, and approaching a target. In general, patrol officers are not carrying extreme loads, however increased fat-free mass and reduced fat mass will increase the officer's ability to perform explosive movements in time critical situations during load carriage.

14.2.3 Body Composition and Risk of Injury

Injury rates among LEO are higher than in other first responder populations (Reichard and Jackson 2010). Despite a paucity of literature investigating the influence of body composition on risk of injury among LEO, body weight status has been found to be associated with injuries. Specifically, LEO with a BMI greater than 35 kg/m² were three times more likely to report back pain compared to officers with a normal BMI (18–25 kg/m²; Nabeel et al. 2007). Greater fat mass increases anthropometric dimensions in the trunk and thighs, thus placing additional stress on the musculoskeletal system and requires the individual to alter movement patterns to accommodate these factors (Cavuoto and Nussbaum 2014). In addition, obese individuals possess lesser strength and aerobic fitness relative to body mass, which may increase risk of injury (Capodaglio et al. 2010). Furthermore, Capodaglio et al. (2010) indicate that obesity leads to the development of disability via decreased lower extremity strength and balance, diminished upper body strength and dexterity (Tunceli et al. 2006), and loss of lean mass (Borsello 1998). Despite a lack of research demonstrating a causal link between body composition and injury occurrence in LEO, it seems reasonable to speculate that weight management is important for reducing the risk of injuries among LEO.

14.2.4 Effects of Exercise on Body Composition, Physical Fitness, and Occupational Performance

Exercise training is one strategy to enhance body composition, physical fitness, and occupational performance among LEO. A recent study of 55 cadets determined the effect of basic training on physical fitness outcomes. Physical fitness assessments were conducted at 8 and 16 weeks of training (Crawley et al. 2016). Significant improvements were noted in agility, lower-body peak power, sit-ups, push-ups, and half-mile shuttle run across the full 16 weeks, however most of these improvements occurred within the first 8 weeks with minimal fitness outcome improvements during the second 8-week period, suggesting that academies and active duty exercise regimens should utilize periodized training programs to enhance fitness attributes over an extended period of time. Unfortunately, changes in body composition were not reported in this study. Stamford et al. (1978) evaluated body composition and demonstrated that despite making improvements in physical fitness and body composition during 4 months of the academy, these improvements reverted to baseline levels after 12 months of active duty. Likewise, Rossomanno et al. (2012) demonstrated that a 6-month supervised training intervention significantly reduced BMI and body weight, while also improving performance on an occupational physical ability test in active duty LEO. Unfortunately, these trends were reversed at a 12-month follow-up assessment, while no exercise supervision was provided. The fact that many officers increase body mass and lose physical fitness over their career is not surprising as officers face many of the same barriers to performing regular exercise as the general population, namely lack of time and/or motivation to exercise (Sallis and Hovell 1990). Collectively, these findings suggest that municipalities should provide individualized and occupationally relevant periodized exercise programs, on-duty exercise time, fitness facilities, and qualified supervision (i.e., tactical strength and conditioning professionals) to enhance exercise adherence, body composition, and occupational physical ability.

14.3 FIRE SUPPRESSION

14.3.1 Body Composition and Health Outcomes

CVD is one of the most prominent health concerns in the fire service with sudden cardiac death as the leading cause of on-duty fatalities among firefighters (Fahy et al. 2014). Although numerous factors contribute to CVD risk, obesity is one of the most common risk factors identified in the fire service. One study reported that 44.7% of firefighters were classified as obese according to body mass index or BMI (>30 kg/m²) or relative body fat (≥25% body fat for men and ≥32% body fat for women) (Fahy et al. 2011). Increased BMI among firefighters and first responders was associated with greater arterial stiffness, peripheral blood pressure, unfavorable metabolic profiles, and lower exercise tolerance (Fahs et al. 2009; Tsismenakis et al. 2009). Unfortunately, obesity rates among firefighters increase while in the fire service. Soteriades et al. (2005) reported that the prevalence of obesity among 332 firefighters increased from 35% to 40% over a 5-year period. In addition, body mass among normal weight firefighters increased by 1.1 pounds, whereas the body mass of obese firefighters (BMI $\geq$ 35 kg/m^2) increased by 1.9 pounds per year (Soteriades et al. 2005). The findings from these studies highlight the importance for implementation of wellness programs focused on appropriate dietary intake, regular exercise, and frequent medical examinations.

14.3.2 Body Composition and Occupational Performance

Body composition is associated with simulated fire-ground performance in firefighters (Davis et al. 1982; Williford et al. 1999; Michaelides et al. 2008, 2011; Calavalle et al. 2013). Michaelides et al. (2011) evaluated the relationship between physical fitness measures and occupational performance. The investigators reported that relative body fat was the strongest and negative predictor of occupational performance (Michaelides et al. 2011). In addition, BMI and waist circumference were also inversely correlated with simulated occupational performance (Michaelides et al. 2011). Similarly, Williford et al. (1999) found that relative body fat was positively correlated and LBM was inversely correlated to time to complete a simulated fire-ground test (Williford et al. 1999). Finally, Calavalle et al. (2013) conducted a study employing principle component analysis and ascertained that 19.6% of the total variance on a stair climbing test was explained by the effect of body fat. In general, excess body fat augments the external load, and thus increases the metabolic cost of a given activity, decreases aerobic performance (Cureton and Sparling 1980), and reduces the firefighter's ability to perform load carriage tasks over extended periods of time.

Figure 14.1 describes the relationship between external load carriage relative to body mass. Firefighters have unique physical demands because of the weight of their personal protective ensemble (PPE). This includes their self-contained breathing apparatus, or SCBA (compressed air) and helmet, bunker coat and pants, hood, and gloves. Of course, once all this equipment has been donned, there is an expectation to perform hard work. External loads easily approach 50 pounds or more. Physical size, particularly LBM plays a significant role in physical work capacity (PWC)

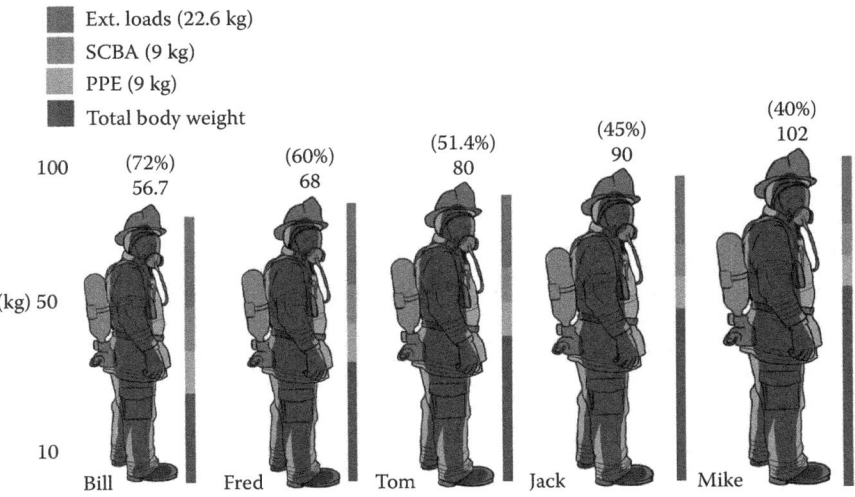

FIGURE 14.1 (**See color insert.**) Body weight as a percentage of total load for firefighters. (Copyright 2016, Paul O. Davis.)

when heavy objects need to be moved horizontally and vertically, with a clear advantage in favor of larger individuals. In the example above, Mike is carrying 40% of his body weight compared to Bill at 72%, meaning that Bill must have a much higher relative level of fitness.

The University of Maryland's School of Public Health-Sports Medicine Center embarked on a FEMA-funded study (Dotson et al. 1977) to explain the underlying constructs and variability in structural fire suppression. Five political jurisdictions surrounding the District of Columbia agreed to participate by donating on-duty time of 100 randomly selected firefighters who were representative of the demographics of age. There were no female firefighters in these fire departments at the time of the testing.

The participants underwent a battery of human performance laboratory tests for oxygen uptake kinetics, lactate production, body composition, and muscular fitness. At a second appointment at the Maryland Fire Rescue Institute, they underwent a simulated set of five linked fire-ground criterion tasks while wearing their PPE and breathing with the assistance of the SCBA.

Subject's time for the completion of the criterion task test (CTT) including climbing stairs under load, hoisting, simulated forcible entry with hand tools, and the "rescue" of a victim were recorded and correlated against their laboratory measures employing canonical correlation and multiple regression analysis.

The Maryland study would answer several questions about job performance and employment opportunity law. First, the expected, positive relationship between advancing age and time to perform the CTT, with further inspection of the data revealed body composition to be the likely culprit rather than age alone.

Table 14.1, sorted by elapsed time to perform the CTT and arbitrarily assigned fitness classifications from excellent to poor based upon group averages, is highly instructive. The lean body weight for each of the groups is nearly the same but the amount of body fat differs by classification. Adipose tissue is a reservoir of potential energy to fuel aerobic activity. However, increasing amounts of body fat have a strong negative correlation with performance requiring body movement, thus it is no more than ballast and does not effectively contribute to performance of the weight-supported tasks.

To put this into perspective, the SCBA unit, which is the heaviest component in the PPE exacts the greatest metabolic demand of all the worn equipment. For many of the firefighters, they are in essence carrying two SCBA units: one on their back, the other with excess adipose tissue. This

TABLE 14.1
Fitness Classifications and Measurements of 100 Firefighters

	Excellent	Good	Average	Fair	Poor
Age, year	28	28.3	31.4	37.9	46.1
Height, cm	175	176	176	178	177
Weight, kg	77.8	79.2	82.1	86.9	93.5
Lean body, kg	66	65.8	65	64	66
Body fat, %	14.8	18.1	20.3	25	28.5
Fat, kg	11.8	14.9	17.1	22.7	27.1
Grip strength, kg	2.9	48.9	47.7	45.9	43.1
Chin ups, reps	9	7.3	5.2	4.2	0.9
Push-ups, reps	28.3	23.3	17.7	15	10.2
Sit-ups, reps	28.3	23.3	17.7	15	10.2
Peak VO$_2$[a]	45.2	43.1	39.2	35.2	34.9
CTT[b] (min:secs)	05:40	05:44	06:50	07:53	10:45

[a] Peak oxygen consumption (mL kg min^{-1}).
[b] Criterion task test.

excess fat has a deleterious effect on stamina since the calculation of aerobic capacity in such set-tings needs to take into account the total mass that has to be moved, divided into the absolute oxygen uptake value (ml/kg/min).

Were we able to maintain body composition at or near that at the point of hiring, the regression seen in this table would flatten out considerably. Another finding hidden in the dataset is that of the variability of age. While the downward trend is clear, an analysis of covariance allowed us to tease out the top performers. In many cases, firefighters in their 40's out-performed colleagues 20 years their junior. Physiologically, they appeared significantly younger (e.g., more fit) than their chrono-logical age, demonstrating that personal fitness is a trait that can be controlled by an individual.

14.3.3 Body Composition and Risk of Injury

Body composition has been linked with risk of injury among firefighters. Jahnke et al. (2013) dem-onstrated that firefighters who were classified as obese (body mass index: BMI ≥ 30 kg/m^2) were 5.2 times more likely to suffer a musculoskeletal injury compared to firefighters classified as normal weight (BMI = 18.5–24.9 kg/m^2). Poplin et al. (2016) developed a comprehensive model, based on multiple fitness attributes, to predict risk of firefighter injury. The model was composed of highly reliable fitness constructs and included flexibility, total grip strength, percentage body fat, and rest-ing heart rate. The findings from this study revealed that the least fit firefighters (based on the above attributes) were 1.82 times more likely to become injured compared to the most fit firefighters. Furthermore, the least fit firefighters were 2.90 times more likely to suffer a sprain or strain com-pared to the most fit firefighters. Although there is not enough causal data to implicate body fat's role in injury occurrence, it is certainly a factor that increases a firefighter's risk of injury and thus weight management and overall physical fitness should be a priority for firefighters and their departments.

14.3.4 Effects of Exercise Training on Body Composition and Occupational Performance/Risk of Injury

Physical fitness conditioning is a recognized need to prepare for the demands of structural fire suppression, and expected results follow in those programs that adhere to the known constructs of exercise frequency, intensity, and duration. Between two groups of firefighters who participated in a 12-week physical training program, firefighters who exercised improved muscular and cardiovas-cular fitness and body composition, but these outcomes did not equate to improvements in move-ment quality (i.e., functional movement screen score) and occupational low-back loading (Beach et al. 2014). The authors concluded that firefighters who are physically fit are better able to perform essential job tasks, but short-term improvements in physical fitness may not necessarily translate into reduced risk of lower back injury (Beach et al. 2014). Furthermore, controlled studies consis-tently demonstrate improvements in virtually all occupational performance predictors. Pawlak et al. (2015) evaluated the effect of a novel exercise program on body composition, physical fitness, and occupational performance outcomes in career firefighters. A supervised exercise group performed circuit-training exercise using standard firefighter equipment while a control group maintained their exercise behaviors. The 12-week training program demonstrated superior improvements in the supervised circuit-training group in cardiorespiratory, body composition (decreased fat mass, % fat, and body mass), and occupational performance outcomes. Despite an increase in peak relative oxygen uptake in the supervised exercise group, there was no improvement in peak absolute oxygen uptake. Thus, these findings suggest that the favorable reduction in body mass increased the relative oxygen uptake measure. Therefore, body composition may have indirectly improved occupational performance by improving the metabolic efficiency of the firefighters.

Peterson et al. (2008) conducted a 9-week training intervention comparing the effects of undu-lating versus traditional (linear) periodization strategies on physical fitness, anthropometric, and occupational performance outcomes in young firefighter trainees. The findings indicated that both training strategies improved strength, power output, and occupational performance, despite no changes in body mass, and chest, biceps, or thigh circumferences. Although body composition was not assessed, the stability of anthropometric outcomes coupled with improved power measures may suggest that neural adaptations and metabolic conditioning were primarily responsible for the improvement in occupational performance.

Roberts et al. (2002) also conducted a 16-week exercise training intervention with firefighter recruits and reported a significant increase in lean tissue mass (mean gain = 0.9 kg) and decrease in fat-mass (1.6 kg). The combined aerobic and resistance training intervention also improved aerobic capacity, muscular endurance, and flexibility. No measure of occupational performance was conducted in this study. Although not directly evaluated, it is likely that the improved occupational performance reported in some of the described training interventions was likely due to a combination of improved body composition and physical fitness attributes (i.e., cardiorespiratory endurance, muscular strength, and endurance).

Although there are numerous types of training regimens for firefighters, high intensity training (HIT) has attracted a number of adherents within the fire service. To document benefits within this cohort, a self-reported study of 625 firefighters found that those who engaged in HIT training were half as likely to be classified as obese and twice as likely to meet fitness recommendations of 12 metabolic equivalents (METs; Jahnke et al. 2015). Thus, participation in a self-directed or organized/commercial training program (e.g., CrossFit, P90X, Insanity) may enhance body composition and physical fitness outcomes in firefighters.

14.4 CONTRIBUTORS OF OBESITY AMONG INDUSTRIAL ATHLETES: DIETARY HABITS, PHYSICAL INACTIVITY, STRESS, AND SLEEP RESTRICTION

There are numerous contributors to unfavorable body composition among firefighters and LEO. A brief summary of several contributors is provided herein. Dietary knowledge and intake is one likely contributor. In general, most career firefighters do not follow a specific dietary plan and indicate that they would like additional information on healthy eating (Yang et al. 2015). Research indicates that firefighters tend to prefer the nutritional composition of the Mediterranean diet over Paleo, Atkins, and Esselsteyn Engine 2 (low-fat, strictly plant-based) diets (Yang et al. 2015). Furthermore, compared to normal weight counterparts, obese firefighters reported less nutritional knowledge and were more likely to feel that they receive insufficient nutritional information (Yang et al. 2015). These findings suggest that practitioners and municipalities should provide educational resources to enhance firefighters' dietary knowledge and assist with implementation of dietary modifications.

Physical inactivity is another contributor to obesity, as it has been found to be associated with obesity among industrial populations (Can and Hendy 2014). Unpublished data indicate that structural firefighters and campus LEO do not perform adequate amounts of physical activity to obtain health benefits (Koebke 2012; Morris 2012). Furthermore, LEOs typically decrease physical activity levels during their career (Sorensen et al. 2000). Can and Hendy (2014) reported that the weekly duration of cardiovascular and resistance training activity is inversely associated with BMI among LEOs. Interestingly, when comparing occupations, Leischik et al. (2015) found that German firefighters were about 28% more active than LEOs, and relative body fat was nearly 4% higher in LEOs (17.7 ± 6.2% vs. 21.4 ± 5.6%).

Additional contributors to obesity among firefighters and LEOs include psychological stress and shift work. These occupations are associated with repeated exposure to trauma (Jahnke et al. 2016) and increased levels of stress and anxiety (Nelson and Smith 2016). Increased exposure to stress may increase the consumption of comfort foods (Dallman 2003). Furthermore, increased stress may alter hippocampus function, which is associated with the regulation of body mass and food intake (Davidson et al. 2005). Thus, individuals experiencing greater perceived stress may have a reduced ability to control excessive food intake. Shift work, especially afternoon and evening shifts, has been associated with inadequate sleep quality and quantity (Lombardi et al. 2014;

Fekedulegn et al. 2016). Insufficient sleep duration has been associated with increased levels of obesity (Gangwisch et al. 2005), as sleep restriction promotes increased appetite potentially via hormonal alterations (Spiegel et al. 1999, 2004). In addition, working longer hours on third shift is associated with increased BMI and waist circumferences in male LEOs (Gu et al. 2012). In summary, there are numerous factors associated with unfavorable body composition among firefighters and LEOs. Considerations should be made at the organizational and personal levels to address these issues and suggestions are provided in the following section.

14.5 PRACTICAL APPLICATIONS

Body composition has substantial implications regarding the health, performance, and safety of industrial athletes. It is important that the industrial athlete achieves and maintains an appropriate body composition to optimize these outcomes and enhance career longevity and post-career quality of life. Organizational policies should be implemented to assist industrial athletes in achieving suitable body composition and overall wellness. For instance, municipalities should allow employees to exercise on-duty and provide qualified supervision to enhance compliance and reduce risk of injury while exercising. Exercise training for LEOs and firefighters should target a variety of fitness attributes as are required to perform occupational tasks. Specifically, resistance training should be incorporated to stimulate the hypertrophy of skeletal muscle tissue to enhance LBM. Similarly, aerobic and muscular endurance exercise should be incorporated to increase energy expenditure and decrease fat mass. Furthermore, operators should be provided with educational materials and/or workshops on healthy dietary intake, stress reduction strategies, and proper sleep hygiene. Collectively, these practices may enhance body composition and help to develop the *Industrial Athlete*.

Figure 14.2 illustrates these points. From one of the very few controlled, longitudinal studies (Kasch et al. 1990), the changes in aerobic fitness were tracked over 20 years, the typical period of employment in public safety. Virtually no decline in year-to-year repeated measures of aerobic fitness was observed in the chronic exercise group compared to other sedentary populations that showed 10% per decade or greater in aerobic fitness.

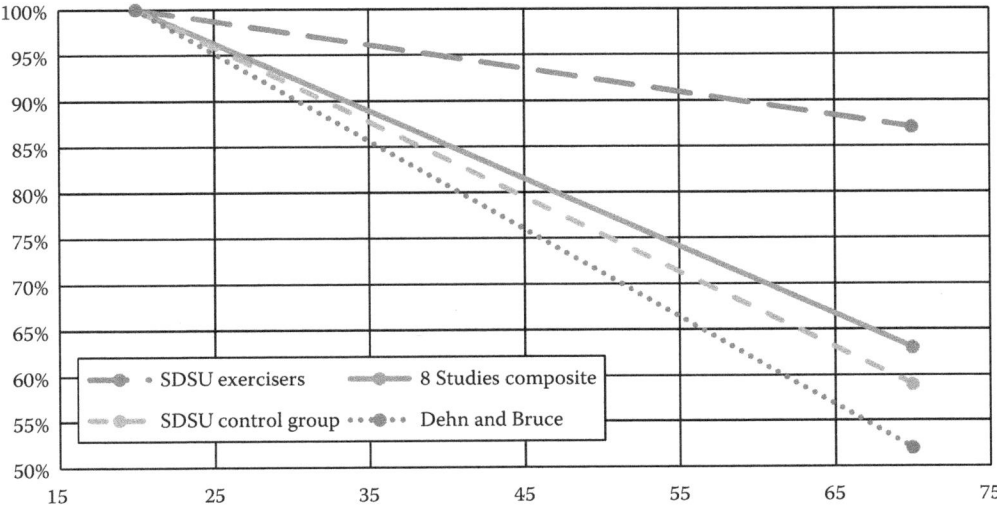

FIGURE 14.2 Decline in maximal oxygen uptake with age in men. (Adapted from data of Kasch, F. W. et al. 1990. *Phys Sportsmed* 18:73–88.)

Once hired ("on the job") the knowledge, skills, and abilities (KSAs) of emergency service personnel rapidly ascend. The age-associated decline in aerobic fitness in sedentary populations is approximately 1% per year. A person hired at the minimum entry-level standard will fall below that standard without intervention through a regular program of physical activity. Figure 14.3 shows the regression lines for the uninterrupted decay in fitness estimated at 10% per decade, compared to the ascendency of job-related KSAs. These findings demonstrate that knowledge of required job behaviors grows asymptotically with experience while job-related fitness declines. Employment of individuals who minimally meet the entry-level physical performance standards without a mandatory conditioning program virtually assures a workforce that is limited in performance. For this reason, it makes sense to hire individuals who exceed the minimum standards by a very large margin. Longitudinal studies have demonstrated that virtually no loss of aerobic fitness takes place within a cohort of regularly exercising adults over the typical span of gainful employment.

A frequent theme in the professional literature of public safety performance is the general lack of fitness as evidenced by the number of line-of-duty heart attacks and musculoskeletal injuries (Kales et al. 2007). Gadesam et al. (2010) found that aerobic fitness had a stronger association with thrombotic risk markers than fatness and Poplin et al. (2014) demonstrated that greater aerobic fitness was associated with reduced risk of musculoskeletal injury. The descriptive data in most of these studies strongly suggest a need for hiring physically capable first responders and for mandatory maintenance fitness throughout employment.

For an occupation with above average metabolic and strength demands, public safety employee cohort data reveal a mediocre workforce. The preponderance of the literature focuses on the usual range of physiological constructs including aerobic and muscular fitness and estimates of body composition. The fitness constructs underpinning work performance do not reside in all members of the applicant pool. Initial awareness that physical size, specifically stature, was an important characteristic in the performance of occupational tasks resulted in use of minimum heights in the hiring criteria. Realization that total body weight played a role prompted public safety organizations to "borrow" insurance company height and weight nomograms (charts) in a crude attempt to identify ideal body sizes and mitigate risk associated with obesity. Human body composition assessment has evolved from simple lean and fat models (e.g., densitometry and anthropometry) with imprecision for an individual to more complex multi-component models (e.g., dual x-ray absorptiometry) with increased cost and less concern about validity.

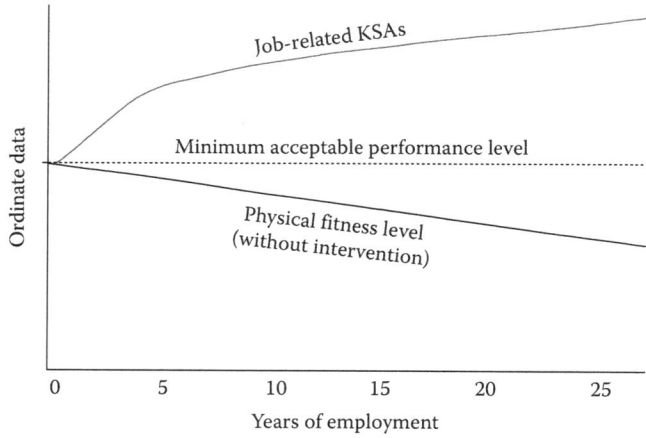

FIGURE 14.3 Trends in job-related knowledge, skills, and aptitudes (KSA's) compared to fitness of emergency personnel over time. (Copyright 2016, Paul O. Davis.)

The potential problem of adverse consequences of poor body composition and fitness on public safety performance begins at the point of hire. Incredibly, many public safety organizations have no employment-based screening standards, and many that do, place little importance on meaningful work-related predictors. Body composition as a single predictor for hiring presents problems when individuals who may exceed any specific evaluation standard or cut-point are clearly capable of performing the essential physical functions. Importantly, body composition is a significant contributor to the explained variance in any type of ambulation involved in public safety employment. For this reason, running tests for law enforcement have inherent validity. Likewise, stair climbing, particularly while under load (e.g., safety equipment or simulated weight of an injured victim) will aid in selection of the best prospects for employment.

Some key issues to consider in optimizing body composition, health, and performance of public safety workers include

- Identify realistic, valid job-related criteria that focus on replication of arduous and critical essential functions. Work sample tests are one example.
- Place the onus of responsibility on the employee to maintain personal fitness as a condition of employment.
- Body composition is only one of a number of important fitness constructs. Incorporate regular assessments of body composition with the same method or techniques to monitor changes and provide science-based interventions to maintain healthy body composition. Simple measurement protocols (i.e., waist circumference) with trained and certified test administrators provide valid, longitudinal data and direction of change.
- Place the onus of responsibility on the employee to maintain personal fitness as a condition of employment. Remediation of deficits in work-related physical performance and/or trends in body composition toward excess fatness or loss of lean mass is required.

REFERENCES

Beach, T. A., D. M. Frost, S. M. McGill, and J. P. Callaghan. 2014. Physical fitness improvements and occupational low-back loading—An exercise intervention study with firefighters. *Ergonomics* 57:744–63.

Beck, A. Q., J. L. Clasey, J. W. Yates, N. C. Koebke, T. G. Palmer, and M. G. Abel. 2015. Relationship of physical fitness measures vs. occupational physical ability in campus law enforcement officers. *J Strength Cond Res* 29:2340–50.

Borsello, O. 1998. *Obesità: un trattamento multidimen sionale [Obesity: A Multi-Disciplinary Treatment].* Milano, Italy: Ed Kurtis.

Boyce, R., G. Jones, C. Lloyd, and E. Boone. 2008. A longitudinal observation of police: Body composition changes over 12 years with gender and race comparisons. *J Exerc Physiol Online* 11:1–13.

Calavalle, A. R., D. Sisti, G. Mennelli et al. 2013. A simple method to analyze overall individual physical fitness in firefighters. *J Strength Cond Res* 27:769–75.

Calvert, G. M., J. W. Merling, and C. A. Burnett. 1999. Ischemic heart disease mortality and occupation among 16- to 60-year-old males. *J Occup Environ Med* 41:960–66.

Can, S. H. and H. M. Hendy. 2014. Behavioral variables associated with obesity in police officers. *Ind Health* 52:240–47.

Capodaglio, P. C., G. Brunani, A. Vismara, L. Villa, V. Capodaglio, and E. Maria. 2010. Functional limitations and occupational issues in obesity: A review. *Int J Occup Saf Ergon* 16:507–23.

Carlton, S. D., P. D. Carbone, M. Stierli, and R. Orr. 2014. The impact of occupational load carriage on the mobility of the tactical police officer. *J. Aust. Strength Cond* 21:32–7.

Cavuoto, L. A. and M. A. Nussbaum. 2014. Influences of obesity on job demands and worker capacity. *Curr Obes Rep* 3:341–47.

Charles, L. E., C. M. Burchfiel, K. Sarkisian et al. 2015. Leptin, adiponectin, and heart rate variability among police officers. *Am J Hum Biol* 27:184–91.

Crawley, A. A., R. A. Sherman, W. R. Crawley, and L. M. Cosio-Lima. 2016. Physical fitness of police academy cadets: Baseline characteristics and changes during a 16-week academy. *J Strength Cond Res* 30:1416–24.

Cureton, K. J. and P. B. Sparling. 1980. Distance running performance and metabolic responses to running in men and women with excess weight experimentally equated. *Med Sci Sports Exerc* 12:288–94.

Dallman, M. F. 2003. Chronic stress and obesity: A new view of "comfort food." *Proc Natl Acad Sci USA* 100:11696–701.

Da Silva, F. C., S. S. Hernandez, E. Gonçalves, B. A. Arancibia, T. L. Da Silva, and R. Da Silva. 2014. Anthropometric indicators of obesity in policeman: A systematic review of observational studies. *Int J Med Environ Health* 17:891–901.

Davidson T. L., S. E. Kanoski, E. K. Walls, and L. E. Jarrard. 2005. Memory inhibition and energy regulation. *Physiol Behav* 86:731–46.

Davis, P. O., C. O. Dotson, and D. L. Santa Maria. 1982. Relationship between simulated fire-fighting tasks and physical performance measures. *Med Sci Sports Exerc* 14:65–71.

Dawes, J. J., R. M. Orr, C. L. Elder, and C. J. Rockwell. 2014. Association between body fatness and measures of muscular endurance among part-time SWAT officers. *J Aust Strength Cond* 22:33–7.

Dawes, J. J., R. M. Orr, C. L. Siekaniec, A. A. Vanderwoude, and R. Pope. 2016. Associations between anthropometric characteristics and physical performance in male law enforcement officers: A retrospective cohort study. *Ann Occup Environ Med* 28:26.

Dotson, C. O., D. L. Santa Maria, P. O. Davis, and R. A. Schwartz. 1977. *The Development of Job-Related Physical Performance Examination for Firefighters*. Washington, D.C.: GPO, U.S. Fire Administration.

Fahs, C. A., D. L. Smith, G. P. Horn et al. 2009. Impact of excess body weight on arterial structure, function, and blood pressure in firefighters. *Am J Cardiol* 104:1441–45.

Fahy, R. F., P. R. LeBlanc, and J. L. Molis. 2011. *Firefighter Fatalities in the United States-2010*. Quincy, MA: National Fire Protection Association.

Fahy, R. F., P. R. LeBlanc, and J. L. Molis. 2014. *Firefighter Fatalities in the United States-2013*. Quincy, MA: National Fire Protection Association.

Fekedulegn, D., C. M. Burchfiel, L. E. Charles, T. A. Hartley, M. E. Andrew, and J. M. Violanti. 2016. Shift work and sleep quality among urban police officers: The BCOPS study. *J Occup Environ Med* 58:e66–71.

Gadesam, R. R., C. Skrifvars, B. Garrett et al. 2010. Aerobic fitness strongly associated with thrombotic risk markers than fatness in firefighters. *J Am Coll Cardiol* 29:55; A173.E1621.

Gangwisch, J. E., D. Malaspina, B. Boden-Albala, and S. B. Heymsfield. 2005. Inadequate sleep as a risk factor for obesity: Analyses of the NHANES I. *Sleep* 28:1289–96.

Gu, J. K., L. E. Charles, C. M. Burchfiel et al. 2012. Long work hours and adiposity among police officers in a US northeast city. *Occup Environ Med* 54:1374–81.

Hartley, T. A., C. M. Burchfiel, D. Fekedulegn, M. E. Andrew, S. S. Knox, and J. M. Violanti. 2011. Associations between police officer stress and the metabolic syndrome. *Int J Emerg Ment Health* 13:243–56.

Hasan-Ali, H., N. A. Abd El-Mottaleb, H. B. Hamed, and A. Abd-Elsayed. 2011. Serum adiponectin and leptin as predictors of the presence and degree of coronary atherosclerosis. *Coron Artery Dis* 22:264–69.

Haskell, W. M., N. Brachfeld, R. A. Bruce et al. 1989. Determination of occupational working capacity in patients with ischemic heart disease. *J Am Coll Cardiol* 14:1025–34.

Jahnke, S. A., M. L. Hyder, C. K. Haddock, J. Jitnarin, R. S. Day, and W. S. Carlos-Poston. 2015. High-intensity fitness training among a national sample of male career firefighters. *Saf Health Work* 6:71–4.

Jahnke, S. A., W. S. Poston, C. K. Haddock, and N. Jitnarin. 2013. Obesity and incident injury among career firefighters in the central United States. *Obesity* 21:1505–8.

Jahnke, S. A., W. S. Poston, C. K. Haddock, and B. Murphy. 2016. Firefighting and mental health: Experiences of repeated exposure to trauma. *Work* 53:737–44.

Kales, S. N., E. S. Soteriades, C. A. Christophi, and D. C. Christiani. 2007. Emergency duties and deaths from heart disease among firefighters in the United States. *N Engl J Med* 356:1207–15.

Kasch, F. W., J. L. Boyer, S. P. Van Camp, L. S. Verity, and J. P. Wallace. 1990. The effect of physical activity and inactivity on aerobic power in older men: A longitudinal study. *Phys Sportsmed* 18:73–88.

Koebke, N. 2012. Assessment of cardiovascular disease risk factors and physical activity levels in university law enforcement officers. *Master's thesis*. University of Kentucky.

Leischik, R., P. Foshag, M. Straub et al. 2015. Aerobic capacity, physical activity and metabolic risk factors in firefighters compared with police officers and sedentary clerks. *PLoS ONE* 10(7):e0133113. http://www.ncbi.nlm.nih.gov/pmc/articles/PMC4506022/pdf/pone.0133113.pdf.

Lemon, P. W. R. and R. T. Hermiston. 1977. The human energy cost of fire-fighting. *J Occup Med* 19:558–62.

Lewinski, W. J., J. L. Dysterheft, N. D. Dicks, and R. W. Pettitt. 2015. The influence of officer equipment and protection on short sprinting performance. *Appl Ergon* 47:65–71.

Lombardi, D. A., K. Jin, C. Vetter et al. 2014. The impact of shift starting time on sleep duration, sleep quality, and alertness prior to injury in the People's Republic of China. *Chronobiol Int*. 31:1201–8.

Michaelides, M. A., K. M. Parpa, L. J. Henry, G. B. Thompson, and B. S. Brown. 2011. Assessment of physical fitness aspects and their relationship to firefighters' job abilities. *J Strength Cond Res* 25:956–65.

Michaelides, M. A., K. M. Parpa, J. Thompson, and B. Brown. 2008. Predicting performance on a firefighter's ability test from fitness parameters. *Res Q Exerc Sport* 79:468–75.

Morris, C. 2012. Evaluation of cardiovascular disease risk factors and physical activity patterns of firefighters. *Master's thesis*. University of Kentucky.

Moulson-Litchfield, M. and P. S. Freedson. 1986. Physical training programs for public safety personnel. *Clin Sports Med* 5:571–87.

Nabeel, I., B. A. Baker, M. P. McGrail Jr, and T. J. Flottemesch. 2007. Correlation between physical activity, fitness, and musculoskeletal injuries in police officers. *Minn Med* 90:40–3.

Nelson, K. V. and A. P. Smith. 2016. Occupational stress, coping and mental health in Jamaican police officers. *Occup Med (Lond)* 66:488–91. 2016 Apr 30. pii: kqw055. [Epub ahead of print].

Pawlak, R., J. L. Clasey, T. Palmer, T. B. Symons, and M. G. Abel. 2015. The effect of a novel tactical training program on physical fitness and occupational performance in firefighters. *J Strength Cond Res* 29:578–88.

Peterson, M. D., D. J. Dodd, B. A. Alvar, M. R. Rhea, and M. Favre. 2008. Undulation training for development of hierarchical fitness and improved firefighter job performance. *J Strength Cond Res* 22:1683–95.

Poplin, G. S., D. J. Roe, J. L. Burgess, W. F. Peate, and R. B. Harris. 2016. Fire fit: Assessing comprehensive fitness and injury risk in the fire service. *Int Arch Occup Environ Health* 89:251–59.

Poplin, G. S., D. J. Roe, W. Peate, R. B. Harris, and J. L. Burgess. 2014. The association of aerobic fitness with injuries in the fire service. *Am J Epidemiol* 179:149–55.

Reichard, A. A. and L. L. Jackson. 2010. Occupational injuries among emergency responders. *Am J Ind Med*. 53:1–11.

Rhodes, E. C. and D. W. Farenholtz. 1992. Police officer's physical abilities test compared to measures of physical fitness. *Can J Sport Sci* 17:226–33.

Ricciardi, R., P. A. Deuster, and L. A. Talbot. 2007. Effects of gender and body adiposity on physiological responses to physical work while wearing body armor. *Mil Med* 172:743–48.

Roberts, M. A., J. O'Dea, A. Boyce, and E. T. Mannix. 2002. Fitness levels of firefighter recruits before and after a supervised exercise training program. *J Strength Cond Res* 16:271–77.

Rossomanno, C. I., J. E. Herrick, S. M. Kirk, and E. P. Kirk. 2012. A 6-month supervised employer-based minimal exercise program for police officers improves fitness. *J Strength Cond Res* 26:2338–44.

Sallis, J. F. and M. F. Hovell. 1990. Determinants of exercise behavior. *Exerc Sport Sci Rev* 18:307–30.

Sorensen, L., J. Smolander, V. Louhevaara, O. Korhonen, and P. Oja. 2000. Physical activity, fitness and body composition of Finnish police officers: A 15-year follow-up study. *Occup Med* 50:3–10.

Soteriades, E. S., R. Hauser, I. Kawachi, D. Liarokapis, D. C. Christiani, and S. N. Kales. 2005. Obesity and cardiovascular disease risk factors in firefighters: A prospective cohort study. *Obes Res* 13:1756–63.

Spiegel, K., R. Leproult, and E. Van Cauter. 1999. Impact of sleep debt on metabolic and endocrine function. *Lancet* 354:1435–39.

Spiegel, K., E. Tasali, P. Penev, and E. Van Cauter. 2004. Brief communication: Sleep curtailment in healthy young men is associated with decreased leptin levels, elevated ghrelin levels, increased hunger and appetite. *Ann Intern Med* 141:846–50.

Spitier, D. L., G. Jones, J. Hawkins, and L. Dudka. 1987. Body composition and physiological characteristics of law enforcement officers. *Br J Sports Med* 21:154–57.

Stamford, B. A., A. Weltman, R. J. Moffatt, and C. Fulco. 1978. Status of police officers with regard to selected cardio-respiratory and body compositional fitness variables. *Med Sci Sports Exerc* 10:294–97.

Tsismenakis A. J., C. A. Christophi, J. W. Burress, A. M. Kinney, M. Kim, and S. N. Kales. 2009. The obesity epidemic and future emergency responders. *Obesity* 17:1648–50.

Tsuji, H., M. G. Larson, F. J. Venditti Jr et al. 1996. Impact of reduced heart rate variability on risk for cardiac events. The Framingham Heart Study. *Circulation* 94:2850–55.

Tunceli, K., K. Li, and L. K. Williams. 2006. Long-term effects of obesity on employment and work limitations among U.S. adults, 1986 to 1999. *Obesity* 14:1637–46.

Violanti, J. M., D. Fekedulegn, M. E. Andrew, L. E. Charles, T. A. Hartley, and C. M. Burchfiel. 2011. Adiposity in policing: Mental health consequences. *Int J Emerg Ment Health* 13:257–66.

Williford, H. N., W. J. Duey, M. S. Olson, R. Howard, and N. Wang. 1999. Relationship between fire-fighting suppression tasks and physical fitness. *Ergonomics* 42:1179–86.

Yang, J., A. Farioli, M. Korre, and S. N. Kales. 2015. Dietary preferences and nutritional information needs among career firefighters in the United States. *Glob Adv Health Med.* 4:16–23.

Section IV

Moderating Factors

15 Dietary Protein and Physical Training Effects on Body Composition and Performance

Michaela C. Devries, Sara Y. Oikawa, and Stuart M. Phillips

CONTENTS

15.1 INTRODUCTION

Skeletal muscle is a vital tissue supporting locomotion and performance for both athletic and functional tasks. Skeletal muscle health can be optimized through performance of both resistance and aerobic exercise and consumption of adequate amounts of protein. When performed regularly, the combination of activity and protein consumption can enhance both athletic and functional performance across the lifespan. Skeletal muscle mass increases in the early years of life and plateaus thereafter, but begins to decline in the fourth or fifth decade of life at a rate of ~0.8% per year (Goodpaster et al. 2006). Furthermore, states of energy restriction for weight loss can also induce a reduction in skeletal muscle mass (Krieger et al. 2006). Declines in muscle mass can negatively impact muscle strength as well as athletic and functional performance both in young and older adults and thus strategies to offset these declines are advantageous. In this chapter, we discuss the role protein and exercise (both aerobic and resistance) play in the optimization of muscle mass and performance under normal conditions (i.e., young, healthy individuals) as well as during periods of acute (i.e., weight loss) and chronic (i.e., aging) muscle catabolism.

15.2 ROLE OF PROTEIN QUALITY AND PROTEIN DOSE ON SKELETAL MUSCLE MASS

Both the quality of protein and the quantity (dose) of protein can affect the rates of muscle protein synthesis (MPS) and muscle protein breakdown (MPB). As such, these variables can affect gains or losses in muscle mass. Thus, here we discuss the influence of both protein quality and protein dose on changes in muscle mass.

15.2.1 ROLE OF PROTEIN QUALITY

Proteins differ in their quality based on their essential amino acid (EAA) content and digestibility (Food and Agriculture Organization of the United Nations (FAO) 2013) as summarized in Table 15.1. Protein quality has been previously defined using the protein digestibility-corrected amino acid score (PDCAAS), which classifies proteins according to their EAA content and level of digestibility relative to a "gold standard" reference protein, which is egg protein (Food and Agriculture Organization of the United Nations (FAO) 2013). Amino acid digestibility is crucial as undigested dietary proteins may be unabsorbed or poorly absorbed and excreted rather than being absorbed in the small intestine and contributing to lean mass accrual or other amino acid-requiring metabolic processes (Rasmussen et al. 2000). Using PDCAAS, proteins with the highest digestibility and quality scores are given a maximum value of 1.0 and include casein, soy, whey, and egg proteins (Hoffman and Falvo 2004). More recently in 2013, FAO recommended the adoption of, as a superior method to PDCAAS, the digestible indispensable amino acid score (DIAAS) to assess protein quality. The DIAAS improves upon the PDCAAS as it is able to distinguish between proteins that were previously classed at an equivalent value by the PDCAAS such as whey, soy, and casein proteins which were all given a score of 1.0 (Rutherfurd et al. 2015). The DIAAS score differs from the PDCAAS as it samples protein digestibility at the distal ileum rather than from fecal matter and also allows for measurement of the digestibility of individual amino acids rather than that of crude protein. Thus, using the DIAAS, proteins that were "undervalued" using

TABLE 15.1
Comparison of Protein Quality Characteristics of Commonly Consumed Proteins

	Whey	Casein	Soy	MPC	Pea	Collagen	Rice
Complete protein	Yes	Yes	Yes	Yes	No	No	No
Limiting AA	–	–	Met + Cys	–	Met + Cys	Trp	Lys
Amino acid content (g/25 g protein)							
Leucine	3.0	2.3	1.5	2.5	2.6	0.8	1.7
ΣEAA	12.4	11.0	9.0	12.1	10.3	3.8	6.5
% EAA	49.6%	44.0%	36.0%	48.4%	41.2%	15.2%	26.0%
PDCAAS	1.0	1.0	1.0	1.0	0.893	0.0	0.419
DIAAS	1.09	1.12	0.906	1.18	0.822	0.0	0.371

Note: DIAAS, Digestible indispensable amino acid score; EAA, essential amino acids; Limiting AA, limiting amino acid (i.e., amino acid less than egg—PDCAAS—or less than the test protein—DIAAS); Lys, lysine; Met, methionine; MPC, milk protein concentrate; PDCAAS, protein digestibility-corrected amino acid score; Trp, tryptophan.

the PDCAAS (whey and casein) now have quality scores of 1.18 and 1.09, respectively while soy protein is now scored at a lower value of 0.91 (Rutherfurd et al. 2015). The revised quality scores are reflective of the higher EAA and ileal digestibility of whey and casein protein in comparison to soy protein. While it is not the limiting amino acid in the protein, it is worth acknowledging that the leucine content of some of these proteins is quite disparate. The relevance of this is that leucine has been shown to be a potent stimulator of MPS via the mechanistic target of rapamycin complex 1 (mTORC1), a 280 kDa serine/threonine kinase known to activate key translation initiation factors involved in regulating MPS (Churchward-Venne et al. 2012). In fact, increasing the leucine content of a lower protein dose has been shown to restore rates of postprandial MPS to that seen with four-times higher protein doses (Churchward-Venne et al. 2012). Additionally, the amino acid content of whey is more readily available to support peripheral tissues after ingestion whereas with soy and casein protein ingestion, a greater percentage of amino acids are directed to splanchnic extraction (Rasmussen et al. 2000). Furthermore, whey protein supplementation results in a higher amino acid peak and stimulation of MPS compared with casein due to its rapid absorption kinetics (Rasmussen et al. 2000). The ability of amino acids to be rapidly available are crucial to driving the processes of MPS as rises in intracellular and extracellular amino acid concentrations regulate the rate of protein building (Bohe et al. 2003).

15.2.2 ROLE OF PROTEIN DOSE

Along with the consideration of protein quality, protein dose is crucial when attempting to maximize MPS. Protein doses are typically described as protein intake per kg body mass per day (g/kg/day). The current recommended dietary allowance (RDA) for protein consumption is 0.8 g protein/kg/day for healthy adults over the age of 18 years; however, a recommended per-meal dose has not been formalized. In healthy younger adults (18–55 years), ~20 grams or 0.24 g/kg/meal of high-quality protein has been shown to be optimal to maximally stimulate MPS in the postprandial and postexercise states (Tipton et al. 1999; Moore et al. 1999, 2015). Doses exceeding this amount do not result in a further increase in MPS, but do increase rates of amino acid oxidation and urea production (Tipton et al. 1999). These results are explained by what has been termed the "muscle full effect" (Bohe et al. 2001), which describes that an upper limit of amino acid delivery must be achieved before amino acids are not used as a substrate for MPS and instead are diverted into processes involving amino acid oxidation (Tipton et al. 1999).

When selecting a protein supplement for the purposes of enhancing or maintaining lean mass it is important to make adjustments for protein dose based on protein quality (Figure 15.1). Previous research has shown that at rest, ~2–3 g of leucine per protein-containing meal is necessary to induce a leucinemia (and increase intracellular leucine concentration) that would maximally stimulate MPS (Tang et al. 2009; Norton et al. 2012), which is often referred to as the "leucine threshold." Therefore, in order to receive an adequate amount of leucine from a protein supplement to maximally stimulate MPS it is important to know the leucine content of the supplement and adjust accordingly. For example, to achieve a leucine dose of 2.5 g, it would be necessary to consume 23 g of whey protein, 31 g of soy protein, or 38 g of wheat protein (Devries and Phillips 2015). When translated into a mixed meal or leucine derived from food sources, doses such as 874 mL of milk, 5 eggs, or 641 g (12.8 servings) of bread would be necessary to acquire 2.5 of leucine. Interestingly, exercise, particularly resistance exercise (RE), appears to reduce the leucine threshold and impart an increased sensitivity to protein (leucine) in young, healthy adults such that less protein is required for a maximal stimulation of MPS, the same is likely true in older adults (Tang et al. 2009).

15.3 RESISTANCE EXERCISE AND PROTEIN CONSUMPTION EFFECTS ON BODY COMPOSITION

Changes in skeletal muscle size are underpinned, in part, by the feeding- and loading-driven changes in MPS and MPB. In the postabsorptive state, MPB exceeds MPS resulting in a state of

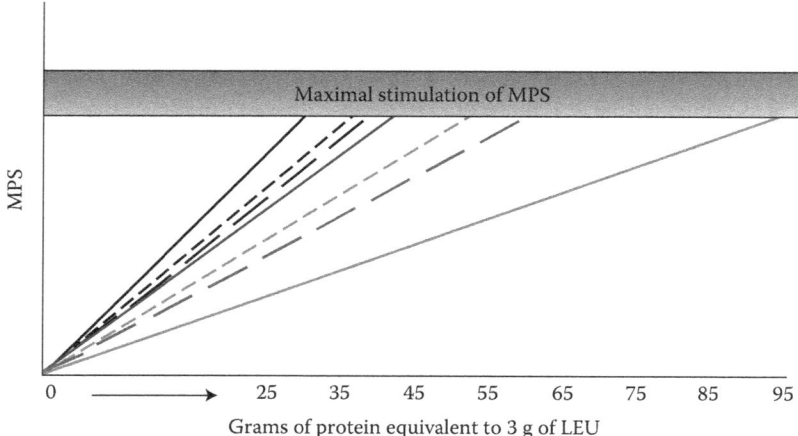

FIGURE 15.1 Doses of protein required to reach maximal stimulation of MPS based on leucine content of 3 g. Lines from left to right are the approximate amounts of whey protein isolate, pea protein, MPC, micellar casein, rice protein, soy protein, and collagen peptide.

net catabolism. Young healthy men and women who consume adequate daily protein on a per-meal basis fluctuate between periods of negative and positive protein balance which remain roughly equal throughout the day resulting in the maintenance of lean body mass (LBM) (Biolo et al. 1995). Changes in the rates of MPS in response to a bout of acute fasted-state RE have been examined with several variations in training stimulus and when performed over the long term, result in lean mass accretion. RE adaptations are a response to mechanical overload. These adaptations occur as a result of chronic RE through the increase in muscle fiber cross-sectional area (CSA) and increases in maximal strength, but are extremely variable ranging 0%–56% and 10%–149%, respectively (Hubal et al. 2005); however, these adaptations can be optimized when nutritional stimulation are combined with RE over a prolonged period (Hartman et al. 2007; Miller et al. 2014). When a sufficient, high-quality dose of protein is consumed following RE there is a synergistic interaction between post-meal hyperaminoacidemia and the contractile stimulus to further augment MPS (Biolo et al. 1995; Glynn et al. 2010). Thus, RE serves to "sensitize" skeletal muscle to the anabolic impact of protein feeding. As such, repeated bouts of RE and protein ingestion often lead to expansion of the skeletal muscle protein pool and thus skeletal muscle hypertrophy. Doses as low as 5 g of high-quality protein are able to significantly increase MPS in healthy young men following RE, however much like in the rested state, do not exert greater effects at doses larger than 20 g or 0.25–0.3 g/kg/meal (Moore et al. 2009, 2015).

Protein ingestion has the ability to maximize the acute MPS response following RE though it is ultimately the sum of frequent episodic bouts of heightened anabolism resulting from chronic resistance training (RT) that are fundamental for the augmentation of lean mass. Several studies have examined the influence of chronic protein supplementation on changes in body composition and performance (Kerksick et al. 2006; Willoughby et al. 2007; Hoffman et al. 2009; Josse et al. 2011) and have shown that protein ingestion enhances RT-induced increases in LBM and strength. Protein quality, as mentioned previously, is crucial to maximize gains in skeletal muscle mass when combined with a potent anabolic stimulus such as RE. The consumption of whey protein has been shown to elicit the greatest responses in muscular hypertrophy and strength when consumed immediately following a bout of exercise over a chronic training period (Volek et al. 2013). Similarly, when participants consumed either soy protein, fluid milk (whey protein and casein protein), or an isoenergetic control, participants consuming milk were able to significantly increase muscle fiber CSA in both type I and type II fibers as well as fat-free-bone-free mass as indicated by dual-energy x-ray absorptiometry (Hartman et al. 2007).

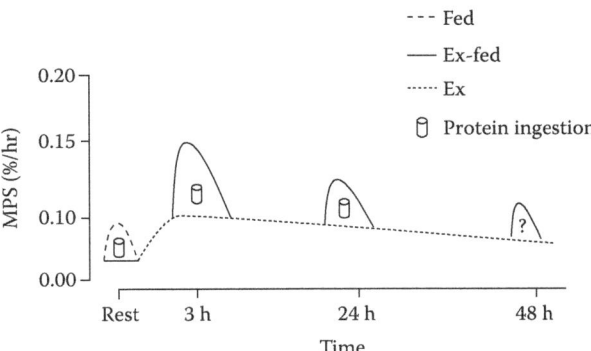

FIGURE 15.2   RE stimulates a prolonged elevation of MPS that can remain elevated for ≥24 hour (dashed lines). Thus, we propose that protein ingestion at any point during this enhanced period of "anabolic potential" will be additive to these already elevated exercise mediated rates (solid line). (Reprinted from Churchward-Venne, T. A. et al. 2012. Nutritional regulation of muscle protein synthesis with resistance exercise: Strategies to enhance anabolism. *Nutr Metab (Lond)* 9:40, http://nutritionandmetabolism.biomedcentral.com/articles/10.1186/1743-7075-9-40.)

Although it is known that protein ingestion enhances RE-induced rates of MPS, the timing of protein ingestion has been shown to mediate the MPS response. Immediate postexercise consumption of high-quality protein serves as an effective strategy to enhance MPS greater than RE alone (Biolo et al. 1997; Tipton et al. 1999; Moore et al. 2009). Timing of protein consumption is of importance as exercise-induced stimulation of MPS is the greatest following exercise (Kumar et al. 2009). This concept has been termed the "anabolic window" wherein a dose of protein, and subsequent hyperaminoacidemia, will have a potent stimulatory effect when consumed in close temporal proximity following the performance of exercise. The duration of this anabolic window is heavily debated, however. For example, it is known that postexercise rates of MPS following a bout of RE last for up to 48 hours (Burd et al. 2010); thus, protein consumed anytime within this window would elicit an enhanced MPS response [(Churchward-Venne et al. 2012), Figure 15.2]. Thus, in our view "immediate" postexercise provision is not necessary to augment gains in muscle mass (Schoenfeld et al. 2013).

15.4   EFFECTS OF EXERCISE AND PROTEIN ON MUSCLE STRENGTH, POWER, AND PERFORMANCE

While muscle mass is important, particularly in the context of aging, it is also important to consider the impact that dietary protein may have on improving muscle function. Thus, in this section we discuss the impact of protein supplementation on muscle function.

15.4.1   PROTEIN CONSUMPTION DURING RESISTANCE TRAINING IMPROVES MUSCLE STRENGTH

Chronic consumption of protein during a period of RT not only increases LBM, but also induces greater gains in muscle strength and power when compared with placebo or isoenergetic carbohydrate supplement (Burke et al. 2001; Cermak et al. 2012; Pasiakos et al. 2015; Snijders et al. 2015). A meta-analysis of studies investigating the effect of supplemental protein on muscle strength gains during prolonged RT (>6 weeks) showed that leg press one repetition maximum (1 RM) increased to a greater extent when supplemental protein was consumed during the training period (Cermak et al. 2012). Importantly, the greater strength gains with protein supplementation were similar in young and older individuals, indicating that protein supplementation can be used to enhance strength gains during RT across the lifespan. However, another systematic review of protein intervention trials found that a minimum training duration of at least 8 weeks is necessary for an effect of protein supplementation on muscle strength gains to become apparent, with no differences between protein and its comparator being found with training durations less than 4 weeks (Pasiakos et al. 2015). The aforementioned systematic review (Pasiakos et al. 2015) only recruited subjects under the age of 50 years and so the minimum RT program duration where differences in protein intake induce greater gains in strength in older adults is not known, but is likely similar.

The benefits of protein supplementation on strength gains are more pronounced in trained as compared with untrained individuals (Cermak et al. 2012; Pasiakos et al. 2015). One reason why the effects of protein supplementation to enhance strength gains in untrained individuals may be blunted is due to neural adaptations that occur at the onset of RT (Moritani and deVries 1979). At the onset of RT the increases in strength are neuromuscular or "skill" oriented and strongly outweigh the effect of protein supplementation and improvements in LBM as a driver of strength (Rasch and Morehouse 1957). However, as the duration and/or frequency of training increases, a benefit of protein supplementation on muscle strength becomes more apparent (Pasiakos et al. 2015). The temporal effect of protein supplementation to enhance muscle strength gains as RT progresses is in line with findings that greater gains (>4-fold) in LBM in response to protein supplementation are seen in trained versus untrained individuals (Cermak et al. 2012). Together these findings suggest that the increase in muscle strength that results from protein supplementation during RT corresponds to the increase in LBM, which is supported by data from a previous study showing that ~76% of the improvements in strength following a period of RT were attributable to muscle hypertrophy (Cribb et al. 2007).

The effect of the timing of protein consumption during a period of RT on muscle strength is another important factor to consider. Consuming protein in the postexercise "anabolic window" has been shown to induce greater gains in muscle strength (Andersen et al. 2005; Candow et al. 2006; Coburn et al. 2006; Josse et al. 2011) and performance (Andersen et al. 2005) following a period of RT as compared with placebo. However, a recent meta-analysis has brought into question the importance of consuming protein in the peri-workout period, showing that protein timing did not induce greater increases in muscle strength (Schoenfeld et al. 2013). In fact, no relationship between daily protein intake and strength gains was found (Schoenfeld et al. 2013). As detailed above, given that anabolic sensitivity is enhanced for up to 48 hours following a bout of RE (Burd et al. 2010), it is not surprising that consumption of protein in the 1–2 hours peri-workout period did not result in greater gains in muscle strength; however, the lack of relationship between overall protein intake and muscle strength gains during RT found in this meta-analysis are perplexing (Schoenfeld et al. 2013). Thus, while it is pragmatic to begin the recovery process as soon as exercise is complete the provision of immediate protein to stimulate MPS is not an absolute requirement.

As is the case for muscle hypertrophy, the type of protein consumed can also influence the strength gains induced by RT. A study by Cribb et al. (2006) found that whey protein supplementation during a 12-week RT protocol induced greater gains in strength as compared with casein protein. Furthermore, a study by Hartman et al. (2007) found that consumption of 35 g of milk protein (consisting of whey and casein proteins) postexercise during 12 weeks of RT resulted in greater increases in LBM with a trend toward a greater increase in muscle strength as compared with soy protein (p = 0.08). However, not all trials have found differential effects of different proteins on muscle strength (Candow et al. 2006; Joy et al. 2013). A possible explanation for the lack of beneficial effect of whey, as compared with other forms of supplemental protein, during RT in these studies may be due to the already high pre-intervention consumption of dietary protein by participants in the trial [i.e. 25% of energy intake (Joy et al. 2013) or 1.6–1.9 g/kg BW/day (Candow et al. 2006)].

15.4.2 Protein Consumption during Resistance Training or Sport-Specific Training Improves Muscle Performance

Protein consumption during an RT program or a program of sport-specific training improves muscle performance. When isoenergetic protein or carbohydrate (CHO) were consumed for 14 weeks before and after thrice weekly RT sessions, greater increases in squat jump performance were found in the protein-consuming group in comparison to the control group (Andersen et al. 2005). Similarly, whey protein consumption before and after combined anaerobic and RT induced greater gains in strength and agility, but not vertical or broad jump performance in elite female basketball players as compared with a CHO control (Taylor et al. 2016). Furthermore, elite judo athletes undergoing pre-season training (consisting of endurance, speed, and RT) who received soy protein supplementation (0.5 g/kg/day) for 4 weeks had greater gains in maximal aerobic capacity ($VO_{2\,peak}$) and maximum power output during a Wingate bike test (measure of peak anaerobic power) as compared with a training-only control group (Laskowski and Antosiewicz 2003). Importantly, when training continued for 3 months without protein supplementation no difference in aerobic or anaerobic capacity were seen between the two groups suggestive of the importance of continued protein supplementation to maintain performance enhancements. The enhancements in performance tasks with protein consumption in athletes could lead to improved event performance/finishes and indicate that protein supplementation may be an advantageous ergogenic strategy for elite athletes.

15.5   AEROBIC EXERCISE AND PROTEIN CONSUMPTION EFFECTS ON BODY COMPOSITION

It has been proposed that protein requirements for endurance athletes should be similar to those of a recreationally active population (Moore 2015). Nonetheless, requirement in the sense of off-setting deficiency is not the same concept as protein to promote optimal adaptation. Thus, an elevated (i.e., greater than the RDA) protein intake appears to be required in order to optimally adapt and perform maximally during endurance exercise training. Ingestion of both CHO prior to or following and protein following endurance exercise are necessary to enhance muscle glycogen resynthesis and aid in the remodeling of skeletal muscle proteins, respectively. For example, when consuming a mixed CHO and protein beverage, levels of plasma insulin were higher than when consuming an isocaloric CHO beverage following 2 hours of recovery from endurance exercise, which is indicative of an environment that would promote greater rates of muscle glycogen repletion. Results confirming this hypothesis have, however, been mixed with many studies lacking statistical power and using conditions where CHO delivery has not been optimal (McLellan et al. 2014). Fluid milk has also been examined as a cost-effective and convenient alternative to protein supplementation in endurance athletes as it contains both CHO as well as high-quality proteins (whey and casein) that optimize aminoacidemia; however, as with previous studies examining the acute effects of protein consumption with aerobic bouts, much conflicting evidence exists (McLellan et al. 2014).

Nitrogen balance studies in endurance training (ET) men have shown that endurance exercise results in similar rates of protein turnover as RE, which result from a greater breakdown and oxidation of amino acids (Forslund et al. 1999; Tarnopolsky 2004). Thus, despite a lesser need for amino acids for muscle building (hypertrophy) with endurance exercise, amino acids are required following endurance exercise to remodel skeletal muscle through increases in mitochondrial protein synthesis (augmenting aerobic capacity) (Moore 2015) and increases in myofibrillar protein synthesis to increase force-generating capacity. It has been proposed that individuals who engage in chronic ET require protein intakes between 1.2 and 1.7 g/kg/day in comparison to the RDA of 0.8 g/kg/day (Moore 2015). Currently, a limited number of published studies exist surrounding the effects of prolonged protein supplementation on body composition or performance when combined with chronic ET. Knowing the potentiating effects of protein supplementation when combined with RE on MPS, it could be hypothesized that the consumption of high-quality protein following ET could possibly result in a more efficient repair/remodeling of protein structures within muscle with a possible increase in mitochondrial density due to the effects of amino acids on mitochondrial protein synthesis. No study has addressed these effects at both the recreational or elite athlete level.

15.6 EFFECTS OF EXERCISE AND INCREASED PROTEIN INTAKE DURING WEIGHT LOSS

Diet (energy restriction) and exercise alone or in combination are integral to weight loss. Typical energy restriction diets not only induce decreases in total body weight, but also in lean mass (~20%–25% of total weight loss) (Krieger et al. 2006), which is mostly due to loss of LBM (Weinheimer et al. 2010). This is obviously not ideal given the important role skeletal muscle plays in glucose storage, metabolic rate, locomotion, and performance. Furthermore, given the relationship between LBM and resting metabolic rate, the progressive loss of lean mass and ensuing decrease in resting metabolic rate that accompanies typical weight loss can eventually lead to an inability to lose weight and/or induce weight regain (Westerterp-Plantenga et al. 2009). The decline in LBM during weight loss is at least in part due to energy restriction-induced declines in myofibrillar MPS (Areta et al. 2014). Recent evidence has evaluated the effectiveness of different types of diet and exercise regimes to promote "high quality" weight loss, defined as weight loss with a high ratio of fat to LBM loss. Energy restriction regimes incorporating higher protein intakes and/or RT have been shown to attenuate the loss of LBM while maximizing the loss of fat mass (FM) during weight loss (Clark 2015).

15.6.1 HIGHER PROTEIN-CONTAINING DIETS PROMOTE "HIGH QUALITY" WEIGHT LOSS AND IMPROVED WEIGHT MAINTENANCE

Higher protein diets are defined as diets providing 25%–35% of energy intake (Clifton and Keogh 2007) and have been found to promote greater losses in body weight and FM and attenuate the loss of LBM during energy restriction as compared with standard protein diets [12%–18% energy intake (Ein) (Clifton and Keogh 2007)] (Krieger et al. 2006; Wycherley et al. 2012; Pasiakos et al. 2013). A recent meta-analysis of trials comparing high (30% Ein) versus standard (17% Ein) protein intakes during energy restriction found that higher protein diets induced more favorable changes in body composition as evidenced by greater losses in total body mass and FM as well as an attenuated loss in LBM in the high protein diet group (Wycherley et al. 2012). Importantly, in this meta-analysis , while the higher protein diets provided ~30% of Ein from protein, given that these diets were energy restricted, the mean relative protein intake in the higher-protein group was 1.25 g/kgBW/day, which is in line with the protein intake of much the general population under the age of 55 during energy balance [~1.3 g/kgBW/day (Fulgoni 2008)]. Thus, energy restricted, higher protein diets truly represent diets that maintain habitual protein intakes while reducing CHO and/or fat intake. Given the importance of LBM to resting metabolic rate (Müller et al. 2013), the maintenance of LBM during weight loss is key to successful weight loss and maintenance and highlights the importance of consuming higher protein during energy restriction.

Consumption of a higher protein diet during weight maintenance following weight loss may also be advantageous, decreasing the propensity for weight regain. In overweight/obese adults who had undergone 8 weeks of energy restriction to induce an 11 kg reduction in body weight, weight regain in the subsequent 12 months was lower in those consuming an *ad libitum* higher protein (23% Ein) as compared with *ad libitum* lower protein (16% Ein) diet (Aller et al. 2014). Similarly, during 6 months of weight maintenance following a 7.5% decrease in total body weight, subjects who had a higher protein intake (1.3 g/kgBW/day) regained less body weight (0.8 kg vs. 3.0 kg) than those who had a lower protein intake [1.06 g/kgBW/day, (Lejeune et al. 2005)]. Furthermore, during weight maintenance FM and waist circumference continued to decrease and LBM increased in the higher protein group such that the weight regain in the higher protein group was completely attributed to an increase in LBM (Lejeune et al. 2005). In contrast, FM in the lower protein group increased and constituted over 50% (1.7 kg) of the weight that was regained (Lejeune et al. 2005). These findings highlight the importance of sustained higher protein intakes to promote weight maintenance and improved body composition following weight loss.

There are several mechanisms by which higher protein diets promote higher quality weight loss including an attenuated decline in resting energy expenditure (REE) that accompanies weight loss (Whitehead et al. 1996), which may promote further weight loss and/or aid in the prevention of weight regain. Indeed, higher protein consumption during weight maintenance following weight loss has also been shown to attenuate the decline in REE in overweight/obese young adults (Ebbeling et al. 2012). The maintenance of REE with higher protein diets is the result of a direct effect of protein to increase diet-induced energy expenditure (Westerterp et al. 1999), which in turn increases REE [~3%, (Mikkelsen et al. 2000)] as well as the maintenance of LBM via protein-induced stimulation of MPS (Hector et al. 2015).

Higher protein diets also likely promote greater weight loss through their satiating effect, whereby they reduce hunger and *ad libitum* food intake (Skov et al. 1999). In fact, as compared with the American Heart Association (AHA) phase I diet, a low-glycemic index, low-fat, high-protein diet consumed *ad libitum* for 6 days resulted in a 25% decrease in energy intake (Dumesnil et al. 2001). The decreased energy intake induced by the higher protein diet resulted in a 2.3 kg loss in body weight over the 6-day intervention period, compared with no loss with AHA diet (Dumesnil et al. 2001). In a longer-term trial, Weigle et al. (2005) showed that a higher protein-containing diet (~30% of total energy intake as protein) induced greater satiety when compared with an isocaloric lower protein diet (15%). Furthermore, when the participants were instructed to consume the higher protein diet *ad libitum* for 12 weeks they consumed ~500 kcal less per day as compared with their usual weight maintenance diet, and total body mass and FM decreased by 4.9 and 3.7 kg, respectively over the *ad libitum* eating period.

The type of protein consumed is also an important consideration. Higher protein intake during weight loss sustains LBM through maintained stimulation of MPS. As detailed above, higher quality proteins such as whey protein, have the greatest ability to stimulate MPS (Tang et al. 2009; Burd et al. 2012; Yang et al. 2012a) and thus might be able to prevent the decline in fasted and/or fed state MPS that is seen with energy restriction (Pasiakos et al. 2010). Indeed, whey protein supplementation during 2 weeks of energy restriction was able to attenuate the decline in feeding-induced MPS (−9%) as compared to soy (−28%) and CHO (−31%) supplementation (Hector et al. 2015), which may result in greater lean mass retention during weight loss. In fact, as compared with a control diet, whey protein was better able to promote weight and FM loss, whereas soy protein was not, when incorporated into an *ad libitum* diet in overweight/obese adults (Baer et al. 2011). Furthermore, higher quality proteins can stimulate MPS to a greater extent with lower doses (Yang et al. 2012b), which would allow for optimal stimulation to occur with a lower energy intake, which is of importance when one is trying to maintain LBM while inducing an energy deficit.

15.6.2 EXERCISE-INDUCED WEIGHT LOSS AND RESISTANCE TRAINING-INDUCED LEAN MASS RETENTION

Exercise is another strategy that can induce an energy deficit to promote weight loss. The American College of Sports Medicine Position Stand (Donnelly et al. 2009) states that, at a population level, >150 minutes/week of physical activity can induce modest weight loss and that physical activity of 225–420 minutes/week can induce substantial weight loss. Both aerobic exercise and RE can induce weight loss; however, aerobic exercise has been shown to induce greater losses in total body mass and FM whereas RE attenuates declines in LBM (Willis et al. 2012). A recent meta-analysis found that both ET and RT can induce weight loss; however, the analysis indicated that RT was better than ET to preserve LBM during weight loss (Clark 2015). The meta-analysis also reported that high intensity exercise, which for RT meant 2–4 sets of 6–10 repetitions at ≥75% 1 RM and for ET meant either intervals or steady-states exercise with intensities ≥70% of VO_2peak, had a greater effect on changes in body composition than lower intensities (Clark 2015).

As a fundamentally anabolic stimulus, RT is better able to preserve LBM during weight loss because it stimulates myofibrillar MPS (Wilkinson et al. 2008; Burd et al. 2010; Bell et al. 2015), whereas aerobic exercise stimulates mitochondrial MPS (Wilkinson et al. 2008). Indeed, the reduction in myofibrillar MPS induced by energy restriction can be rescued by RE (Areta et al. 2014). Intriguingly, data from our laboratory has shown that low-loads lifted to failure induce greater increases in myofibrillar MPS (Burd et al. 2010) and similar gains in LBM during RT (Mitchell et al. 2012; Morton et al. 2016), suggesting that lower-loads lifted to failure should be at least as effective as higher-load RE in the maintenance of LBM during weight loss. However, this conclusion is discordant to the data from the meta-analysis discussed above where heavier loads had more favorable effects on body composition (Clark 2015). Studies investigating the use of lower-loads lifted to failure during energy deficit are needed to establish whether lower-loads can be an effective strategy to prevent lean mass loss during weight loss. Interestingly, recent data has shown that high-intensity interval training (HIIT) can also stimulate myofibrillar MPS, though not to the same magnitude as RE, in older men (Bell et al. 2015), suggesting that HIIT may also be effective at maintaining lean mass during weight loss.

Exercise also plays a critical role in the maintenance of weight loss. In fact, a descriptive study examining factors contributing to sustained weight loss found that those individuals who had maintained weight loss for at least 5 years reported high levels of physical activity, expending ~2800 kcal/week through physical activity (Klem et al. 1997). There appears to be a minimally effective dose of activity whereby those who perform greater amounts of physical activity are more successful at maintaining weight loss such that those performing >200 minutes/week of physical activity experience very little weight regain (Jakicic et al. 2003, 2008). Together these findings indicate that exercise is an important strategy to promote weight loss and prevent weight regain.

15.6.3 THE COMBINATION OF HIGHER PROTEIN INTAKE AND EXERCISE DURING ENERGY DEFICIT IS BETTER THAN EITHER MODALITY ALONE

The effects of diet and exercise in combination to promote weight loss are better than either modality alone. Several studies have shown that the consumption of higher protein paired with exercise training during an energy deficit induces greater FM loss and lean mass preservation. Josse et al. (2011) found that higher protein (30% Ein), high dairy (15% Ein) consumption plus combined aerobic and RT during 16 weeks of energy deficit induced greater losses in FM than those in the adequate protein (15% Ein), medium dairy (7.5% Ein) or adequate protein (15% Ein), low dairy (<2% Ein) groups in overweight/obese women. Furthermore, those in the higher protein group not only maintained, but gained lean mass during the intervention period; whereas those in the adequate protein, medium dairy group maintained lean mass and those in the adequate protein, low dairy group lost lean mass (Josse et al. 2011). The findings from this study show not only the importance of higher protein diets to promote high-quality weight loss, but the importance of protein quality whereby despite equal protein intakes, those who consumed high-quality dairy protein maintained lean mass during weight loss whereas those who maintained their usual dairy intake (<2% Ein) lost lean mass during weight loss (Josse et al. 2011). Similarly, Longland et al. (2016) found that consumption of 2.4 g protein/kgBW/day along with intense exercise training during significant energy deficit (~40% reduction Ein) was more effective than 1.2 g protein/kgBW/day at inducing losses in FM and gains in LBM. Importantly, lean mass was maintained and FM lost in the group consuming 1.2 g protein/kgBW/day (Longland et al. 2016), indicating protein consumption at the lower level was appropriate to offset the declines in LBM induced by energy deficit. However, the group consuming 2.4 g protein/kgBW/day actually gained 1.2 kg of lean mass, which shows that even higher protein intakes would be required, in combination with resistive exercise, to allow lean mass gain. Furthermore, a recent meta-analysis showed that the combination of diet and ET enhanced total weight loss and the combination of diet and RT enhanced FM loss and retention of LBM (Clark 2015). Taken together these findings suggest that higher protein intakes paired with exercise training during energy deficit are ideal for promoting FM loss while preventing lean mass losses.

15.7 EFFECT OF EXERCISE AND PROTEIN ON THE MAINTENANCE OF MUSCLE MASS AND STRENGTH IN AGING

Aging is characterized by a progressive loss of muscle mass and strength and function termed sarcopenia (Cruz-Jentoft et al. 2010). Low levels of muscle mass increase the risk of falls (Landi et al. 2012; Scott et al. 2014) and decrease the ability to perform activities of daily living [ADL (Velazquez Alva Mdel et al. 2013; da Silva Alexandre et al. 2014)], resulting in a loss of independence and a decreased quality of life. As such, strategies to enhance retention of muscle mass, strength, and functional performance in aging adults is of utmost importance. Strategies involving increasing protein intake, RE, and their combination have been shown to improve muscle health in this population.

15.7.1 Older Adults Should Consume More Protein to Attenuate Lean Mass Losses That Accompany Aging

Consumption of protein increases MPS and decreases MPB and in a weight-stable individual results in maintenance of muscle mass over time. With aging the MPS response to protein feeding is blunted and whereas it has been shown that 0.24 g protein/kgBW is needed to maximally stimulate MPS in younger men, 0.4 g protein/kgBW is needed to maximally stimulate MPS in older men (Moore et al. 2015). As a result, older adults require greater amounts of protein to maintain muscle mass and it has been recommended that they consume between 1.0 and 1.5 g protein/kgBW/day (Wolfe et al. 2008; Bauer et al. 2013). Unfortunately, older adults are not consuming this level of protein and in fact, 40% are not meeting the RDA (0.8 g/kgBW/day) and 10% of older women are not even consuming protein at the level of the estimated average requirement (0.66 g/kg/day; EAR) (Houston et al. 2008; Volpi et al. 2013).

Higher protein intakes in older adults have been shown to be protective against weight loss (Stookey et al. 2005) and loss of lean mass (Houston et al. 2008). Furthermore, when protein (15 g at breakfast and lunch) was supplemented into the diet of frail older adults for 24 weeks there were improvements in muscle strength and physical performance (Tieland et al. 2012). Given the blunted MPS response to protein feeding in older adults, protein quality is an especially important consideration. Studies from our laboratory (Burd et al. 2012; Yang et al. 2012b) have shown whey protein to be superior to casein and soy proteins in acutely increasing MPS in response to feeding in older adults, which over time could lead to a greater attenuation of lean mass loss. Indeed, while 20 g of whey protein was able to increase MPS rates above basal levels, with no further increase with 40 g, up to 40 g of soy protein was unable to increase MPS rates above basal levels in older adults (Yang et al. 2012b). Similarly, ingestion of 20 g of whey protein resulted in a 65% greater MPS response than 20 g of micellar casein protein in older men (Burd et al. 2012). Taken together with the fact that many older adults are not consuming adequate amounts of protein to maintain lean mass, these findings suggest that protein supplements, particularly whey protein supplements, or protein enriched foods may be an effective strategy to offset lean mass losses that accompany aging.

How protein is consumed throughout the day is also an important consideration. In North America (and much of Europe), adults typically consume protein in a skewed manner throughout the day with suboptimal "doses" being consumed at breakfast and lunch and the majority (~75%) of protein being consumed at dinner (Berner et al. 2013). As a result, even if an older adult is consuming adequate amounts of protein for their age (i.e., at least 1.0 g/kgBW/day), the distribution of protein is such that MPS will only rise slightly, if at all, in response to breakfast and lunch and the protein consumed above the 0.4 g/kgBW threshold to maximally stimulate MPS at the dinner meal, while maximally stimulatory for MPS, is more than is required. Recent recommendations state that older adults should consume protein in a balanced manner throughout the day (~30 g/meal) in order to repeatedly increase MPS throughout the day (Paddon-Jones and Rasmussen 2009; Bauer et al. 2013). Indeed, employing this method a recent study showed that balanced consumption of protein throughout the day was better able to maintain rates of MPS during energy restriction than a skewed protein intake in older adults (Murphy et al. 2015). Not all studies have shown that balanced protein distribution is superior to a skewed distribution (Arnal et al. 1999; Bouillanne et al. 2013); however, these findings are not surprising given that the per-meal doses of protein provided to the balanced group were suboptimal (<20 g/meal). Together, these findings suggest that older adults require a greater amount of protein (1.0–1.5 g/kgBW/day) than their younger counterparts and this protein should be consumed in a balanced manner (~0.4 g/kgBW/meal) throughout the day to help maintain LBM (Murphy et al. 2016). Furthermore, consideration should be given to the quality of protein consumed as greater per-meal doses of lower quality proteins (>0.4 g/kgBW/meal) would be required to induce similar increases in MPS when compared with higher quality proteins (Murphy et al. 2016).

15.7.2 RESISTANCE TRAINING IS AN INTEGRAL STRATEGY TO INCREASE MUSCLE MASS AND STRENGTH IN OLDER ADULTS

The primary adaptations induced by RT are increases in muscle mass and strength. Despite a progressive decline in muscle mass and strength with aging, significant gains in these outcomes as well as functional performance are achieved in older adults upon adoption of an RT regime (Liu and Latham 2009; Peterson et al. 2010, 2011; Steib et al. 2010; Tschopp et al. 2011; Cruz-Jentoft et al. 2014 Silva et al. 2014), decreasing the risk of falls, fractures, and loss of independence. Furthermore, RT in older adults has been deemed safe (Liu and Latham 2009; Tschopp et al. 2011), which together with its effectiveness has led to the recommendation that progressive RT be performed by older adults to prevent sarcopenia (Peterson and Gordon 2011; Cruz-Jentoft et al. 2014). Unfortunately, most older adults do not meet the current recommendations for RT (Kraschnewski et al. 2014).

One of the main effects of RT is to induce muscle hypertrophy. Given the progressive loss of muscle mass that occurs with aging, the ability of RT to attenuate this loss is an attractive health strategy. In fact, while normal aging is associated with an ~0.8%/year decline in LBM (Phillips 2009), 12 weeks of RT has been shown to increase leg lean mass by 6% (Verdijk et al. 2009). A meta-analysis that included data from 49 studies and 1328 subjects found that RT was able to induce a 1.1 kg increase in LBM in older adults between the ages of 50–83 years (Peterson et al. 2011). A subsequent meta-regression revealed that of the training variables assessed (training intensity, volume, and frequency), only training volume was a significant predictor of LBM changes, with greater training volumes inducing greater gains in LBM (Peterson et al. 2011). Importantly, age was determined to be a significant predictor of LBM change as well with older men and women gaining less LBM in response to RT (Peterson et al. 2011), indicating that while RT can attenuate the decline in muscle mass that accompanies aging, it cannot completely overcome biological aging. This is not to say that the very old (i.e., >85 years) will not benefit from RT, but that they will not respond as readily as those in their early aging (i.e., 65–85) years. However, as compared with age-matched, sedentary individuals, the resistance trained very old would still be at a lower risk for sarcopenia, falls, and loss of independence.

A full review of the mechanism by which RT increases LBM is beyond the scope of this chapter and the reader is directed to the following reviews (Phillips 2009; Atherton et al. 2015). Briefly, however, with RE a mechanical overload stress is applied to the muscle, which triggers a signaling cascade that results in an increase in MPS. In older adults a single bout of RE increases myofibrillar MPS for at least 48 hours (Bell et al. 2015), which when repeated over numerous bouts (training) results in muscle hypertrophy. Traditionally, it has been suggested that moderate loads (70%–85% 1 RM) lifted for 8–12 repetitions per set for 1–3 sets should be performed to induce the greatest increase in LBM (Kraemer et al. 2002). However, recent work has challenged this dogma, at least in young individuals, by showing that low-loads (30% 1 RM) when lifted to failure induce similar increases in myofibrillar MPS immediately following exercise and result in a more sustained MPS response (24 hours) than high-loads (90% 1 RM) (Burd et al. 2010). Furthermore, when applied over a period of RT, a similar muscle hypertrophic response is seen with low- and high-loads when lifted to failure (Mitchell et al. 2012). These findings are in line with the meta-analysis conducted by Peterson et al. (2011) who showed that training volume, but not intensity (i.e., heavier vs. lighter loads) was a significant predictor of lean mass gains in response to RT. These findings have implications for the development of RT strategies to increase LBM in older adults, given that lifting low, as compared with high, loads may be preferred by older adults, particularly if they have any musculoskeletal injury or disorder, putting them at a lower risk for injury.

Importantly, the increase in LBM induced by RT in older adults is accompanied by improvements in muscle strength and functional performance. Strength gains in the magnitude of ~25%–35% are typically found following a period of progressive RT in older adults (Peterson et al. 2010). Given the established relationship between leg strength and survival in older adults (Newman et al. 2006), the improvement in muscle strength is one of the most important adaptations to RT. Furthermore, improvements in gait speed, walking distance, balance, and other functional performance tasks (i.e., timed up-and-go, chair rise) are also found following RT (Liu and Latham 2009; Peterson et al. 2010, 2011a; Steib et al. 2010; Howe et al. 2011; Tschopp et al. 2011; Cruz-Jentoft et al. 2014; Silva et al. 2014) and are directly related to the ability to perform ADL and maintain independence. Together, the advantageous effects of RT on muscle mass, strength and functional performance in older adults provide firm evidence supporting the important role of RT in the maintenance of muscle health in older adults. Unfortunately, as noted above, most older adults do not meet the current recommendations for RT (Kraschnewski et al. 2014). Thus, knowledge translation and behavioral modification strategies to increase participation in RT in this population are needed.

15.7.3 The Combination of Higher Protein Intakes and Resistance Training Is Better than Either Modality Alone to Enhance Muscular Health of Older Adults

Similar to our previous message in weight loss, combined RT and higher protein intakes in older adults act in a synergistic manner, resulting in greater adaptations than either strategy alone. In fact, it has been found that, compared to placebo, the addition of protein either via supplementation or incorporation into the habitual diet during RT induces greater increases in LBM and strength in older adults (Cermak et al. 2012). Protein quality remains important here as well with ingestion of whey protein inducing a greater increase in MPS following a bout of RE in older adults as compared to soy (Yang et al. 2012b) and casein (Burd et al. 2012) proteins. Indeed, while 20 and 40 g of whey protein increased MPS rates in older adults following a bout of RE, an increase in MPS above basal levels was only seen with soy protein when 40 g was consumed (Yang et al. 2012a, b). While not confirmed in older adults, this difference in MPS response to different protein sources has been shown to align with the muscle hypertrophic response to protein consumption during RT (Hartman et al. 2007; Wilkinson et al. 2007), with consumption of milk (a 1:4 blend of whey and casein protein) inducing a greater increase in MPS postexercise and a greater increase in LBM following training as compared with isonitrogenous soy protein. These findings indicate that older adults should consume at least 20 g of whey protein (or at least 40 g of soy protein) following a bout of RE in order to induce an appreciable MPS response. Furthermore, given that 40 g of whey protein induced a greater MPS response than 20 g, consumption of 40 g of whey protein following RE may lead to even greater increases in muscle mass in older adults during RT. Additionally, given that the MPS response to 40 g of whey protein was greater than that of 40 g of soy protein it is likely that higher doses of soy protein would induce a greater MPS response and thus to induce an optimal MPS response following RE it is likely that upward of 60 g (or more) of soy protein would be needed. Given the lower appetite and protein intakes of older adults, these findings highlight the logistical issues that surround the use of lower quality proteins to support muscle hypertrophy in older adults during RT. In summary, these findings emphasize the importance of adequate protein consumption and RT to the optimization of muscle mass, strength, and functional performance in older adults. Unfortunately, as noted above, older adults are not consuming protein at the levels recommended here and nor are they participating in RE and thus are not realizing the potential to have full muscle health. The incorporation of increased protein intake and/or RT could have a profound effect on the health of older adults, decreasing risk of sarcopenia, improving functional performance, preventing falls, and maintaining independence.

15.8 CONCLUSION

Skeletal muscle mass is an integral tissue vital for locomotion, athletic performance, and the ability to perform ADL. Exercise is key to the optimal function of skeletal muscle with aerobic activities enhancing muscle endurance and RE enhancing muscle strength, both of which can have a profound impact on athletic and functional performance. The consumption of protein acts in a synergistic manner enhancing the muscles response to exercise. The maintenance of muscle mass during weight loss and aging is crucial to optimal health and can be achieved by increasing protein consumption and performing RE. As such, exercise training and adequate protein consumption should be encouraged particularly in older persons.

REFERENCES

Aller, E., T. Larsen, H. Claus et al. 2014. Weight loss maintenance in overweight subjects on ad libitum diets with high or low protein content and glycemic index: The DIOGENES trial 12-month results. *Int J Obes (Lond)* 38:1511–7.

Andersen, L. L., G. Tufekovic, M. K. Zebis et al. 2005. The effect of resistance training combined with timed ingestion of protein on muscle fiber size and muscle strength. *Metabolism* 54:151–6.

Areta, J., L. Burke, D. Camera et al. 2014. Reduced resting skeletal muscle protein synthesis is rescued by resistance exercise and protein ingestion following short-term energy deficit. *Am J Physiol Endocrinol Metab* 306:E989–97.

Arnal, M., L. Mosoni, Y. Boirie et al. 1999. Protein pulse feeding improves protein retention in elderly women. *Am J Clin Nutr* 69:1202–08.

Atherton, P. J., B. E. Phillips, and D. J. Wilkinson. 2015. Exercise and regulation of protein metabolism. In *Progress in Molecular Biology and Translational Science*, ed. C. Bouchard, 75–98. The Netherlands, UK: Caister Academic Press.

Baer, D., K. Stote, D. Paul, G. Harris, W. Rumpler, and B. Clevidence. 2011. Whey protein but not soy protein supplementation alters body weight and composition in free-living overweight and obese adults. *J Nutr* 141:1489–94.

Bauer, J., G. Biolo, T. Cederholm et al. 2013. Evidence-based recommendation for optimal dietary protein intake in older people: A position paper from the PROT-AGE Study Group. *J Am Med Dir Assoc* 14:542–59.

Bell, K. E., C. Seguin, G. Parise, S. K. Baker, and S. M. Phillips. 2015. Day-to-day changes in muscle protein synthesis in recovery from resistance, aerobic, and high-intensity interval exercise in older men. *J Gerontol A Biol Sci Med Sci* 70:1024–9.

Berner, L., G. Becker, M. Wise, and J. Doi. 2013. Characterization of dietary protein among older adults in the United States: Amount, animal sources, and meal patterns. *J Acad Nutr Diet* 113:809–15.

Biolo, G., S. P. Maggi, B. D. Williams, K. D. Tipton, and R. R. Wolfe. 1995. Increased rates of muscle protein turnover and amino acid transport after resistance exercise in humans. *Am J Physiol Endocrinol Metab* 268:E514–20.

Biolo, G., K. D. Tipton, S. Klein, and R. R. Wolfe. 1997. An abundant supply of amino acids enhances the metabolic effect of exercise on muscle protein. *Am J Physiol Endocrinol Metab* 273:E122–9.

Bohe, J., A. Low, R. R. Wolfe, and M. J. Rennie. 2001. Latency and duration of stimulation of human muscle protein synthesis during continuous infusion of amino acids. *J Physiol* 532:757–79.

Bohe, J., A. Low, R. R. Wolfe, and M. J. Rennie. 2003. Human muscle protein synthesis is modulated by extracellular, not intramuscular amino acid availability: A dose-response study. *J Physiol* 552:315–24.

Bouillanne, O., E. Curis, B. Hamon-Vilcot et al. 2013. Impact of protein pulse feeding on lean mass in malnourished and at-risk hospitalized elderly patients: A randomized controlled trial. *Clin Nutr* 32:186–92.

Burd, N., D. West, A. Staples et al. 2010. Low-load high volume resistance exercise stimulates muscle protein synthesis more than high-load low volume resistance exercise in young men. *PLoS One* 5:e12033.

Burd, N. A., Y. Yang, D. R. Moore, J. Tang, M. Tarnopolsky, and S. Phillips. 2012. Greater stimulation of myofibrillar protein synthesis with ingestion of whey protein isolate v. micellar casein at rest and after resistance exercise in elderly men. *Br J Nutr* 108:958–62.

Burke, D., P. Chilibeck, K. Davidson, D. Candow, J. Farthing, and T. Smith-Palmer. 2001. The effect of whey protein supplementation with and without creatine monohydrate combined with resistance training on lean tissue mass and muscle strength. *Int J Sport Nutr Exerc Metab* 11:349364.

Candow, D., N. Burke, T. Smith-Palmer, and D. Burke. 2006. Effect of whey and soy protein supplementation combined with resistance training in young adults. *Int J Sport Nutr Exerc Metab* 16:233–44.

Cermak, N., P. Res, L. de Groot, H. Saris, and L. van Loon. 2012. Protein supplementation augments the adaptive response of skeletal muscle to resistance-type exercise training: A meta-analysis. *Am J Clin Nutr* 96:1454–64.

Churchward-Venne, T. A., N. Burd, and S. Phillips. 2012. Nutritional regulation of muscle protein synthesis with resistance exercise: Strategies to enhance anabolism. *Nutr Metab (Lond)* 9:40.

Clark, J. 2015. Diet, exercise or diet with exercise: Comparing the effectiveness of treatment options for weight-loss and changes in fitness for adults (18–65 years old) who are overfat, or obese; systematic review and meta-analysis. *J Diabetes Metab Disord* 14:31.

Clifton, P. and J. Keogh. 2007. Metabolic effects of high-protein diets. *Curr Atheroscler Rep* 9:472–8.

Coburn, J., D. Housh, T. Housh et al. 2006. Effects of leucine and whey protein supplementation during eight weeks of unilateral resistance training. *J Strength Cond Res* 20:284–91.

Cribb, P., A. Williams, M. Carey, and A. Hayes. 2006. The effect of whey isolate and resistance training on strength, body composition, and plasma glutamine. *Int J Sport Nutr Exerc Metab* 16:494–509.

Cribb, P., A. Williams, C. Stathis, M. Carey, and A. Hayes. 2007. Effects of whey isolate, creatine, and resistance training on muscle hypertrophy. *Med Sci Sports Exer* 39:298–307.

Cruz-Jentoft, A., J. Baeyens, J. Bauer et al. 2010. Sarcopenia: European consensus on definition and diagnosis: Report of the European Working Group on Sarcopenia in Older People. *Age Ageing* 39:412–23.

Cruz-Jentoft, A. J., F. Landi, S. M. Schneider et al. 2014. Prevalence of and interventions for sarcopenia in ageing adults: A systematic review. Report of the International Sarcopenia Initiative (EWGSOP and IWGS). *Age Ageing* 43:748–59.

da Silva Alexandre, T., Y. de Oliveira Duarte, J. Ferreira Santos, R. Wong, and M. Lebrao. 2014. Sarcopenia according to the European Working Group on sarcopenia in older people (EWGSOP) versus dynapenia as a risk factor for disability in the elderly. *J Nutr Health Aging* 18:547–53.

Devries, M. C. and S. M. Phillips. 2015. Supplemental protein in support of muscle mass and health: Advantage whey. *J Food Sci 80 Suppl* 1:A8–15.

Donnelly, J., S. Blair, J. Jakicic et al. 2009. American College of Sports Medicine position stand. Appropriate physical activity intervention strategies for weight loss and prevention of weight regain for adults. *Med Sci Sports Exer* 41:459–71.

Dumesnil, J., J. Turgeon, A. Tremblay et al. 2001. Effect of a low-glycaemic index—low-fat—high-protein diet on the atherogenic metabolic risk profile of abdominally obese men. *Br J Nutr* 86:557–68.

Ebbeling, C., J. Swain, H. Feldman et al. 2012. Effects of dietary composition on energy expenditure during weight-loss maintenance. *JAMA* 307:2627–34.

Food and Agriculture Organization of the United Nations (FAO). 2013. Dietary protein quality evaluation in human nutrition. *FAO Food Nutr Paper* 92:1–67. http://www.fao.org/ag/humannutrition/35978–02317b979a686a57aa4593304ffc17f06.pdf.

Forslund, A. H., A. E. El-khoury, R. M. Olsson, A. M. Sjodin, L. Hambraeus, and V. R. Young. 1999. Effect of protein intake and physical activity on 24-h pattern and rate of macronutrient utilization. *Am J Physiol* 276:E964–76.

Fulgoni, V. 2008. Current protein intake in America: Analysis of the National Health and Nutrition Examination Survey, 2003–2004. *Am J Clin Nutr* 87:1554S–7S.

Glynn, E. L., C. S. Fry, M. J. Drummond et al. 2010. Muscle protein breakdown has a minor role in the protein anabolic response to essential amino acid and carbohydrate intake following resistance exercise. *Am J Physiol Regul Integr Comp Physiol* 299:R533–40.

Goodpaster, B., S. Park, T. Harris et al. 2006. The loss of skeletal muscle strength, mass, and quality in older adults: The health, aging and body composition study. *J Gerontol A Biol Sci Med Sci* 61:1059–64.

Hartman, J., J. E. Tang, S. Wilkinson et al. 2007. Consumption of fat-free fluid milk after resistance exercise promotes greater lean mass accretion than does consumption of soy or carbohydrate in young, novice, male weightlifters. *Am J Clin Nutr* 86:373–81.

Hector, A. J., G. Marcotte, T. A. Churchward-Venne et al. 2015. Whey protein supplementation preserves postprandial myofibrillar protein synthesis during short-term energy restriction in overweight and obese adults. *J Nutr* 145:246–52.

Hoffman, J. R. and M. J. Falvo. 2004. Protein—Which is best? *J Sports Sci Med* 3:118–30.

Hoffman, J. R., N. A. Ratamess, C. P. Tranchina, S. L. Rashti, J. Kang, and A. D. Falgenbaum. 2009. Effect of protein-supplement timing on strength, power, and body-composition changes in resistance-trained men. *Int J Sport Nutr Exerc Metab* 19:172–85.

Houston, D., B. Nicklas, J. Ding et al. 2008. Dietary protein intake is associated with lean mass change in older, community-dwelling adults: The health, aging, and body composition (Health ABC) study. *Am J Clin Nutr* 87:150–5.

Howe, T., L. Rochester, F. Neil, D. Skelton, and C. Ballinger. 2011. Exercise for improving balance in older people. *Cochrane Database Syst Rev* 11:CD004963.

Hubal, M. J., H. Gordish-Dressman, P. D. Thompson et al. 2005. Variability in muscle size and strength gain after unilateral resistance training. *Med Sci Sports Exerc* 37:964–72.

Jakicic, J., B. Marcus, K. Gallagher, M. Napolitano, and W. Lang. 2003. Effect of exercise duration and intensity on weight loss in overweight, sedentary women: A randomized trial. *JAMA* 290:1323–30.

Jakicic, J., B. Marcus, W. Lang, and C. Janney. 2008. Effect of exercise on 24-month weight loss maintenance in overweight women. *Arch Intern Med* 168:1550–9.

Josse, A., S. Atkinson, M. Tarnopolsky, and S. Phillips. 2011. Increased consumption of dairy foods and protein during diet- and exercise-induced weight loss promotes fat mass loss and lean mass gain in overweight and obese premenopausal women. *J Nutr* 141:1626–34.

Joy, J., R. Lowery, J. Wilson et al. 2013. The effects of 8 weeks of whey or rice protein supplementation on body composition and exercise performance. *Nutr J* 12:86. doi: 10.1186/1475-2891-12-86.

Kerksick, C. M., C. J. Rasmussen, S. Lancaster et al. 2006. The effects of protein and amino acid supplementation on perofrmance and training adaptations during ten weeks of resistance training. *J Strength Cond Res* 20:643–53.

Klem, M., R. Wing, M. McGuire, H. Seagle, and J. Hill. 1997. A descriptive study of individuals successful at long-term maintenance of substantial weight loss. *Am J Clin Nutr* 66:239–46.

Kraemer, W., K. Adams, E. Cafarelli et al. 2002. American College of Sports Medicine position stand. Progression models in resistance training for healthy adults. *Med Sci Sports Exerc* 34:364–80.

Kraschnewski, J., C. Sciamanna, J. Ciccolo, E. Lehman, C. Candotti, and N. Ballentine. 2014. Is exercise used as medicine? Association of meeting strength training guidelines and functional limitations among older US adults. *Prev Med* 66:1–5.

Krieger, J., H. Sitren, M. Daniels, and B. Langkamp-Henken. 2006. Effects of variation in protein and carbohydrate intake on body mass and composition during energy restriction: A meta-regression. *Am J Clin Nutr* 83:260–74.

Kumar, V., P. Atherton, K. Smith, and M. J. Rennie. 2009. Human muscle protein synthesis and breakdown during and after exercise. *J Appl Physiol* 106:2026–39.

Landi, F., R. Liperoti, A. Russo et al. 2012. Sarcopenia as a risk factor for falls in elderly individuals: Results from the il SIRENTE study. *Clin Nutr* 31:652–8.

Laskowski, R. and J. Antosiewicz. 2003. Increased adaptability of young judo sportsmen after protein supplementation. *J Sports Med Phys Fitness* 43:342–6.

Lejeune, M., E. Kovacs, and M. Westerterp-Plantenga. 2005. Additional protein intake limits weight regain after weight loss in humans. *Br J Nutr* 93:281–9.

Liu, C. and N. Latham. 2009. Progressive resistance strength training for improving physical function in older adults. *Cochrane Database Syst Rev* 3:CD002759.

Longland, T., S. Oikawa, C. Mitchell, M. Devries, and S. Phillips. 2016. Higher compared with lower dietary protein during an energy deficit combined with intense exercise promotes greater lean mass gain and fat mass loss: A randomized trial. *Am J Clin Nutr* 103:738–46.

McLellan, T. M., S. M. Pasiakos, and H. R. Lieberman. 2014. Effects of protein in combination with carbohydrate supplements on acute or repeat endurance exercise performance: A systematic review. *Sports Med* 44:535–50.

Mikkelsen, P., S. Toubro, and A. Astrup. 2000. Effect of fat-reduced diets on 24-h energy expenditure: Comparisons between animal protein, vegetable protein and carbohydrate. *Am J Clin Nutr* 72:1135–41.

Miller, P. E., D. D. Alexander, and V. Perez. 2014. Effects of whey protein and resistance exercise on body composition: A meta-analysis of randomized controlled trials. *J Am Coll Nutr* 33:163–75.

Mitchell, C., T. Churchward-Venne, D. West et al. 2012. Resistance exercise load does not determine training-mediated hypertrophic gains in young men. *J Appl Physiol* 113:71–7.

Moore, D. R. 2015. Nutrition to support recovery from endurance exercise: Optimal carbohydrate and protein replacement. *Curr Sports Med Rep* 14:294–300.

Moore, D. R., T. A. Churchward-Venne, O. Witard et al. 2015. Protein ingestion to stimulate myofibrillar protein synthesis requires greater relative protein intakes in healthy older versus younger men. *J Gerontol A Biol Sci Med Sci* 70:57–62.

Moore, D. R., M. J. Robinson, J. L. Fry et al. 2009. Ingested protein dose response of muscle and albumin protein synthesis after resistance exercise in young men. *Am J Clin Nutr* 89:161–8.

Moritani, T. and H. deVries. 1979. Neural factors versus hypertrophy in the time course of muscle strength gain. *Am J Phys Med* 58:115–30.

Morton, R., S. Oikawa, C. Wavell et al. 2016. Neither load nor systemic hormones determine resistance training-mediated hypertrophy or strength gains in resistance-trained young men. *J Appl Physiol* 121:129–38.

Müller, M., Z. Wang, S. Heymsfield, B. Schautz, and A. Bosy-Westphal. 2013. Advances in the understanding of specific metabolic rates of major organs and tissues in humans. *Curr Opin Clin Nutr Metab Care* 16:501–8.

Murphy, C., T. A. Churchward-Venne, C. Mitchell et al. 2015. Hypoenergetic diet-induced reductions in myofibrillar protein synthesis are restored with resistance training and balanced protein ingestion in older men. *Am J Physiol Endocrinol Metab* 308:E734–43.

Murphy, C., S. Oikawa, and S. Phillips. 2016. Dietary protein to maintain muscle mass in aging: A case for per-meal protein recommendations. *J Frailty Aging* 5:49–58.

Newman, A., V. Kupelian, M. Visser et al. 2006. Strength, but not muscle mass, is associated with mortality in the health, aging and body composition study cohort. *J Gerontol A Biol Sci Med Sci* 61:72–7.

Norton, L. E., G. J. Wilson, D. K. Layman, C. J. Moulton, and P. J. Garlick. 2012. Leucine content of dietary proteins is a determinant of postprandial skeletal muscle protein synthesis in adult rats. *Nutr Metab* 9:67.

Paddon-Jones, D. and B. B. Rasmussen. 2009. Dietary protein recommendations and the prevention of sarcopenia. *Curr Opin Clin Nutr Metab Care* 12:86–90.

Pasiakos, S., J. Cao, L. Margolis et al. 2013. Effects of high-protein diets on fat-free mass and muscle protein synthesis following weight loss: A randomized controlled trial. *FASEB J* 27:3837–47.

Pasiakos, S., T. McLellan, and H. Liberman. 2015. The effects of protein supplements on muscle mass, strength, and aerobic and anaerobic power in healthy adults: A systematic review. *Sports Med* 45:111–31.

Pasiakos, S., L. Vislocky, J. Carbone et al. 2010. Acute energy deprivation affects skeletal muscle protein synthesis and associated intracellular signaling proteins in physically active adults. *J Nutr* 140:745–51.

Peterson, M., A. Sen, and P. Gordon. 2011. Influence of resistance exercise on lean body mass in aging adults: A meta-analysis. *Med Sci Sports Exerc* 43:249–58.

Peterson, M. D. and P. M. Gordon. 2011. Resistance exercise for the aging adult: Clinical implications and prescription guidelines. *Am J Med* 124:194–8.

Peterson, M. D., M. R. Rhea, A. Sen, and P. M. Gordon. 2010. Resistance exercise for muscular strength in older adults: A meta-analysis. *Ageing Res Rev* 9:226–37.

Phillips, S. 2009. Physiologic and molecular bases of muscle hypertrophy and atrophy: Impact of resistance exercise on human skeletal muscle (protein and exercise dose effects). *Appl Physiol Nutr Metab* 34:403–10.

Rasch, P. and L. Morehouse. 1957. Effect of static and dynamic exercises on muscular strength and hypertrophy. *J Appl Physiol* 11:29–34.

Rasmussen, B. B., K. D. Tipton, S. L. Miller, S. E. Wolf, and R. R. Wolfe. 2000. An oral essential amino acid-carbohydrate supplement enhances muscle protein anabolism after resistance exercise. *J Appl Physiol* 88:386–92.

Rutherfurd, S. M., A. C. Fanning, B. J. Miller, and P. J. Moughan. 2015. Protein digestibility-corrected amino acid scores and digestible indispensable amino acid scores differentially describe protein quality in growing male rats. *J Nutr* 145:372–9.

Schoenfeld, B., A. Aragon, and J. Krieger. 2013. The effect of protein timing on muscle strength and hypertrophy: A meta-analysis. *J Int Soc Sports Nutr* 10:53. doi: 10.1186/1550-2783-10-53.

Scott, D., A. Hayes, K. Sanders, D. Aitken, P. Ebeling, and G. Jones. 2014. Operational definitions of sarcopenia and their associations with 5-year changes in falls risk in community-dwelling middle-aged and older adults. *Osteoporosis Int* 25:187–93.

Silva, N. L., R. B. Oliveira, S. J. Fleck, A. C. M. P. Leon, and P. Farinatti. 2014. Influence of strength training variables on strength gains in adults over 55 years-old: A meta-analysis of dose–response relationships. *J Sci Med Sport* 17:337–44.

Skov, A., S. Toubro, B. Ronn, L. Holm, and A. Astrup. 1999. Randomized trial on protein vs carbohydrate in ad libitum fat reduced diet for the treatment of obesity. *Int J Obes Relat Metab Disord* 23:528–36.

Snijders, T., P. T. Res, J. S. Smeets et al. 2015. Protein ingestion before sleep increases muscle mass and strength gains during prolonged resistance-type exercise training in healthy young men. *J Nutr* 145:1178–84.

Steib, S., D. Schoene, and K. Pfeifer. 2010. Dose-response relationship of resistance training in older adults: A meta-analysis. *Med Sci Sports Exerc* 42:902–14.

Stookey, J., L. Adair, and B. Popkin. 2005. Do protein and energy intakes explain long-term changes in body composition? *J Nutr Health Aging* 9:5–17.

Tang, J. E., D. R. Moore, G. W. Kujbida, M. A. Tarnopolsky, and S. M. Phillips. 2009. Ingestion of whey hydrolysate, casein, or soy protein isolate: Effects on mixed muscle protein synthesis at rest and following resistance exercise in young men. *J Appl Physiol* 107:987–92.

Tarnopolsky, M. 2004. Protein requirements for endurance athletes. *Nutrition* 20:662–8.

Taylor, L., C. Wilborn, M. Roberts, A. White, and K. Dugan. 2016. Eight weeks of pre- and postexercise whey protein supplementation increases lean body mass and improves performance in Division III collegiate female basketball players. *Appl Physiol Nutr Metab* 41:249–54.

Tieland, M., O. van de Rest, M. Dirks et al. 2012. Protein supplementation improves physical performance in frail elderly people: A randomized, double-blind, placebo-controlled trial. *J Am Med Dir Assoc* 13:720–6.

Tipton, K. D., A. A. Ferrando, S. M. Phillips, D. Doyle, and R. R. Wolfe. 1999. Postexercise net protein synthesis in human muscle from orally administered amino acids. *Am J Physiol* 276 E628–34.

Tschopp, M., M. K. Sattelmayer, and R. Hilfiker. 2011. Is power training or conventional resistance training better for function in elderly persons? A meta-analysis. *Age Ageing* 40:549–56.

Velazquez Alva Mdel, C., M. Irigoyen Camacho, J. Delgadillo Velazquez, and I. Lazarevich. 2013. The relationship between sarcopenia, undernutrition, physical mobility and basic activities of daily living in a group of elderly women of Mexico City. *Nutr Hosp* 28:514–21.

Verdijk, L. B., R. A. Jonkers, B. G. Gleeson, M. Beelen, K. Meijer, and H. H. Savelberg. 2009. Protein supplementation before and after exercise does not further augment skeletal muscle hypertrophy after resistance training in elderly men. *Am J Clin Nutr* 89:608–16.

Volek, J., B. Volk, A. Gómez et al. 2013. Whey protein supplementation during resistance training augments lean body mass. *J Am Coll Nutr* 32:122–35.

Volpi, E., W. Campbell, J. Dwyer et al. 2013. Is the optimal level of protein intake for older adults greater than the recommended dietary allowance? *J Gerontol A Biol Sci Med Sci* 68:677–81.

Weigle, D., P. Breen, C. Matthys et al. 2005. A high-protein diet induces sustained reductions in appetite, ad libitum caloric intake, and body weight despite compensatory changes in diurnal plasma leptin and ghrelin concentrations. *Am J Clin Nutr* 82:41–8.

Weinheimer, E., L. Sands, and W. Campbell. 2010. A systematic review of the separate and combined effects of energy restriction and exercise on fat-free mass in middle-aged and older adults: Implications for sarcopenic obesity. *Nutr Rev* 68:375–88.

Westerterp-Plantenga, M., A. Nieuwenhuizen, D. Tome, D. Soenen, and K. Westerterp. 2009. Dietary protein, weight loss, and weight maintenance. *Annu Rev Nutr* 29:21–41.

Westerterp, K., S. Wilson, and A. Rolland. 1999. Diet-induced thermogenesis measured over 24 h in a respiration chamber: Effect of diet composition. *Int J Obes Relat Metab Disord* 23:287–92.

Whitehead, J., G. McNeill, and J. Smith. 1996. The effect of protein intake on 24-h energy expenditure during energy restriction. *Int J Obes Relat Metab Disord* 20:727–32.

Wilkinson, S., S. Phillips, P. Atherton et al. 2008. Differential effects of resistance and endurance exercise in the fed state on signalling molecule phosphorylation and protein synthesis in human muscle. *J Physiol* 586:3701–17.

Wilkinson, S., M. Tarnopolsky, M. MacDonald, J. Macdonald, D. Armstrong, and S. Phillips. 2007. Consumption of fluid skim milk promotes greater muscle protein accretion after resistance exercise than does consumption of an isonitrogenous and isoenergetic soy-protein beverage. *Am J Clin Nutr* 85:1031–40.

Willis, L., C. Slentz, L. Bateman et al. 2012. Effects of aerobic and/or resistance training on body mass and fat mass in overweight or obese adults. *J Appl Physiol* 113:1831–7.

Willoughby, D. S., J. R. Stout, and C. D. Wilborn. 2007. Effects of resistance training and protein plus amino acid supplementation on muscle anabolism, mass, and strength. *Amino Acids* 32:467–77.

Wolfe, R., S. Miller, and K. Miller. 2008. Optimal protein intake in the elderly. *Clin Nutr* 27:675–84.

Wycherley, T., L. Moran, P. Clifton, M. Noakes, and G. Brinkworth. 2012. Effects of energy-restricted high-protein, low-fat compared with standard-protein, low fat diets: A meta-analysis of randomized controlled trials. *Am J Clin Nutr* 96:1281–98.

Yang, Y., L. Breen, N. A. Burd et al. 2012a. Resistance exercise enhances myofibrillar protein synthesis with graded intakes of whey protein in older men. *Br J Nutr* 108:1780–8.

Yang, Y., T. A. Churchward-Venne, N. A. Burd, L. Breen, M. Tarnopolsky, and S. Phillips. 2012b. Myofibrillar protein synthesis following ingestion of soy protein isolate at rest and after resistance exercise in elderly men. *Nutr Metab* 9:57.

16 Influence of Dietary Supplements on Body Composition

Col. Karl E. Friedl

CONTENTS

Dis-moi ce que tu manges, je te dirai ce que tu es
[Tell me what you eat and I will tell you what you are]

Brillat-Savarin, 1826

16.1 INTRODUCTION

We are what we eat in a more literal way than previously believed. For example, the composition of fatty acids stored in adipose tissue is associated with the composition of fat in one's diet (Field et al. 1985; Malcom et al. 1989; Van Staveren et al. 1986). On a grosser level, chronic energy intake (and expenditure) habits in a healthy person are reflected in body weight, lean mass, and adiposity. This energy intake is reflected in consistent patterns of change in body composition components in normal overfed or malnourished individuals, with lean mass and fat mass generally moving along a line together, as originally described by Forbes (1993; Figure 16.1). The macronutrient composition of the diet (i.e., fat, carbohydrate, and protein components) is generally thought to differentially affect

343

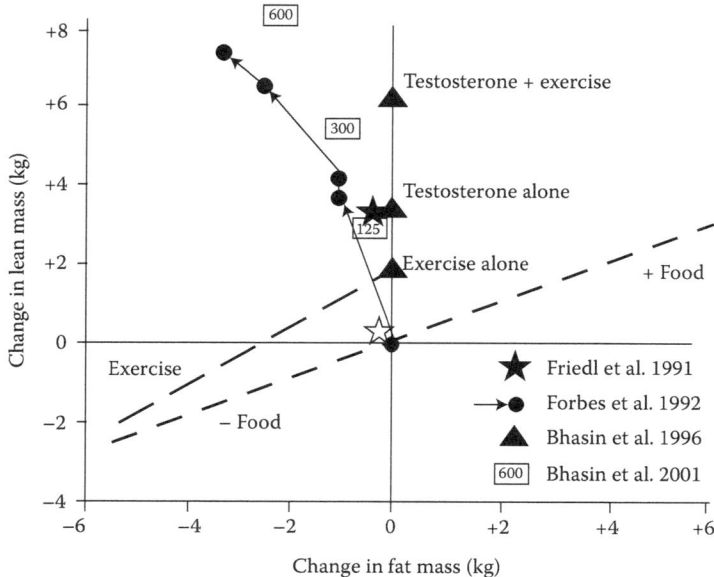

FIGURE 16.1 The "companionship of fat and lean" was described by Forbes in a keynote lecture at the 1992 *In Vivo Body Composition Symposium* (Forbes 1993). Supplements are used with the intention of skewing this relationship in favor of preserving or preferentially increasing lean mass over fat mass. Four studies with administration of testosterone enanthate (TE) to healthy young men are plotted to show the effects of dose, duration of administration, and concurrent exercise. Friedl et al. (1991) showed that 100 mg/week for 6 weeks was a "replacement" dose with no effect (star symbol), while 300 mg/week of TE or nandrolone decanoate produced significant lean mass gain (filled star symbol). Forbes et al. (1992), using K40 counting, reported progressive fat loss with 200 mg/week of TE over 12 weeks. Bhasin et al. (1996), using underwater weighing, showed the effect of 600 mg/week TE over 10 wks with and without exercise. Bhasin et al. (2001), using UWW and DXA, showed the dose effects of TE administered over 20 weeks.

body weight and adiposity; however, this has been difficult to demonstrate in longitudinal weight loss studies (de Souza et al. 2012) or in current metabolic models (Hall 2010). The specific influence of protein intake is the topic of a separate chapter in this book and has also been reviewed elsewhere by Stefan Pasiakos (Pasiakos 2015, Pasiakos et al. 2015a,b). Nutritional ergogenic aids have been explored as a means to modify body composition for fat reduction in overweight individuals and as anabolic enhancers in body builders and athletes. Generally, the goal of these supplements has been to promote weight loss with preservation of the lean mass, or to produce a preferential gain of lean mass by moving off the normal path of weight gain, such as the effect of anabolic hormones (Figure 16.1). The influence of dietary supplements on major components of body composition such as adipose, bone, and muscle tissues, including their topography, is the topic of this chapter.

16.2 DIETARY SUPPLEMENTS AND BODY COMPOSITION EFFECT CLAIMS

16.2.1 THE SUPPLEMENT SPECTRUM

Human metabolism does not run amok with every meal because our normally ingested food is processed, absorbed, and managed by the body in a highly regulated system of metabolic checks and balances. This can be illustrated with the example of carnitine which has been touted as a "fat burner" because L-carnitine has a known role in normal fatty acid oxidation in the mitochondria. Carnitine has been heavily marketed for this purpose as a dietary supplement. In fact, in normal healthy individuals, carnitine is limited in absorption from the gastrointestinal tract and its effects on fatty acid transport are offset by inhibitory biochemical pathways (Friedl and Moore 1992). If this did not happen, out-of-control mitochondrial oxidative activity would conceivably damage intracellular components. Marketing claims that are not well supported by scientific evidence are often made more compelling by testimonials such as the fact that the Italian soccer team won the World Soccer Cup in 1982 while using the product.

There are, however, longer term shifts in the balance between accretion and loss of components such as water, fat, or bone mineral, which can be influenced by specific nutrients, vitamins, minerals, and other ingested substances. Some of these changes may be produced by herbal supplements but the claimed effects have generally been very difficult to demonstrate (Bucci 2000). Better data are available for purified products such as creatine (Hultman et al. 1996), and the best validated changes in body composition are produced by certain drugs and hormones such as sympathomimetics and sex steroid hormones (Astrup et al. 1991; Bhasin et al. 2001). The line between dietary supplements and drugs distinguishes products that are freely available over the counter from products that are FDA regulated for medical and health safety purposes. Dietary supplements were formally defined under the 1994 Dietary Supplement Health and Education Act (DSHEA). The DSHEA legislation protects the marketing of useless dietary supplements and bizarre combinations of substances with claims about effects on performance and body composition so long as the claims do not involve prevention or treatment of a disease. For the discussion in this chapter, this distinction between drugs and supplements is a softer divide because there are steroid hormones such as dehydroepiandrosterone that are not regulated products and there are some dietary supplement claims that have a pharmacological nature such as claims to dramatically increase testosterone levels (Baulieu et al. 2000; Friedl et al. 1992).

16.2.2 DIETARY SUPPLEMENTS WITH CLAIMS AS ANABOLIC DRUG REPLACEMENTS

The creative claims of endocrine-based effects of dietary supplements are entertaining but are also easily debunked. For example, there are plant species that produce ecdysone-related substances to disrupt the physiology of their natural pest enemies. Ecdysone is a potent hormone involved in insect molting (ecdysis) and pupation. There are no known effects of insect molt hormones in humans, nor are there any known receptors for ecdysone action in humans; nevertheless, creative marketers easily conjure images of ecdysone-consuming body builders with Hulk-like cartoon characters and superhuman growth increases. At least one human study empirically tested these plant-derived ecdysone-based supplement claims and found no effects on body composition (Wilborn et al. 2006).

A classic target of dietary supplement claims has been promotion of testosterone actions without directly providing FDA-regulated testosterone products. These products have no effects on body composition because the products actually have none of the claimed effects on testosterone, except perhaps in some cases where methyl testosterone was illegally added to the product (Friedl et al. 1992). A range of plant-derived saponins have been marketed as "testosterone replacers" with the explanation that these are the same raw materials used in the manufacture of corticosteroids and sex steroids. A big breakthrough in affordable production of steroid hormones came about in the 1940s when Russell Marker converted diosgenin, a saponin obtained from a Mexican yam species, to progesterone and other steroid hormones; however, his process requires acetic anhydride and 200°C temperatures. Conversion of saponins to steroids in the human body has not been demonstrated. At best, this would be no better than increasing cholesterol intake, with the rationale that cholesterol is also in the pathway for steroid biosynthesis and might increase testosterone synthesis rates. Many other "testosterone replacer" products have similar fascinating fairy tales with a few thin threads of misconstrued science (Neychev and Mitev 2005; Brown et al. 2006).

As one more example, boron is heavily marketed as a dietary supplement for boosting male testosterone levels. There is no published research that supports any such effects but there is a body of literature demonstrating high levels of boron associated with male impotence and causing testicular lesions in rats. The basis for the marketing claims originated from a single paper published by an ultratrace mineral researcher, Forrest Nielsen (Friedl et al. 1992). In a careful study of post-menopausal women, Nielsen restricted dietary boron and this reduced already very low levels of sex steroids, including testosterone; when he restored normal intakes, he observed a return to the baseline levels of testosterone (Nielsen et al. 1987). This return to baseline represented a "doubling" of testosterone from the boron deficient diet reduction (serum levels of testosterone of women in the study declined from 0.6 to 0.3 ng/dL with dietary boron restriction, but testosterone levels in normal men are 1000 times higher). These data on postmenopausal women were then extrapolated by supplement manufacturers to claim that boron supplements will triple normal testosterone levels within 2 weeks in normal young men. Boron supplements do no such thing in men or women and have no demonstrated effects on muscle mass.

16.2.3 DIETARY SUPPLEMENTS WITH WEIGHT LOSS CLAIMS

A wide variety of dietary supplements have been promoted for weight loss. This class of supplements includes botanical products (either herbs or their extracts) with a mechanistic basis for a weight loss effect (e.g., *Garcinia cambogia*) and/or an empirical basis for weight regulation in animal studies (e.g., *Coleus forskohlii*), or an anecdotal efficacy based on traditional practices (e.g., *Hoodia gordonii*). Melinda Manore has provided an authoritative review of these products, dividing them by likely mechanisms (Manore 2012). Four main categories of products block absorption of fat or carbohydrates, stimulate thermogenesis, moderate appetite, or work through very specific metabolic pathways to change body composition. Manore concludes that, at best, these supplements produce only small weight losses even when used in conjunction with healthy lifestyle habits, and the metabolic stimulants which may have more profound effects are simply too dangerous to use as weight loss supplements (Manore 2012). Ultimately, none of these products has gained sufficient evidence of efficacy to claim weight loss applications (Heymsfield et al. 1998; Blom et al. 2011; Manore 2012; Astell et al. 2013; Rios-Hoyo and Gutierrez-Salmean 2016). Although the applications for weight loss may seem compelling based on mechanisms of action and even animal data, careful human trials seem to be consistently disappointing. For example, hydroxycitric acid may competitively inhibit lipogenesis and is found in *Garcinia cambogia*, a herbal supplement marketed for weight loss, but in careful human trials, this promising herbal product did not produce changes in weight or adiposity (Heymsfield et al. 1998).

Another group of botanicals have specific and potent actions that are better understood since some of these are the origins of well-known pharmaceuticals such as caffeine, ephedrine (e.g., Ma Huang), yohimbine, and synephrine (e.g., bitter orange) products which clearly do influence human energy metabolism. The supplements can be difficult to study because of the variations in potency and bioavailability of the active ingredients, and also because of the complex combinations of metabolic stimulants (Schaneberg and Khan 2004). Because of their dangers with medically unsupervised use, some of these products, such as ephedrine-containing supplements, have been banned in the United States.

Despite the difficulties of conducting a human study that demonstrates the efficacy of natural products in body composition change, there are a few dietary supplements that have been demonstrated to specifically influence human energy metabolism (e.g., caffeine and ephedrine) and muscle size (e.g., creatine), as will be further discussed in this chapter. There are more potent pharmacological preparations with well-known effects, as well. To date, there are few demonstrated effects of most dietary supplements on body composition.

16.3 PHYSIOLOGICAL REGULATION OF BODY COMPOSITION COMPONENTS

Dietary supplements may influence energy balance but they may also work through endocrine mechanisms. For example, sex steroid hormones also have important influences on fat, muscle, and bone mineral placement. In studies of the effects of dietary supplements on body composition, it may be important to also take into account changes in total body water or shifts in body water compartments. These assessments may involve some methodological challenges, where normal assumptions about the makeup of fat-free mass may not be appropriate. Study designs have also become more complicated as other influences such as concurrent exercise, and even mode of exercise, may have important interactions with nutrition and dietary supplements and body composition outcomes.

16.3.1 HYDRATION CHANGES AND BODY COMPOSITION ARTIFACTS

Large changes in energy balance even without the use of dietary supplements produce marked regionally specific changes in fat, muscle, and bone. These are evident in studies of semi-starvation in healthy normal individuals (Keys et al. 1950; Friedl et al. 1993, 1994, 1997a). It is important to note that dramatic changes such as rapid weight loss can produce changes that complicate body composition assessments with commonly used techniques. Rapid weight loss includes an increase in water retention as first detected by Ancel Keys and his team in the Minnesota Starvation Experiment through the increased swelling of joints. In subsequent studies involving extreme weight loss in army soldiers, there was an estimated shift in water content of the fat-free mass that increased from 73% to over 80%. This produces an artifact in both the interpretations of density from underwater weighing and in the attenuation coefficients in dual x-ray absorptiometry (DXA), producing incorrect estimates of lean mass (Figure 16.2).

Shifts in body water are not limited to energy deficiency but likely occur in other settings such as rapid muscular hypertrophy produced with anabolic substances such as growth hormone, androgens, and creatine. Dietary supplements that interfere with anabolic hormone secretion or actions may have the opposite effects on osmoregulation (Rosen et al. 1993; De Boer et al. 2009). The artifacts produced in standard methods by the increase in hydration of the lean mass require some concurrent measurements for a multicomponent body composition analysis. This would include

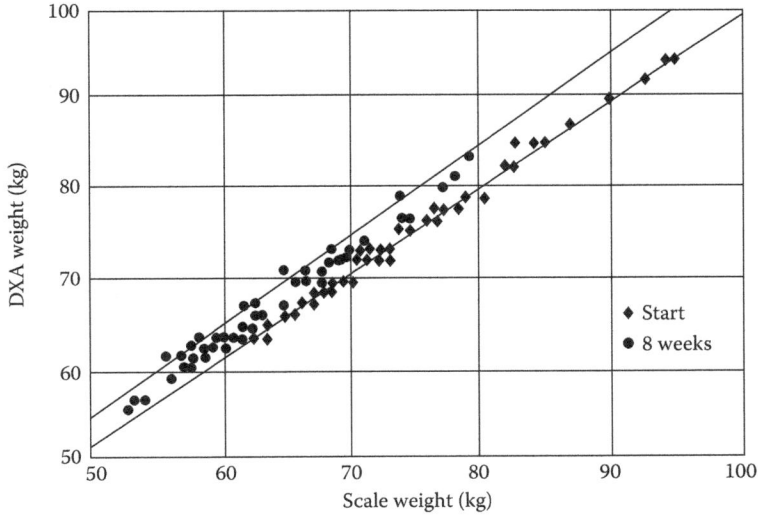

FIGURE 16.2 Comparison of the relationship between DXA-measured body weight and gravimetrically determined body weight in healthy young men before and after 8 weeks of semi-starvation with nearly complete loss of body fat stores (Friedl et al. 1994). There is good agreement between the assessments at baseline but semi-starvation increased hydration of the lean mass from an estimated 73% to over 80% and produced ~3 kg overestimates of body tissue in the DXA assessment. (Reprinted from Friedl, K.E. 1997b. Military application of body composition assessment technologies. In *Emerging Technologies for Nutrition Research: Potential for Assessing Military Performance Capability*, eds. S. J. Carlson-Newberry and R. B. Costello, 81–126. Washington, DC: National Academy Press, with permission from National Academy Press.)

measurement of the water compartments such as total body water and extracellular water with isotopic or bioelectrical impedance methods. More innovative approaches might use whole body laser scanning for physical measurement of body volumes correcting DXA-derived body volumes (Wilson et al. 2013).

16.3.2 INFLUENCE OF ENERGY BALANCE ON BODY COMPOSITION TOPOGRAPHY

Modest weight loss produced through dietary restriction and increased exercise affects specific fat depots differently. Abdominal and gluteal adipose cells are more labile than other sites such as thigh adipose cells. This has been demonstrated in biopsied adipose from these three sites in Norwegian military cadets at the end of 5 days with no food and an enormous physical demand that included no organized sleep (Rognum et al. 1982). In these healthy young men losing 3.4 kg body weight (including 2.7 kg of fat mass), there was a significant triglyceride depletion in abdominal and gluteal adipose cells, but the thigh fat demonstrated no change. In a more protracted semi-starvation model, fit lean soldiers participating in the 8th-week U.S. Army Ranger course, lost a mean of 12.1 kg and demonstrated a 10 cm mean reduction in abdominal circumference (Friedl et al. 1994). From DXA regional analysis, there was a greater reduction in muscle mass in arms (−11.7%) than in legs (−2.5%), while fat loss was more profound (−65%) and proportionally reduced in both the arms and legs (Friedl et al. 1993).

As highlighted by Forbes (1993), fat and lean are companions during weight gain and weight loss and tend to change together, except in special cases such as the administration of anabolic hormones or "nutrient partitioning" agents (Figure 16.1). However, the location and changes of these stored or mobilized depots is sexually dimorphic. With abdominal fat computed tomography (CT) slices, Kvist has demonstrated that as adiposity increases in men, there is a straight line increase in intra-abdominal fat, but this site is protected against significant fat deposition in women and the first ~30 kg of fat are preferentially stored extra-abdominally (Kvist et al. 1988). There are also important genetic modifiers of fat deposition, as noted by Matsuzawa in CT scans of healthy young sumo wrestlers, with a distinct minority subgroup that deposits fat intra-abdominally despite their intense training (Matsuzawa et al. 1992).

These are important considerations in the assessment of effects of dietary supplements because they are typically used in conjunction with weight loss diets and exercise programs which themselves produce characteristic changes in body composition.

16.3.3 ENDOCRINE REGULATION OF BODY COMPOSITION TOPOGRAPHY

The effects of sex steroids, notably testosterone and estrogen, on fat, muscle, and bone distributions are well known. For example, adipose tissue has been described as behaving as a single organ yet there are well-described regional differences that are highly regulated by hormones such as the sex steroids and glucocorticoids, as well as hormones that are important in pregnancy such as prolactin (Rebuffé-Scrive et al. 1985; Rebuffé-Scrive et al. 1986). Well-described hormonal influences on body composition provide obvious markers to an endocrinologist (as one component of characteristic facies) such as fat accumulation on the shoulder region (Cushing's syndrome), characteristically narrow shoulders in men (Klinefelter's syndrome), specific characteristics of bone overgrowth (acromegaly), and large weight loss including loss of bone and muscle (hyperthyroidism), etc. These diseases of excessive hormonal response signify extremes of hormonal actions when normal regulatory systems fail.

Supplement manufacturers and some individual consumers assume that dietary supplements can influence these regulatory systems to enhance desired effects without creating a disease condition. The evidence does not generally support a simple continuum of effect, where more hormonal action produces more benefit. The benefits of replacement hormone treatment for a deficiency such as adult onset growth hormone deficiency include some reduction in body fat and modest increase in lean mass, but these replacement effects do not translate to simply more goodness when an additional level of hormone is provided to normal individuals. In the typical feedback system of normal hormonal regulation, excess hormone suppresses endogenous hormone secretion and, as doses increase, it may also produce unintended effects through crossover stimulation of other hormone receptors (Jänne 1990).

There are intriguing possibilities for dietary supplement interactions in some of the endocrine regulatory pathways, but these have yet to be clearly demonstrated. For example, supplements that produce a calming or "antistress" effect could conceivably reduce abdominal fat through interactions with glucocorticoid receptors, where abdominal fat accretion is a recognized biomarker of chronic stress activation (Ljung et al. 1996, 2000). Such antistress claims have not been well researched or demonstrated for products ranging from lavender metabolites to ayurvedic spice mixtures.

16.4   DIETARY SUPPLEMENT EFFECTS ON BODY COMPOSITION

16.4.1   NUTRIENT PARTITIONING AGENTS: IF IT WORKS FOR BEEF AND PORK PRODUCTION, WHAT DOES IT DO FOR HUMAN ATHLETES?

Sympathomimetic drugs including so called nutrient partitioning agents developed for meat production also found their way into human use, with athletes testing positive for clenbuterol use at various international competitions (Ricks et al. 1984; Rothwell and Stock 1985; Prather et al. 1995). In the push for new antiobesity drugs, beta-3 agonists have been considered. However, the paucity of beta-3 receptors and the role of brown adipose tissue in weight management in humans are still poorly understood and differ from the responses of another species (Weyer et al. 1999). This would presumably be more desirable than the beta-2 agonists which have significant chronotropic and other undesirable cardiovascular effects (Huckins and Lemons 2013). The beta-2 agonists are approved for human use in the United States in inhaled form because they provide significant benefits to asthmatics; these doses and formulations may not produce the body composition changes that have been anecdotally reported with higher doses in oral form used by body builders and athletes. There may even be antagonistic effects of exercise on the clenbuterol-stimulated increase in muscle mass (Kearns et al. 2001). In animal studies, the beta-2 agonists promote protein accretion primarily through suppression of protein degradation (Costelli et al. 1995), and also accelerate fat metabolism (Kearns et al. 2001). This suggests therapeutic potential at least in human applications for cancer cachexia and aging-related muscle wasting. Only anecdotal data exists for human body composition and physical performance effects.

This fat burning action is similar to the "fat burning" effect reported in humans with caffeine and ephedrine, especially through a synergistic action when administered together (Daly et al. 1993; Liu et al. 1995). The use of ephedrine in the United States is prohibited because of previous misuse by athletes and serious cardiovascular side effects. Because of the likely but poorly characterized effects to promote lean mass accretion in humans, these drugs are carefully monitored in elite athletic competition. Caffeine is no longer banned from most sports testing but high dose use is still monitored.

16.4.2   BUILDING MUSCLE MASS: DEPARTURES FROM TYPICAL FAT FREE MASS AND FAT MASS RELATIONSHIPS

A range of products have been promoted for their anabolic effects. In addition to the sympathomimetics discussed in the previous section, this ranges from potent hormones including growth hormone, growth factors, and androgens; creatine and protein supplements; and myostatin inhibitors.

16.4.2.1   Growth Hormone

In a much cited study, 24 growth hormone deficient men and women treated with growth hormone for 6 months demonstrated substantial anabolic and lipolytic effects (Salomon et al. 1989). There was no change in body weight in the hormone-treated group. The placebo group also demonstrated no changes in body composition, but it gained an average 5.5 kg of lean mass and lost an average of 5.7 kg fat mass. Circulating levels of insulin-like growth factor 1 (IGF-1) were tripled during the growth hormone treatment. In a 10-year follow up, 10 of the patients with continued growth hormone treatment were compared to 11 that stopped treatment, and a control group from the same era. The results demonstrated sustained increased muscle mass (measured by total body potassium and CT cross-sectional views of the thigh) (Gibney et al. 1999). In studies of healthy fit men and women without growth hormone deficiency, Crist and his colleagues demonstrated similar effects of growth hormone administration (Crist et al. 1988, 1991). Using underwater weighing, they estimated progressive increases in fat-free mass and concurrent declines in fat mass averaging 1.3 kg after 18 weeks of treatment (Crist et al. 1991). Growth hormone administration to healthy individuals consistently increases circulating IGF-1 concentrations but the thyroid axis has also been reported to be suppressed. Both of these effects may contribute to muscle protein accretion (Crist et al. 1991; Sgro et al. 2010).

It should be noted that growth hormone (GH) is an osmoregulatory hormone, affecting fluid compartments in the body. In replacement treatments, growth hormone dose was reduced by 50% when the patients developed significant fluid retention or hypertension (Salomon et al. 1989). Growth hormone administration specifically increases the extracellular water compartment, at least in growth hormone deficient adults. This has been measured with bioelectrical impedance and by deuterium and bromide dilution techniques (Janssen et al. 1997; van Marken Lichtenbelt et al. 1997). Charles Kochakian, a pioneer in anabolic hormone research once described the muscle hypertrophy that occurred in both growth hormone and testosterone-treated rats as easily differentiated by a soft squishy feel in the growth hormone-treated animals compared to a hard muscle feel in the testosterone-treated animals (Kochakian 1988). The changes in both cases, include some portion of increased protein synthesis and net muscle protein accretion, and some element of increased hydration of the lean mass.

Dietary supplements are touted for growth hormone releasing capabilities. This likely stems from the standard clinical test for growth hormone insufficiency which is based on a hormone challenge test using arginine infusion. The levels of amino acids that must be ingested to provoke a measureable increase in growth hormone secretion are generally not well tolerated and, in any case, may not be greater than the spikes in growth hormone and IGF-1 that can be produced with an intense bout of resistance exercise (Bucci et al. 1990; Kraemer et al. 1991; Chromiak and Antonio 2002).

16.4.2.2 Androgens

At a macro level, the changes in muscle size produce male pattern hypertrophy emphasizing the upper body. Bhasin put to rest the question of whether or not supra-physiological levels of testosterone in normal men could increase muscle mass in healthy young men just as it did in hypogonadal men (Bhasin et al. 2001). Increases in fat-free mass were dose dependent with up to an average of nearly 8 kg gain at the 600 mg/week dose of testosterone enanthate for 20 weeks (Bhasin et al. 2001) (Figure 16.1). Body composition changes were assessed in the same studies using DXA, underwater weighing, and MRI scans of leg muscles. Changes in fat mass are less consistently reported in any studies of androgen administration to healthy men. In previous studies such as one reported by Forbes et al., testosterone treatment causes an apparent lean mass gain and fat mass loss (Forbes et al. 1992) (Figure 16.1). However, these changes are largely temporary, with a return toward the original body composition following drug cessation (Friedl et al. 1990; Forbes et al. 1992). Such observations suggest that the rapid changes may involve intracellular fluid retention. However, in Bhasin's studies, body water, measured by deuterium dilution, averaged around 74% of the fat free mass, with nonstatistical increases at highest doses of testosterone, suggesting that the weight gains were primarily associated with protein accretion (Bhasin et al. 2001). Circulating IGF-1 levels demonstrate dose-dependent increases with testosterone administration.

Androgens also influence lipolysis, affecting lipoprotein lipase activity; however, studies with androgen administration consistently demonstrate weight gain and increased lean mass but do not consistently report a decline in body fat (Friedl et al. 1990, 1991). Per Marin has conducted studies on the role of testosterone and its key metabolite, dihydrotestosterone (DHT), on abdominal fat in obese men, finding that testosterone administration may specifically reduce intra-abdominal fat (as measured by CT), while DHT administration tends to increase it (Marin et al. 1993; Marin 1995). In contrast, androgen supplementation has no effect on femoral fat depots (Marin et al. 1995). It should be noted that adipose tissue is also the site of aromatization of testosterone to estrogen, a potential confounder in the interpretation of effects. The main lipolytic effect of testosterone administration is on intra-abdominal fat (e.g., omental adipose tissue) and it may actually increase fat storage in subcutaneous abdominal fat (Marin et al. 1996). One effect of androgen supplements on abdominal fat may be to help block or reverse the effect of cortisol from chronic stress. Abdominal adipocytes appear to be more sensitive to glucocorticoid stimulation and, in animal studies, abdominal fat has been reduced by treatment with glucocorticoid inhibition, using the progestogen, RU-486 (Blouin et al. 2009).

Bhasin has proposed a sensible unifying hypothesis that a key site of androgen action is via stem cells, shifting in favor of a myogenic lineage and away from an adipogenic lineage (Bhasin et al. 2003). This helps to explain multiple observations about the effects of androgens on body composition including specific effects on muscle fiber hypertrophy (Sinha-Hakim et al. 2002).

16.4.2.3 Creatine

Creatine supplements provide substrate for the substrate rate-limited short burst strength performance, increasing muscle phosphocreatine stores as an energy buffer, but this also serves as an energy carrier as well as serving an important role in maintaining adenosine triphosphate/adenosine diphosphate (ATP/ADP) ratios (Greenhaff 2001). An ingested creatine dose of 20 g/day increases muscle creation concentration by 20% (Hultman et al. 1996). Typical doses of creatine supplement use are equivalent to what would be obtained in several kilograms of red meat ingestion; thus, the effects of this dietary supplementation are not easily duplicated with normal diet. Supplementation typically increases body weight by 1–2 kg. While this was initially assumed to be increased muscle mass, it is now apparent that the weight increase is largely body water. It was also assumed that since the creatine is stored intramuscularly, the increased water retention would also be primarily reflected in an increase in the intracellular water compartment. While this seemed to be true, especially based on some bioelectrical impedance studies, measurement with deuterium and sodium bromide dilution techniques have not established a differential shift in the increased water compartments (Ziegenfuss et al. 1998; Powers et al. 2003).

16.4.3 Vitamin D and Bone Mineral Accretion—Only Effective in Deficiency?

Dietary supplements are heavily marketed for bone health purposes. These include products that are known to be important for bone mineral accretion such as calcium and Vitamin D. Sex steroids increase bone mineral density in various bone measurement sites for aging men and women with declining testosterone and estrogen levels that are at risk for osteoporotic fractures (Khosla et al. 1998; Snyder et al. 1999; Cauley et al. 2003; Cauley 2015). Even low-dose oral contraceptive use appears to produce some benefits to bone mineral density, measured by DXA over 2 years of drug administration in a randomized controlled study of collegiate female runners; however, effects were significant only in the subsample of oligomenorrheic/amenorrheic women (Cobb et al. 2007). It could be reasonably expected from the available data that dietary supplements that increase bone mineral accretion based on steroidogenic mechanisms would be most effective in sustaining bone mineral content in individuals with low or declining sex steroid hormone levels. There may also be modest benefits to soft tissue with preservation of lean mass and reduction of fat mass. Specific regional bone changes occur with treatments but these effects have to be carefully separated from weight bearing exercise and other interrelated effects. Bone biology studies have unraveled some of the mysteries of sex steroid actions on bone (Wiren 2005). Most notable are the findings that estrogens inhibit bone resorption, while androgens help to stimulate bone formation and specifically increase bone growth on the periosteal surface, widening bones during development in males (Wiren 2005). However, it has also been observed that androgens may not be anabolic in mature osteoblasts and could even inhibit osteogenesis and compromise bone health in healthy normal men (Wiren et al. 2008).

Phytoestrogens are one category of dietary supplements that have been promoted for bone mineral accretion actions, but these effects have been difficult to demonstrate because of the complexity of such studies. For example, in the Study of Women's Health Across the Nation (SWAN), there was only one of four ethnic groups that had sufficiently high estimated intakes of genistein, an isoflavone phytoestrogen, the Japanese-American participants. Of these women, only the premenopausal group demonstrated an association between genistein intake and bone mineral density (Greendale et al. 2002). This was, however, consistent with other studies of Japanese cohorts where dietary isoflavone intakes are high and these benefits to bone could be demonstrated. This opens the door to more questions about the interaction of genetics, diet, and bone physiology.

Vitamin D is a popular dietary supplement and may be useful to young women, the one group of Americans that have the lowest dietary intakes of Vitamin D and low blood levels, based on National Health and Nutrition Examination Survey (NHANES) data (Ross et al. 2011; Schleicher et al. 2016). Vitamin D and calcium supplementation increases bone mineral content and also reduces stress fracture incidence during military basic training for younger women, many of whom are Vitamin D deficient (Lappe et al. 2008; Lutz et al. 2012). However, more than normal adequate intakes of Vitamin D, as promoted for a myriad of health and performance benefits, is not necessarily more beneficial and carries health risks (Ross et al. 2011). An expert panel convened by the Institute of Medicine (IOM), concluded that Vitamin D is regulated like many other hormones, where massive amounts of supplemental Vitamin D are required to force a pharmacological elevation of blood levels above normal circulating levels to support poorly defined benefit claims (Ross et al. 2011).

16.5   CONCLUSIONS

This chapter attempted to highlight some of the most important influences of supplements on body composition. It must be acknowledged that there are many more known unknowns and especially unknown unknowns in this area than what we think we know, and this is a rich topic for future research. What is currently well known is that most dietary supplements have no effect on body composition despite extensive marketing claims and testimonial puffery. Some of these claims invoke known physiological mechanisms, especially in endocrine regulation of muscle, fat, and bone yet fail to demonstrate actual effects through these mechanisms. Stimulant substances (e.g., caffeine, ephedrine, and synephrine) that are often found in dietary supplement products, actual hormones (and related drugs), and some concentrated food components such as creatine have proven effects on effective body composition change. Measurement of these changes can be complicated by factors that affect interpretation of the results of specific techniques; an important factor is altered hydration status.

ACKNOWLEDGEMENTS

This work was prepared by the author as a paid Fellow in the Knowledge Preservation Program, Oak Ridge Institute for Research and Education, funded by the Biophysics and Biomedical Modeling Division, U.S. Army Research Institute of Environmental Medicine. The editing assistance of Ms Mallory E. Roussel is gratefully acknowledged. The opinions and assertions in this chapter are solely those of the author and do not necessarily represent any official view or position of the Department of the Army.

REFERENCES

Astell, K. J., M. L. Mathai, and X. Q. Su. 2013. A review on botanical species and chemical compounds with appetite suppressing properties for body weight control. *Plant Foods Hum Nutr* 68:213–21.

Astrup, A., S. Toubro, S. Cannon, P. Hein, and J. Madsen. 1991. Thermogenic synergism between ephedrine and caffeine in healthy volunteers: A double-blind, placebo-controlled study. *Metabolism* 40:323–9.

Baulieu, E. E., G. Thomas, S. Legrain et al. 2000. Dehydroepiandrosterone (DHEA), DHEA sulfate, and aging: Contribution of the DHEAge Study to a sociobiomedical issue. *Proc Natl Acad Sci* 97:4279–84.

Bhasin, S., T. W. Storer, N. Berman et al. 1996. The effects of supraphysiologic doses of testosterone on muscle size and strength in normal men. *N Engl J Med* 335:1–7.

Bhasin, S., L. Woodhouse, R. Casaburi et al. 2001. Testosterone dose-response relationships in healthy young men. *Am J Physiol Endocrinol Metab* 281:E1172–81.

Bhasin, S., W. E. Taylor, R. Singh et al. 2003. The mechanisms of androgen effects on body composition: Mesenchymal pluripotent cell as the target of androgen action. *J. Gerontol* 58A:1103–10.

Blom, W. A., S. L. Abrahamse, R. Bradford et al. 2011. Effects of 15-d repeated consumption of *Hoodia gordonii* purified extract on safety, ad libitum energy intake, and body weight in healthy, overweight women: A randomized controlled trial. *Am J Clin Nutr* 94:1171–81.

Blouin, K., A. Veilleux, V. Luu-The, and A. Tchernof. 2009. Androgen metabolism in adipose tissue: Recent advances. *Mol Cell Endocrinol* 301:97–103.

Brillat-Savarin, J. A. 1826. *Physiologie du Gout, ou, Meditations de Gastronomie Transcendante*. Paris: Charpentier, Libraire-Editeur (available through Google Books).

Brown, G. A., M. Vukovich, and D. S. King. 2006. Testosterone prohormone supplements. *Med Sci Sport Exerc* 38:1451–61.

Bucci, L. R. 2000. Selected herbals and human exercise performance. *Am J Clin Nutr* 72:624–36.

Bucci, L., J. F. Hickson, J. M. Pivarnik, I. Wolinsky, J. C. McMahon, and S. D. Turner. 1990. Ornithine ingestion and growth hormone release in bodybuilders. *Nutr Res* 10:239–45.

Cauley, J. A. 2015. Estrogen and bone health in men and women. *Steroids* 99:11–5.

Cauley, J. A., J. Robbins, Z. Chen et al. 2003. Effects of estrogen plus progestin on risk of fracture and bone mineral density: The Women's Health Initiative randomized trial. *J Am Med Assoc* 290:1729–38.

Chromiak, J. A., and J. Antonio. 2002. Use of amino acids as growth hormone-releasing agents by athletes. *Nutr* 18:657–61.

Cobb, K. L., L. K. Bachrach, M. Sowers et al. 2007. The effect of oral contraceptives on bone mass and stress fractures in female runners. *Med Sci Sport Exerc* 39:1464–73.

Costelli, P., C. García-Martínez, M. Llovera et al. 1995. Muscle protein waste in tumor-bearing rats is effectively antagonized by a beta 2-adrenergic agonist (clenbuterol): Role of the ATP-ubiquitin-dependent proteolytic pathway. *J Clin Invest* 95:2367–72.

Crist, D. M., G. T. Peake, P. A. Egan, and D. L. Waters. 1988. Body composition response to exogenous GH during training in highly conditioned adults. *J Appl Physiol* 65:579–84.

Crist, D. M., G. T. Peake, R. B. Loftfield, J. C. Kraner, and P. A. Egan. 1991. Supplemental growth hormone alters body composition, muscle protein metabolism and serum lipids in fit adults: Characterization of dose-dependent and response-recovery effects. *Mech Age Develop* 58:191–205.

Daly, P. A., D. R. Krieger, A. G. Dulloo, J. B. Young, and L. Landsberg. 1993. Ephedrine, caffeine and aspirin: Safety and efficacy for treatment of human obesity. *Int J Obes Related Metab Disord* 17:S73–8.

De Boer, H., G. J. Blok, H. J. Voerman, P. M. De Vries, and E. A. van der Veen. 2009. Body composition in adult growth hormone-deficient men, assessed by anthropometry and bioimpedance analysis. *J Clin Endocrinol Metab* 75:833–7.

de Souza, R. J., G. A. Bray, V. J. Carey et al. 2012. Effects of 4 weight-loss diets differing in fat, protein, and carbohydrate on fat mass, lean mass, visceral adipose tissue, and hepatic fat: Results from the POUNDS LOST trial. *Am J Clin Nut* 95:614–25.

Field, C. J., A. Angel, and M. T. Clandinin. 1985. Relationship of diet to the fatty acid composition of human adipose tissue structural and stored lipids. *Am J Clin Nutr* 42:1206–20.

Forbes, G. B. 1993. The companionship of lean and fat. In *Human Body Composition*, eds. K. J. Ellis and J. D. Eastman, 1–4. New York: Plenum Press.

Forbes, G. B., C. R. Porta, B. E. Herr, and R. C. Griggs. 1992. Sequence of changes in body composition induced by testosterone and reversal of changes after drug is stopped. *J Am Med Assoc* 267:397–9.

Friedl, K. E. 1997a. Variability of fat and lean tissue loss during physical exertion with energy deficit. In *Physiology, Stress, and Malnutrition: Functional Correlates, Nutritional Intervention*, eds. J. M. Kinney and H. N. Tucker, 431–50. New York: Lippincott-Raven Publishers.

Friedl, K. E. 1997b. Military application of body composition assessment technologies. In *Emerging Technologies for Nutrition Research: Potential for Assessing Military Performance Capability*, eds. S. J. Carlson-Newberry and R. B. Costello, 81–126. Washington, DC: National Academy Press.

Friedl, K. E., and R. J. Moore. 1992. Physiology of nutritional supplements. Fat burners: Clenbuterol, Ma Huang, caffeine, L-carnitine, & growth hormone releasers. *Nat Strength Conditioning Assoc J* 14:35–44.

Friedl, K. E., J. R. Dettori, C. J. Hannan Jr., T. H. Patience, and S. R. Plymate. 1991. Comparison of the effects of high dose testosterone and 19-nortestosterone to a replacement dose of testosterone on strength and body composition in normal men. *J Steroid Biochem Mol Biol* 40:607–12.

Friedl, K. E., C. J. Hannan Jr., R. E. Jones, and S. R. Plymate. 1990. HDL-cholesterol is not decreased if an aromatizable androgen is administered. *Metabolism* 39:69–74.

Friedl, K. E., R. J. Moore, and L. J. Marchitelli. 1992. Physiology of nutritional supplements. "Steroid replacers": Let the athlete beware! *Nat Strength Conditioning Assoc J*14:14–9.

Friedl, K. E., R. J. Moore, L. E. Martinez-Lopez et al. 1994. Lower limits of body fat in healthy active men. *J App Physiol* 77:933–40.

Friedl, K. E., J. A. Vogel, R. J. Marchitelli, and S. L. Kubel. 1993. Assessment of regional body composition changes by dual-energy x-ray absorptiometry. In *Human Body Composition*, eds. K. J. Ellis and J. D. Eastman, 99–103. New York: Plenum Press.

Gibney, J., J. D. Wallace, T. Spinks et al. 1999. The effects of 10 years of recombinant human growth hormone (GH) in adult GH-deficient patients. *J Clin Endocrinol Metab* 84:2596–602.

Greendale, G. A., G. FitzGerald, M. H. Huang et al. 2002. Dietary soy isoflavones and bone mineral density: Results from the study of women's health across the nation. *Am J Epidemiol* 155:746–54.

Greenhaff, P. L. 2001. The creatine-phosphocreatine system: There's more than one song in its repertoire. *J Physiol* 537:657.

Hall, K. D. 2010. Predicting metabolic adaptation, body weight change, and energy intake in humans. *Am J Physiol Endocrinol Metab* 298:E449–66.

Heymsfield, S. B., D. B. Allison, J. R. Vasselli, A. Pietrobelli, D. Greenfield, and C. Nunez. 1998. Garcinia cambogia (hydroxycitric acid) as a potential antiobesity agent: A randomized controlled trial. *J Am Med Assoc* 280:1596–600.

Huckins, D. S., and M. F. Lemons. 2013. Myocardial ischemia associated with clenbuterol abuse: Report of two cases. *J Emerg Med* 44:444–9.

Hultman, E., K. Soderlund, J. A. Timmons, G. Cederblad, and P. L. Greenhaff. 1996. Muscle creatine loading in men. *J Appl Physiol* 81:232–7.

Jänne, O. A. 1990. Androgen interaction through multiple steroid receptors. In *Anabolic Steroid Abuse*, eds. G. C. Lin and L. Erinoff, Vol. 102, 178–86. Rockville, MD: U.S. Department of Health and Human Services.

Janssen, Y. J. H., P. Deurenberg, and F. Roelfsema. 1997. Using dilution techniques and multifrequency bioelectrical impedance to assess both total body water and extracellular water at baseline and during recombinant human growth hormone (GH) treatment in GH-deficient adults. *J Clin Endocrinol Metab* 82:3349–55.

Kearns, C. F., K. H. McKeever, K. Malinowski, M. B. Struck, and T. Abe. 2001. Chronic administration of therapeutic levels of clenbuterol acts as a repartitioning agent. *J Appl Physiol* 91:2064–70.

Keys, A., J. Brozek, A. Henschel, O. Michelsen, and H. L. Taylor. 1950. *The Biology of Human Starvation*. Vol. 1–2. Minneapolis: University of Minnesota Press.

Khosla, S., L. J. Melton III, E. J. Atkinson, W. M. O'Fallon, G. G. Klee, and B. L. Riggs. 1998. Relationship of serum sex steroid levels and bone turnover markers with bone mineral density in men and women: A key role for bioavailable estrogen. *J Clin Endocrinol Metab* 83:2266–74.

Kochakian, C. D. 1988. The evolution from "male hormone" to anabolic-androgenic steroids. *Alabama J Med Sci* 25:96–102.

Kraemer, W. J., S. E. Gordon, S. J. Fleck et al. 1991. Endogenous anabolic hormone and growth factor responses to heavy resistance exercise in males and females. *Int J Sport Med* 12:228–35.

Kvist, H., B. Chowdhury, U. Grangård, U. Tylen, and L. Sjöström. 1988. Total and visceral adipose-tissue volumes derived from measurements with computed tomography in adult men and women: Predictive equations. *Am J Clin Nutr* 48:1351–61.

Lappe, J., D. Cullen, G. Haynatzki, R. Recker, R. Ahlf, and K. Thompson. 2008. Calcium and vitamin D supplementation decreases incidence of stress fractures in female Navy recruits. *J Bone Mineral Res* 23:741–9.

Liu, Y. L., S. Toubro, A. Astrup, and M. J. Stock. 1995. Contribution of beta 3-adrenoceptor activation to ephedrine-induced thermogenesis in humans. *Int J Obes Related Metab Disord* 19:678–85.

Ljung, T., B. Andersson, B. Å. Bengtsson, P. Björntorp, and P. Mårin. 1996. Inhibition of cortisol secretion by dexamethasone in relation to body fat distribution: A dose-response study. *Obes Res* 4:277–82.

Ljung, T., G. Holm, P. Friberg et al. 2000. The activity of the hypothalamic-pituitary-adrenal axis and the sympathetic nervous system in relation to waist/hip circumference ratio in men. *Obes Res* 8:487–95.

Lutz, L. J., J. P. Karl, J. C. Rood et al. 2012. Vitamin D status, dietary intake, and bone turnover in female Soldiers during military training: A longitudinal study. *J Int Soc Sport Nutr* 9:38.

Malcom, G. T., A. K. Bhattacharyya, M. Velez-Duran, M. Guzman, M. C. Oalmann, and J. P. Strong. 1989. Fatty acid composition of adipose tissue in humans: Differences between subcutaneous sites. *Am J Clin Nutr* 50:288–91.

Manore, M. M. 2012. Dietary supplements for improving body composition and reducing body weight: Where is the evidence? *Int J Sport Nutr Exerc Metab* 22:139–54.

Marin, P. 1995. Testosterone and regional fat distribution. *Obes Res* 3(4):609S–12S.

Marin, P., S. Holmang, C. Gustafsson et al. 1993. Androgen treatment of abdominally obese men. *Obes Res* 1:245–51.

Marin, P., B. Oden, and P. Bjorntorp. 1995. Assimilation and mobilization of triglycerides in subcutaneous abdominal and femoral adipose tissue *in vivo* in men: Effects of androgens. *J Clin Endocrinol Metab* 80:239–43.

Marin, P., L. Lonn, B. Andersson et al. 1996. Assimilation of triglycerides in subcutaneous and intraabdominal adipose tissues in vivo in men: Effects of testosterone. *J Clin Endocrinol Metab* 81:1018–22.

Matsuzawa, Y., S. Fujioka, K. Tokunaga, and S. Tarui. 1992. Classification of obesity with respect to morbidity. *Exp Biol Med* 200:197–201.

Neychev, V. K., and V. I. Mitev. 2005. The aphrodisiac herb *Tribulus terrestris* does not influence the androgen production in young men. *J Ethnopharmacol* 101:319–23.

Nielsen, F. H., C. D. Hunt, L. M. Mullen, and J. R. Hunt. 1987. Effect of dietary boron on mineral, estrogen, and testosterone metabolism in postmenopausal women. *FASEB J* 1:394–7.

Pasiakos, S. M. 2015. Metabolic advantages of higher protein diets and benefits of dairy foods on weight management, glycemic regulation, and bone. *J Food Sci* 80:A2–7.

Pasiakos, S. M., L. M. Margolis, and J. S. Orr. 2015a. Optimized dietary strategies to protect skeletal muscle mass during periods of unavoidable energy deficit. *FASEB J* 29:1136–42.

Pasiakos, S. M., H. L. McClung, L. M. Margolis et al. 2015b. Human muscle protein synthetic responses during weight-bearing and non-weight bearing exercise: A comparative study of exercise modes and recovery nutrition. *PLOS One* 10:e0140863.

Powers, M. E., B. L. Arnold, and A. L. Weltman et al. 2003. Creatine supplementation increases total body water without altering fluid distribution. *J Athl Training* 38:44–50.

Prather, I. D., D. E. Brown, P. E. North, and J. R. Wilson. 1995. Clenbuterol: A substitute for anabolic steroids? *Med Sci Sport Exerc* 27:1118–21.

Rebuffé-Scrive, M., L. Enk, N. Crona et al. 1985. Fat cell metabolism in different regions in women. Effect of menstrual cycle, pregnancy, and lactation. *J Clin Inves* 75:1973–76.

Rebuffé-Scrive, M., P. Lönnroth, P. Mårin, C. Wesslau, P. Björntorp, and U. Smith. 1986. Regional adipose tissue metabolism in men and postmenopausal women. *Int J Obes* 11:347–55.

Ricks, C. A., R. H. Dalrymple, P. K. Baker, and D. L. Ingle. 1984. Use of a p-agonist to alter fat and muscle deposition in steers. *J Anim Sci* 59:1247–55.

Rios-Hoyo, A., and G. Gutierrez-Salmean. 2016. New dietary supplements for obesity: What we currently know. *Curr Obes Rep* 5:262–70.

Rognum, T. O., K. Rodahl, and P. K. Opstad. 1982. Regional differences in the lipolytic response of the subcutaneous fat depots to prolonged exercise and severe energy deficiency. *Eur J Appl Physiol Occup Physiol* 49:401–8.

Rosen, T., I. Bosaeus, J. Tolli, G. Lindstedt, and B. A. Bengtsson. 1993. Increased body fat mass and decreased extracellular fluid volume in adults with growth hormone deficiency. *Clin Endocrinol* 38:63–71.

Ross, A. C., J. E. Manson, S. A. Abrams et al. 2011. The 2011 report on dietary reference intakes for calcium and vitamin D from the Institute of Medicine: What clinicians need to know. *J Clin Endocrinol Metab* 96:53–8.

Rothwell, N. J., and M. J. Stock. 1985. Modification of body composition by clenbuterol in normal and dystrophic (mdx) mice. *Biosci Rep* 5:755–60.

Salomon, F., R. C. Cuneo, R. Hesp, and P. H. Sonksen. 1989. The effects of treatment with recombinant human growth hormone on body composition and metabolism in adults with growth hormone deficiency. *N Engl J Med* 321:1797–803.

Schaneberg, B. T., and I. A. Khan. 2004. Quantitative and qualitative HPLC analysis of thermogenic weight loss products. *Pharmazie* 59:819–23.

Schleicher, R. L., M. R. Sternberg, A. C. Looker et al. 2016. National estimates of serum total 25-Hydroxyvitamin D and metabolite concentrations measured by liquid chromatography–tandem mass spectrometry in the U.S. population during 2007–2010. *J Nutr* 146:1051–61.

Sinha-Hikim, I., J. Artaza, L. Woodhouse et al. 2002. Testosterone-induced increase in muscle size in healthy young men is associated with muscle fiber hypertrophy. *Am J Physiol Endocrinol Metab* 283:E154–64.

Sgro, P., L. Guidetti, C. Crescioli et al. 2010. Effect of supra-physiological dose administration of rhGH on pituitary-thyroid axis in healthy male athletes. *Reg Peptides* 165:163–7.

Snyder, P. J., H. Peachey, P. Hannoush et al. 1999. Effect of testosterone treatment on bone mineral density in men over 65 years of age 1. *J ClinEndocrinol Metab* 84:1966–72.

van Marken Lichtenbelt, W. D., Y. E. M. Snel, R. J. M. Brummer, and P. F. Koppeschaar. 1997. Deuterium and bromide dilution, and bioimpedance spectrometry independently show that growth hormone-deficient adults have an enlarged extracellular water compartment related to intracellular water. *J Clin Endocrinol Metab* 82:907–11.

Van Staveren, W. A., P. Deurenberg, M. B. Katan, J. Burema, L. C. DeGroot, and M. D. Hoffmans. 1986. Validity of the fatty acid composition of subcutaneous fat tissue microbiopsies as an estimate of the long-term average fatty acid composition of the diet of separate individuals. *Am J Epidemiol* 123:455–63.

Weyer, C., J. F. Gautier, and E. Danforth Jr. 1999. Development of beta 3-adrenoceptor agonists for the treatment of obesity and diabetes—an update. *Diab Metab* 25:11–21.

Wilborn, C. D., L. W. Taylor, B. I. Campbell et al. 2006. Effects of methoxyisoflavone, ecdysterone, and sulfo-polysaccharide supplementation on training adaptations in resistance-trained males. *J Int Soc Sport Nutr* 3:19–27.

Wilson, J. P., B. Fan, J. A. Shepherd. 2013. Total and regional body volumes derived from dual-energy x-ray absorptiometry output. *J Clin Densit* 16:368–73.

Wiren, K. M. 2005. Androgens and bone growth: It's location, location, location. *Curr Opin Pharmacol* 5:626–32.

Wiren, K. M., A. A. Semirale, Z. W. Zhang et al. 2008. Targeting of androgen receptor in bone reveals a lack of androgen anabolic action and inhibition of osteogenesis: A model for compartment-specific androgen action in the skeleton. *Bone* 43:440–51.

Ziegenfuss, T. N., L. M. Lowery, and P. W. R. Lemon. 1998. Acute fluid volume changes in men during three days of creatine supplementation. *J Exerc Physiol* 1:1–9.

17 Diet and Exercise Approaches for Reversal of Exercise-Associated Menstrual Dysfunction

Lynn Cialdella-Kam and Melinda M. Manore

CONTENTS

17.1 INTRODUCTION: ENERGY STATUS

For the female athlete with exercise-associated menstrual dysfunction (ExMD), energy intake (EI) is not adequate to meet the energy demands of exercise, activities of daily living, and menstrual function. Thus, the primary objective is to increase EI to a level that allows normal menstrual function to resume. In young female athletes, the additional energy demands of growth must also be met. This chapter first examines diet and exercise approaches to improve energy status and then discusses the health consequences of chronic energy deficit in athletes.

17.1.1 LOW ENERGY AVAILABILITY

Chronic energy deficits in athletes have been classified utilizing energy availability (EA), defined as dietary EI less exercise energy expenditure (EEE) expressed relative to fat-free mass (FFM, kg). In athletes, EA is classified as suboptimal when it is <45 kcal/kg of FFM/day and has been associated with ExMD at levels of approximately 30 kcal/kg of FFM/day (Loucks 2013). This threshold is based on energy restriction studies conducted in sedentary women to determine whether exercise stress or energy deficit was the driver of menstrual dysfunction and associated hormonal disruptions in active women (Loucks and Callister 1993; Loucks et al. 1998). However, the use of EA in ExMD does have its limitations related to the difficulty in accurately assessing EA measurements (Guebels et al. 2014) and no observed difference in EA based on menstrual status (Cialdella-Kam et al. 2014; Melin et al. 2015). Assessment of EA and related issues will be discussed in this section. Table 17.1 includes terminology related to energy and menstrual status (Thomas et al. 2016) and recommended equations for estimating basal metabolic rate (BMR) in athletes (Thompson and Manore 1996; Millward 2012).

To determine an individual's EA, laboratory assessment of EI, EEE, and body composition is required. Various methods exist to assess each of these components as previously described (Thomas et al. 2016), which are beyond the scope of this chapter. Generally accepted research methods for EA include 7-day weighed food records for dietary intake (Monsen et al. 2008), 7-day activity logs, doubly labeled water, or tracking devices such as heart rate or accelerometers for total energy expenditure (TEE) and EEE (Thomas et al. 2016), indirect calorimetry for resting metabolic

TABLE 17.1
Energy Status Terminology and Equations for BMR

Definition

Energy Status Terminology (Thomas et al. 2016)

Basal metabolic rate (BMR)	Calories required to support bodily functions at rest
Energy availability (EA)	Calories remaining to support metabolic processes and daily living activities after accounting for energy used during exercise
Energy balance (EB)	The difference between caloric intake (EI) and caloric expenditure (TEE)
Energy intake (EI)	Calories obtained from food, fluids, and supplements
Exercise energy expenditure (EEE)	Calories expended during planned physical activity (e.g., exercise training)
Non-exercise thermogenesis (NEAT)	Calories expended during unplanned physical activity (e.g., daily living activities)
Resting metabolic rate (RMR)	Calories required to support bodily functions in relaxed state. This is commonly used instead of BMR as it is more practical to measure. Estimates may be 10% higher than BMR.
Thermic effect of food (TEF)	Calories used to metabolize and store nutrients consumed
Thermic effect of activity (TEA)	Total energy expended during exercise (EEE), spontaneous physical activity (e.g., fidgeting), and daily living activities (NEAT)
Total energy expenditure (TEE)	Calories expended during the day (i.e., the sum of BMR, TEF, and TEA)

Menstrual Status Terminology (Nattiv et al. 2007)

Anovulation	Absence of ovulation during menstrual cycle
Eumenorrhea	Normal menses or cycles every 21–35 days
Luteal suppression	Luteal phase of menstrual cycle shorter than 11 days
Oligomenorrhea	No menses for greater than 35 days
Primary amenorrhea	Age of menarche ≥15 years
Secondary amenorrhea	No menses for greater than 90 days

Equations for BMR (kcal/day)

Harris and Benedict (1918)	BMR (Males) in kcal/day $= 66.47 + (13.75 \times \text{weight in kg}) + (5.00 \times \text{height in cm}) - (6.76 \times \text{age in years})$ BMR (Female) in kcal/day $= 655.1 + (9.56 \times \text{weight in kg}) + (1.85 \times \text{height in cm}) - (4.68 \times \text{age in years})$
Cunningham (1980)	BMR (kcal/day) $= 500 \times (22 \times \text{fat free mass in kg})$ where FFM = fat-free mass in kg

rate (RMR), and dual x-ray absorptiometry (DXA) for body composition (Ackland et al. 2012). However, these research methods are expensive and often impractical in the context of sports nutrition counseling for an individual athlete. Thus, in practice, multiple 24-hour recalls or diet logs for EI and factorial equations and/or metabolic equivalents (METs) for energy expenditures are often employed by registered dietitian nutritionists (RDNs). An example of energy status calculations utilizing this approach is provided in Table 17.2.

When body composition is assessed, RDNs commonly use field tools such as bioelectrical impendence (BIA) and skinfold measurements, but these methods have inherent errors resulting in imperfect estimates of FFM (Ackland et al. 2012). Thus, it is difficult for an RDN in this setting to obtain an accurate estimate of EA. Other issues with EA included no universal definition of exercise. Specifically, the types and intensity of exercise that should be included in EEE calculations are undefined. As a result, EA estimates can vary based on the criteria used for determining the activities to be included in EEE (Guebels et al. 2014). In addition, not all female athletes with low EA experience menstrual dysfunction (Melin et al. 2015; Muia et al. 2016) as discussed in Section 17.3. Therefore, RDN would evaluate biochemical data, food and nutrition history, weight change history, and medical history to identify females potentially at risk for low EA and menstrual dysfunction (Steinmuller et al. 2014). As new technology continues to emerge, more practical and accurate energy assessment methodologies may aid in better EA estimates (Attal et al. 2015; Burke 2015; Evans 2016).

TABLE 17.2

Energy Status Calculation Example for Female Long Distance Runner

Steps	Calculations
Step 1: Calculate BMR Female long distance runner Age: 22 years Height: 1.61 m Weight: 48 kg Body fat %: 16	**Cunningham BMR** (Cunningham 1980) $= [500 \times (22 \times \text{FFM})]$ kcal/day *where* FFM = fat-free mass (kg) calculated as weight in kg − (body fat (%) × weight in kg) $= 500 \times (22 \times 40.3) = 1387$ kcal/day
Step 2: Apply activity factor of 1.8–2.3 (Rodriguez et al. 2009)	Applying an activity factor of 1.9, total energy expenditure (TEE) is then estimated to be: TEE $\approx 1387 \times 1.9 = 2635$ kcal/day
Step 3: Estimate exercise energy expenditure (EEE) using metabolic equivalents (METs)	During week, she runs trains ~75 min/day. Assuming METs of 7.5 (Tudor-Locke et al. 2009), her EEE is as follows: $\text{EEE} \approx \dfrac{\text{BMR} \times \text{METs}}{24 \text{ hour}} \times \text{Ex Duration kcal/d}$ where BMR = basal metabolic rate (kcal/day); METs = metabolic equivalents $\text{EEE} \approx \dfrac{1387 \times 7.5}{24 \text{ hour}} \times 1.25 \text{ hour} = 542 \text{ kcal/day}$
Step 4: Calculate energy balance (EB) and energy availability (EA) Energy intake = 2300 kcal/day based on 24-h recall	EB $\approx$ Energy Intake − TEE kcal/day EB $\approx 2400 - 2635$ kcal/day $= -235$ kcal/day **Interpretation:** Technically, this individual is in a negative energy balance. However, since this is an estimate, the individual would be classified as "in energy balance" (i.e., consuming adequate calories) EA $\approx$ Energy Intake − EEE kcal/day EA $\approx 2400 - 542$ kcal/day $= 1858$ kcal/day or $\text{EA} \approx \dfrac{1858 \text{ kcal/day}}{40 \text{ kg of FFM}} = 46$ kcal/day per kg of FFM **Interpretation:** This individual is meeting energy needs for optimal health and is likely in EB (Thomas et al. 2016)

17.1.2 Energy Deficiency to Clinical Eating Disorders

Chronic low EA can be a result of inadvertent low EI, subclinical disorder eating practices such as intermittent fasting or purging, or clinical eating disorders (Manore et al. 2007). Athletes particularly at risk for low EA are those participating in weight sensitive sports such as gravitational sports (e.g., ski jumping), weight-class sports (e.g., light weight rowing), and aesthetic sports (e.g., gymnastics) (Sundgot-Borgen et al. 2013). Briefly, we will review the spectrum of disordered eating, which spans from healthy eating and exercise practices to subclinical disorders to clinical eating disorders (Sundgot-Borgen et al. 2013).

The most severe forms of disordered eating are the clinical eating disorders: anorexia nervosa (AN), bulimia nervosa (BN), binge eating disorder (BED), and other specified feeding or eating disorder (OSFED) (American Psychiatric Association et al. 2013). Key characteristics of these disorders are described in Table 17.3. Clinical eating disorders are more prevalent in female athletes; however, male athletes are still at risk for eating disorders and suboptimal EI (Strother et al. 2012; Sundgot-Borgen et al. 2013; Mountjoy et al. 2014; Joy et al. 2016). Subclinical disordered eating such as cyclic dieting, purging via vomiting or laxative use, binging (i.e., eating large quantities of food at one time), excessive exercise, and rumination (Sundgot-Borgen et al. 2013; Joy et al. 2016) are more common. However, low EI and availability can also occur inadvertently as result of following a healthy diet (Horvath et al. 2000; Stubbs et al. 2004; Cialdella-Kam et al. 2014; Melin et al. 2016; Hand et al. 2016). A high-fiber diet (i.e., high fruit, vegetable, and whole-grains consumption) can lead to early satiety and thus inadvertently lead to suboptimal EI and low EA.

The female athlete triad refers to the interrelation among EA, bone health, and menstrual function with the recognition that each of its components occur on a spectrum (Joy et al. 2014, 2016). As depicted in Figure 17.1, an athlete may have optimal EA but still experience menstrual disturbances or bone loss.

Menstrual disturbances include mild issues such as light periods and spotting between periods to more severe conditions such as functional hypothalamic amenorrhea (FHA) (Table 17.1). Bone health is based on z-scores that compares an individual's bone mineral density (BMD; e.g., density or strength of bone) to that of controls of same race, sex, and age (Schousboe et al. 2013). Low BMD in athletes is defined as a z-score of −1.0 to −2.0 with osteoporosis (e.g., weak and brittle bones) defined as a z-score <−2.0 (Nattiv et al. 2007). However, athletes typically have higher BMD than normal controls. Thus, an athlete with a z-score of less between 0.0 and −1.0 could be experiencing

---

TABLE 17.3
Clinical Eating Disorders Key Characteristics

Name	Typical Body Weight Status	Key Characteristics
Anorexia nervosa	Underweight	Restrict energy intake resulting in low body weight Intense fear of weight gain Body image distortion
Bulimia nervosa	Normal weight	Recurring episodes of binge eating Inappropriate compensatory behaviors Body image distortion
Binge eating disorder	Overweight	Recurring episodes of binge eating with feelings of guilt, lack of control, embarrassment, or disgust
Other specified feeding or eating disorder	Variable	Have characteristics of clinical eating disorders above but do not meet all criteria

Source: American Psychiatric Association et al. 2013. *Diagnostic and Statistical Manual of Mental Disorders: DSM-5* (5th Ed.). Washington, DC: American Psychiatric Association.

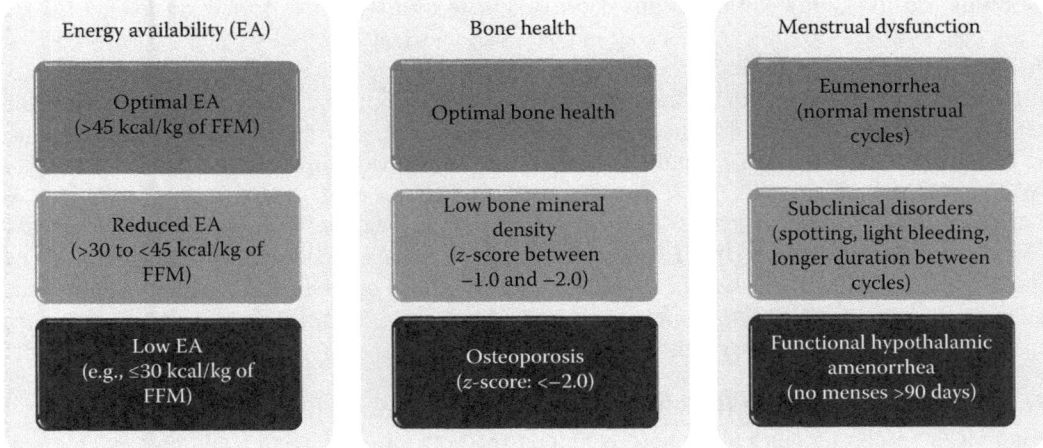

FIGURE 17.1 Female athlete triad represents the interplay among EA, bone health, and menstrual status. Each component occurs on a spectrum of severity. EA can range from optimal EA to low EA with or without clinical eating disorder. Bone health can be in normal status to osteoporosis. Finally, menstrual status ranges from normal menses to FHA. FFM = fat-free mass.

abnormal bone loss. Finally, EA also occurs on a spectrum from optimal EA to low EA that may occur with or without a clinical eating disorder (Nattiv et al. 2007). Treatment for the female athlete triad will be adjusted depending on the severity of each component (Joy et al. 2014; Mountjoy et al. 2014).

17.2 HEALTH RISKS ASSOCIATED WITH LOW EA

Low EA is associated with health concerns beyond menstrual disturbances and bone loss such as nutritional deficiencies, chronic fatigue, frequent injuries and infections, and hormonal disruptions (Mountjoy et al. 2014). Nutritional deficiencies include inadequate intake of energy, carbohydrate, protein, essential fatty acids, and micronutrients such as B-vitamins, vitamin D, and calcium (Manore et al. 2007; Mountjoy et al. 2014). In this section, we explore the impact of nutritional deficiencies and hormonal disruptions on bone health and then summarize other health consequences associated with low EA.

17.2.1 BONE HEALTH IN LOW EA

Bone remolding is essential for maintaining the integrity of bone and occurs in a process that involves the bone multicellular unit (i.e., osteocytes, osteoblast, osteoclast, and bone lining cells) (Florencio-Silva et al. 2015). During this process, osteoclasts break down bone tissue, and osteoblasts lay down new bone matrix (Florencio-Silva et al. 2015). In athletes, osteocytes play an important role since they orchestrate the bone remolding process in response to the mechanical load of exercise (Florencio-Silva et al. 2015). Exercise is an important stimulant for bone remolding and bone health (Kohrt et al. 2004). Thus, athletes typically have higher BMD than matched non-athletes (Torstveit and Sundgot-Borgen 2005; Barkai et al. 2007).

In both male and female athletes, low EA has been associated with increased risk for stress fractures and musculoskeletal injuries (Manore et al. 2007; Mountjoy et al. 2014). As described in Section 17.3, low EI can independently lead to bone loss primarily via its actions through the hormone, leptin. In addition, both macronutrient (i.e., carbohydrate, protein, and fat) and micronutrient (i.e., B-vitamins, calcium, and vitamin D) imbalances can contribute to increased bone resorption (i.e., breakdown of bone) and decreased bone formation (i.e., formation of new bones). In athletes with low EA, dietary fat (acceptable macronutrient distribution range = 20%–35% of total kcal/day) (Institute of Medicine (U.S.). Panel on Macronutrients et al. 2005) and protein (recommend intake = 1.2–2.0 g/kg of body weight [BW]/day) recommendations for athletes are often met (Cialdella-Kam et al. 2014; Viner et al. 2015; Thomas et al. 2016). Carbohydrate intakes, thus, are commonly either less than or at the low end of recommended ranges for athletes (5–10 g/kg of BW/day) (Cialdella-Kam et al. 2014; Viner et al. 2015; Thomas et al. 2016). Carbohydrate intakes at these levels do not appear to have a direct impact on bone health in energy restriction (Santesso et al. 2012). In athletes who restrict EI and/or have low EA, the main concern with low carbohydrate intake is that protein will be used for energy production instead of repair and building of new tissue and bone (Mountjoy et al. 2014; Thomas et al. 2016). Thus, the role of protein in bone is the primary focus of potential macronutrient deficiencies.

17.2.1.1 Protein and Bone Health

Protein is an important nutrient for bone health during both childhood and adulthood. In children, long-term dietary protein intake has been positively linked to bone modeling (Bihuniak and Insogna 2015). In adults, protein intake was initially linked to urinary calcium loss with a loss of approximately 12.5 mg of calcium for every 10 g of protein consumed (Bihuniak and Insogna 2015). Thus, high-protein diets (>2.0 g/kg/day) were believed to be detrimental to bone health (Heaney and Layman 2008; Bihuniak and Insogna 2015). The acid-ash hypothesis was used to explain the calcium loss as a result of a high-protein diet (Fenton et al. 2009). According to this hypothesis, proteins that are high in sulfur-containing amino acids such as meat and fish created a metabolic acid load, and the bone is degraded to serve as a buffer (Fenton et al. 2009). The acidosis created by proteins suppress osteoblasts (i.e., bone formation cells) activity and stimulate osteoclasts (i.e., bone resorption cells) activity and thus resulted in calcium release from the bone (Krieger et al. 2004). However, this concept was challenged when researchers reported a positive relationship between protein intake and bone health (Heaney and Layman 2008). In the Framingham Osteoporosis Study, BMD and protein intake was assessed at baseline and at 4-year follow-up in elderly men and women (age = 74.5 ± 4.4 years) (Hannan et al. 2000). Bone loss at the femoral neck and the lumbar spine was the least in the high-protein quartile group (1.2–2.8 g/kg/day) at the 4-year follow-up (Hannan et al. 2000). After adjusting for risk factors for bone loss such as age, sex, height, weight, weight change, smoking, and alcohol use, the lowest protein quartile (0.2–0.7 g/kg/day) had the greatest bone loss (Hannan et al. 2000). The type of protein (i.e., animal vs. plant protein) may also impact bone. Individuals in the lowest quartile of animal protein intake (1.9%–8.2% of total kcal/day) experienced the greatest bone loss in the femoral neck and lumbar spine (Hannan et al. 2000). To the contrary, others have found that higher plant-based protein intake is positively associated with BMD (Jennings et al. 2016). In addition, certain amino acids intakes such as leucine were associated with higher BMD (Jennings et al. 2016). These findings are consistent with current sports nutrition recommendations. Specifically, in hypocaloric diets, athletes are recommended to consume a higher protein intake (1.5–2.0 g/kg/day) to preserve skeletal muscle and bone mass (Mettler et al. 2010; Sundgot-Borgen et al. 2013; Helms et al. 2014; Murphy et al. 2015). In addition, leucine has been identified as a key amino acid for athletes related to its role in muscle protein synthesis (MPS) (Murphy et al. 2015).

The mechanisms by which dietary protein protects the bone may be by increasing gut calcium absorption and the bioavailability of insulin-like growth factor 1 (IGF-1) (Bihuniak and Insogna 2015). IGF-I is a hormone that stimulates osteoblasts resulting in bone formation (Bihuniak and Insogna 2015) and is discussed in Section 17.3. In both human and rodent models, the relationship between protein intake and calcium homeostasis has been examined. In a paired study design (i.e., women served as their own control), calcium absorption in healthy women was approximately 40% higher on a high-protein diet (2.1 g/kg/day) versus a low-protein diet (0.7 g/kg/day) for 4 days (Kerstetter et al. 2003). In a second study, secondary hyperparathyroidism and impaired intestinal calcium absorption was observed in young healthy women when consuming a diet that met recommended dietary allowance (RDA) for protein of 0.8 g/kg/day for 4 days (Kerstetter et al. 2003). Higher-protein intake (1.0 g/kg/d) was associated with minor changes in calcium homeostasis (Kerstetter et al. 2003). In rats, Gaffney-Stomberg et al. (2010) compared calcium metabolism on a 40% casein diet (high-protein group) versus a 5% casein diet (low-protein group) for 7 days. Despite different protein intakes, no differences were found in bone turnover markers with the exception of serum osteocalcin, which was 20% lower in the high-protein versus low-protein group (Gaffney-Stomberg et al. 2010). Osteocalcin is a protein produced by osteoblast cells in the presence of vitamin K and used as a marker of bone turnover (Lombardi et al. 2015). High levels of osteocalcin may be indicative of bone metabolism disorder such as osteoporosis (Vergnaud et al. 1997; Chapurlat and Confavreux 2016). In addition, rats on the high-protein diet had higher urinary calcium excretion as previously observed but had lower fecal calcium excretion and higher net calcium absorption compared to the low-protein group (Gaffney-Stomberg et al. 2010). Thus, the findings from both human and rodent studies suggest that a low-protein diet (<0.8 g/kg/day) may be more detrimental to the bone than a high-protein diet (>2.0 g/kg/day). Therefore, by consuming a higher-protein intake during periods of energy restriction, athletes can attenuate the rate of muscle (Phillips 2014) and bone loss.

17.2.1.2 Dietary Fat and Bone Health

Athletes with low EA have been reported to meet the Dietary Reference Intakes (DRI) for dietary fat of 20%–35% of total kcal/day (Institute of Medicine (U.S.). Panel on Macronutrients et al. 2005; Cialdella-Kam et al. 2014; Viner et al. 2015; Thomas et al. 2016). The composition of dietary fat intake in athletes and its impact on bone has not been well studied. However, one strategy to reduce EI is to select low energy dense foods (i.e., foods low in kcal/g of food) (Rolls 2012; Manore 2015). A low energy dense diet is likely to have a better fatty acid composition profile (i.e., lower saturated fat intake and higher polyunsaturated [PUFA] fat intake). Dietary fat composition has been reported to have important implications on bone health with low BMD and increased stress fracture risk liked with diets high in saturated fats (i.e., ≥10% of total kcal/day) (Wauquier et al. 2015). Saturated fats negatively affect bone by interfering with intestinal calcium absorption and increasing oxidative stress and inflammation (Wauquier et al. 2015). This proinflammatory environment stimulates osteoclast differentiation and decreases osteoblast differentiation resulting in net bone loss (Wauquier et al. 2015). Bone health, however, in athletes could be low if they have an insufficient intake of n3-PUFAs such as docosahexaenoic acid (DHA) and eicosapentaenoic acid (EPA). n3-PUFAs have a positive on bone through enhancement of gut calcium absorption and attenuation of inflammatory and oxidation stress response (Manore 2015; Wauquier et al. 2015). Thus, it may be important to ensure athletes have adequate intake (AI) of n3-PUFA for bone health; AI for normal healthy adults for α-linoleic acid, a plant-based n-3 PUFA which can be converted to DHA or EPA, is 1.6 g/day for men and 1.1 g/day for women (Institute of Medicine (U.S.). Panel on Macronutrients et al. 2005).

17.2.1.3 Micronutrients and Bone Health

In low EA, dietary intakes of micronutrients such as the bone building nutrients, calcium, and vitamin D may also be inadequate. In competitive cyclists, Viner et al. (2015) determined EA using 3-day food and activity records collected once a month over a season and FFM utilizing DXA. All cyclists had inadequate intake of Vitamin D, approximately 3/4 had low dietary calcium intake, and approximately 20% had low dietary intakes of B6 and B12 (Viner et al. 2015). Despite low intakes of these nutrients, bone health remained stable over the competitive season (Viner et al. 2015). In female athletes with ExMD, dietary intake was sufficient in all females for calcium and all but one for vitamin B12 (Cialdella-Kam et al. 2014). However, vitamin D intake was low in more than half of the athletes (Cialdella-Kam et al. 2014). In this study, only three women with ExMD met the definition of low EA (<30 kcal/kg of FFM/day) with low BMD present at the hip for two women and at the spine for three women (Cialdella-Kam et al. 2014); thus, vitamin D is a nutrient of particular concern. A recent meta-analysis reported that approximately 56% of all athletes examined had vitamin D inadequacy (defined as serum 25(OH)D levels of <80 mmol/L) (Farrokhyar et al. 2015).

Vitamin D with parathyroid hormone (PTH) maintains serum calcium levels within a narrow range (8.5 and 10.5 mg/dL) (Sunyecz 2008; Ross et al. 2011; Peterlik et al. 2013). A decline in serum calcium levels stimulates PTH secretion (Ross et al. 2011), which then acts to restore calcium balance by decreasing urinary calcium excretion, stimulating bone resorption (i.e., releasing calcium from the bone), and activating the enzyme, 1 α-hydroxylase in the kidneys (Balasch 2003; Sunyecz 2008; Ross et al. 2011). Vitamin D is then converted by 1α-hydroxylase from its inactive form, 25-hydroxyvitamin D, to its active form, 1,25 hydroxyvitamin D (calcitriol) (Todd et al. 2015). Calcitriol increases the transcellular active transport of calcium in the duodenum and jejunum resulting in increased calcium absorption in the gut (Ross et al. 2011). In addition, vitamin D may maintain calcium levels by activating bone resorption via receptor activator of nuclear factor kappa-β ligand (RANKL); however, further research is needed to elicit the mechanism (Ross et al. 2011; Takahashi et al. 2014). Both PTH and vitamin D stimulate reabsorption in the renal distal tubule (Ross et al. 2011; Millward 2012). Thus, vitamin D has important role in bone remolding, and inadequate intake has been associated with rickets, osteomalacia (i.e., soft bones), stress fractures, and bone loss (Carmeliet et al. 2015; Todd et al. 2015).

The intake of B-vitamins, which are involved in energy production, may be low in athletes with low EA, particularly those who follow a vegetarian or vegan diet. AI of folate and B12 are essential to maintain normal homocysteine levels, which may have an implication on bone health (van Wijngaarden et al. 2013; Fratoni and Brandi 2015). However, research in athletes is lacking related to the relationship between homocysteine and bone health. In elite university lacrosse players, homocysteine levels were compared in those with a history of stress fractures and those without with no difference found between groups, but it appears that most athletes had normal homocysteine levels (Wakamatsu et al. 2012). More research is needed to understand the role of inadequate B-vitamin intake and bone health.

17.2.1.4   Key Points on Nutrition and Bone Health

In summary, the key concerns in athletes with low EA for bone health are AIs of protein, vitamin D, and calcium. These nutrients have a direct role in bone health modulating gut calcium absorption, bone calcium release, and stimulating IGF-1 release. In addition, n-3 PUFA, may also improve calcium absorption and attenuate inflammation. Finally, the role of B-vitamins has been explored but remains unknown. More research on these nutrients is needed to understand their role in bone health. It is important to note that BMD is typically higher in athletes than nonathletes related to the mechanical stimuli on bone from exercise training (Weaver et al. 2016). Specifically, mechanical load stimulates osteocytes, the mechanosensor cells, which modulates osteoblast and osteoclast activity, leading to bone formation (Rosa et al. 2015; Weaver et al. 2016). Athlete need strong bones to handle the impact of rigorous training programs (McInnis and Ramey 2016). However, low EA alone has been associated with stress fractures and can also result in muscle loss, which can further increase susceptibility to bone loss (Tagliaferri et al. 2015; McInnis and Ramey 2016). Thus, a normal BMD (i.e., z-score >1.0) in an athlete that is lower than expected for their sport may be an early warning sign of stress fracture risk and need for nutrition intervention.

17.2.2   Leptin Disruptions in Low EA

Leptin plays a critical role in energy balance and bone metabolism (Upadhyay et al. 2015). In athletes with low leptin levels, menstrual dysfunction and impaired bone health may occur (Barrack et al. 2013). In addition, leptin affects several hormone signaling pathways including the hypothalamus–pituitary–gonadal (HPG) axis, the hypothalamus–pituitary–thyroid axis, the hypothalamus–pituitary–adrenal axis, and the hypothalamus–pituitary–growth hormone axis. In this section, leptin's role in energy balance will be described, followed by a discussion of how low leptin levels affect each of these axes and bone health.

17.2.2.1 Leptin and Energy Balance

Leptin is a hormone secreted from adipocytes in response to both acute and chronic changes in energy levels (Park and Ahima 2015). Plasma leptin levels correlate well with body fat stores and are representative of long-term energy stores (Park and Ahima 2015). Thus, in AN, an eating disorder characterized by low body fat, leptin levels are low, and leptin's circadian rhythm is disrupted (Probst et al. 2004; Misra and Klibanski 2014; Singhal et al. 2014; Tortorella et al. 2014). Excessive exercise, reported to occur in approximately 31%–80% of those with AN, can further suppress leptin as levels have been inversely correlated to physical activity (Tortorella et al. 2014). In BN, females with a low body mass index (BMI; <20 kg/m^2) have been reported to have lower body fat compared to healthy females (Probst et al. 2004). However, BN patients with BMI between 20 and 25 kg/m^2 had similar body fat percentage to healthy controls, and those with BMI >25 kg/m^2 had higher body fat levels than healthy controls (Probst et al. 2004). Consistent with this, leptin levels have been reported to be low, normal, or increased in BN, and thus leptin is indicative of energy stores (Monteleone and Maj 2013). Leptin levels, however, are affected by the frequency of binge/purge episodes and the duration of BN and thus do not serve as a good indicator of acute energy status (Monteleone and Maj 2013). In athletes with low EA, similar parallels between leptin and energy stores have been found. Specifically, leptin levels do not correspond with EA status in the absence or presence of menstrual dysfunction but are associated with body fat stores (Cialdella-Kam et al. 2014; Melin et al. 2015). Thus, as observed in BN, leptin levels in athletes are more reflective of long-term energy stores than acute caloric deficit (Tataranni et al. 1997).

Leptin disruptions has implications on both appetite and energy expenditure. In healthy individuals, peripheral leptin crosses the blood–brain barrier via transporters and possibly other unidentified methods into the hypothalamus (Parimisetty et al. 2016). Leptin then binds to its long receptor and initiates several downstream pathways including janus kinase/signal tranducers and activators of transcription (JAK-STAT) pathway (Kwon et al. 2016). As a result, orexigenic neuropeptides, neuropeptide Y (NPY), and agouti-related peptide (AgRP) are inhibited, and anorexigenic neuropeptides, pro-opiomelanocortin (POMC), and cocaine- and amphetamine-regulated transcript (CART) are stimulated (Park and Ahima 2015; Kwon et al. 2016). Leptin signaling in the hypothalamus results in decreased appetite and increased energy expenditure (Park and Ahima 2015). Thus, low leptin levels should be beneficial for restoration of energy stores since inhibition on appetite and the stimulation of energy expenditure would be attenuated. Indeed, in athletes with low EA, a decrease in RMR has been reported (Thomas et al. 2016). However, gut hormones such as ghrelin and peptide YY (PYY) also play an important role in appetite signaling. An acute bout of exercise has been associated with gut hormone changes resulting in increased satiety and decreased hunger after exercise (Howe et al. 2014, 2016; Hazell et al. 2016). In athletes with low EA, the gut hormones potentially may have a more potent effect on appetite than the observed reduction in leptin levels, and thus appetite remains suppressed (Barrack et al. 2013). Further research is warranted in the biology of appetite in athletes with low EA.

17.2.2.2 Leptin and Bone

Leptin has both direct and indirect effects on the bone remolding process (Upadhyay et al. 2015). The direct effects of leptin include stimulation on osteoblasts and chondrocytes (i.e., repair and form cartilage), regulation of the pro-osteoblastic bone matrix protein, osteocalcin, and activation of the phosphate-regulating hormone, fibroblast growth factor 23 (FGF23) (Florencio-Silva et al. 2015; Upadhyay et al. 2015). Indirectly, leptin may regulate neuronal signaling, which is beyond the scope of this chapter (Houweling et al. 2015). Several bone-regulating hormones such as estradiol, cortisol, thyroid, and IGF-1 are regulated via leptin-signaling pathways (Upadhyay et al. 2015).

In the next sections, we describe the implications of leptin disruptions on these pathways and the impact on bone.

17.2.2.3 HPG Axis

Low EA has been associated with malfunction of the HPG axis provoking decreased estrogen release and menstrual dysfunction (Stafford 2005; Mountjoy et al. 2014; Melin et al. 2015; Thomas et al. 2016). In healthy women, hypothalamic gonadotropin releasing hormone (GnRH) stimulates the pituitary release of luteinizing hormone (LH), which triggers the production of estrogen and progesterone (Stafford 2005). In low EA, GnRH pulsatility is disrupted and thus results in decreased estrogen release from the ovaries (Stafford 2005; Mountjoy et al. 2014). Leptin is thought to play an important role in the regulation of the GnRH pulse generator (Stafford 2005). Several direct and indirect pathways have been proposed for leptin (Stafford 2005; Vazquez et al. 2015). Currently, leptin appears to regulate the release of kisspeptins from the Kiss1 neurons in the hypothalamus, which in turn regulate the GnRH pulse generator (Vazquez et al. 2015). As noted previously, low leptin levels are not consistently observed in individuals with low EA and menstrual dysfunction (Cialdella-Kam et al. 2014; Melin et al. 2015). Thus, other hormonal disruptions such as high cortisol and high ghrelin among others may contribute to low estrogen levels and menstrual disturbances (Stafford 2005; Pauli and Berga 2010; Maggi et al. 2016). The control of GnRH pulse generator appears to be modulated by several neuropeptides and hormones (Maggi et al. 2016; Vazquez et al. 2015); thus, further research is needed to elucidate the pathway related to menstrual dysfunction and low EA.

Estrogen is an important inhibitor of osteoclast activity as demonstrated by bone loss that parallels estrogen declines during menopause (Lupsa and Insogna 2015). The exact mechanism by which estrogen inhibits osteoclast activity remains unknown, but it may induce Fas/Fas ligand increasing osteoclast apoptosis and stimulate the decoy receptor of RANK, osteoprotegerin (OPG) inhibiting osteoclastogenesis (Kovacic et al. 2010; Florencio-Silva et al. 2015). In addition, estrogen may modulate osteocytes response to mechanical load and attenuate osteoclastogenic cytokines (Florencio-Silva et al. 2015; Klein-Nulend et al. 2015). Estrogen therapy is not recommended as a first line of defense for osteoporosis and may not be effective in restoring bone loss in active women (Barrack et al. 2013; Cosman et al. 2014). Thus, diet and exercise should be adjusted to restore EA as a first line of defense (Kelly and Ronnekleiv 2015).

17.2.2.4 Leptin's Effect on Other Hormones

Leptin-signaling pathways in the hypothalamus modulate cortisol, thyroid hormones, and IGF-1 release. Thus, low leptin levels may contribute to the altered hormonal status in EA such as high cortisol levels and low thyroid and IGF-1 levels. As a result, bone health is further attenuated. Specifically, high cortisol levels lead to increased net bone resorption (Goddard et al. 2015; Mazziotti et al. 2015) and are predictive of lower bone density in AN (Misra and Klibanski 2014). The exact mechanism by which thyroid levels impacts bone has not been elucidated, but thyroid hormones maybe bone promoting via inhibition of osteoclastogenesis and stimulation of bone formation (Bassett and Williams 2016). Hypothyroidism has been associated with increased fracture risk (Vestergaard and Mosekilde 2002). Finally, suppressed IGF-1 levels in low EA alters bone health as IGF-1 has an anabolic effect on bone including osteoblast maturation and differentiation and chondrocyte differentiation (Tahimic et al. 2013). Thus, bone health in low EA is affected by a multitude of factors including inadequate and nutrient intake and hormonal disruptions as previously described. Low EA also is associated with other health risks as summarized below.

17.2.3 OTHER HEALTH RISKS

Low EA have been associated with other health risks beyond those already discussed affecting skeletal muscle, cardiovascular and central nervous systems and altering immune and renal function (Nattiv et al. 2007; Joy et al. 2014; Mountjoy et al. 2014; Gleeson 2016). In this section, we will

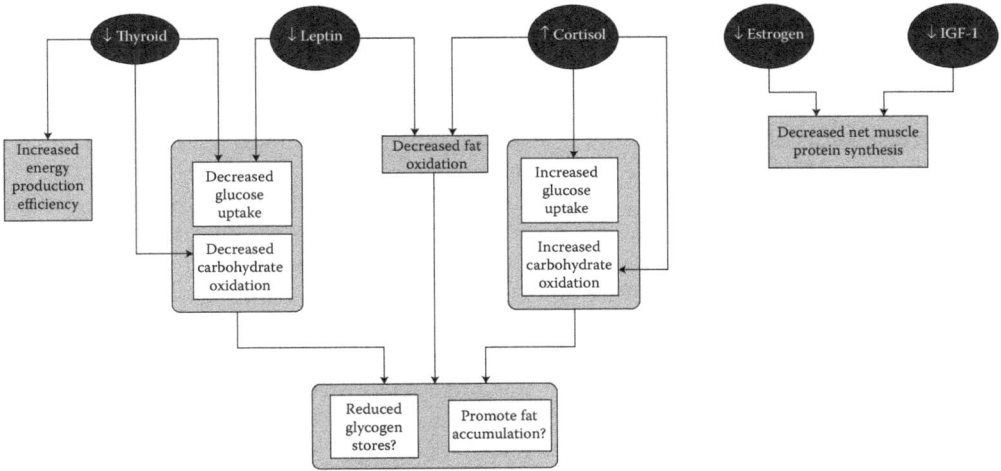

FIGURE 17.2 In low EA, several hormonal disruptions occur including low levels of leptin, estrogen, thyroid, and IGF-1, and high levels of cortisol. As depicted in the figure, these disruptions can alter both substrate utilization and net MPS (i.e., MPS less muscle protein degradation [MPD]) in skeletal muscle. In healthy individuals, leptin normally stimulates fatty acid oxidation, inhibits lipid biosynthesis, and increase glucose uptake primarily though activation of adenosine monophosphate-activated protein kinase (AMPK), which would preserve glycogen stores (Coles 2016). The combination of high cortisol levels and low leptin levels result in increased carbohydrate oxidation and decreased fat oxidation resulting in low glycogen stores and fat accumulation (de Guia and Herziq 2015; Kuo et al. 2015; Coles 2016). Low thyroid levels may confound the effects by changes in gene expression related to decreased glucose uptake and decreased mitochondrial density, but may also offset the effects by increased metabolic efficiencies and decreased carbohydrate oxidation (Salvatore et al. 2014). However, it is likely that glycogen stores would be low and fat oxidation would be attenuated. Estrogen and IGF-1 primarily affect skeletal muscle repair and growth (Velders and Diel 2013; Song 2016). Thus, low estrogen and IGF-1 levels coupled with high cortisol levels can lead to decreased net MPS (Velders and Diel 2013; Kuo et al. 2015; Song 2016).

describe the impact of low EA on skeletal muscle with a focus on the implications of hormonal disruptions. Additional information on other health risks have been addressed in prior review articles (Manore et al. 2007; Nattiv et al. 2007; Barrack et al. 2013; Sundgot-Borgen et al. 2013; Joy et al. 2014; Mountjoy et al. 2014; Thomas et al. 2016).

Skeletal muscle health in low EA is affected by both energy and nutritional insufficiencies and disruptions in hormone levels. Briefly, low EI results in low glycogen stores and impaired MPS, which can be exaggerated by inadequate carbohydrate intake and insufficient or low-quality protein intake (Mountjoy et al. 2014; Thomas et al. 2016). Altered micronutrient status in low EA may also have implications on skeletal muscle health. In particular, vitamin D's role has been explored in skeletal muscle due to the prevalence of vitamin D insufficiencies in athletes, the presence of vitamin D receptors on skeletal muscle cells, and its hormone-like actions; however, further research in this area is warranted to elicit vitamin D's role (von Hurst and Beck 2014; Owens et al. 2015; Todd et al. 2015). Hormonal disruptions observed in low EA may impact substrate utilization, MPS and degradation, and glycogen stores as depicted in Figure 17.2 (Velders and Diel 2013; Salvatore et al. 2014; de Guia and Herziq 2015; Kuo et al. 2015; Coles 2016; Song 2016).

17.3 DIETARY AND EXERCISE INTERVENTIONS IN EXERCISE-INDUCED MENSTRUAL DYSFUNCTION

Diet and exercise interventions for the reversal of ExMD have been examined in a limited number of studies including four case studies (Kopp-Woodroffe et al. 1999; Zanker et al. 2004; Fredericson and Kent 2005; Mallinson et al. 2013), one retrospective chart review (Arends et al. 2012), and one prospective intervention study (Cialdella-Kam et al. 2014). Baseline energy and nutrient intake from three of these studies are presented in Table 17.4 (Kopp-Woodroffe et al. 1999; Arends et al. 2012; Cialdella-Kam et al. 2014); the data from three of the case studies were insufficient to be included in the table (Zanker et al. 2004; Fredericson and Kent 2005; Mallinson et al. 2013). Athletes with menstrual dysfunction had low EA (i.e., <45 g/kg/day).

In two studies, EA (mean EA range = 37–41 kcal/kg FFM/day) has been reported to be similar between athletes with eumenorrhea and ExMD (Cialdella-Kam and Manore 2009; Melin et al. 2015). Thus, some women may be more susceptible to menstrual dysfunction in low EA (levels <45 kcal/kg FFM/day) or other associated imbalances may be contributing to the occurrence. As previously discussed, athletes with menstrual dysfunction are typically meeting the sports nutrition guidelines for carbohydrate, protein, and fat (Table 17.4) with carbohydrates falling at the low end of the range (Thomas et al. 2016). Athletes, in general, preferred to increase EA by increased EI rather than decreased EEE (Kopp-Woodroffe et al. 1999; Arends et al. 2012). In general, EA improvements between approximately 230 and 380 kcal/day appear to be sufficient to resume menstrual status if the athlete also realized an increase in weight gain of 2–5 kg (Kopp-Woodroffe et al. 1999; Arends et al. 2012; Mallinson et al. 2013; Cialdella-Kam et al. 2014). The time to restoration of

---

TABLE 17.4
Diet and Exercise Studies in Active Women with Menstrual Dysfunction[a]

Description	Energy Intake (kcal/day)	Energy Availability (kcal/kg/day)	Carbohydrates (g/kg/day)	Protein (g/kg/day)	Fat (% of total kcal)	Menses Resumed (%)	Time to Resumption of Menses (months)
			Arends et al. (2012)[b]				
Amen ($n = 12$)	2076	NR	5.8[c]	1.7[c]	23[c]	17.6	17.7
Oligo ($n = 38$)	2383	NR	6.1[c]	1.6[c]	23[c]	15.8	14.5
			Cialdella-Kam et al. (2014)[d]				
Amen/Oligo ($n = 8$)	2312	36.7	5.0	1.4	30	88	2.6
			Kopp-Woodroffe et al. (1999)[e]				
Amen ($n = 4$)	1892[c]	25.1[c]	5.5[c]	1.2[c]	23	75	3.8[c]
			Łagowska et al. (2014)[f]				
Amen/Oligo ($n = 31$)	2354	28.3	5.2[c]	1.3[c]	35[c]	0	–

Note: Amen, amenorrheic; Oligo, oligomenorrheic; NR, not reported.

[a] Three case studies were excluded from this table due to lack of energy and nutrition information.

[b] Retrospective study: Athletes worked with sports dietitian to increase EI by ~250–300 kcal/day; some athletes may have decreased EEE.

[c] Estimated based on data presented in article.

[d] Intervention study: Athletes increased EI by 360 kcal/day for 6 months. This study included seven amenorrheic and one oligomenorrheic. All women resumed menses, but one remained anovulatory.

[e] Case study: Two athletes increased EI and two athletes increased EI and decreases energy expenditure. The average change in EA was an increase of approximately 233 kcal/day. One athlete discontinued the study at week 12 prior to resumption of menses.

[f] Intervention study: Athletes increased EI by approximately 234 kcal/day for 3 months. This study included five amenorrheic and 26 oligomenorrheic athletes. Improvement in reproductive hormones was realized, but there was no change in menstrual status at 3 months.

menses varied among participants (Table 17.4), which may be associated with duration of menstrual dysfunction (Cialdella-Kam et al. 2014) with one 3-month intervention study reporting no change in menstrual status with increase in EI (Łagowska et al. 2014). In addition, some athletes may not restore menses on diet and exercise interventions alone and require pharmacological interventions (Kopp-Woodroffe et al. 1999; Arends et al. 2012). Thus, it is important that sports dietitians and physicians work together in resolving menstrual dysfunction in athletes. In summary, strategies for improving and identifying low EA in athletes are as follows (Arends et al. 2012; Sundgot-Borgen et al. 2013; Cialdella-Kam et al. 2014; Mountjoy et al. 2014):

1. Educate athletes on the signs or symptoms of low EA such as menstrual disturbances, frequent illness and injuries, chronic fatigue, underperformance, and depressed mood state.
2. Improve EA by
   a. Increasing EI via inclusion of energy dense foods and drinks such as smoothies, meal replacement shakes, trail mix, and fruit with nut butter and/or
   b. Decreasing EEE by taking a day off or reducing training intensity; athletes, however, may be reluctant to do this.
3. Ensure adequate vitamin D (600–2000 IU/day) and calcium (1000–1500 mg/day) intakes to support bone health.
4. Engage a multidisciplinary team for optimal care of athletes with low EA.

It is important to monitor the athlete's progress working in a team of professionals including physicians, coaches, athletic trainers, psychologists, and sports dietitians as appropriate. The team can help identify athletes who may need interventions that go beyond diet and exercise.

17.4 CONCLUSIONS AND PERSPECTIVES

Low EA in athletes is associated with menstrual dysfunction, impaired bone health, and hormonal disruptions among other health risks. Dietary interventions that increase EI by 250–350 kcal/day may be effective in improving EA and subsequently restoring menstrual status. However, some athletes may require further interventions and thus a multidisciplinary team should be engaged for the care of the athlete with low EA. In addition, some athletes experience ExMD and health consequences in the presence of low EA whereas others do not. Further research is warranted to identify other factors that may affect an individual's sensitivity to low EA and those particularly at risk.

REFERENCES

Ackland, T. R., T. G. Lohman, J. Sundgot-Borgen et al. 2012. Current status of body composition assessment in sport: Review and position statement on behalf of the ad hoc research working group on body composition health and performance, under the auspices of the I.O.C. Medical Commission. *Sports Med* 42:227–49.

American Psychiatric Association, and American Psychiatric Association. DSM-5 Task Force. 2013. *Diagnostic and Statistical Manual of Mental Disorders: DSM-5* (5th Ed.). Washington, DC: American Psychiatric Association.

Arends, J. C., M. Y. Cheung, M. T. Barrack, and A. Nattiv. 2012. Restoration of menses with nonpharmacologic therapy in college athletes with menstrual disturbances: A 5-year retrospective study. *Int J Sport Nutr Exerc Metab* 22:98–108.

Attal, F., S. Mohammed, M. Dedabrishvili, F. Chamroukhi, L. Oukhellou, and Y. Amirat. 2015. Physical human activity recognition using wearable sensors. *Sensors (Basel)* 15:31314–38.

Balasch, J. 2003. Sex steroids and bone: Current perspectives. *Hum Reprod Update* 9:207–222.

Barkai, H. S., J. F. Nichols, M. J. Rauh, M. T. Barrack, M. J. Lawson, and S. S. Levy. 2007. Influence of sports participation and menarche on bone mineral density of female high school athletes. *J Sci Med Sport* 10:170–9.

Barrack, M. T., K. E. Ackerman, and J. C. Gibbs. 2013. Update on the female athlete triad. *Curr Rev Musculoskelet Med* 6:195–204.

Bassett, J. H. and G. R. Williams. 2016. Role of thyroid hormones in skeletal development and bone maintenance. *Endocr Rev* 37:135–87.

Bihuniak, J. D. and K. L. Insogna. 2015. The effects of dietary protein and amino acids on skeletal metabolism. *Mol Cell Endocrinol* 410:78–86.

Burke, L. M. 2015. Dietary assessment methods for the athletes: Pros and cons of different methods. *Sports Sci. Exchange* 28:1–6.

Carmeliet, G., V. Dermauw, and R. Bouillon. 2015. Vitamin D signaling in calcium and bone homeostasis: A delicate balance. *Best Pract Res Clin Endocrinol Metab* 29:621–31.

Chapurlat, R. D. and C. B. Confavreux. 2016. Novel biological markers of bone: From bone metabolism to bone physiology. *Rheumatology (Oxford)* 55:1714–25. doi: 10.1093/rheumatology/kev410.

Cialdella-Kam, L., C. P. Guebels, G. F. Maddalozzo, and M. M. Manore. 2014. Dietary intervention restored menses in female athletes with exercise-associated menstrual dysfunction with limited impact on bone and muscle health. *Nutrients* 6:3018–39.

Cialdella-Kam, L. C. and M. M. Manore. 2009. Macronutrient needs of active individuals: An update. *Nutr Today* 44:104–11.

Coles, C. A. 2016. Adipokines in healthy skeletal muscle and metabolic disease. *Adv Exp Med Biol* 900:133–60.

Cosman, F., S. J. de Beur, M. S. LeBoff et al. 2014. Clinician's guide to prevention and treatment of osteoporosis. *Osteoporos Int* 25:2359–81.

Cunningham, J. J. 1980. A reanalysis of the factors influencing basal metabolic rate in normal adults. *Am J Clin Nutr* 33:2372–4.

de Guia, R. M. and S. Herzig. 2015. How do glucocorticoids regulate lipid metabolism? *Adv Exp Med Biol* 872:127–44.

Evans, D. 2016. MyFitnessPal. *Br J Sports Med*. doi: 10.1136/bjsports-2015-095538.

Farrokhyar, F., R. Tabasinejad, D. Dao et al. 2015. Prevalence of vitamin D inadequacy in athletes: A systematic-review and meta-analysis. *Sports Med* 45:365–78.

Fenton, T. R., A. W. Lyon, M. Eliasziw, S. C. Tough, and D. A. Hanley. 2009. Meta-analysis of the effect of the acid-ash hypothesis of osteoporosis on calcium balance. *J Bone Miner Res* 24:1835–40.

Florencio-Silva, R., G. R. Sasso, E. Sasso-Cerri, M. J. Simoes, and P. S. Cerri. 2015. Biology of bone tissue: Structure, function, and factors that influence bone cells. *Biomed Res Int* 2015:421746.

Fratoni, V. and M. L. Brandi. 2015. B vitamins, homocysteine and bone health. *Nutrients* 7:2176–92.

Fredericson, M. and K. Kent. 2005. Normalization of bone density in a previously amenorrheic runner with osteoporosis. *Med Sci Sports Exerc* 37:1481–6.

Gaffney-Stomberg, E., B. H. Sun, C. E. Cucchi et al. 2010. The effect of dietary protein on intestinal calcium absorption in rats. *Endocrinology* 151:1071–8.

Gleeson, M. 2016. Immunological aspects of sport nutrition. *Immunol Cell Biol* 94:117–23.

Goddard, G. M., A. Ravikumar, and A. C. Levine. 2015. Adrenal mild hypercortisolism. *Endocrinol Metab Clin North Am* 44:371–9.

Guebels, C. P., L. C. Kam, G. F. Maddalozzo, and M. M. Manore. 2014. Active women before/after an intervention designed to restore menstrual function: Resting metabolic rate and comparison of four methods to quantify energy expenditure and energy availability. *Int J Sport Nutr Exerc Metab* 24:37–46.

Hand, T. M., S. Howe, L. Cialdella-Kam, C. P. Hoffman, and M. Manore. 2016. A pilot study: Dietary energy density is similar between active women with and without exercise-associated menstrual dysfunction. *Nutrients* 8(4):230. doi: 10.3390/nu8040230.

Hannan, M. T., K. L. Tucker, B. Dawson-Hughes, L. A. Cupples, D. T. Felson, and D. P. Kiel. 2000. Effect of dietary protein on bone loss in elderly men and women: The Framingham Osteoporosis Study. *J Bone Miner Res* 15:2504–12.

Harris, J. A. and F. G. Benedict. 1918. A biometric study of human basal metabolism. *Proc Natl Acad Sci USA* 4:370–3.

Hazell, T. J., H. Islam, L. K. Townsend, M. S. Schmale, and J. L. Copeland. 2016. Effects of exercise intensity on plasma concentrations of appetite-regulating hormones: Potential mechanisms. *Appetite* 98:80–8.

Heaney, R. P. and D. K. Layman. 2008. Amount and type of protein influences bone health. *Am J Clin Nutr* 87:1567s–70s.

Helms, E. R., C. Zinn, D. S. Rowlands, and S. R. Brown. 2014. A systematic review of dietary protein during caloric restriction in resistance trained lean athletes: A case for higher intakes. *Int J Sport Nutr Exerc Metab* 24:127–38.

Horvath, P. J., C. K. Eagen, N. M. Fisher, J. J. Leddy, and D. R. Pendergast. 2000. The effects of varying dietary fat on performance and metabolism in trained male and female runners. *J Am Coll Nutr* 19:52–60.

Houweling, P., R. N. Kulkarni, and P. A. Baldock. 2015. Neuronal control of bone and muscle. *Bone* 80:95–100.

Howe, S. M., T. M. Hand, D. E. Larson-Meyer, K. J. Austin, B. M. Alexander, and M. M. Manore. 2016. No effect of exercise intensity on appetite in highly-trained endurance women. *Nutrients* 8(4):223. doi: 10.3390/nu8040223.

Howe, S. M., T. M. Hand, and M. M. Manore. 2014. Exercise-trained men and women: Role of exercise and diet on appetite and energy intake. *Nutrients* 6:4935–60.

Institute of Medicine (U.S.). Panel on Macronutrients, and Institute of Medicine (U.S.). Standing Committee on the Scientific Evaluation of Dietary Reference Intakes. 2005. *Dietary Reference Intakes for Energy, Carbohydrate, Fiber, Fat, Fatty Acids, Cholesterol, Protein, and Amino Acids.* Washington, DC: National Academies Press.

Jennings, A., A. MacGregor, T. Spector, and A. Cassidy. 2016. Amino acid intakes are associated with bone mineral density and prevalence of low bone mass in women: Evidence from discordant monozygotic twins. *J Bone Miner Res* 31:326–35.

Joy, E., M. J. De Souza, A. Nattiv et al. 2014. 2014 female athlete triad coalition consensus statement on treatment and return to play of the female athlete triad. *Curr Sports Med Rep* 13:219–32.

Joy, E., A. Kussman, and A. Nattiv. 2016. 2016 update on eating disorders in athletes: A comprehensive narrative review with a focus on clinical assessment and management. *Br J Sports Med* 50:154–62.

Kelly, M. J. and O. K. Ronnekleiv. 2015. Minireview: Neural signaling of estradiol in the hypothalamus. *Mol Endocrinol* 29:645–57.

Kerstetter, J. E., K. O. O'Brien, and K. L. Insogna. 2003. Dietary protein, calcium metabolism, and skeletal homeostasis revisited. *Am J Clin Nutr* 78(3 Suppl):584s–92s.

Klein-Nulend, J., R. F. van Oers, A. D. Bakker, and R. G. Bacabac. 2015. Bone cell mechanosensitivity, estrogen deficiency, and osteoporosis. *J Biomech* 48:855–65.

Kohrt, W. M., S. A. Bloomfield, K. D. Little, M. E. Nelson, and V. R. Yingling. 2004. Physical activity and bone health. *Med Sci Sports Exerc* 36:1985–96.

Kopp-Woodroffe, S. A., M. M. Manore, C. A. Dueck, J. S. Skinner, and K. S. Matt. 1999. Energy and nutrient status of amenorrheic athletes participating in a diet and exercise training intervention program. *Int J Sport Nutr* 9:70–88.

Kovacic, N., D. Grcevic, V. Katavic, I. K. Lukic, and A. Marusic. 2010. Targeting Fas in osteoresorptive disorders. *Expert Opin Ther Targets* 14:1121–34.

Krieger, N. S., K. K. Frick, and D. A. Bushinsky. 2004. Mechanism of acid-induced bone resorption. *Curr Opin Nephrol Hypertens* 13:423–36.

Kuo, T., A. McQueen, T. C. Chen, and J. C. Wang. 2015. Regulation of glucose homeostasis by glucocorticoids. *Adv Exp Med Biol* 872:99–126.

Kwon, O., K. W. Kim, and M. S. Kim. 2016. Leptin signalling pathways in hypothalamic neurons. *Cell Mol Life Sci* 73:1457–77.

Łagowska, K., K. Kapczuk, Z. Friebe, and J. Bajerska. 2014. Effects of dietary intervention in young female athletes with menstrual disorders. *J Int Soc Sports Nutr* 11:21–21.

Lombardi, G., S. Perego, L. Luzi, and G. Banfi. 2015. A four-season molecule: Osteocalcin. Updates in its physiological roles. *Endocrine* 48:394–404.

Loucks, A. B. 2013. Energy balance and energy availability. In R. J. Maughan (ed.) *The Encyclopaedia of Sports Medicine*, 72–87. John Wiley, West Sussex, UK.

Loucks, A. B. and R. Callister. 1993. Induction and prevention of low-T3 syndrome in exercising women. *Am J Physiol* 264(5 Pt 2):R924–30.

Loucks, A. B., M. Verdun, and E. M. Heath. 1998. Low energy availability, not stress of exercise, alters LH pulsatility in exercising women. *J Appl Physiol (1985)* 84:37–46.

Lupsa, B. C. and K. Insogna. 2015. Bone health and osteoporosis. *Endocrinol Metab Clin North Am* 44:517–30.

Maggi, R., A. M. Cariboni, M. M. Marelli et al. 2016. GnRH and GnRH receptors in the pathophysiology of the human female reproductive system. *Hum Reprod Update* 22:358–81.

Mallinson, R. J., N. I. Williams, M. P. Olmsted, J. L. Scheid, E. S. Riddle, and M. J. De Souza. 2013. A case report of recovery of menstrual function following a nutritional intervention in two exercising women with amenorrhea of varying duration. *J Int Soc Sports Nutr* 10:34.

Manore, M. M. 2015. Weight management for athletes and active individuals: A brief review. *Sports Med* 45(Suppl 1):S83–92.

Manore, M. M., L. C. Kam, and A. B. Loucks. 2007. The female athlete triad: Components, nutrition issues, and health consequences. *J Sports Sci* 25(Suppl 1):S61–71.

Mazziotti, G., S. Chiavistelli, and A. Giustina. 2015. Pituitary diseases and bone. *Endocrinol Metab Clin North Am* 44:171–80.

McInnis, K. C. and L. N. Ramey. 2016. High-risk stress fractures: Diagnosis and management. *PM R* 8(3 Suppl):S113–24.

Melin, A., A. B. Tornberg, S. Skouby et al. 2016. Low-energy density and high fiber intake are dietary concerns in female endurance athletes. *Scand J Med Sci Sports* 26:1060–71. doi: 10.1111/sms.12516.

Melin, A., A. B. Tornberg, S. Skouby et al. 2015. Energy availability and the female athlete triad in elite endurance athletes. *Scand J Med Sci Sports* 25(5):610–22.

Mettler, S., N. Mitchell, and K. D. Tipton. 2010. Increased protein intake reduces lean body mass loss during weight loss in athletes. *Med Sci Sports Exerc* 42:326–37.

Millward, D. J. 2012. A new approach to establishing dietary energy reference values. *Curr Opin Clin Nutr Metab Care* 15:413–7.

Misra, M. and A. Klibanski. 2014. Endocrine consequences of anorexia nervosa. *Lancet Diabetes Endocrinol* 2:581–92.

Monsen, E. R., L. Van Horn, and American Dietetic Association. 2008. *Research: Successful Approaches* (3rd Ed.). Chicago, IL: American Dietetic Association.

Monteleone, P. and M. Maj. 2013. Dysfunctions of leptin, ghrelin, BDNF and endocannabinoids in eating disorders: Beyond the homeostatic control of food intake. *Psychoneuroendocrinology* 38:312–30.

Mountjoy, M., J. Sundgot-Borgen, L. Burke et al. 2014. The IOC consensus statement: Beyond the Female Athlete Triad—Relative Energy Deficiency in Sport (RED-S). *Br J Sports Med* 48:491–7.

Muia, E. N., H. H. Wright, V. O. Onywera, and E. N. Kuria. 2016. Adolescent elite Kenyan runners are at risk for energy deficiency, menstrual dysfunction and disordered eating. *J Sports Sci* 34:598–606.

Murphy, C. H., A. J. Hector, and S. M. Phillips. 2015. Considerations for protein intake in managing weight loss in athletes. *Eur J Sport Sci* 15:21–8.

Nattiv, A., A. B. Loucks, M. M. Manore, C. F. Sanborn, J. Sundgot-Borgen, and M. P. Warren. 2007. American College of Sports Medicine position stand. The female athlete triad. *Med Sci Sports Exerc* 39:1867–82.

Owens, D. J., W. D. Fraser, and G. L. Close. 2015. Vitamin D and the athlete: Emerging insights. *Eur J Sport Sci* 15:73–84.

Parimisetty, A., A. C. Dorsemans, R. Awada, P. Ravanan, N. Diotel, and C. Lefebvre d'Hellencourt. 2016. Secret talk between adipose tissue and central nervous system via secreted factors—An emerging frontier in the neurodegenerative research. *J Neuroinflamm* 13:67. doi: 10.1186/s12974-016-0530-x.

Park, H. K. and R. S. Ahima. 2015. Physiology of leptin: Energy homeostasis, neuroendocrine function and metabolism. *Metabolism* 64:24–34.

Pauli, S. A. and S. L. Berga. 2010. Athletic amenorrhea: Energy deficit or psychogenic challenge? *Ann NY Acad Sci* 1205:33–8.

Peterlik, M., E. Kallay, and H. S. Cross. 2013. Calcium nutrition and extracellular calcium sensing: Relevance for the pathogenesis of osteoporosis, cancer and cardiovascular diseases. *Nutrients* 5:302–27.

Phillips, S. M. 2014. A brief review of higher dietary protein diets in weight loss: A focus on athletes. *Sports Med* 44(Suppl 2):S149–53.

Probst, M., M. Goris, W. Vandereycken, G. Pieters, J. Vanderlinden, and H. Van Coppenolle. 2004. Body composition in bulimia nervosa patients compared to healthy females. *Eur J Nutr* 43:288–96.

Rodriguez, N. R., N. M. Di Marco, and S. Langley. 2009. American College of Sports Medicine position stand. Nutrition and athletic performance. *Med Sci Sports Exerc* 41:709–31.

Rolls, B. J. 2012. Dietary strategies for weight management. *Nestle Nutr Inst Workshop Ser* 73:37–48.

Rosa, N., R. Simoes, F. D. Magalhaes, and A. T. Marques. 2015. From mechanical stimulus to bone formation: A review. *Med Eng Phys* 37:719–28.

Ross, A. Catharine, and Institute of Medicine (U.S.). Committee to Review Dietary Reference Intakes for Vitamin D and Calcium. 2011. *DRI, Dietary Reference Intakes Calcium, Vitamin D*. Washington, DC: National Academies Press.

Salvatore, D., W. S. Simonides, M. Dentice, A. M. Zavacki, and P. R. Larsen. 2014. Thyroid hormones and skeletal muscle—New insights and potential implications. *Nat Rev Endocrinol* 10:206–14.

Santesso, N., E. A. Akl, M. Bianchi et al. 2012. Effects of higher- versus lower-protein diets on health outcomes: A systematic review and meta-analysis. *Eur J Clin Nutr* 66:780–8.

Schousboe, J. T., J. A. Shepherd, J. P. Bilezikian, and S. Baim. 2013. Executive summary of the 2013 International Society for Clinical Densitometry Position Development Conference on bone densitometry. *J Clin Densitom* 16:455–66.

Singhal, V., M. Misra, and A. Klibanski. 2014. Endocrinology of anorexia nervosa in young people: Recent insights. *Curr Opin Endocrinol Diabetes Obes* 21:64–70.

Song, Y. 2016. Function of membrane-associated proteoglycans in the regulation of satellite cell growth. *Adv Exp Med Biol* 900:61–95.

Stafford, D. E. 2005. Altered hypothalamic–pituitary–ovarian axis function in young female athletes: Implications and recommendations for management. *Treat Endocrinol* 4:147–54.

Steinmuller, P. L., L. J. Kruskall, C. A. Karpinski, M. M. Manore, M. A. Macedonio, and N. L. Meyer. 2014. Academy of nutrition and dietetics: Revised 2014 standards of practice and standards of professional performance for registered dietitian nutritionists (competent, proficient, and expert) in sports nutrition and dietetics. *J Acad Nutr Diet* 114:631–41.e43.

Strother, E., R. Lemberg, S. C. Stanford, and D. Turberville. 2012. Eating disorders in men: Underdiagnosed, undertreated, and misunderstood. *Eat Disord* 20:346–55.

Stubbs, R. J., D. A. Hughes, A. M. Johnstone et al. 2004. Rate and extent of compensatory changes in energy intake and expenditure in response to altered exercise and diet composition in humans. *Am J Physiol Regul Integr Comp Physiol* 286:R350–8.

Sundgot-Borgen, J., N. L. Meyer, T. G. Lohman et al. 2013. How to minimise the health risks to athletes who compete in weight-sensitive sports review and position statement on behalf of the Ad Hoc Research Working Group on Body Composition, Health and Performance, under the auspices of the IOC Medical Commission. *Br J Sports Med* 47:1012–22.

Sunyecz, J. A. 2008. The use of calcium and vitamin D in the management of osteoporosis. *Ther Clin Risk Manag* 4:827–36.

Tagliaferri, C., Y. Wittrant, M. J. Davicco, S. Walrand, and V. Coxam. 2015. Muscle and bone, two interconnected tissues. *Ageing Res Rev* 21:55–70.

Tahimic, C. G., Y. Wang, and D. D. Bikle. 2013. Anabolic effects of IGF-1 signaling on the skeleton. *Front Endocrinol (Lausanne)* 4:4–6. doi: 10.3389/fendo.2013.00006.

Takahashi, N., N. Udagawa, and T. Suda. 2014. Vitamin D endocrine system and osteoclasts. *BoneKey Rep* 3:495. doi: 10.1038/bonekey.2013.229.

Tataranni, P. A., M. B. Monroe, C. A. Dueck et al. 1997. Adiposity, plasma leptin concentration and reproductive function in active and sedentary females. *Int J Obes Relat Metab Disord* 21:818–21.

Thomas, D. T., K. A. Erdman, and L. M. Burke. 2016. Position of the Academy of Nutrition and Dietetics, Dietitians of Canada, and the American College of Sports Medicine: Nutrition and athletic performance. *J Acad Nutr Diet* 116:501–28.

Thompson, J. and M. M. Manore. 1996. Predicted and measured metabolic rate of male and female endurance athletes. *J Am Diet Assoc* 96:30–4.

Todd, J. J., L. K. Pourshahidi, E. M. McSorley, S. M. Madigan, and P. J. Magee. 2015. Vitamin D: Recent advances and implications for athletes. *Sports Med* 45:213–29.

Torstveit, M. K. and J. Sundgot-Borgen. 2005. Low bone mineral density is two to three times more prevalent in non-athletic premenopausal women than in elite athletes: A comprehensive controlled study. *Br J Sports Med* 39:282–7.

Tortorella, A., F. Brambilla, M. Fabrazzo et al. 2014. Central and peripheral peptides regulating eating behaviour and energy homeostasis in anorexia nervosa and bulimia nervosa: A literature review. *Eur Eat Disord Rev* 22:307–20.

Tudor-Locke, C., T. L. Washington, B. E. Ainsworth, and R. P. Troiano. 2009. Linking the American Time Use Survey (ATUS) and the compendium of physical activities: Methods and rationale. *J Phys Act Health* 6:347–53.

Upadhyay, J., O. M. Farr, and C. S. Mantzoros. 2015. The role of leptin in regulating bone metabolism. *Metabolism* 64:105–13.

van Wijngaarden, J. P., E. L. Doets, A. Szczecinska et al. 2013. Vitamin B12, folate, homocysteine, and bone health in adults and elderly people: A systematic review with meta-analyses. *J Nutr Metab* 2013:486186.

Vazquez, M. J., A. Romero-Ruiz, and M. Tena-Sempere. 2015. Roles of leptin in reproduction, pregnancy and polycystic ovary syndrome: Consensus knowledge and recent developments. *Metabolism* 64:79–91.

Velders, M. and P. Diel. 2013. How sex hormones promote skeletal muscle regeneration. *Sports Med* 43:1089–100.

Vergnaud, P., P. Garnero, P. J. Meunier, G. Breart, K. Kamihagi, and P. D. Delmas. 1997. Undercarboxylated osteocalcin measured with a specific immunoassay predicts hip fracture in elderly women: The EPIDOS Study. *J Clin Endocrinol Metab* 82:719–24.

Vestergaard, P. and L. Mosekilde. 2002. Fractures in patients with hyperthyroidism and hypothyroidism: A nationwide follow-up study in 16,249 patients. *Thyroid* 12:411–9.

Viner, R. T., M. Harris, J. R. Berning, and N. L. Meyer. 2015. Energy availability and dietary patterns of adult male and female competitive cyclists with lower than expected bone mineral density. *Int J Sport Nutr Exerc Metab* 25:594–602.

von Hurst, P. R. and K. L. Beck. 2014. Vitamin D and skeletal muscle function in athletes. *Curr Opin Clin Nutr Metab Care* 17:539–45.

Wakamatsu, K., K. Sakuraba, Y. Suzuki et al. 2012. Association between the stress fracture and bone metabolism/quality markers in lacrosse players. *Open Access J Sports Med* 3:67–71.

Wauquier, F., L. Leotoing, C. Philippe, M. Spilmont, V. Coxam, and Y. Wittrant. 2015. Pros and cons of fatty acids in bone biology. *Prog Lipid Res* 58:121–45.

Weaver, C. M., C. M. Gordon, K. F. Janz et al. 2016. The National Osteoporosis Foundation's position statement on peak bone mass development and lifestyle factors: A systematic review and implementation recommendations. *Osteoporos Int* 27:1281–386.

Zanker, C. L., C. B. Cooke, J. G. Truscott, B. Oldroyd, and H. S. Jacobs. 2004. Annual changes of bone density over 12 years in an amenorrheic athlete. *Med Sci Sports Exerc* 36:137–42.

Index

A

Abdominal adipocytes, 351
Abdominal adipose cells, 348
Abdominal adiposity, 117
    abdominal obesity reduction, 117–119
    effects of exercise amount and intensity on WC,
        117–119
Abdominal circumference method, 8, 16, 296
Abdominal fat, 296, 298
    accretion, 349
    effect of androgen supplements on, 351
Abdominal obesity reduction, 117–119
Abdominal SAT (ASAT), 117
    exercise-induced reduction in VAT *vs.*, 119–121
Accelerometry, 71
Accuracy, 15
Acid-ash hypothesis, 362
Acromiale, 90–91
Activities of daily living (ADL), 333, 335
Adaptive response of bone to mechanical loading, 137
Adenosine diphosphate (ADP), 351
Adenosine monophosphate-activated protein kinase
    (AMPK), 367
Adenosine triphosphate (ATP), 351
Adequate intake (AI), 52, 363
ad hoc working group, 164
    ad hoc Research Working Group, 150
    International Olympic Committee *Ad Hoc* Working
        Group, 96–97
    IOC, 236
Adipokines, 130
Adiponectin, 261
Adipose tissue (AT), 3, 109, 268–269, 348, 351
    distribution, 122–124
    exercise and regional variation in AT reduction,
        119–122
    relationships with bone during growth, 139–140
Adiposity, 129
    and activity in general population, 79
    effect of, 136
    training for sport and adiposity in youth athletes,
        79–80
ADL, *see* Activities of daily living
ad libitum diet, 330–331
Adolescence, 73, 74, 136
ADP, *see* Adenosine diphosphate; Air displacement
    plethysmography
Adult(s), 133, 135
    female athletes, 259
    onset growth hormone deficiency, 348–349
Aerobic
    capacity, 172
    endurance exercise regimens, 140
    exercise, 8, 315, 329, 331–332
    fitness, 309–310, 315–316
    performance, 296
    processes, 172

    training, 134
Aesthetics, 259
    aesthetically judged sports, 235
    sports, 103, 236, 237, 251–253, 257–258
Age/aging
    age-related body fat standards, 295
    combination of higher protein intakes and RT,
        335–336
    exercise and protein effect on maintenance of muscle
        mass and strength, 333
    older adults consuming protein to attenuate lean mass
        losses, 333–334
    RT, 334–336
    strength athletes, 214–215
Agouti-related peptide (AgRP), 365
AHA, *see* American Heart Association
AI, *see* Adequate intake
Air displacement, 29
Air displacement plethysmography (ADP), 15, 19–20,
    100–101, 195, 301
Air Force, 292
Allometric scaling, 215
Alpine skiers, 173
Amenorrhea, 259, 264, 268
American football, 100, 224–225
American Heart Association (AHA), 331
Amino acid, 325, 329
    digestibility, 324–325
    oxidation, 325
Aminoacidemia, 329
A-Mode ultrasound, *see* Amplitude mode ultrasound
AMPK, *see* Adenosine monophosphate-activated protein
    kinase
Amplitude mode ultrasound (A-Mode ultrasound),
    196–197
AN, *see* Anorexia nervosa
Anabolic
    drug replacements, dietary supplements with claims
        as, 345–346
    hormone research, 350
    substances, 347
    window, 327–328
Analysis of variance (ANOVA), 15
Anatomical heights, 90–91
Androgens, 350–351
"Android" phenotype, 122
Anorexia, 259
    anorexia-related hypogonadal conditions, 268
Anorexia nervosa (AN), 259, 264, 360
ANOVA, *see* Analysis of variance
Anovulation, 260, 264–265
Anterior superior iliac spine (ASIS), 90
Anthropometrically based body fat
    army experience with 30 years of body fat standards,
        298–300
    basis for military body fat standards, 295–298
    development of service-specific anthropometric
        equations, 288–295